Cancer and Chronic Conditions

Bogda Koczwara
Editor

Cancer and Chronic Conditions

Addressing the Problem of Multimorbidity in Cancer Patients and Survivors

Springer

Editor
Bogda Koczwara, AM
Flinders Centre for Innovation in Cancer
Flinders University
Bedford Park, SA
Australia

ISBN 978-981-10-1843-5 ISBN 978-981-10-1844-2 (eBook)
DOI 10.1007/978-981-10-1844-2

Library of Congress Control Number: 2016945773

Printed on acid-free paper

This Springer imprint is published by Springer Nature
The registered company is Springer Science+Business Media Singapore Pte Ltd.

Foreword

It is such a surprise that a book like this has not been written before.

Cancer does not occur in a vacuum. Just as our lives are complex and multi-layered, so are our individual medical situations with many cancer patients already experiencing other diseases and conditions, often with no seeming connection to their cancer. Dealing with the fallout of a cancer diagnosis and treatment is difficult enough on its own, but when it occurs against a backdrop of other illnesses, the degree of difficulty can become overwhelming.

The cancer world is becoming increasingly sophisticated with deeper knowledge about the disease, more high-tech detection approaches, improved treatments and the commitment towards improved statistics and outcomes. Large amounts of money are spent on driving research across the cancer spectrum. We celebrate incremental steps in new knowledge and its application, and so we should!

Within all the closely watched cancer statistics and clinical discussions sit ordinary people—cancer patients—who have been thrust into the alien world of oncology and just want to get better. The statistics and graphs actually mean very little to an individual who will not know on which part of the survival curve he or she sits until ultimately survival or death occurs.

The trouble is that a lot can go on in the meantime, including simply living with all the complications and complexities that go with it.

Cancer never sits in its own separate space, not to a patient anyway, even though sometimes it can feel like an all-encompassing presence. There are other bits of life that need to be taken account of, including decisions about treatment for example, which will also have an impact on other people close to us. In the breast cancer area which is what I know, a mother might decide to put off her breast reconstruction operation until she has all her young children at school and relatively independent, physically at least; or a rural woman might opt for mastectomy rather than breast-conserving surgery because she cannot manage to live away from the property for 6 weeks of radiotherapy; another young woman might well decide to change her chemotherapy regime to protect future fertility prospects. Consideration about our individual social situation can certainly change the way we approach cancer treatment.

Twenty-plus years ago, when I was diagnosed with cancer, there was not so much attention given to an individual's life circumstances. The focus was squarely on the tumour with minimal consideration directed towards social needs or emotional well-being. Increasingly, since that time, an individual's circumstances and setting have been acknowledged as an important pathway to best managing a person with cancer—so that what is happening in the heart and in the head is taken into account as well as how the tumour or disease is clinically presenting. Psychosocial clinical practice guidelines are a strong acknowledgement of this.

Despite a movement towards considering the whole patient, many people with cancer would still say their doctors' treatment approaches did not focus sufficiently on their holistic care. And that is just within the cancer realm!

From the patient's perspective, navigating the oncology world is tricky at best. It is imperative to ensure you have the best team caring for you and that the advice you are given is accurate and reflects best practice. But who, apart from yourself, has your whole situation uppermost in considerations? Who is going to actively consider decisions and their impact on other areas of an individual's health, especially when these needs are also complex and ever-changing? How do we best consider and manage the situation when the cancer treatment aimed at helping us survive causes long-term damage to our organs or results in a life-threatening non-cancer condition?

If researchers, clinicians, policy makers and the like are to take strides and really make a difference in assisting cancer patients with comorbidities or multimorbidities, then this would be a very positive and welcome step. It will take far more than goodwill and commitment, but this is an excellent start. It will require collaboration and I suggest a completely new way of looking at how we approach cancer and those most directly affected by the disease. It will also need agreed system change with processes and policies. Perhaps more than anything, it will require champions and trailblazers.

If we are to make real progress, we need people whose vision can take in wide horizons. We know this will not be easy. As patients, we are looking for practitioners who are not only specialists, but also subspecialists, and by definition, this makes collaboration across other areas of medicine and science so much more challenging.

This book is not able to provide simple solutions; it marks a starting point. It raises issues for consideration and discussion. It highlights the challenges for researchers, clinicians and policy makers. Most importantly, it is an acknowledgement that if we are to genuinely meet the complex needs of people affected by cancer, in the short and long terms, then we have to ask questions, consider other perspectives, collaborate, work on the big picture and look with new eyes as much as possible from the patient's perspective.

Lyn Swinburne, AM
Breast Cancer Survivor and Advocate
Founder of Breast Cancer Network Australia

Preface

The great progress in cancer control could not have been possible without the single-minded focus on cancer, almost at exclusion of anything else. To control cancer, one should not to be distracted by the side effects of treatment and often sheer physical and mental exhaustion that accompanies cancer and its treatment. Only by putting these aside, one can grasp a chance of changing the course of this terrible disease.

But as an oncologist who has treated patients for nearly a quarter of the century, I face the sobering truth that while the frontiers in the war against cancer are advancing every day, the lay of the land is defined by more than cancer alone. It takes a few years after the cancer diagnosis before one can embrace the joy of cancer survivorship, but also face the tragedy of long-standing consequences of cancer treatment, and the question of could have these been prevented? With more cancers becoming treatable and treatments better tolerated, we need to learn to better balance the benefits and risks of treatment in light of coexisting conditions that the patient is already dealing with.

As cancer is becoming a chronic condition itself and the prevalence of chronic conditions in the Western population at the all-time high, this book aims to answer some of the questions related to the interface of cancer and comorbidity that an oncology practitioners face every day—how does comorbidity impact on cancer treatment and its outcomes and how can we deliver better care that addresses both cancer and the comorbid conditions? In some cases, where evidence is not yet well established, the authors define questions as the basis for future research.

My thanks go to all the contributors of the book who brought with them tremendous diversity of perspectives and fields truly reflective of the complexity of the topic and who, through coming together in this project, serve as nidus of the multidisciplinary collaboration in this field.

Most importantly, my deepest thanks go to my family for their unwavering patience and support during the development of the book. I could not have done it without them.

Bedford Park, SA, Australia

Bogda Koczwara, AM

Contents

1 **What Is Comorbidity?** 1
Diana Sarfati and Jason Gurney

2 **How Do We Measure Comorbidity?** 35
Diana Sarfati

3 **Cancer, Chronic Conditions and Social Disadvantage—The Perfect Storm** 71
Janelle V. Levesque, Afaf Girgis and Paul R. Ward

4 **Impact of Comorbidity on Cancer Screening and Diagnosis** 105
Steven T. Fleming, Diana Sarfati, Gretchen Kimmick, Nancy Schoenberg and Ruth Cunningham

5 **Impact of Comorbidity on Treatment Decision Making and Outcomes** 131
Jae Jin Lee and Martine Extermann

6 **The Impact of Cancer and Chronic Conditions on Caregivers and Family Members** 159
Sylvie D. Lambert, Janelle V. Levesque and Afaf Girgis

7 **Prevention of Chronic Conditions and Cancer** 203
Alexandra McCarthy, Tina Skinner, Michael Fenech and Shelley Keating

8 **Chronic Condition Management Models for Cancer Care and Survivorship** 241
Sharon Lawn and Malcolm Battersby

9 **The Management of Polypharmacy in People with Cancer and Chronic Conditions** 261
Justin P. Turner, Ross A. McKinnon and J. Simon Bell

10 Breaking the Silos: Integrated Care for Cancer *and* Chronic Conditions 287
Lauren J. Cortis, Paul R. Ward, Ross A. McKinnon and Bogda Koczwara

11 Advocacy in Cancer and Chronic Conditions—Challenges and Opportunities 315
Paul Grogan and Sanchia Aranda

12 Research Considerations in Patients with Cancer and Comorbidity 341
Marjan van den Akker, Laura Deckx, Rein Vos and Christiane Muth

13 The Cost of Cure: Chronic Conditions in Survivors of Child, Adolescent, and Young Adult Cancers 371
Christina Signorelli, Joanna E. Fardell, Claire E. Wakefield, Kate Webber and Richard J. Cohn

14 Chronic Conditions and Cancer in Older Adults 421
Arduino A. Mangoni, Kimberley Ruxton, Anna Rachelle Mislang and Laura Biganzoli

15 Chronic Conditions and Cancer at the End of Life 455
David C. Currow and Jane L. Phillips

Chapter 1
What Is Comorbidity?

Diana Sarfati and Jason Gurney

Abstract Comorbidity is "*any distinct additional clinical entity that has existed or that may occur during the clinical course of a patient that has the index disease under study*". It is related to, but distinct from other constructs such as multimorbidity, functional status, disability, allostatic load, frailty, burden of disease and patient complexity. As populations age, the prevalence of chronic disease increases. As a consequence, many people live with, rather than die from chronic health conditions. Cancer is often a chronic disease itself, and is also more prevalent among the elderly. This confluence in timing means that many cancer patients (if not most) live with at least one other chronic disease, although the prevalence of comorbidity varies markedly across populations with different types of cancer. There are several reasons why cancer and comorbidity co-exist; cancer and other long-term conditions share common risk factors, some chronic conditions or their treatments are causally related to cancer and there may be some instances where there are common physiological pathways between cancer and other conditions.

Keywords Comorbidity · Cancer · Complexity · Chronic disease

Key Points

- The presence of chronic disease—comorbidity—in addition to cancer is now the norm rather than the exception.
- While comorbidity is common among cancer populations, the precise prevalence of comorbidity is difficult to determine; however, it is clear that the prevalence of comorbidity varies considerably by cancer site.
- There is substantial evidence of differing comorbidity burden between population sub-groups, with those in ethnic minority groups and those living in poverty or deprivation carrying a greater burden.

D. Sarfati (✉) · J. Gurney
Department of Public Health, University of Otago Wellington,
7343 Wellington, New Zealand
e-mail: diana.sarfati@otago.ac.nz

B. Koczwara (ed.), *Cancer and Chronic Conditions*,
DOI 10.1007/978-981-10-1844-2_1

- The reasons why cancer and comorbidity coexist are multiple and varied. Cancer and other long-term conditions share many risk factors; there are also many examples where specific comorbid conditions or their treatments may be involved in the aetiology of cancer, or vice versa. There may also be common genetic or physiological links between some chronic conditions and cancer.

1.1 What Is Comorbidity?

> Management of patients with several chronic diseases is now the most important task facing health services in developed counties, which presents a fundamental challenge to the single-disease focus that pervades medicine.
>
> – Chris Salisbury, The Lancet [1]

As populations age, the prevalence of chronic disease increases. Almost all chronic diseases are more common among the elderly than younger adults, and are not life threatening in the short term. Consequently, many people live with, rather than die from chronic health conditions.

Cancer is often a chronic disease itself, and is also more prevalent among the elderly. Via a natural convergence in the timing of peak occurrence, concomitant chronic disease—which we term *comorbidity*—in addition to cancer is now the norm rather than the exception. This confluence has the potential to profoundly impact affected individuals [2–5].

Comorbidity results in increased risk of hospitalisation, adverse effects of treatment, multiple competing demands on both patient and health care professionals, high health care costs, reduced quality of life and higher mortality [4–15]. Despite this, much of the research and planning relating to cancer and cancer care assume a single disease paradigm. For example, patients with comorbidity are often excluded from randomised controlled trials, which means that it is difficult to generalise the findings of such trials to those with chronic health problems, or to predict the difficulties or complications from treatment that such patients may face [16–19]. Partly as a consequence of this, clinical practice guidelines tend to be very poor at addressing the needs of older patients with comorbidity [18, 20, 21]. Health care service providers, policy makers and researchers need to be able to respond adequately to the requirements of individuals with complex health needs [15, 22].

Despite the importance of comorbidity in the care of cancer patients, there is no consensus about how to define it, and even less on how to measure it. To add to the confusion, there are multiple other constructs that are related to—but distinct from—comorbidity.

1.2 The Evolution of the Concept of Comorbidity

In 1970 Feinstein noted that "*although patients with more than one diagnosed disease are frequently encountered in modern medical practice, the inter-relationships and effects of multiple diseases have not received suitable taxonomic attention in clinical science*" [6]. Feinstein argued that this "*neglect of comorbidity*" had many detrimental effects, although his focus was largely on defining comorbidity in order to ensure comparability between study groups in studies of treatment effectiveness, and to ensure that *statistics* relating to disease were accurate. Feinstein defined comorbidity as "*any distinct additional clinical entity that has existed or that may occur during the clinical course of a patient that has the index disease under study*". He noted the importance of comorbid disease in terms of its potential effects on diagnosis, treatment and outcomes of patients. Subsequent work by Kaplan and Feinstein in 1974 [23] resulted in possibly the first attempt to measure comorbidity as a separate construct in its own right. They found that comorbidity was related to increased risk of mortality, and higher severity of comorbidity with increased risk among patients with diabetes mellitus.

During the 1980s and early 1990s, the measurement of comorbidity developed into two distinct branches: diagnostic-based risk (or case-mix) adjustment systems, and clinically-based comorbidity indices. These approaches differed both in the underlying assumptions and constructs relating to comorbidity, and in the approaches that were used to measure comorbidity. While this dichotomy is clearly distinguishable, it is important to note that both approaches have been used in a variety of study types with varying aims and objectives [3, 24–29].

1.3 Diagnostic-Based Risk (or Case-Mix) Adjustment Systems

These were developed largely in the United States in response to the need to allocate health care resources in managed care environments where populations were enrolled in health care organisations where there was pressure to develop systems which could predict future cost and utilisation of healthcare.

These systems were based on routinely collected data that could be applied to large populations, and often included factors other than comorbidity. The concept of comorbidity for these tended to be focused on conditions or categories of conditions that were associated with increased health service utilisation or health care costs [25, 28, 29].

The ACG system developed at John Hopkins University is an example of a diagnosis-based risk adjustment system. It was developed in response to the recognition of the increasing costs of health care, the rapid expansion of managed and capitated care in the US, and an increasing emphasis on ambulatory care [28, 29]. This system uses administrative data to categorise individuals into groups

(ACGs or Adjusted Clinical Groups) with similar health resource use expectations, based on specified individual or categories of conditions as well as patient factors such as age and sex [28, 29]. This system has been used in a number of settings, primarily for health care management purposes, including setting capitation rates and profiling the efficiency of health care organisations and clinicians [25–34].

1.4 Clinically-Based Comorbidity Indices

Clinically-based comorbidity indices were developed primarily for clinicians and researchers to assess the role of comorbidity in outcomes for their patients, often in the context of clinical or epidemiological studies.

They employ a range of approaches and data sources in an attempt to optimise the measurement of comorbidity [24, 35, 36]. Comorbidity in this context tends to be focused on conditions that have an impact on patient outcomes, most commonly mortality.

The best known example of a clinically-based comorbidity index is the Charlson Comorbidity Index (CCI) developed by Mary Charlson and colleagues in 1987 [37]. The Charlson index includes seventeen conditions (in 19 categories) which are allocated a weight of 1–6, depending on their association with 1-year mortality. For each individual, these weights are summed to give an overall score. A higher score indicates a higher the level of comorbidity.

The Charlson index has been validated and used in a huge variety of clinical and research settings, and has been adapted for use with administrative data [38–41] and for use with patient self-reporting [42–44]. Subsequently, a number of approaches to measure comorbidity have been developed [2, 24, 35, 36, 45]. These are described in detail in the next chapter, but in general can be divided into three categories:

- Simple counts of conditions [46–48].
- Weighted indices that adjust for seriousness of conditions [23, 37, 49–51].
- Systems that depend on models involving varying numbers of individual conditions [52–54].

Data sources used to estimate comorbidity have also varied, including administrative data, medical charts, physical examination, personal interviews and self-reporting [3, 8, 45, 55].

1.5 Recent Evolution Relating to the Concept of Comorbidity

In October 2003, the National Institute on Aging (NIA) Geriatrics and Clinical Gerontology Program convened a taskforce on comorbidity. The objective of this taskforce was to '*explore conceptual and methodological complexities of comorbidity*' [14].

There was general consensus that comorbidity was a complex and heterogeneous concept, and that no single measure would be likely to adequately serve all research and clinical purposes. The taskforce determined that the definition and measurement of comorbidity depended on the objective that was being addressed, the setting and population(s) of interest, the extent to which comorbid conditions inter-relate, and the severity and timing of conditions. The conclusion, then, was that more research was needed on the measurement and impact of comorbidity, but that a balance needed to be maintained on advancing the conceptual and theoretical aspects of comorbidity on one hand, and not losing sight of the practical issues of measuring comorbidity on the other.

Subsequent work has tended to shift into more complex conceptualisations of comorbidity. For example, Karlamangla et al. [56] suggested a categorisation of comorbidity that was based on body systems (i.e. mental function, sensory, pain, voice and speech functions, and movement, skin, cardiovascular, haematological, immunological, respiratory, digestive, metabolic, endocrine, GU/reproductive/sexual, and neuromusculoskeletal systems). They suggested each could be classified on a spectrum ranging from high-functioning, through subclinical abnormalities and through to clinically-manifest disease of various severities. For example, in the endocrine system, abnormal fasting blood glucose levels may be categorised as a subclinical abnormality, where overt diabetes mellitus controlled by diet may be considered disease on the less severe end of the spectrum, while insulin dependent diabetes mellitus with complications may be on the more severe end of the spectrum. The authors also suggested that interactions between domains could be included; for example, the known synergies between hypertension and diabetes could be included in the estimate of overall patient comorbidity, although it was unclear how this would be achieved. In this way, sub-clinical disease could be explicitly recognised, disease clusters would be accounted for, the system would not depend solely on diagnosed disease and high functioning would be measured as well as low functioning. Whilst these aims are laudable, the collection of data required for such a measurement tool would be intensive, expensive and often not feasible.

In their narrative review, Valderas et al. [12] attempted to 'define and measure the concept of comorbidity'. They identified four distinctions that could be made in relation to comorbidity. The first three are related to the definition of comorbidity itself:

1. The requirement to be clear about what a comorbid entity is, and how these can be identified and defined.
2. The relative importance of the primary condition, and given the co-existence of multiple conditions, which can be considered primary.
3. The chronology of the conditions—i.e. are they co-occurring, and does the order in which they occur affect genesis, prognosis or treatment.

The fourth distinction highlighted was that related to 'expanded conceptualisations' relating to comorbidity. Such conceptualisations, expanded on below, included those of *multimorbidity*, where no single condition is considered primary; *burden of disease,* which includes elements of multimorbidity and functional status; and *patient complexity,* which expands this idea further into other factors which may influence patient outcomes and healthcare resource requirements, such as socioeconomic status, lack of social support or language difficulties. Other related constructs not explicitly included in the paper by Valderas et al. include allostatic load, disability and frailty [57–60].

1.6 Constructs Related to Comorbidity

The multiple constructs related to comorbidity are further described below.

1.7 Multimorbidity

Multimorbidity is the "*the co-occurrence of multiple chronic or acute diseases and medical conditions within one person*" [61]. It is distinct from comorbidity in that the latter implies an index disease under study. The concept of multimorbidity shifts the focus from a single disease paradigm to one where the causes and effects of multiple combined conditions are explored.

Multimorbidity is a particularly useful concept in the context of primary care, where practitioners are responsible for the overall health of their patients rather than the management of a single disease entity [62]. However more recently, there have been strong calls to reorient the health system in general away from a single-disease orientation [1, 18, 19, 63]. Much of the research on multimorbidity has focused on the epidemiology and effects of multimorbidity. For example, van der Akker et al. [64] used data from a network of family health practitioners in the Netherlands to identify permanent, chronic or recurrent conditions. They found that 29.7 % of the population had two or more conditions, and that multimorbidity was more common among older people, women and those with lower education, or those who did not have private health insurance. There was also evidence that certain conditions tended to cluster. They concluded that this clustering of diseases was likely to be due to a combination of *causal* mechanisms, such as common genetic, immunological, environmental or behavioural risk factors, or *artefactual* mechanisms, particularly chance clustering, or detection bias where a patient is more likely to have a second condition diagnosed because of health service contact related to a first condition.

More recently, Barnett et al. analysed data from primary care databases in the United Kingdom for 1.75 million patients [65]. They found that nearly a quarter of all patients had more than one chronic condition, that the likelihood of multimorbidity increased with increasing deprivation, and that whilst multimorbidity was more common among those aged over 65 years, in absolute terms there were more people under 65 years with multimorbidity.

Multimorbidity, like comorbidity, has been found to be associated with an increased risk of disability, poor functional status, higher health care expenditure, polypharmacy, and complications of care [18, 19, 42, 63, 65–71].

1.8 Functional (or Performance) Status

Functional limitations are defined as limitations in performance at the level of the whole organism or person [58]. Functional status is broader than this, and is the ability or otherwise to carry out everyday tasks. Scrag (2008) articulately describes it as "*captur [ing] much of what seasoned clinicians ascertain in an instant as they watch a patient enter a room, rise from a chair, or clamber onto an exam table*" [72].

The presence of chronic disease is directly related to functional status. Pain and stiffness in arthritis, shortness of breath in chronic respiratory disease, and dysphasia or dyspraxia as a result of a stroke, all lead to a loss of ability to carry out everyday tasks. Functional status is measured by the ability or otherwise to carry out such tasks, and is often related to both the presence and the consequences of chronic disease [73]. Assessment of functional status may be based on self-reporting or proxy reporting of ability to carry out specified tasks; for example the World Health Organisation performance status instrument (WHO-PS) or the physical functioning scale of the SF-36, or physical performance tests such as ability to open and close fasteners, gait speed, ability to climb stairs or rise from a chair [74]. Functional status is a predictor of morbidity, mortality, length of hospital stay and hospital charges independent of other characteristics, including age and comorbidity [9, 75–77]. The measurement of functional status as an outcome is also useful in determining the impact of the consequences of chronic disease.

1.9 Disability

Disability is closely related to the concept of functional status. It is defined as a "*limitation in performance of socially defined roles and tasks within a sociocultural and physical environment*" [58]. Functional impairments can lead to disability, but the extent to which this occurs depends on the physical, social and psychological environments in which people live [60]. Environments can be more or less disabling. For example, an individual with severe arthritis may be considerably less disabled if they have access to mobility aids, and aids to assist with tasks requiring dexterity.

Disability, like functional status, is most commonly assessed using self-reported difficulty in specific tasks, and these are assessed in the clinical setting by screening tools such as Activities of Daily Living (ADLs) and Instrumental Activities of daily Living (IADLs) [57].

1.10 Allostatic Load

While disability takes explicit account of a person's environment, allostatic load is a purely physiological measure of ill-health. It is a measure of cumulative, chronic physiological dysfunction across multiple body systems [59]. Seeman's hypothesis was that organisms must adapt body systems to alter their internal milieu in response to environmental challenges. When these adaptive responses are no longer able to cope with such challenges, progressive dysregulation occurs and can be measured. Allostatic load is related to, but is not the same as comorbidity. Chronic disease may result in a cumulative physiological burden which results in an increase of the allostatic load. Seeman et al. see the measure of allostatic load as an indicator that an individual may be decompensating as a result of various internal and external challenges including comorbid disease:

> No single form of comorbidity occurs with high frequency, but rather a multiplicity of diverse combinations are observed (e.g. osteoarthritis and diabetes, colon cancer, coronary heart disease, depression and hypertension). This diversity underscores the need for an early warning system of biomarkers that can signal early signs of dysregulation across multiple physiological systems [59].

Allostatic load was initially measured using 10 biological parameters, which are physiologically related to a number of homeostatic metabolic processes, such as the hypothalamic-pituatary-adrenal axis, the sympathetic nervous system, and the cardiovascular system. The parameters were systolic and diastolic blood pressure, waist/hip ratio, serum high density lipoprotein and total cholesterol, plasma glycosylated haemoglobin, serum dihydroepiandrosterone, 12 h cortisol excretion and urinary norepinephrine and epinephrine excretion [59]. In later work, serum fibrinogen, C-reactive protein and interleukin 6, all measures of chronic inflammation, were added to the measure of allostatic load [59, 78].

In the development of the measure of allostatic load, each of these parameters was measured in a group of 70–79 year olds. Each parameter was categorised into quartiles, and the number of parameters for each individual that fell into the highest risk quartile was summed to give a total score. Higher scores were cross-sectionally and longitudinally related to all-cause mortality, cardiovascular disease, and a poorer cognitive and physical functioning, and frailty [59, 78, 79].

1.11 Frailty

Frailty has been defined as a "*physiologic state of increased vulnerability to stressors that results from decreased physiologic reserves, and … dysregulation, of multiple physiologic systems*" [57]. Frailty is considered a physiological syndrome related to, but separate from comorbidity and disability [57, 80]. Frailty is characterised by weakness, decreased endurance and slowed performance. It is related to poor nutrition, concurrent chronic disease, loss of muscle mass, reduced metabolic rate, decreased activity and energy expenditure [81]. It has been measured in a variety of ways, for example, Fried (2001) categorised those with frailty as having a combination of any three of unintentional weight loss, weakness, poor endurance, slowness or low physical activity [81], whereas Baldaucci used age greater than 85 years, high ADL score, three or more comorbidities and the diagnosis of a geriatric syndrome (any one of delirium, dementia, depression, osteoporosis, incontinence, falls, etc.) [80, 82]. Frailty is strongly related to increasing age and is most common in the very elderly. It has also been found to be more common among cancer patients than similarly aged patients without cancer [83]. Frailty may cause disability independently of coexisting disease and may be caused by comorbidity [57]. Frailty is strongly associated with adverse outcomes including disability, mortality and dependency [57, 80, 81, 84–86].

1.12 Burden of Disease/Illness

Burden of disease (in this context) expands the concept of multimorbidity to include the functional status of individuals. Burden of disease is a combined measure of the number of chronic diseases, their severity and their impact on functional status [9]. It is therefore a measure of chronic disease, and its impact on the individual concerned. There is no gold standard measure for burden of disease. The first attempt to measure this construct was in 1995 by Greenfield et al. [87]. Their aim was to measure a "*composite illness-based measure of risk for substantial declines in health*" (Total Illness Burden Index or TIBI). They did this by identifying the presence of chronic disease divided into categories (such as pulmonary disease, heart disease, stroke and neurological disease, gastrointestinal disease, other cancers, arthritis, eye problems, hearing problems, hypertension, diabetes mellitus and arthritis) among a cohort of patients. For each category or condition, they assessed the likely impact on functional status, both through clinician assessment and through statistical assessment of the association of each, with outcomes such as the physical functioning scale of the SF-36 instrument. TIBI scores have been associated with poorer outcomes in general, and among cancer patients specifically [87, 88].

Mandelblatt (2001) assessed burden of disease by examining the separate roles of comorbidity and functional status, as well as life-expectancy and self-rated health on treatment patterns and outcomes, for a cohort of older women with early stage breast cancer [9]. They posited that biological aging and the effects of chronic disease would result in physiological dysregulation, which is in turn a determinant of functional status and disability (Fig. 1.1). These three components of total illness burden (number of chronic conditions, physiological dysregulation and functional status) would then impact on life expectancy and other health outcomes. They found that whilst these separate constructs were correlated with each other, the strength of the correlation varied considerably, suggesting that each was capturing a different dimension of illness burden. However, they also found that, even in

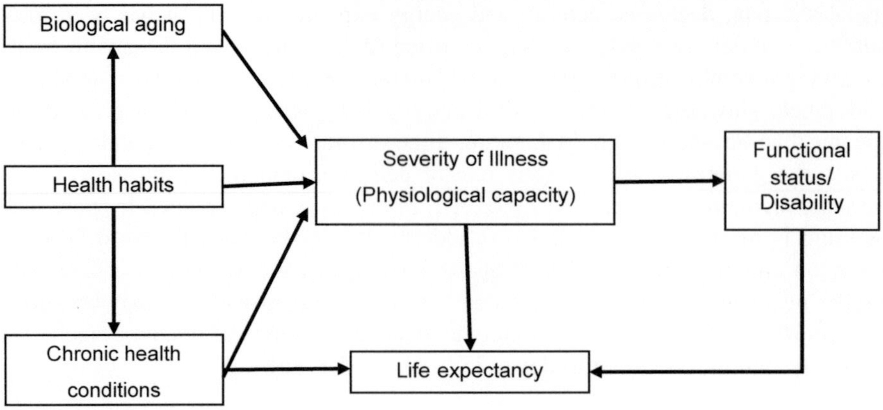

Fig. 1.1 Conceptual model of total illness burden. *Source* Buchner and Wagner (1992); cited in Mandleblatt et al. [9]

combination, these variables did not explain much of the variance in number of treatments received among this cohort of patients. Interestingly, this group of patients were healthier than average breast cancer patients, so the authors concluded that their estimates of the effects of burden of illness on cancer treatment were likely to be somewhat conservative.

Clinically, total illness burden may be measured using instruments such as the Comprehensive Geriatric Assessment (CGA) tool. This tool provides data on patient functional status, comorbidity, polypharmacy, existence of geriatric syndromes, nutritional status, social support and psychological status [89–93]. Studies that have used the CGA tool among older patients with cancer have found that people who score poorly on CGA tend to have poorer survival, higher levels of treatment toxicity, and higher mortality [85, 94–96].

1.13 Complexity

Complexity is the broadest related construct [97, 98], as it includes all determinants of health at an individual level. These include a broad range of factors including, but not limited to socioeconomic, cultural, and environmental factors that are likely to impact on patient care and outcomes.

Safford (2007) developed a graphical model of patient complexity that involved a series of vectors, each relating to individual determinants of health, and each with a force and magnitude resulting either in increasing or decreasing complexity (Fig. 1.2) [97]. The concept of complexity reflects the intricate interactions between a multitude of factors that impact on care and outcomes at an individual level. The presence of chronic disease is one of these, but it is only one part of a highly complex and dynamic system [98, 99].

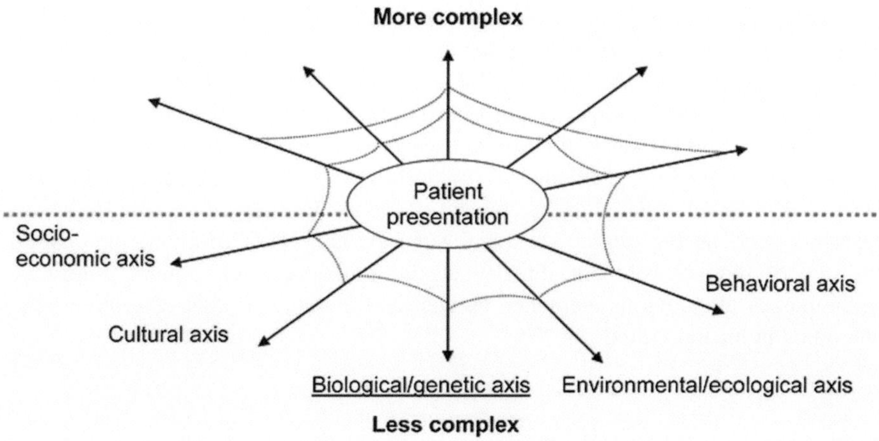

Fig. 1.2 Vector model of complexity. *Source* Safford et al. [97]

1.14 How Are the Comorbidity-Related Constructs Linked?

There is considerable overlap between these inter-related concepts, and the boundaries between them are blurred.

Figure 1.3 is amended and expanded from Valderas et al. [12]. It shows the close relationship between *comorbidity* and *multimorbidity*, the difference being that

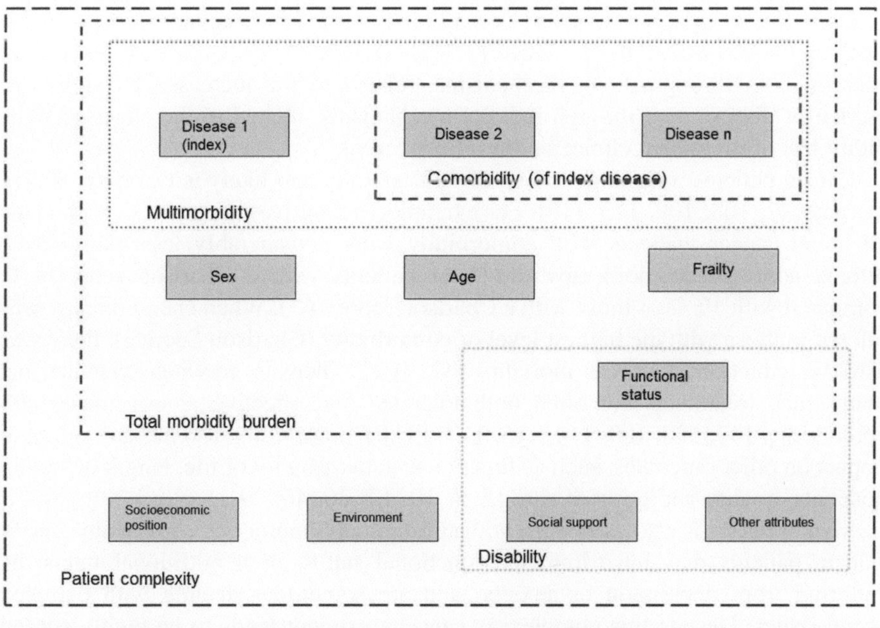

Fig. 1.3 Comorbidity and related constructs. Expanded from Valderas et al. [12]

comorbidity is measured in relation to a primary index disease, whilst multimorbidity is a total measure of all diseases occurring concurrently in an individual. In this figure, *functional status* and *frailty* are represented as separate constructs, but clearly they are both strongly related to each other and to other factors, particularly increasing age and presence of chronic disease. *Total morbidity burden* is a broader concept encompassing elements of comorbidity, frailty and functional status. *Disability* is closely related to the concept of functional status, but includes broader elements such as the degree of social support, and other disabling or enabling features of the environment. Finally at the broadest level, patient complexity encompasses all previous elements, as well as other factors that determine health outcomes in an individual.

1.15 Why Should We Focus on Comorbidity in Cancer?

There are many reasons why it is important for cancer researchers and clinicians alike to pay attention to comorbidity. We have outlined some of these reasons below.

Comorbidity is common. The exact prevalence of comorbidity among cancer patients varies both by cancer site and by the method used to measure comorbidity; but regardless, comorbidity is common among cancer patients [3, 100, 101]. For example, in New Zealand 70 % of those with colon cancer and 72 % of those with lung cancer have at least one comorbid condition [47, 102, 103]. As the population ages, comorbidity will become even more common.

Comorbidity affects outcomes. Comorbidity has a major negative effect on the likelihood of survival from cancer [2, 47, 51, 103–112]. Comorbidity acts on survival both through direct mechanisms, related to the increased physiological burden of disease, and through indirect mechanisms, related to the effects comorbidity has on treatment choice and/or effectiveness.

Cancer patients with comorbidity are substantially less likely to be offered active therapy [47, 108, 109, 113–116]. For example, among New Zealanders with stage III colon cancer, patients with comorbidity were considerably less likely to be offered adjuvant chemotherapy (84 % of patients with a Charlson score of 0, compared with 19 % of those with a Charlson score of 3). When chemotherapy was offered to those with the highest level of comorbidity (Charlson Score 3), there was a 60 % reduction in excess mortality [47, 102]. There is growing evidence that many such treatments are often both tolerated and effective among those with comorbidity [47, 108, 109, 114, 115, 117–121]. Comorbidity also has an important impact on other outcomes, such as functional status, quality of life, length of stay in hospitals, quality and costs of care [5, 8, 10, 12, 26, 46, 99].

Mental illness is also associated with substantially poorer outcomes from cancer. Cancer patients may have impaired functional status, poor nutritional status, be suffering from depression or anxiety, and are sometimes dealing with complex social issues. Despite this complexity, cancer treatment tends to be highly silo'ed and delivered in specialised units that are focused, unsurprisingly, on the treatment of cancer.

The impact of comorbidity is modifiable. There is evidence that focusing at a clinical level on more complex patients with comorbidity can result in benefits in terms of both improved outcomes and satisfaction with care for patients [13, 57, 97, 122]. Systems can be redesigned to optimise healthcare processes for complex patients, and from a policy perspective, incorporating complexity of patient mix into quality measurements and performance profiling, results in a more comprehensive understanding of health service quality and processes [1, 5, 15, 18, 19, 63].

As we will see in the next section, comorbidity is common among cancer populations. Despite this fact, there is a scarcity of evidence about how to manage these patients. Patients with comorbidity are routinely excluded from randomised controlled trials that are designed to identify the benefits and harms of cancer treatment, and there is lack of consensus on how best to manage these patients. Clinicians are left to weigh up the benefits and potential harms of treatment strategies for themselves, without evidence to inform them.

1.16 How Common Is Comorbidity in Cancer?

Whilst there is general agreement that comorbidity is common among cancer patients, it is remarkably difficult to state with any certainly how common it is. This is because the prevalence of comorbidity varies, sometimes dramatically, depending on the measure of comorbidity used, the data available, the study population, and the cancer site.

In their review of the impact of comorbidity on chemotherapy use and outcomes among patients with solid tumours, Lee et al. reported a wide prevalence range for comorbidity of 0.4–90 % among cancer patients [100]. Data from the New Zealand context suggests that approximately half of all cancer patients have at least one other chronic condition recorded, and a third have two or more [123, 124]. In their Annual Report to the Nation on the Status of Cancer, Edwards et al. reported that approximately 40 % of U.S. cancer patients have at least one comorbid condition [101].

Not surprisingly, studies that use a more inclusive measure of comorbidity demonstrate a higher prevalence of comorbidity than those that use a more restrictive approach. For example, Tammemagi et al. used an extensive and inclusive approach to identify comorbid conditions from computerised medical records in their cohort of patients with breast cancer, and found that 72 % had at least one condition [118]. This compares with Gonzalez et al., who used data extracted only from routine discharge abstracts and found that 13 % of women with breast cancer had at least one Charlson index-related comorbid condition [125]. Even if the approach to measuring comorbidity is limited to a single comorbidity index, the Charlson index, there is still a large range of prevalence estimates. Most studies that use the Charlson index report that 10–75 % of cancer patients have at least one Charlson index-related condition [47, 125–132]. The variation is largely due to characteristics of the study population and the data collected. For example, studies that are restricted to older patients generally demonstrate higher levels of comorbidity. Comorbidity also tends to be higher among patients with certain cancers, particularly smoking-related cancers such as lung, head and neck and bladder cancers [105]. Studies based on administrative data, often, but not always, report lower levels of comorbidity than those based on medical notes review or self-reporting [40, 110, 133–136].

Is comorbidity more or less common among cancer patients compared to the general population? There is universal agreement that comorbidity is common among cancer patients in general. However, it is less clear whether cancer patients have higher rates of comorbidity than similarly aged non-cancer populations. Some authors have noted generally similar prevalence rates of comorbid conditions among cancer patients compared with non-cancer populations [137, 138]. In contrast, other studies have reported that cancer patients have somewhat higher levels of comorbidity than the general population [101, 139, 140]. Two studies compared the self-reported prevalence of conditions from the US National Health Interview Study among those with a history of cancer to those without [139, 140]. Hewitt et al. found that among those aged over 65 years, 3.9 % of cancer patients reported having three or more chronic medical conditions, compared with 2.3 % of those without a history of cancer [140]. Similarly, Smith et al. found that, with the exception of patients with melanoma, non-Hodgkin's lymphoma and prostate cancer, cancer patients were more likely to report two or more conditions than those without cancer [139]. More recently, Edwards et al. reported that 40 % of lung, breast, colorectal and prostate cancer patients had at least one comorbid condition compared to 31 % of time period-, age- and sex-matched individuals from the general population [101].

By contrast, there are two studies that have reported that cancer patients actually have lower levels of comorbidity than age matched controls. The first study, by Repetto et al., compared cancer patients to patients admitted to hospital medical or geriatric services who would be expected to have higher levels of multimorbidity than people of a similar age in the general population [141], while the second study, by Piccirillo et al., compared comorbidity data extracted from hospital notes for cancer patients with self-reported national data on similar conditions. Both these sets of authors concluded that the differences between the cancer and non-cancer populations were likely to reflect inadequacies in the data comparison [142].

One obvious reason for inconsistencies in the comparison of the comorbidity burden between cancer and non-cancer populations is likely to be that the prevalence of comorbidity varies considerably by cancer site. In their matched case-control study of men with newly diagnosed cancer, Driver et al. found that the overall (modified Charlson) comorbidity scores were similar for men with and without cancer [143]. However, they found that there was variation by cancer type: in particular, men who had been diagnosed with potentially screen-detected cancers (such as prostate cancer and melanoma) had lower comorbidity scores than age-matched population controls, whilst those with smoking-related cancers had higher scores [143]. Other studies have also found a similar pattern [101, 144, 145].

As well as variation in terms of the general burden of comorbidity, there is also natural variation in the types of comorbidities that patients are affected by, according the cancer type. In some instances, there is a clear association between the kind of comorbidity and the cancer type: for example, in the New Zealand context, more than half of liver cancer patients have cirrhosis of the liver [146]. Unsurprisingly, recent data from the U.S. suggests that more than a third (34 %) of lung cancer patients also have Chronic Obstructive Pulmonary Disorder (COPD) compared to just 10 % of breast cancer patients [101].

Tables 1.1, 1.2, 1.3, and 1.4 show a range of prevalence estimates for the most common conditions for patients with lung, breast, colorectal and prostate cancers, respectively. They show that there is variation in prevalence estimates of specific conditions even within cancer sites. For example, estimates of the prevalence of diabetes among colorectal cancer patients range between 6 and 18 %, of hypertension between 16 and 47 % and of chronic respiratory disease between 5 and 22 %. As with global comorbidity measures, these variations are a function of the study populations, the data collected and the definitions used for specific comorbid conditions. These tables do usefully show that the most common concomitant conditions include hypertension, respiratory disease, heart disease, cerebrovascular disease, previous cancer, arthritis and diabetes. They also show that the prevalence of some comorbid conditions varies between sites, for example respiratory conditions are (unsurprisingly) particularly high among patients with lung cancer, with estimates ranging from 15 to 47 % compared with prostate (1–30 %), colorectal cancer (5–22 %) and breast (all 3–14 % except for one outlier at 52 %).

1.17 Cancer, Comorbidity and Disparity

The prevalence of long term health conditions is not evenly distributed across the population. Disparities in health occur across many axes, including gender, socioeconomic position, geography and sexual orientation. However, health inequities between people of different ethnicity and/or different socioeconomic status are perhaps the largest and most persistent [147, 148].

Comorbidity is generally more common among ethnic minority and Indigenous populations, and among those with higher levels of poverty or deprivation, both within the general population and within cancer populations. The causes of these disparities are related to the uneven distribution of determinants of health, and deficits in health care systems and infrastructures (expanded in Chap. 1.3) [149–151]. For example, the indigenous populations of Australia, New Zealand, the U.S. and Canada, all have a higher prevalence of comorbidity, and are more likely to have multiple, complex comorbidity than non-Indigenous people [147, 152–154].

These patterns are echoed in cancer populations. For example, in the New Zealand colon cancer context only 23 % of Māori had no recorded comorbidity

Table 1.1 Prevalence of specific conditions among patients with prostate cancer from selected studies (%)

Paper	Driver (2010)	Janssen-Heijnen (2005)	Janssen-Heijnen (2005)	Klabunde (2007)	Piccirillo (2008)	Fleming (2006)	Fleming (2006)	Fan (2002)	Putt (2009)	Putt (2009)	Edwards (2014)
Age range (years)	40–84	65–79	80+	66+	All	67+, White men	67+, Black men	All	65+, White men	65+, Black men	65+
Data source	From Dr	Medical notes	Medical notes	Admin data	Medical notes	Admin data	Admin data	Self-report	Admin data	Admin data	Admin data
Hypertension	19	17	12		37	55	88	59	40	58	
Other cancer		9	14		6	9	11	13			
CHF/heart disease		24	27	10	2	13	20	9	4	6	6
COPD/respiratory	21	12	15	16	8	26	30	24	1	13	10
Diabetes		8	9	19	10	16	27	24	14	23	13
Cerebrovascular disease				7	3	11	12		2	4	4
Angina					13			31			
Previous MI				3	7			22			2
PVD				5		13	17		6	7	3
Arthritis	20							59			

Table 1.2 Prevalence of specific conditions among patients with colorectal cancer from selected studies (%)

Paper	Driver (2010)	Janssen-Heijnen (2005)	Janssen-Heijnen (2005)	Gross (2006)	Klabunde (2007)	Klabunde (2007)	Ogle (2000)	Piccirillo (2008)	Sarfati (2009)	Edwards (2014)
Age range (years)	40–84	65–79 males	65–79 females	67+	66+ males	66 + Females	All (colon)	All	>25 (colon)	65+
Data source	From Dr	Medical notes	Medical notes	Admin data	Admin data	Admin data	Self-report	Medical notes	Medical notes	Admin data
Hypertension	16	21	25				47	41	38	
Other cancer		15	14					14	5	
CHF/heart disease	15	28	14	19	4	5		5	11	12
COPD/respiratory	19	15	8	21	5	5	15	12	22	13
Diabetes		10	14	18	6	7	6	16	16	17
Cerebrovascular disease				10	2	2	7	5	7	7
Angina								12	12	
Previous MI					1	<1		8	8	2
PVD				7	2	2			4	4
Arthritis	15						5			

Table 1.3 Prevalence of specific conditions among patients with lung cancer from selected studies (%)

Paper	Driver (2010)	Janssen-Heijnen (2005)	Janssen-Heijnen (2005)	Klabunde (2007)	Klabunde (2007)	Ogle (2000)	Piccirillo (2008)	Tammemagi (2003)	Blanco (2008)	Colinet (2005)	Stevens (2008)	Edwards (2014)
Age range (years)	40–84	65–79 males	65–79 females	66 males	66 females	All	All	All	>70	All	All	65+
Data source	From Dr	Medical notes	Medical notes	Admin data	Admin data	Self-report	Medical notes	Computerised medical records	Medical notes	Medical notes	Medical notes	Admin data
Hypertension	16	15	21			37	38					
Other cancer		16	16				18	1.2	13	12		
CHF/heart disease	21	34	22	7	5		5	8				12
COPD/respiratory	28	24	24	19	15	37	29	29	42	44	47	34
Diabetes		10	12	8	5	5	11		16	9	13	15
Cerebrovascular disease				4	3	9	5		12			7
Angina							14					
Previous MI				2	2		10					3
PVD				4	2			10				7
Arthritis						5						

Table 1.4 Prevalence of specific conditions among patients with female breast cancer from selected studies (%)

Paper	Janssen-Heijnen (2005)	Harlan (2009)	Klabunde (2007)	Patnaik (2011)	Piccirillo (2008)	Fleming (1999)	Mandelblatt (2001)	Satariano (1994)	Wang (2000)	Edwards (2014)
Age range (years)	65–79	All	66+	66+	All	67+	67+	40–84	20+	65+
Data source	Medical notes	Medical notes	Admin data		Medical notes	Admin data	Medical records	Medical records	Admin records	Admin data
Hypertension	29	28			35	69	48	44		
Other cancer	10			16	12	9	10	6		
CHF/heart disease	12	1.2	6	7		25			1	7
COPD/respiratory	6	10	7	9	8	52	14	5	3	10
Diabetes	13	8	11	13	10	32	11	8	4	15
Cerebrovascular disease			4	4	3	16		3	1	5
Angina		1			4	8				
Previous MI		1.4	1	2	3			1	1	1
PVD			2	3		15			<1	3
Arthritis		14					34	21		

compared with 37 % of non-Māori [102]. Māori colon cancer patients also had more than twice the risk of diabetes, heart failure, respiratory disease and renal disease than non-Māori, and were 80 % more likely to have three or more comorbid conditions [102]. In the U.S., Black lung cancer patients were more likely to have at least one comorbid condition that impacts on survival (65 % vs. 59 %) [111], while only 14 % of Black breast cancer patients had no recorded comorbidity compared to 34 % of White patients [118]. In Australia, only 50 % of Indigenous cancer patients had no recorded comorbidity compared to 69 % of non-Indigenous cancer patients, and were three times more likely to have diabetes (30 % vs. 10 %) [155].

Cancer patients of lower socioeconomic status (SES) are also at increased risk of comorbidity. For example, Schrijvers et al. observed that breast cancer patients from a low SES background were nearly three and a half times more likely to have at least one comorbidity compared to breast cancer patients from a high SES background, even after adjusting for age [156]. Louwman et al. observed that cancer patients from a low SES backgrounds were at 50 % higher risk of serious comorbidity compared to those with high SES across a considerable range of cancer types—with a particularly high prevalence of cardiovascular and cerebrovascular disease, COPD, diabetes and gastrointestinal disease [157].

Comorbidity has been shown to be in part responsible for ethnic and socioeconomic disparities in cancer survival. For example, a study by Hill et al. showed that a third of the disparity in colon cancer survival between Māori and non-Māori New Zealanders was due to comorbidity [102]. Similarly, Shepphard et al. found that comorbidity was the most important factor in explaining the three fold poorer survival among First Nations women with breast cancer in Canada, compared with non-Indigenous women [158]. Even for a given level of comorbidity, comorbidity may affect some groups of patients differently to others. For example, in Australia, Indigenous cancer patients with diabetes had an overall survival disadvantage compared to Indigenous cancer patients without diabetes, with an all-cause Hazard Ratio (HR) = 1.4 (95 % CI 1.1–1.8) adjusted for age, sex and cancer site [159]. Fewer non-Indigenous cancer patients had diabetes, and those that had diabetes showed no difference in survival compared to their counterparts without diabetes.

In the US, the evidence relating to the impact of comorbidities on ethnic/racial inequalities in outcomes is somewhat inconsistent. Several authors have found that comorbidity partially or completely explains such disparities [118, 160–165], while others have concluded that comorbidity may not be important in this regard [166–168].

1.18 Why Do Cancer and Comorbidity Coexist?

We have established that cancer and comorbidity commonly occur together—but why is this so? The principal reasons for this co-occurrence vary by (and within) cancer types, but the cause of this association might be attributed to one or more of the following.

1.18.1 Common Conditions Occur Commonly

The primary drivers of comorbidity patterns among cancer patients are the same as those that drive patterns of multimorbidity in the community at large. Thus the underlying pattern of comorbidity in the general population (for example, cardiovascular disease, metabolic disease and mental health disorders) are common to both cancer and non-cancer populations [65, 66, 101].

1.18.2 Cancer and Comorbid Conditions Share Many Common Risk Factors

The strongest single driver of the co-occurrence of cancer and other chronic conditions is increasing age. Smoking, poor diet, lack of physical activity, obesity and alcohol abuse are all risk factors for a range of common non-cancer conditions, including diabetes, hypertension, respiratory, cardiovascular and peripheral vascular disease and liver disease. They are also risk factors for many cancers, including cancers of lung, bladder, head and neck, colorectum, liver and breast [169].

In their Annual Report to the Nation on the Status of Cancer, Edwards et al. [101] compared the prevalence of comorbidity among cancer patients to that of the general (age-matched) population. Compared with the general population, they observed a similar prevalence of comorbidity for older breast and prostate cancer patients (30–32 % of those aged 66 years and over), considerably higher comorbidity prevalence among lung cancer patients (53 %), with colorectal cancer patients intermediate between the two (41 %). These results (and those of others [101, 123, 143–145]) suggest that the wide spectrum of comorbidity prevalence among cancer patients is informative with respect to the question of why cancer and comorbidity coexist: at one end of the spectrum—the lung cancer end—we have patients who are diagnosed with cancers that are strongly associated with risk factors (like particularly smoking), which are in turn also strongly associated with the development of other chronic conditions, such as COPD. At the other end of the spectrum—the breast and prostate cancer end—are patients diagnosed with cancers that are not strongly associated with such risk factors.

1.18.3 Comorbidity May Increase or Decrease Predisposition to Cancer

There are a number of chronic conditions, in particular chronic infections, diseases of the immune system and diabetes, which are causally associated with an increased risk of cancer. For example, Hepatitis B can cause chronic liver disease which is strongly associated with hepatocellular carcinoma, and tuberculosis patients have an increased risk of lung cancer [170]. Conditions associated with immune suppression (such as HIV/AIDS) or dysregulation of the immune system (such as rheumatoid arthritis) are associated with a number of cancers [171–173]. HIV/AIDS is related to Kaposi's Sarcoma, Hodgkin's disease and anal cancers [171] and rheumatoid arthritis is associated with non-Hodgkin's lymphoma and other haematological malignancies [172, 173]. The exact mechanisms through which these associations occur have yet to be fully clarified, but are likely to be multifactorial [173].

We know that the presence of diabetes is associated with an increased risk of several cancers, including colorectal, pancreatic, liver, endometrial and bladder cancers [173–176]. Whilst in part, these associations may be related to common risk factors between diabetes and cancer (such as obesity), there is also evidence that there are specific biological pathways that directly link diabetes with cancer [173, 175, 176]. Type II diabetes is caused (in part) by insulin resistance, which in turn is associated with hyperinsulinaemia (high circulating levels of insulin) and high levels of other insulin-like growth factors, which promote cellular proliferation and affect programmed cell death (apoptosis), increasing the risk of cancer development. In addition to hyperinsulinaemia and hyperglycaemia, chronic inflammation is also thought to be an important neoplastic factor in the link between diabetes and cancer [177].

Whilst patients with diabetes are at increased risk of a number of cancers, they are also at lower risk of lung, and prostate cancers and Hodgkins disease [176, 177]. It is not known why this is the case, but it is postulated to be due to changes in hormone profiles, growth factors and steroids. Patients with hypothyroidism have also been found to have lower rates of breast cancer [173].

1.18.4 Treatment for Comorbidity May Increase or Decrease the Risk of Cancer

As well as the direct effect of long term conditions on cancer risk, medications used to treat such conditions may impact on risk. For example, long term use of immunosuppressive medications, such as those that might be taken by renal failure patients following transplant, are associated with an increased risk of cancer development [178–181]. In contrast, the use of Non-Steroidal Anti-Inflammatory (NSAID) drugs, such as those used chronically among arthritis sufferers, is associated with a reduced risk of colorectal cancer [182–184]. In addition, there is some evidence that metformin, an hypoglycaemic medication commonly used in the management of diabetes, is associated with a reduced incidence of cancer among diabetic patients [177, 185]. However, it is possible that the latter association is at least partly exaggerated by a methodological problem known as immortal time bias [178–181, 186].

1.18.5 Treatment for Cancer May Cause or Exacerbate Comorbidity

As well as comorbidity affecting cancer outcomes, the inverse can also be true, wherein treating a cancer can impact on comorbidity outcomes. Therapies for cancer can increase the risk of developing a comorbid condition, including cardiovascular, musculoskeletal, metabolic or other complications. For example, hormonal treatment for breast and prostate cancer will affect the metabolism and may, in turn, lead to associated complications of diabetes control, and an increased risk of osteoporosis [187]. Some forms of chemotherapy (anthracyclines), as well as anti-HER2 therapies, have been associated with cardiac failure [188], while androgen deprivation therapy for prostate cancer is associated with a greater risk of cardiovascular problems and worsening of pre-existing cardiac disease [189, 190].

It is likely that the impact of cancer treatment on the development or exacerbation of comorbid disease is greatest amongst those who are at highest risk of developing these conditions in the first place, or those who already have some pre-existing (likely related) comorbid disease. However, we really do not know how much cancer and its treatment impacts on patient comorbidity, for the reasons given earlier. Patients with significant comorbidity are generally excluded from clinical trials, and also because data pertaining to cancer patients tends to focus on cancer-specific outcomes rather than broader health outcomes.

1.18.6 There May Be Common Genetic or Physiological Pathways Between Cancer and Comorbidities

A possible example of this is the inverse relationship between neurodegenerative disorders (such as Alzheimer's and Parkinson's disease) and cancer [191–198]. For example, Roe et al. [196] found that there was both a low risk of cancer among Alzheimer's disease patients (HR = 0.31; 012–0.86) and low risk of Alzheimer's disease among cancer patients (HR = 0.57; 0.36–0.90) after adjustment for demographic, smoking and other factors.

Neurodegenerative diseases are related to neuronal loss and cellular destruction, while cancer is a disease of unchecked cellular proliferation. At the cellular level, there is a fine balance between mechanisms that repair DNA and promote cell growth, and those that stop cellular replication and induce apoptosis. The hypothesis relating to the negative correlation between cancer and neurodegenerative disorders is that if the balance favours cell growth and repair, then an individual may be protected from neurodegenerative disorders but may be at increased risk of cancer; whilst if the balance favours effective inhibition of cell growth and replication the opposite will be true [198]. However it is also possible that these associations are at least in part related to methodological problems in the studies that have investigated them, including immortality bias.

1.19 Future Directions for Practice or Research

We have outlined some suggested areas of future practice and/or novel research below:

- There is a need to monitor, at a national and international level, the prevalence of comorbidity among cancer populations, and disparities within these populations. Ongoing collection of comorbidity data among cancer populations (perhaps as a legislated part of regional and national cancer registers) would have multiple benefits, for example, there is a paucity of information regarding how the prevalence and impact of comorbidity is changing over time. As will be discussed in the next chapter, there are methods of measuring comorbidity using routinely-available datasets that would make such monitoring possible.
- There is also a need for further research on how specific comorbid conditions or their treatments interact to either increase or decrease the risk of cancer. Such research would require large, high quality, population-level datasets in order to be informative, particularly for those comorbid conditions and/or cancers that are not highly prevalent.
- There is a need for a greater understanding of the role of genes in determining the predisposition to certain comorbid conditions, and how this predisposition relates (either directly or indirectly) with the development of cancer. The advent of population-level genome data in combination with population-level routine healthcare data will assist in potentially ground-breaking discoveries in this area.
- Finally, there is a general need for the inclusion of more comorbid patients in clinical trials. Our understanding of whether cancer treatment might cause or exacerbate comorbidity is limited by the fact that there is a tendency for patients with comorbidity to be excluded from clinical trials. The exclusion of such patients ignores clinical reality, where many (if not most, in some cancer contexts) cancer patients live with at least one comorbid condition. Stratification of comorbid patients into treatment arms is one mechanism of overcoming this problem.

References

1. Salisbury C (2012) Multimorbidity: redesigning health care for people who use it. Lancet 380 (9836):7–9
2. Extermann M (2000) Measurement and impact of comorbidity in older cancer patients. Crit Rev Oncol Hematol 35(3):181–200
3. Extermann M (2000) Measuring comorbidity in older cancer patients. Eur J Cancer 36 (4):453–471
4. Satariano WA, Silliman RA (2003) Comorbidity: implications for research and practice in geriatric oncology. Crit Rev Oncol Hematol 48(2):239–248
5. Sarfati DBK, Jackson C (2016) The impact of comorbidity on cancer and its treatment. CA Cancer J Clin (in press)

6. Feinstein A (1970) The pre-therapeutic classification of co-morbidity in chronic disease. J Chron Dis 23:455–469
7. Fortin M, Bravo G, Hudon C et al (2006) Relationship between multimorbidity and health-related quality of life of patients in primary care. Qual Life Res 15(1):83–91
8. Gijsen R, Hoeymans N, Schellevis FG, Ruwaard D, Satariano WA, van den Bos GA (2001) Causes and consequences of comorbidity: a review. J Clin Epidemiol 54(7):661–674
9. Mandelblatt JS, Bierman AS, Gold K et al (2001) Constructs of burden of illness in older patients with breast cancer: a comparison of measurement methods. [Erratum appears in Health Serv Res. 2007 Oct; 42(5):2088 Note: Maserejan, N [corrected to Maserejian, N]]. Health Serv Res 36(6 Pt 1):1085–1107
10. Parekh AK, Barton MB (2010) The challenge of multiple comorbidity for the US health care system. JAMA 303(13):1303–1304
11. Valderas JM, Starfield B, Roland M (2007) Multimorbidity's many challenges: a research priority in the UK. BMJ 334(7604):1128
12. Valderas JM, Starfield B, Sibbald B, Salisbury C, Roland M (2009) Defining comorbidity: implications for understanding health and health services. Ann Fam Med 7(4):357–363
13. Wagner EH, Austin BT, Von Korff M (1996) Organizing care for patients with chronic illness. Milbank Q 74(4):511–544
14. Yancik R, Ershler W, Satariano W, Hazzard W, Cohen HJ, Ferrucci L (2007) Report of the national institute on aging task force on comorbidity. J Gerontol A Biol Sci Med Sci 62 (3):275–280
15. Institute of Medicine (2013) Delivering high-quality cancer care: charting a new course for a system in crisis. The National Academies Press, Washington, DC
16. Fortin M, Dionne J, Pinho G, Gignac J, Almirall J, Lapointe L (2006) Randomized controlled trials: do they have external validity for patients with multiple comorbidities? Ann Fam Med 4(2):104–108
17. Starfield B (2006) Threads and yarns: weaving the tapestry of comorbidity. Ann Fam Med 4 (2):101–103
18. Mangin D, Heath I, Jamoulle M (2012) Beyond diagnosis: rising to the multimorbidity challenge. BMJ 344:e3526
19. Tinetti ME, Fried TR, Boyd CM (2012) Designing health care for the most common chronic condition–multimorbidity. [Erratum appears in JAMA. 2012 Jul 18;308(3):238]. JAMA 307 (23):2493–2494
20. Vitry AI, Zhang Y (2008) Quality of Australian clinical guidelines and relevance to the care of older people with multiple comorbid conditions. Med J Aust 189(7):360–365
21. Boyd CM, Darer J, Boult C, Fried LP, Boult L, Wu AW (2005) Clinical practice guidelines and quality of care for older patients with multiple comorbid diseases: implications for pay for performance. JAMA 294(6):716–724
22. van Weel C, Schellevis FG (2006) Comorbidity and guidelines: conflicting interests. Lancet 367(9510):550–551
23. Kaplan MH, Feinstein AR (1974) The importance of classifying initial co-morbidity in evaluating the outcome of diabetes mellitus. J Chronic Dis 27(7–8):387–404
24. de Groot V, Beckerman H, Lankhorst GJ, Bouter LM (2003) How to measure comorbidity. a critical review of available methods. J Clin Epidemiol 56(3):221–229
25. Duckett SJ, Agius PA (2002) Performance of diagnosis-based risk adjustment measures in a population of sick Australians. Aust N Z J Public Health 26(6):500–507
26. Perkins AJ, Kroenke K, Unutzer J et al (2004) Common comorbidity scales were similar in their ability to predict health care costs and mortality. J Clin Epidemiol 57(10):1040–1048
27. Reid RJ, MacWilliam L, Verhulst L, Roos N, Atkinson M (2001) Performance of the ACG case-mix system in two Canadian provinces. Med Care 39(1):86–99
28. Starfield B, Weiner J, Mumford L, Steinwachs D (1991) Ambulatory care groups: a categorization of diagnoses for research and management. Health Serv Res 26(1):53–74

29. Weiner JP, Starfield BH, Steinwachs DM, Mumford LM (1991) Development and application of a population-oriented measure of ambulatory care case-mix. Med Care 29 (5):452–472
30. Chang H-Y, Weiner JP (2010) An in-depth assessment of a diagnosis-based risk adjustment model based on national health insurance claims: the application of the Johns Hopkins adjusted clinical group case-mix system in Taiwan. BMC Med 8:7
31. Fowles JB, Weiner JP, Knutson D, Fowler E, Tucker AM, Ireland M (1996) Taking health status into account when setting capitation rates: a comparison of risk-adjustment methods. JAMA 276(16):1316–1321
32. Greene BR, Barlow J, Newman C (1996) Ambulatory care groups and the profiling of primary care physician resource use: examining the application of case mix adjustments. J Ambul Care Manag 19(1):86–89
33. Orueta JF, Lopez-De-Munain J et al (1999) Application of the ambulatory care groups in the primary care of a European national health care system: does it work? Med Care 37(3): 238–248
34. Tucker AM, Weiner JP, Honigfeld S, Parton RA (1996) Profiling primary care physician resource use: examining the application of case mix adjustment. J Ambul Care Manag 19 (1):60–80
35. Hall SF (2006) A user's guide to selecting a comorbidity index for clinical research. J Clin Epidemiol 59(8):849–855
36. Sarfati D (2012) Review of methods to measure comorbidity in cancer populations: no gold standard exists. J Clin Epidemiol 65:924–933
37. Charlson M, Pompei P, Ales K, Mackenzie C (1987) A new method for classifying prognostic comorbidity in longitudinal studies: development and validation. J Chronic Dis 40:373–383
38. Deyo RA, Cherkin DC, Ciol MA (1992) Adapting a clinical comorbidity index for use with ICD-9-CM administrative databases. J Clin Epidemiol 45(6):613–619
39. Romano PS, Roos LL, Jollis JG (1993) Adapting a clinical comorbidity index for use with ICD-9-CM administrative data: differing perspectives. J Clin Epidemiol 46(10):1075–1079 Discussion 81-90
40. Romano PS, Roos LL, Jollis JG (1993) Further evidence concerning the use of a clinical comorbidity index with ICD-9-CM administrative data. J Clin Epidemiol 46(10):1085–1090
41. Quan H, Sundararajan V, Halfon P et al (2005) Coding algorithms for defining comorbidities in ICD-9-CM and ICD-10 administrative data. Med Care 43(11):1130–1139
42. Byles JE, D'Este C, Parkinson L, O'Connell R, Treloar C (2005) Single index of multimorbidity did not predict multiple outcomes. J Clin Epidemiol 58(10):997–1005
43. Fan VS, Au D, Heagerty P, Deyo RA, McDonell MB, Fihn SD (2002) Validation of case-mix measures derived from self-reports of diagnoses and health. J Clin Epidemiol 55 (4):371–380
44. Katz JN, Chang LC, Sangha O, Fossel AH, Bates DW (1996) Can comorbidity be measured by questionnaire rather than medical record review? Med Care 34(1):73–84
45. Lash TL, Mor V, Wieland D, Ferrucci L, Satariano W, Silliman RA (2007) Methodology, design, and analytic techniques to address measurement of comorbid disease. J Gerontol A Biol Sci Med Sci 62(3):281–285
46. Davis P, Lay-Yee R, Fitzjohn J et al (2002) Co-morbidity and health outcomes in three Auckland hospitals. N Z Med J 115(1153):211–215
47. Sarfati D, Hill S, Blakely T et al (2009) The effect of comorbidity on the use of adjuvant chemotherapy and survival from colon cancer: a retrospective cohort study. BMC Cancer 9:116
48. Verbrugge LM, Lepkowski JM, Konkol LL (1991) Levels of disability among US adults with arthritis. J Gerontol 46(2):S71–S83
49. Fleming ST, Rastogi A, Dmitrienko A, Johnson KD (1999) A comprehensive prognostic index to predict survival based on multiple comorbidities: a focus on breast cancer. Med Care 37(6):601–614

50. Greenfield S, Kaplan SH, Ware JE Jr, Yano EM, Frank HJ (1988) Patients' participation in medical care: effects on blood sugar control and quality of life in diabetes. J Gen Intern Med 3(5):448–457
51. Piccirillo JF, Tierney RM, Costas I, Grove L, Spitznagel EL Jr (2004) Prognostic importance of comorbidity in a hospital-based cancer registry. JAMA 291(20):2441–2447
52. Elixhauser A, Steiner C, Harris DR, Coffey RM (1998) Comorbidity measures for use with administrative data. Med Care 36(1):8–27
53. Holman CD, Preen DB, Baynham NJ, Finn JC, Semmens JB (2005) A multipurpose comorbidity scoring system performed better than the Charlson index. J Clin Epidemiol 58 (10):1006–1014
54. Tammemagi CM, Neslund-Dudas C, Simoff M, Kvale P (2003) Impact of comorbidity on lung cancer survival. Int J Cancer 103(6):792–802
55. Humphries KH, Rankin JM, Carere RG, Buller CE, Kiely FM, Spinelli JJ (2000) Co-morbidity data in outcomes research: are clinical data derived from administrative databases a reliable alternative to chart review? J Clin Epidemiol 53(4):343–349
56. Karlamangla A, Tinetti M, Guralnik J, Studenski S, Wetle T, Reuben D (2007) Comorbidity in older adults: nosology of impairment, diseases, and conditions. J Gerontol A Biol Sci Med Sci 62(3):296–300
57. Fried LP, Ferrucci L, Darer J, Williamson JD, Anderson G (2004) Untangling the concepts of disability, frailty, and comorbidity: implications for improved targeting and care. J Gerontol A Biol Sci Med Sci 59(3):255–263
58. Nagi SZ (1976) An epidemiology of disability among adults in the United States. Milbank Mem Fund Quart Health Soc 54(4):439–467
59. Seeman TE, Singer BH, Rowe JW, Horwitz RI, McEwen BS (1997) Price of adaptation–allostatic load and its health consequences. MacArthur studies of successful aging. [Erratum appears in Arch Intern Med 1999 Jun 14;159(11):1176]. Arch Intern Med 157(19):2259–2268
60. Verbrugge LM, Jette AM (1994) The disablement process. Soc Sci Med 38(1):1–14
61. van den Akker M, Buntinx F, Knottnerus JA (1996) Comorbidity or multimorbidity: what's in a name. A review of literature. Eur J Gen Pract 2:65–70
62. Fortin M, Soubhi H, Hudon C, Bayliss EA, van den Akker M (2007) Multimorbidity's many challenges. BMJ 334(7602):1016–1017
63. Haggerty JL (2012) Ordering the chaos for patients with multimorbidity. BMJ 345:e5915
64. van den Akker M, Buntinx F, Metsemakers JF, Roos S, Knottnerus JA (1998) Multimorbidity in general practice: prevalence, incidence, and determinants of co-occurring chronic and recurrent diseases. J Clin Epidemiol 51(5):367–375
65. Barnett K, Mercer SW, Norbury M, Watt G, Wyke S, Guthrie B (2012) Epidemiology of multimorbidity and implications for health care, research, and medical education: a cross-sectional study. Lancet 380(9836):37–43
66. Britt HC, Harrison CM, Miller GC, Knox SA (2008) Prevalence and patterns of multimorbidity in Australia. Med J Aust 189(2):72–77
67. Noel PH, Parchman ML, Williams JW Jr et al (2007) The challenges of multimorbidity from the patient perspective. J Gen Intern Med 22(Suppl 3):419–424
68. Tooth L, Hockey R, Byles J, Dobson A (2008) Weighted multimorbidity indexes predicted mortality, health service use, and health-related quality of life in older women. J Clin Epidemiol 61(2):151–159
69. van den Akker M, Buntinx F, Roos S, Knottnerus JA (2001) Problems in determining occurrence rates of multimorbidity. J Clin Epidemiol 54(7):675–679
70. Guthrie B, Payne K, Alderson P, McMurdo MET, Mercer SW (2012) Adapting clinical guidelines to take account of multimorbidity. BMJ 345:e6341
71. Smith SM, Soubhi H, Fortin M, Hudon C, O'Dowd T (2012) Managing patients with multimorbidity: systematic review of interventions in primary care and community settings. BMJ 345:e5205

72. Schrag D (2008) Enhancing cancer registry data to promote rational health system design. J Natl Cancer Inst 100(6):378–379
73. Lash TL, Mor V, Wieland D, Ferrucci L, Satariano WA, Silliman R (2004) Methodology, design an analytic techniques to address measurement of comorbid disease. The National Institute on Aging's Comorbidity Taskforce, White Paper
74. Guralnik JM, Ferrucci L (2003) Assessing the building blocks of function: utilizing measures of functional limitation. Am J Prev Med 25(3 Suppl 2):112–121
75. Pompei P, Charlson ME, Ales K, MacKenzie CR, Norton M (1991) Relating patient characteristics at the time of admission to outcomes of hospitalization. J Clin Epidemiol 44 (10):1063–1069
76. Wedding U, Rohrig B, Klippstein A, Pientka L, Hoffken K (2007) Age, severe comorbidity and functional impairment independently contribute to poor survival in cancer patients. J Cancer Res Clin Oncol 133(12):945–950
77. Parmelee PA, Thuras PD, Katz IR, Lawton MP (1995) Validation of the cumulative illness rating scale in a geriatric residential population. J Am Geriatr Soc 43(2):130–137
78. Gruenewald TL, Seeman TE, Karlamangla AS, Sarkisian CA (2009) Allostatic load and frailty in older adults. J Am Geriatr Soc 57(9):1525–1531
79. Seeman TE, McEwen BS, Rowe JW, Singer BH (2001) Allostatic load as a marker of cumulative biological risk: MacArthur studies of successful aging. Proc Natl Acad Sci USA 98(8):4770–4775
80. Balducci L (2007) Aging, frailty, and chemotherapy. Cancer Control 14(1):7–12
81. Fried LP, Tangen CM, Walston J et al (2001) Frailty in older adults: evidence for a phenotype. J Gerontol A Biol Sci Med Sci 56(3):M146–M156
82. Balducci L, Stanta G (2000) Cancer in the frail patient. A coming epidemic. Hematol Oncol Clin North America 14(1):235–250
83. Mohile SG, Xian Y, Dale W et al (2009) Association of a cancer diagnosis with vulnerability and frailty in older medicare beneficiaries. J Natl Cancer Inst 101(17):1206–1215
84. Balducci L, Extermann M (2000) Management of the frail person with advanced cancer. Crit Rev Oncol Hematol 33(2):143–148
85. Pal SK, Katheria V, Hurria A (2010) Evaluating the older patient with cancer: understanding frailty and the geriatric assessment. CA Cancer J Clin 60(2):120–132
86. Koroukian SM, Murray P, Madigan E (2006) Comorbidity, disability, and geriatric syndromes in elderly cancer patients receiving home health care. J Clin Oncol 24(15):2304–2310
87. Greenfield S, Sullivan L, Dukes KA, Silliman R, D'Agostino R, Kaplan SH (1995) Development and testing of a new measure of case mix for use in office practice. Med Care 33(4 Suppl):AS47–AS55
88. Litwin MS, Greenfield S, Elkin EP, Lubeck DP, Broering JM, Kaplan SH (2007) Assessment of prognosis with the total illness burden index for prostate cancer: aiding clinicians in treatment choice. Cancer 109(9):1777–1783
89. Puts MT, Hardt J, Monette J, Girre V, Springall E, Alibhai SM (2012) Use of geriatric assessment for older adults in the oncology setting: a systematic review. J Natl Cancer Inst 104(15):1133–1163
90. Puts MT, Santos B, Hardt J et al (2014) An update on a systematic review of the use of geriatric assessment for older adults in oncology. Ann Oncol 25(2):307–315
91. Wildiers H, Heeren P, Puts M et al (2014) International society of geriatric oncology consensus on geriatric assessment in older patients with cancer. J Clin Oncol 32(24): 2595–2603
92. Extermann M, Hurria A (2007) Comprehensive geriatric assessment for older patients with cancer. J Clin Oncol 25(14):1824–1831
93. Ramjaun A, Nassif MO, Krotneva S, Huang AR, Meguerditchian AN (2013) Improved targeting of cancer care for older patients: a systematic review of the utility of comprehensive geriatric assessment. J Geriatr Oncol 4(3):271–281

94. Brunello A, Sandri R, Extermann M (2009) Multidimensional geriatric evaluation for older cancer patients as a clinical and research tool. Cancer Treat Rev 35(6):487–492
95. Extermann M (2003) Studies of comprehensive geriatric assessment in patients with cancer. Cancer Control 10(6):463–468
96. Girones R, Torregrosa D, Diaz-Beveridge R (2010) Comorbidity, disability and geriatric syndromes in elderly breast cancer survivors. Results of a single-center experience. Crit Rev Oncol Hematol 73(3):236–245
97. Safford MM, Allison JJ, Kiefe CI (2007) Patient complexity: more than comorbidity. The vector model of complexity. J Gen Intern Med 22(Suppl 3):382–390
98. Schaink A, Kuluski K, Lyons R et al (2012) A scoping review and thematic classification of patient complexity: offering a unifying framework. J Comorbidity 2:1–9
99. Nardi R, Scanelli G, Corrao S, Iori I, Mathieu G, Amatrian RC (2007) Co-morbidity does not reflect complexity in internal medicine patients. Eur J Intern Med 18(5):359–368
100. Lee L, Cheung WY, Atkinson E, Krzyzanowska MK (2011) Impact of comorbidity on chemotherapy use and outcomes in solid tumors: a systematic review. J Clin Oncol 29 (1):106–117
101. Edwards BK, Noone AM, Mariotto AB et al (2014) Annual report to the nation on the status of cancer, 1975–2010, featuring prevalence of comorbidity and impact on survival among persons with lung, colorectal, breast, or prostate cancer. Cancer 120(9):1290–1314
102. Hill S, Sarfati D, Blakely T et al (2010) Survival disparities in Indigenous and non-indigenous New Zealanders with colon cancer: the role of patient comorbidity, treatment and health service factors. J Epidemiol Comm Health 64:117–123
103. Stevens W, Stevens G, Kolbe J, Cox B (2008) Ethnic differences in the management of lung cancer in New Zealand. J Thorac Oncol 3(3):237–244
104. Baldwin L-M, Dobie SA, Billingsley K et al (2005) Explaining black-white differences in receipt of recommended colon cancer treatment. J Natl Cancer Inst 97(16):1211–1220
105. Coebergh JW, Janssen-Heijnen ML, Razenberg PP (1998) Prevalence of co-morbidity in newly diagnosed patients with cancer: a population-based study. Crit Rev Oncol Hematol 27 (2):97–100
106. Fleming ST, Pearce KA, McDavid K, Pavlov D (2003) The development and validation of a comorbidity index for prostate cancer among black men. J Clin Epidemiol 56(11):1064–1075
107. Gross CP, Guo Z, McAvay GJ, Allore HG, Young M, Tinetti ME (2006) Multimorbidity and survival in older persons with colorectal cancer. J Am Geriatr Soc 54(12):1898–1904
108. Hall WH, Jani AB, Ryu JK, Narayan S, Vijayakumar S (2005) The impact of age and comorbidity on survival outcomes and treatment patterns in prostate cancer. Prostate Cancer Prostatic Dis 8(1):22–30
109. Lemmens VE, Janssen-Heijnen ML, Verheij CD, Houterman S, Repelaer van Driel OJ, Coebergh JW (2005) Co-morbidity leads to altered treatment and worse survival of elderly patients with colorectal cancer. Br J Surg 92(5):615–623
110. Newschaffer CJ, Bush TL, Penberthy LT (1997) Comorbidity measurement in elderly female breast cancer patients with administrative and medical records data. J Clin Epidemiol 50 (6):725–733
111. Tammemagi CM, Neslund-Dudas C, Simoff M, Kvale P (2004) In lung cancer patients, age, race-ethnicity, gender and smoking predict adverse comorbidity, which in turn predicts treatment and survival. J Clin Epidemiol 57(6):597–609
112. Yates JW (2001) Comorbidity considerations in geriatric oncology research. CA Cancer J Clin 51(6):329–336
113. Baldwin L-M, Klabunde CN, Green P, Barlow W, Wright G (2006) In search of the perfect comorbidity measure for use with administrative claims data: does it exist? Med Care 44 (8):745–753
114. Etzioni DA, El-Khoueiry AB, Beart RW (2008) Rates and predictors of chemotherapy use for stage III colon cancer. Cancer 113:3279–3289
115. Gross CP, McAvay GJ, Guo Z, Tinetti ME (2007) The impact of chronic illnesses on the use and effectiveness of adjuvant chemotherapy for colon cancer. Cancer 109(12):2410–2419

116. Stevens W, Stevens G, Kolbe J, Cox B (2007) Lung cancer in New Zealand: patterns of secondary care and implications for survival. J Thorac Oncol 2(6):481–493
117. Cronin DP, Harlan LC, Potosky AL, Clegg LX, Stevens JL, Mooney MM (2006) Patterns of care for adjuvant therapy in a random population-based sample of patients diagnosed with colorectal cancer. Am J Gastroenterol 101(10):2308–2318
118. Tammemagi C, Nerenz D, Neslund-Dudas C, Feldkamp C, Nathanson D (2005) Comorbidity and survival disparities among black and white patients with breast cancer. JAMA 294 (14):1765–1772
119. Velanovich V, Gabel M, Walker EM et al (2002) Causes for the undertreatment of elderly breast cancer patients: tailoring treatments to individual patients. J Am Coll Surg 194(1): 8–13
120. Yancik R, Wesley MN, Ries LA, Havlik RJ, Edwards BK, Yates JW (2001) Effect of age and comorbidity in postmenopausal breast cancer patients aged 55 years and older. JAMA 285 (7):885–892
121. Bradley CJ, Dahman B, Anscher M (2014) Prostate cancer treatment and survival: evidence for men with prevalent comorbid conditions. Med Care 52(6):482–489
122. Redelmeier DA, Tan SH, Booth GL (1998) The treatment of unrelated disorders in patients with chronic medical diseases. N Engl J Med 338(21):1516–1520
123. Sarfati D, Gurney J, Lim B et al (2013) Identifying important comorbidity among cancer populations using administrative data: prevalence and impact on survival. Asia Pac J Clin Oncol. doi:10.1111/ajco.12130
124. Sarfati D, Gurney J, Stanley J et al (2014) Cancer-specific administrative data-based comorbidity indices provided valid alternative to Charlson and NHI indices. J Clin Oncol 67 (5):586–595
125. Gonzalez EC, Ferrante JM, Van Durme DJ, Pal N, Roetzheim RG (2001) Comorbid illness and the early detection of cancer. South Med J 94(9):913–920
126. Coebergh JW, Janssen-Heijnen ML, Post PN, Razenberg PP (1999) Serious co-morbidity among unselected cancer patients newly diagnosed in the southeastern part of The Netherlands in 1993–1996. J Clin Epidemiol 52(12):1131–1136
127. Cronin-Fenton DP, Norgaard M, Jacobsen J et al (2007) Comorbidity and survival of Danish breast cancer patients from 1995 to 2005. Br J Cancer 96(9):1462–1468
128. Iversen LH, Norgaard M, Jacobsen J, Laurberg S, Sorensen HT (2009) The impact of comorbidity on survival of Danish colorectal cancer patients from 1995 to 2006–a population-based cohort study. Dis Colon Rectum 52(1):71–78
129. Janssen-Heijnen MLG, Houterman S, Lemmens VEPP, Louwman MWJ, Maas HAAM, Coebergh JWW (2005) Prognostic impact of increasing age and co-morbidity in cancer patients: a population-based approach. Crit Rev Oncol Hematol 55(3):231–240
130. Janssen-Heijnen MLG, Smulders S, Lemmens VEPP, Smeenk FWJM, van Geffen HJAA, Coebergh JWW (2004) Effect of comorbidity on the treatment and prognosis of elderly patients with non-small cell lung cancer. Thorax 59(7):602–607
131. Miller DC, Taub DA, Dunn RL, Montie JE, Wei JT (2003) The impact of co-morbid disease on cancer control and survival following radical cystectomy. J Urol 169(1):105–109
132. Patnaik JL, Byers T, Diguiseppi C, Denberg TD, Dabelea D (2011) The influence of comorbidities on overall survival among older women diagnosed with breast cancer. J Natl Cancer Inst 103(14):1101–1111
133. Kieszak SM, Flanders WD, Kosinski AS, Shipp CC, Karp H (1999) A comparison of the Charlson comorbidity index derived from medical record data and administrative billing data. J Clin Epidemiol 52(2):137–142
134. Malenka DJ, McLerran D, Roos N, Fisher ES, Wennberg JE (1994) Using administrative data to describe casemix: a comparison with the medical record. J Clin Epidemiol 47 (9):1027–1032
135. Sarfati D, Hill S, Purdie G, Dennett E, Blakely T (2010) How well does routine hospitalisation data capture information on comorbidity in New Zealand? NZ Med J 123 (1310):50–61

136. van Doorn C, Bogardus ST, Williams CS, Concato J, Towle VR, Inouye SK (2001) Risk adjustment for older hospitalized persons: a comparison of two methods of data collection for the Charlson index. J Clin Epidemiol 54(7):694–701
137. Harlan LC, Klabunde CN, Ambs AH et al (2009) Comorbidities, therapy, and newly diagnosed conditions for women with early stage breast cancer. J Cancer Surviv 3(2):89–98
138. Zeber JE, Copeland LA, Hosek BJ, Karnad AB, Lawrence VA, Sanchez-Reilly SE (2008) Cancer rates, medical comorbidities, and treatment modalities in the oldest patients. Crit Rev Oncol Hematol 67(3):237–242
139. Smith AW, Reeve BB, Bellizzi KM et al (2008) Cancer, comorbidities, and health-related quality of life of older adults. Health Care Finan Rev 29(4):41–56
140. Hewitt M, Rowland JH, Yancik R (2003) Cancer survivors in the United States: age, health, and disability. J Gerontol A Biol Sci Med Sci 58(1):82–91
141. Repetto L, Venturino A, Vercelli M et al (1998) Performance status and comorbidity in elderly cancer patients compared with young patients with neoplasia and elderly patients without neoplastic conditions. Cancer 82(4):760–765
142. Piccirillo JF, Costas I, Claybour P, Borah A, Gorove L, Jeffe D (2003) The measurement of comorbidity by cancer registries. J Reg Mgmt 30(1):8–14
143. Driver JA, Yung R, Gaziano JM, Kurth T (2010) Chronic disease in men with newly diagnosed cancer: a nested case-control study. Am J Epidemiol 172(3):299–308
144. Jorgensen TL, Hallas J, Friis S, Herrstedt J (2012) Comorbidity in elderly cancer patients in relation to overall and cancer-specific mortality. Br J Cancer 106(7):1353–1360
145. Cho H, Mariotto A, Mann B, Klabunde CN, Feuer E (2013) Assessing non-cancer-related health status of US cancer patients: other-cause survival and comorbidity prevalence. Am J Epidemiol 178(3):339–349
146. Chamberlain J, Sarfati D, Cunningham R, Koea J, Gurney J, Blakely T (2013) Incidence and management of hepatocellular carcinoma among Māori and non-Māori New Zealanders. Aust N Z J Public Health 37:520–526
147. Robson B, Harris R (eds) (2007) Hauora: maori standards of health IV. A study of the years 2000–2005. Te Ropu Rangahau Hauora a Eru Pomare, Wellington
148. Robson B, Purdie G, Cormack D (2010) Unequal impact: maori and non-maori cancer statistics by deprivation and rurality 2002–2006. Ministry of Health, Wellington
149. Knaul F, Frank J, Shulman L (2011) For the global task force on expanded access to cancer care and control in developing countries. Closing the cancer divide: a blueprint to expand access in low and middle income countries. Harvard Global Equity Initiative, Boston, MA
150. Coleman MP (2014) Cancer survival: global surveillance will stimulate health policy and improve equity. Lancet 383(9916):564–573
151. Steinberg ML (2008) Inequity in cancer care: explanations and solutions for disparity. Semin Radiat Oncol 18(3):161–167
152. Valery PC, Coory M, Stirling J, Green AC (2006) Cancer diagnosis, treatment, and survival in Indigenous and non-Indigenous Australians: a matched cohort study. Lancet 367 (9525):1842–1848
153. Centers for Disease Control (2013) CDC health disparities and inequalities report—United States. MMWR 62(Suppl 3):1–187
154. King M (2011) Chronic diseases and mortality in Canadian aboriginal peoples: learning from the knowledge. Prev Chronic Dis 8(1):A07
155. Moore SP, Green AC, Bray F et al (2014) Survival disparities in Australia: an analysis of patterns of care and comorbidities among indigenous and non-indigenous cancer patients. BMC Cancer 14(1):1
156. Schrijvers CTM, Coebergh JWW, Mackenbach JP (1997) Socioeconomic status and comorbidity among newly diagnosed cancer patients. Cancer 80(8):1482–1488
157. Louwman WJ, Aarts MJ, Houterman S, Van Lenthe FJ, Coebergh JWW, Janssen-Heijnen MLG (2010) A 50 % higher prevalence of life-shortening chronic conditions among cancer patients with low socioeconomic status. Br J Cancer 103(11):1742–1748

158. Sheppard AJ, Chiarelli AM, Marrett LD, Nishri ED, Trudeau ME (2011) Stage at diagnosis and comorbidity influence breast cancer survival in first nations women in Ontario Canada. Cancer Epidemiol Biomark Prev 20(10):2160–2167
159. Martin JH, Coory MD, Valery PC, Green AC (2009) Association of diabetes with survival among cohorts of Indigenous and non-Indigenous Australians with cancer. Cancer Causes Control 20(3):355–360
160. Putt M, Long JA, Montagnet C et al (2009) Racial differences in the impact of comorbidities on survival among elderly men with prostate cancer. Med Care Res Rev 66(4):409–435
161. Allard JE, Maxwell GL (2009) Race disparities between black and white women in the incidence, treatment, and prognosis of endometrial cancer. Cancer Control 16(1):53–56
162. Braithwaite D, Tammemagi CM, Moore DH et al (2009) Hypertension is an independent predictor of survival disparity between African-American and white breast cancer patients. Int J Cancer 124(5):1213–1219
163. Holmes L Jr, Chan W, Jiang Z, Ward D, Essien EJ, Du XL (2009) Impact of androgen deprivation therapy on racial/ethnic disparities in the survival of older men treated for locoregional prostate cancer. Cancer Control 16(2):176–185
164. Yang R, Cheung MC, Byrne MM et al (2010) Do racial or socioeconomic disparities exist in lung cancer treatment? Cancer 116(10):2437–2447
165. Cook LS, Nelson HE, Cockburn M, Olson SH, Muller CY, Wiggins CL (2013) Comorbidities and endometrial cancer survival in Hispanics and non-Hispanic whites. Cancer Causes Control 24(1):61–69
166. Curtis E, Quale C, Haggstrom D, Smith-Bindman R (2008) Racial and ethnic differences in breast cancer survival: how much is explained by screening, tumor severity, biology, treatment, comorbidities, and demographics? Cancer 112(1):171–180
167. Coker AL, Eggleston KS, Du XL, Ramondetta L (2009) Ethnic disparities in cervical cancer survival among Medicare eligible women in a multiethnic population. Int J Gynecol Cancer 19(1):13–20
168. Hines RB, Shanmugam C, Waterbor JW et al (2009) Effect of comorbidity and body mass index on the survival of African-American and Caucasian patients with colon cancer. Cancer 115(24):5798–5806
169. Adami HO, Hunter D, Trichopoulos D (eds) (2008) Textbook of cancer epidemiology, 2nd edn. Oxford University Press, New York
170. Wu C-Y, Hu H-Y, Pu C-Y et al (2011) Pulmonary tuberculosis increases the risk of lung cancer: a population-based cohort study. Cancer 117(3):618–624
171. Hensel M, Goetzenich A, Lutz T et al (2011) HIV and cancer in Germany. Dtsch 108 (8):117–122
172. Chen Y-J, Chang Y-T, Wang C-B, Wu C-Y (2011) The risk of cancer in patients with rheumatoid arthritis: a nationwide cohort study in Taiwan. Arthritis Rheum 63(2):352–358
173. Extermann M (2007) Interaction between comorbidity and cancer. Cancer Control 14(1): 13–22
174. Friberg E, Orsini N, Mantzoros CS, Wolk A (2007) Diabetes mellitus and risk of endometrial cancer: a meta-analysis. Diabetologia 50(7):1365–1374
175. Bartosch-Harlid A, Andersson R (2010) Diabetes mellitus in pancreatic cancer and the need for diagnosis of asymptomatic disease. Pancreatology 10(4):423–428
176. Tabares-Seisdedos R, Dumont N, Baudot A et al (2011) No paradox, no progress: inverse cancer comorbidity in people with other complex diseases. Lancet Oncology 12(6):604–608
177. Giovannucci E, Harlan DM, Archer MC et al (2010) Diabetes and cancer: a consensus report. Diabetes Care 33(7):1674–1685
178. Dantal J, Hourmant M, Cantarovich D et al (1998) Effect of long-term immunosuppression in kidney-graft recipients on cancer incidence: randomised comparison of two cyclosporin regimens. Lancet 351(9103):623–628
179. Gallagher MP, Kelly PJ, Jardine M et al (2010) Long-term cancer risk of immunosuppressive regimens after kidney transplantation. J Am Soc Nephrol 21(5):852–858

180. Hernández Vallejo G, Jiménez Romero C, De Vicente JC (2005) Incidence and risk factors for cancer after liver transplantation. Crit Rev Oncol Hematol 56(1 SPEC. ISS.):87–99
181. Jensen P, Hansen S, Moller B et al (1999) Skin cancer in kidney and heart transplant recipients and different long-term immunosuppressive therapy regimens. J Am Acad Dermatol 40(2 I):177–186
182. Din FVN, Theodoratou E, Farrington SM et al (2010) Effect of aspirin and NSAIDs on risk and survival from colorectal cancer. Gut 59(12):1670–1679
183. Flossmann E, Rothwell PM, British Doctors Aspirin T, The UKTIAAT (2007) Effect of aspirin on long-term risk of colorectal cancer: consistent evidence from randomised and observational studies. Lancet 369(9573):1603–1613
184. Huls G, Koornstra JJ, Kleibeuker JH (2003) Non-steroidal anti-inflammatory drugs and molecular carcinogenesis of colorectal carcinomas. Lancet 362(9379):230–232
185. Kasznicki J, Sliwinska A, Drzewoski J (2014) Metformin in cancer prevention and therapy. Ann Trans Med 2(6):57
186. Suissa S, Azoulay L (2012) Metformin and the risk of cancer: time-related biases in observational studies. Diabetes Care 35(12):2665–2673
187. Haugnes HS, Aass N, Fossa SD et al (2007) Components of the metabolic syndrome in long-term survivors of testicular cancer. Ann Oncol 18(2):241–248
188. Smith LA, Cornelius VR, Plummer CJ et al (2010) Cardiotoxicity of anthracycline agents for the treatment of cancer: systematic review and meta-analysis of randomised controlled trials. BMC Cancer 10:337
189. Carver JR, Shapiro CL, Ng A et al (2007) American society of clinical oncology clinical evidence review on the ongoing care of adult cancer survivors: cardiac and pulmonary late effects. J Clin Oncol 25(25):3991–4008
190. Patnaik JL, Byers T, DiGuiseppi C, Dabelea D, Denberg TD (2011) Cardiovascular disease competes with breast cancer as the leading cause of death for older females diagnosed with breast cancer: a retrospective cohort study. Breast Cancer Res 13(3):R64
191. Driver JA, Kurth T, Buring JE, Gaziano JM, Logroscino G (2007) Prospective case-control study of nonfatal cancer preceding the diagnosis of Parkinson's disease. Cancer Causes Control 18(7):705–711
192. Driver JA, Kurth T, Buring JE, Gaziano JM, Logroscino G (2008) Parkinson disease and risk of mortality: a prospective comorbidity-matched cohort study. Neurology 70(16 Pt 2):1423–1430
193. Driver JA, Logroscino G, Buring JE, Gaziano JM, Kurth T (2007) A prospective cohort study of cancer incidence following the diagnosis of Parkinson's disease. Cancer Epidemiol Biomarkers Prev 16(6):1260–1265
194. Olsen J, Friis S, Frederiksen K, McLaughlin J, Mellemkjaier L, Moller H (2005) Atypical cancer pattern in patients with Parkinson's disease. Br J Cancer 92:201–205
195. Roe CM, Behrens MI, Xiong C, Miller JP, Morris JC (2005) Alzheimer disease and cancer. Neurology 64(5):895–898
196. Roe CM, Fitzpatrick AL, Xiong C et al (2010) Cancer linked to Alzheimer disease but not vascular dementia. Neurology 74(2):106–112
197. West AB, Dawson VL, Dawson TM (2005) To die or grow: Parkinson's disease and cancer. Trends Neurosci 28(7):348–352
198. Yashin AI, Ukraintseva SV, Akushevich IV, Arbeev KG, Kulminski A, Akushevich L (2009) Trade-off between cancer and aging: what role do other diseases play? Evidence from experimental and human population studies. Mech Ageing Dev 130(1–2):98–104

Chapter 2
How Do We Measure Comorbidity?

Diana Sarfati

Abstract This chapter reviews methods used to measure comorbidity in the context of cancer; summarising methods, identifying contexts in which they have been used and assessing the validity, reliability and feasibility of each approach. Measures of comorbidity are categorised according to whether they are based on individual conditions or simple counts, on dysfunction/function of organ systems, on conditions that have been weighted and combined into indices or based on alternative approaches. Twenty-one separate approaches are described. Content and face validity of the measures varied but tended to be higher for those developed for cancer populations. Some evidence supporting criterion validity of all approaches was found. Where reported, reliability tended to be moderate to high. Some approaches tended to score well on all aspects, but were resource intensive in terms of data collection. There is no gold standard approach to measuring comorbidity in the context of cancer. All summary approaches require simplifying assumptions and, by necessity, result in loss of information. Approaches vary in their strengths and weaknesses, with the choice of measure depending on the study question, population studied and data available.

Keywords Comorbidity · Neoplasms · Multimorbidity · Measurement · Validity · Reliability

List of abbreviations

ACE-27	Adult Comorbidity Evaluation-27
ACG	Adjusted Clinical Groups
ASA	American Society of Anesthesiologists
CCI	Charlson Comorbidity Index
CDS	Chronic Disease Score
CIRS	Cumulative Illness Rating Scale
ICED	Index of Coexistent Disease

D. Sarfati (✉)
Department of Public Health, University of Otago Wellington,
Wellington 7343, New Zealand
e-mail: diana.sarfati@otago.ac.nz

B. Koczwara (ed.), *Cancer and Chronic Conditions*,
DOI 10.1007/978-981-10-1844-2_2

KFI	Kaplan-Feinstein Index
MACSS	Multipurpose Australian Comorbidity Scoring System
NCI	National Cancer Institute
SCI	Simplified Comorbidity Index
TIBI	Total Illness Burden Index
WUHNCI	Washington University Head and Neck Comorbidity Index
PBCI	Pharmacy-based Comorbidity Index

Key Points

- There is no single measure of comorbidity that is optimal for all purposes.
- All summary measures of comorbidity require simplifying assumptions, which results in loss of information.
- There are four broad approaches to measuring comorbidity identified in the literature; individual conditions or condition counts, organ-based systems, weighted indices or other miscellaneous approaches.
- The choice of comorbidity measure depends on the study question, the population studied and the data available.

2.1 Introduction

Given the importance of comorbidity, it is important to consider how we quantify it, particularly in the context of cancer-related studies. However, the underlying construct of comorbidity is difficult, if not impossible, to measure. This is partly due to the limitations of data, but also to the complexity of this underlying entity.

For this reason and despite the importance of comorbidity, there is little consensus about the best approach to measuring it [1]. The difficulties in measuring comorbidity arise from several factors:

- *The definition and importance of comorbidity depends on the definition of the primary condition*. For example, different concomitant conditions are likely to be important in terms of their impact on outcomes for patients with breast cancer, compared to those with congestive heart failure. For this reason, a number of authors have suggested that disease-specific indices are preferable to general ones [2–4].
- *Defining what a comorbid condition is can be difficult* [5–7]. For example, conditions may be defined as specific entities such as angina, peripheral vascular disease or previous myocardial infarction, or may be aggregated to a group of related conditions such as 'cardiovascular disease'. Even when conditions are clearly defined, their importance is likely to vary depending on other factors, such as the timing and severity of conditions [8].

- *Understanding the combined effects of multiple conditions is difficult.* Conditions may or may not have a synergistic effect on each other, and if such an effect is present, it may be additive or multiplicative. Gross et al. found that the effects of combinations of comorbidities on survival among cancer patients were complex and difficult to predict [9].
- *The best approach to measuring comorbidity may also be affected by the outcome that is being investigated* [10, 11]. For example, Preen et al. found that focusing on conditions present at current admission, or the year previously, was most effective for assessing the impact of comorbidity on mortality, while reviewing a five-year lookback period for comorbidity was better for assessing readmission rates [11].

This section reviews approaches to measuring comorbidity in the context of cancer studies. It summarises the various approaches used to measure comorbidity, indicates the context in which each has been used, and assesses the validity of each approach. This section is an updated and extended version of work published previously [1].

Data relating to each index or measure are presented in relation to:

1. *A general description of the measure or index.* This includes the original purpose of the index or measure, a description of the process through which comorbid conditions were identified, whether severity was accounted for, whether and how conditions were combined to form an index and the extent to which the index has been used in the context of cancer patients.
2. *Content and face validity.* Both these measures relate to the degree to which a measure actually evaluates the construct that it purports to measure [12]. Content validity assesses the extent to which a measure includes all relevant items and face validity assesses the extent to which the measure makes sense, given what is known about the construct and the factors used to measure it. These are qualitative assessments, which include the degree to which the measure is relevant to cancer, whether all important conditions are included and how these conditions have been selected, whether other important factors are included, such as severity of conditions and whether the measure can be 'individualised' for specific study purposes.
3. *Criterion validity* relates to the extent to which an index or measure performs in the expected way [12]. Specifically it is the extent to which a measure correlates with some other measure of the construct under study. Criterion validity can be either concurrent or predictive.
   (a) *Concurrent validity* refers to the degree to which the measure correlates with another measure taken at the same time. In relation to comorbidity, this will usually be another validated measure of comorbidity.

(b) *Predictive validity* is the extent to which the measure is able to predict future outcomes of interest, such as cancer survival or receipt of treatment.

4. *Reliability* is "*the extent to which repeated measurements of a stable phenomenon by different people at different times and places get similar results*" [13]. Reliability depends on the simplicity, clarity and ease of use of the scale, as well as the quality of the data and training of the abstractors. Interrater reliability can be reported as a percentage of agreement between abstractors, Spearman's correlation coefficient or a kappa (k) statistic. Where there are more than two abstractors/raters, an interclass correlation coefficient (ICC) is used [12]. Both the k statistic and the ICC are in a range between 0 and 1. Reliability coefficients are considered to be fair to moderate when they exceed 0.40 and moderate to good when they exceed 0.75 [2].
5. *Feasibility* includes the simplicity, cost, time and effort required to use the measure.

Table 2.1 summarises the key characteristics of twenty-one separate approaches used to measure comorbidity among cancer populations in order of the date of the first paper in which each measure or index appears, the population characteristics in which each was developed, the sources of data used, and the method for item generation for each approach.

Table 2.2 summarises the scoring approaches for each measure of comorbidity, including the number of items, the severity scale, the score range (if relevant), and the distribution of each index or measure.

Following these tables is a description of the different approaches used to measure comorbidity; individual conditions or simple condition counts, organ-based approaches, weighted indices and other approaches.

2.2 Individual Conditions or Counts of Conditions

The simplest approach to measuring comorbidity is to measure the prevalence of individual conditions, and to either include them separately in models or to simply combine them by summing the total number of conditions [27, 39–45].

The total count of conditions depends on how conditions are defined, and which are included in the count. There are several examples where authors have identified individual conditions using an explicit process in the context of cancer.

Satariano et al. [21] identified seven conditions (myocardial infarction, other types of heart disease, diabetes, other forms of cancer, and respiratory, gallbladder and liver conditions) that were associated with all-cause mortality, breast cancer mortality or mortality from other causes after adjustment for age, stage and other comorbid conditions among a cohort of patients with breast cancer. These seven were combined in a simple unweighted index based on the number of conditions present. The Satariano index has also been modified for use with administrative data

Table 2.1 Summary of sources of data for development of measures of comorbidity

Index name	Author (year)	Purpose	Population developed	Initial data sources used	Alternative data sources	Item generation
CIRS	Linn (1968) [14]	Measure of physical impairment	?	Clinical notes data	No	Judgement
KFI	Kaplan and Feinstein (1974) [15]	Measure of comorbidity among diabetic patients	188 men with diabetes	Clinical notes data	No	Judgement
Charlson	Charlson (1987) [16]	To develop a 'prognostic taxonomy' for comorbid conditions	608 general medical patients	Clinical notes data	Administrative data, Patient questionnaire	Empirical
ACGs	Weiner (1991) [17]	To predict resource use in HMOs	16,000 HMO enrollees	Administrative data	No	Empirical
CDS/Rx-Risk	Von Korff (1992) Clark (1995) [18, 19]	To predict resource use in HMOs	122,911 enrollees in a Health Maintenance Organization	Pharmaceutical data	No	Judgement and empirical
ICED	Greenfield (1993) [20]	To measure impact of comorbidity and physical functioning	356 patients undergoing total hip replacement	Clinical notes data	No	Judgement
Satariano	Satariano (1994) [21]	To assess comorbidity in breast cancer patients	936 breast cancer patients	Clinical notes data	Administrative data	Judgement and empirical
TIBI/TIBI-CaP	Greenfield (1995) Litwin (2007) [22, 23]	To measure total burden of disease	1738 general patients and 2894 prostate cancer patients	Patient symptom report	No	Judgement and empirical
NIA/NCI collaborative study	Yancik (1996) [24]	To investigate comorbidity burden among older cancer patients	7600 cancer patients	Clinical notes data	No	Empirical

(continued)

Table 2.1 (continued)

Index name	Author (year)	Purpose	Population developed	Initial data sources used	Alternative data sources	Item generation
Elixhauser	Elixhauser (1998) [25]	To measure comorbidity using administrative data	1,779,167 adult acute care hospital patients	Administrative data	No	Judgement and empirical
Comprehensive prognostic index	Fleming (1999) [26]	To develop site specific measures of comorbidity for breast and prostate cancers	848 breast cancer patients	Administrative data	No	Judgement and empirical
NCI comorbidity index	Klabunde (2000) and (2007) [27, 28]	To measure comorbidity among cancer patients using administrative data	14,429 prostate and 7472 breast cancer patients	Administrative data	No	Judgement and empirical
ASA	Reid (2001) [29]	To assess acute operative risk	Surgical patients	Clinical notes data	May be obtained from administrative data	N/A
Alcohol-tobacco related comorbidities index	Reid (2002) [30]	To assess comorbidity among patients with head and neck cancers	9386 head and neck cancer patients	Administrative data	No	Known associations with smoking/alcohol
Washington University head and neck comorbidity index	Piccirillo (2002) [31]	To assess comorbidity among patients with head and neck cancers	1094 head and neck cancer patients	Clinical notes data	Administrative data	Empirical
ACE-27	Picirillo (2003) [32]	To assess comorbidity among cancer patients	11,906 cancer patients	Clinical notes data	Administrative data	Judgement
Tammemagi	Tammemagi (2003) and (2005) [33, 34]	To assess comorbidity among breast and lung cancer patients	1155 lung and 906 breast cancer patients	Administrative data	No	Empirical

(continued)

Table 2.1 (continued)

Index name	Author (year)	Purpose	Population developed	Initial data sources used	Alternative data sources	Item generation
SCI	Colinet (2005) [35]	To assess comorbidity among patients with lung cancer	735 patients with lung cancer	Clinical notes data	No	Judgement
Elixhauser	van Walraven (2009) [36]	To combine Elixhauser conditions into index	228,565 adult acute care hospital patients	Administrative data	No	Judgement and empirical
C3 index	Sarfati (2014) [37]	To assess comorbidity using administrative data in cancer populations	14,096 cancer patients	Administrative data	No	Judgement and empirical
PBCI	Sarfati (2014) [38]	To assess comorbidity using community pharmaceutical data in cancer populations	14,096 cancer patients	Administrative data	No	Judgement and empirical

Table reproduced and amended with permission from Sarfati et al. [1]

Table 2.2 Scoring approaches for measures of comorbidity

Index name	System or condition based	Items	Severity	Scoring method	Score range	Distribution
CIRS	System	13 or 14 systems	0–4, based on clinical judgment	Summative	0–56	Normal (skewed to right)
KFI	System	12 systems	1–3, based on severity of most severe condition	Highest score of single item	1–3	Uniform
Charlson	Condition	17 conditions (in 19 categories)	1–6; based on impact on 1-year mortality (RR)	Sum of weighted conditions	0–33	Skewed to right
ACGs	Condition	93 mutually exclusive ACGs	Incorporated into ACGs based on impact on resource use	Variable	N/A	N/A
CDS/Rx-Risk	Condition	Variable	Based on association with resource use	Sum of weights	0–50+	Skewed to right
ICED	System	14 systems 10 functional	0–4 for comorbidity and 0–2 for function	Combined highest scores of two dimensions	0–3	Uniform
Satariano	Condition	7 conditions	Unweighted	Condition count	0–7	Not specified
TIBI/TIBI-CaP	System	15/11 sub-dimensions	Weighted by clinicians and empirically	Sum of weighted sub-dimension scores	−21 to 77 and 0–23	Skewed to right
NIA/NCI collaborative study	Condition	24 major categories of conditions	Unweighted	N/A	N/A	N/A
Elixhauser	Condition	30 conditions	Conditions included individually	N/A	N/A	N/A

(continued)

Table 2.2 (continued)

Index name	System or condition based	Items	Severity	Scoring method	Score range	Distribution
Comprehensive Prognostic Index	Condition	11 categories with 34 subcategories	Based on impact on 1-year mortality (RR)	Multiplicative	0–14.8	Skewed to right
NCI comorbidity index	Condition	12 conditions (in 14 categories)	Based on impact on 2-year non-cancer mortality (β)	Summing β coefficients	Various	Skewed to right
ASA	Overall health status	N/A	N/A	Overall assessment of health status	1–6	Skewed to right
Alcohol-tobacco related comorbidities index	Condition	11 conditions	Unweighted	Simple count	0–11	Skewed to right
Washington University head and neck comorbidity index	Condition	7 conditions	Based on impact on 5-year mortality (β)	Summing β coefficients	0–15	Skewed to right
ACE-27	Condition	27 conditions	1–3, based on severity of most severe condition	Highest score of single item	1–3	Uniform
Tammemagi	Condition	19 and 77 for lung and breast respectively	Unweighted	Condition count	0–19 and 0–77	Skewed to right
SCI	Condition	7 comorbidity categories	Based on impact on mortality (β)	Summing β coefficients	0–20	Not specified
Elixhauser	Condition	21 conditions	Based on impact on in-hospital mortality (β)	Summing β coefficients	−19 to 89	Skewed to right
C3	Condition	42 conditions	Based on impact on non-cancer mortality	Summing β coefficients	−0.13 to >15	Skewed to right
PBCI	Condition	19 conditions	Based on impact on non-cancer mortality	Summing β coefficients	0–11.6	Skewed to right

Table reproduced and amended with permission from Sarfati et al. [1]

[46], and for use in combination with measures of performance, functional status, depression and cognitive status in the Comprehensive Geriatric Assessment tool [47].

Yancik et al. [24] reported on the *NIA/NCI Collaborative Study* on Comorbidity and Cancer (NIA/NCI SEER study). This was a collaboration between the National Institutes of Aging (NIA) and the National Cancer Institute (NCI) and investigated the comorbidity burden of older people with cancer. Their aim was to assess the extent to which these conditions affect diagnosis, treatment and survival from cancer. The total sample consisted of more than 7600 people, aged 65 years or older, with diagnosed cancers of breast, cervix, ovary, prostate, colon, stomach and bladder. They used data from the SEER program, relating to incident cancers linked to standardised data on comorbidity, abstracted from medical notes by trained registrars. Data on comorbidity were collected from the period four months prior to diagnosis until diagnosis, and each condition was coded according to severity, with these categories collapsed into two, based on whether or not the patient was receiving active management for the specified condition. A group of high severity conditions was specified in subsequent papers (including chronic obstructive pulmonary disease, diabetes requiring insulin, high severity heart disease, previous malignant cancer and renal failure) [48]. Conditions were treated separately in most descriptive and multivariable analyses, but were combined as a simple count in some [48].

Tammemagi et al. [34] carried out a study to investigate the effect of comorbidity on lung cancer survival, and to assess the extent to which these effects were mediated by differences in receipt of treatments. Data on comorbidities were classified using a system developed by the US Department of Health and Human Services in which ICD 9 diseases are collapsed into 259 homogenous groups, of which 56 categories were considered in this study. The authors identified 19 conditions which predicted survival among lung cancer patients. The authors combined comorbidities by using a simple count. Subsequently, Tammemagi et al. applied a similar approach to a cohort of 906 breast cancer patients [33].

Elixhauser et al. [25] developed a measure of comorbidity using administrative data for general (not cancer specific) use. The main focus of this work was to identify those pre-existing conditions recorded in administrative data that had an effect on major short term patient outcomes (cost of care, length of hospital stay and in-hospital mortality). Using administrative data, Elixhauser et al. excluded the primary reason for hospitalisation and only included secondary conditions that were not related to the Diagnosis-related group (DRG) of the primary condition. They excluded diagnoses that could have been due to complications of treatment or conditions that were likely to have a trivial impact on resource use or outcomes. There was a final list of 30 comorbidities, which was tested to assess the impact of each condition on cost, length of stay, and in-hospital mortality. There was no attempt made to combine these conditions into a summary index, except as a simple comorbidity count. However more recently, van Walraven et al. [36] modified the Elixhauser system to allow it to be expressed as a summary score.

The effect of individual specific comorbid conditions has also been assessed in cancer patient populations. The most commonly assessed single condition in this context is diabetes mellitus, which is generally found to have a negative impact on outcomes from cancer [9, 45, 49–51].

2.3 Content and Face Validity

The validity of using individual conditions or condition counts varies with different studies, the approach used to identify relevant conditions, and the number of conditions included. The content and face validity will be higher in studies where conditions have been specifically identified due to their likely importance for cancer patients [21, 24, 34]. Where conditions are added together in a simple unweighted index, the implicit assumption is made that all conditions are equally important in their relationship to outcomes, which is unlikely to be the case.

2.4 Criterion Validity

2.4.1 Concurrent

Comorbidity counts tend to be correlated with other measures of comorbidity where such comparisons are made [33, 39, 52].

2.4.2 Predictive

Results are variable depending on how individual conditions are treated. Generally higher comorbidity counts are related to lower receipt of treatment and/or poorer outcomes [9, 27, 39, 41, 42, 44, 53]. For example, Satariano et al. found that comorbidity as measured by their index was strongly associated with an increased risk of all-cause mortality, and non-breast cancer mortality [21]. Subsequently, higher Satariano index scores were found to be associated with poorer colon cancer survival, whether medical records, administrative data, or both were used [46]. For the NIA/NCI index, patients with comorbidity were less likely to receive aggressive treatment and had poorer survival compared with other patients [24, 48, 54]. Among cancer patients, the Elixhauser system has been found to be associated with lower receipt of treatments for cancer and worse cancer-specific, non-cancer related and all-cause survival [55–57]. Tammemagi's approach to measuring comorbidity was better at predicting all-cause and competing mortality than the Charlson index or simple comorbidity counts [33, 34].

2.5 Reliability

Newschaffer et al. found that the Satariano index had an excellent inter-rater reliability with a kappa score of 0.955 ($p < 0.001$) [46]. No reliability data have been reported for the NIA/NCI approach. Reliability is generally not relevant for those approaches that are based on administrative data, because, within a given study, data are extracted in a standardised way from electronically stored records.

2.6 Feasibility

Approaches which require notes review are more time consuming and require training, however in many cases these could be converted to administrative data based systems [46].

2.7 Organ-Based Approaches

These approaches assess the impact of comorbidity on the function (*or dysfunction*) *of body organs or systems* (*such as the respiratory, cardiovascular, gastrointestinal and renal systems*).

The earliest example of this, and one of the earliest attempts to measure comorbidity in general, is the *cumulative illness rating scale* (*CIRS*). CIRS is a measure of physical impairment based on assessment of organ dysfuntion [14]. Each of 13 independent body systems (cardiac, vascular, respiratory, ear/nose and throat, upper GI, lower GI, liver, renal, other genitourinary, musculoskeletal, neurological, endocrine/metabolic and psychiatric) are rated according to the severity of organ dysfunction on a Likert scale (0-none, 1-mild, 2-moderate, 3-severe, 4-extremely severe). A single illness may impact on more than one organ system and can therefore be counted more than once. For example, a stroke may impair neurological, vascular and musculoskeletal systems. Scores can be kept separate for each organ system or summed to give a total score. Information for the calculation of a CIRS score is collected by clinical review, with the developers of the index commenting that assessment for the CIRS should be '*based on an adequate and complete medical examination and health history*'. CIRS was modified by Miller et al. to form CIRS-G, which was specifically created to be used in geriatric populations [58]. Subsequent minor modifications have been made for geriatric psychiatric populations and for use with acute conditions [59, 60]. CIRS has been used to identify the negative impact of comorbidity on cancer survival in general [61, 62], and for a number of specific cancers, including laryngeal cancer [63, 64], prostate cancer [65], and colorectal cancer [66].

Kaplan and Feinstein [15] were particularly interested in the role of comorbidity among adult diabetic patients. They classified comorbid conditions as being either 'vascular' or 'non-vascular', the former considered potentially related to diabetes. As a measure of severity, they classified each condition as being 'cogent', if it might be expected to adversely affect the individual's life expectancy, or 'non-cogent', if the condition could be controlled, had no direct effects on vital organs or was related to a single episode in the past. Cogent conditions were further classified according to their severity with grade 1 being slight decompensation of vital systems, and grade 3 being recent full decompensation of vital systems, or chronic conditions that threatened life. The analysis was carried out in a categorical manner, so that individuals were variously categorised as having cogent or non-cogent comorbidity; vascular or non-vascular cogent conditions, and according to the highest grade of any single condition. The KFI has been used in a number of studies, both by itself and as a comparison to other indices, including in relation to breast [46], head and neck [64] and prostate cancer [65].

Piccirillo et al. modified the Kaplan-Feinstein Index, initially into the Modified Medical Comorbidity Instrument and then into the *Adult Comorbidity Evaluation-27 (ACE-27) index* [32, 67, 68]. The purpose was specifically to assess comorbidity in the context of cancer. Cancer registry personnel were trained to collect comorbidity data, and define it according to protocols [69]. Twenty-seven conditions that occurred reasonably frequently and were considered to have a negative impact on prognosis were included [67]. The ACE-27 was initially assessed using newly diagnosed patients from one of six hospitals between 1999 and 2002, for whom ACE-27 data were available (n = 11,906) [32]. The ACE-27 system grades specific comorbid conditions into three grades, according to severity in the same way as the KFI. Once all an individual's comorbid conditions are identified and classified, an overall ranking is assigned based on the severity of the single most severe condition, except where there were two or more conditions in different body systems that have a grade 2 (moderate) severity, in which case the overall score is grade 3 (severe). More recently, work has been done to convert the ACE-27 into a claims-based index using ICD codes to differentiate the severity of individual conditions [70]. Picirrillo et al. assessed ACE-27 among 17,712 patients admitted for prostate, respiratory tract, breast, digestive system, gynaecological, urinary or head and neck cancers at a single academic cancer specialist centre [67]. ACE-27 has also been used successfully in a number of other cancer-related studies [54, 70–76].

The *Index of Coexistent Disease* combines two dimensions; a measure of comorbid disease severity and a measure of functional impairment [20]. The index is a modified version of an earlier (unnamed) comorbidity index that had been used to assess the role of comorbidity in the receipt of treatment among older patients with breast or prostate cancers [77, 78]. The earlier index included three dimensions:

1. A measure of severity of comorbid conditions
2. A measure of acute exacerbations of these conditions
3. A measure of functional impairment.

However, the index was later modified to exclude the acute aspect of comorbid conditions [20]. The severity of comorbidity is assessed for each of 14 organ systems (organic heart disease, ischemic heart disease, primary arrhythmias, congestive heart failure, hypertension, cerebrovascular accident, peripheral vascular disease, diabetes mellitus, respiratory problems, malignancies, hepatobiliary disease, renal disease, arthritis, and gastro-intestinal disease) which are rated on a five-point scale, ranging from no co-existent disease to severe uncontrolled disease based on explicit criteria. The degree of physical impairment due to these and other conditions within 10 functional areas (circulation, respiration, neurological, mental status, urinary, fecal, feeding, ambulation, transfer, vision hearing and speech) are graded on a three point scale from no impairment to severe/serious impairment. Individuals are then classified according to the highest grade for any of the categories in each of the comorbidity and functional impairment dimensions. Finally, these two dimensions are combined into a four-point ordinal scale indicating no, mild, moderate or severe coexistent disease as per Table 2.3 [79]. Data are required from clinical notes (ideally including nursing, medical, and laboratory findings). The ICED (or its immediate precursor) has been used for assessment of the role of comorbidity in treatment and survival for breast, [39, 78] prostate [77, 80, 81] and head and neck cancers [63, 64].

The *Total Illness Burden Index* (*TIBI*) was developed as a measure of case-mix for use in comparisons between hospitals, treatments or health care organisations [22]. It is based on a patient report of symptoms and was designed to be a measure of impact on poor health, on functional status and on quality of life outcomes, not mortality or costs of care. It is, therefore, not strictly speaking a measure of comorbidity, but a measure of impact of illness burden on patients. TIBI has subsequently been adapted specifically for use among men with prostate cancer

Table 2.3 Scoring system for the index of coexistent disease (OECD)

Highest comorbidity severity score (0–3)	Highest functional status score (0–2)	ICED level (0–3)
0	0	0
0	1	0
1	0	1
2	0	1
1	1	2
2	1	2
3	Any	3
Any	2	3

(TIBI-CaP) [23, 82]. In this instrument, 84 items are included in 11 sub-dimensions for which severity scores are calculated, based on patient symptom reports. The sub-dimensions are also weighted according to the greatest expected clinical impact on the patient [23, 82]. A subset of TIBI (the cardiopulmonary index) has been used to assess patient outcomes among breast cancer patients [39, 52].

2.8 Content and Face Validity

The content and face validity of the organ-based approaches varies depending on the purpose for which they were developed and the approach that was used to categorise individuals into severity categories. For example, the KFI was constructed to investigate the complications of diabetes, so cancer was not the focus. It does include a measure of severity, but is highly simplified with only three ordinal categories. It provides explicit criteria for both conditions and severity, but it is not clear whether all relevant conditions for cancer are included in the index, for example, diabetes and dementia were not included. Both the KFI and the ICED require major simplifying assumptions in the scoring system, with a variety of comorbidity and functional status score combinations being treated as equivalent.

CIRS was also not developed specifically for cancer. It allows for a variety of approaches for measuring overall illness, for example, the 'Illness Severity Scale' is based on an average of all the CIRS items, while the 'Co-morbidity Index', is a count of the number of items with moderate or severe impairment [83]. The overall total impairment score assumes that each organ system has an equal impact on the individual, so while there is a measure of severity within each organ system, there is no attempt to measure the potentially differential impact of dysfunction in the different systems.

Both ICED and TIBI include elements of functional status. TIBI, in particular, was designed to investigate the impact of illness on physical functioning. The conditions that it weights highly are likely to be those with a large impact on physical functioning, and these may differ from conditions that impact treatment choice or survival from cancer. Some authors argue that as comorbidity and functional status are distinct constructs, they should not be combined [84, 85], it is not clear whether the method used to combine the two scores is optimal or even appropriate.

In this group of indices, ACE-27 has the highest content and face validity, because it was developed specifically to evaluate the role of comorbidity in the context of cancer. Consideration was given to ensure that all relevant conditions were included. There are clear criteria for the inclusion of conditions, and their severity. However, a number of highly simplifying assumptions are made regarding both the equivalence of severity ratings across conditions and the effect of multiple conditions.

2.9 Criterion Validity

2.9.1 Concurrent

A number of studies have shown that there is correlation between CIRS, KFI, ICED and other comorbidity indices (particularly CCI) [16, 46, 64, 65]. CIRS scores based on medical notes review were found to be closely correlated with those based on autopsy, which is considered the gold standard, and supports (concurrent) criterion validity [86]. TIBI has been found to be more closely correlated with the Charlson and Satariano indices calculated from patient interview, than with those from medical records review [52]. ACE-27 has been found to be significantly correlated with CCI and ASA score [87].

2.9.2 Predictive

Newschaffer et al. found that unlike the Charlson and Satariano indices, KFI scores were poor predictors of survival for breast cancer patients and did not improve the ability of models to predict survival over baseline models that did not include measures of comorbidity [46]. Similarly, Castro et al. found that KFI was not an independent predictor of all-cause mortality among 90 laryngeal patients [63]. In contrast, Hall et al. compared KFI with Charlson, ICED and CIRS, and found the KFI performed best in terms of predicting survival [64]. Boulos et al. found that KFI predicted non-prostate cancer related mortality among a group of men with prostate cancer, and accounted for a statistically significant proportion of the variance in non-prostate cancer death [65].

ICED has been found to be associated with higher all-cause mortality among patients with head and neck cancer. ICED has also been shown to be (slightly) more effective at predicting non-cancer death or all-cause mortality among prostate cancer patients, when compared to CIRS, KFI or CCI [65, 81] and more strongly associated with treatment received for early breast cancer in comparison to CCI [39].

CIRS has been found to be associated with higher risk of mortality, readmission, and poorer cancer and non-cancer survival in a number of studies [14, 62–66, 88]. In one small study that compared the performance of comorbidity indices in predicting all-cause mortality among 90 patients with laryngeal cancer, only CIRS was found to be an independent risk factor [63].

TIBI-CaP scores were found to be related to non-cancer mortality among prostate cancer patients after adjustment for sociodemographic factors [23, 89]. A number of studies have shown an association between higher ACE-27 grades and poorer all-cause and cancer-specific survival [32, 54, 67, 71–74, 76]. In the earliest of these papers, Piccirillo et al. found that there was a relationship between severity of comorbidity based on ACE-27 and higher all-cause mortality [32]. For all cancers combined, hazard ratios increased with increasing severity having been adjusted for age, sex, ethnicity and stage of tumour [HR for mild 1.1 (0.9–1.2), moderate 1.3 (1.1–1.5) and severe 1.9 (1.7–2.2)] compared with patients with no comorbidity. Subsequent work by the same authors also supports the predictive validity of ACE-27 [67, 71–74].

2.10 Reliability

In studies that have assessed the reliability of these indices with the exception of TIBI, all have found moderate or high levels of interrater reliability, with k or ICC scores almost all in the range of 0.55 and 0.85 [13, 46, 58, 65, 79, 80, 88, 90–92]. Inter-relater reliability has been reported to be particularly high for ACE-27, with kappa scores tending to be greater than 0.8 [69]. The reliability of TIBI has not been reported.

2.11 Feasibility

These indices have all been designed to require clinical note review and training for abstractors, except for TIBI which requires patient interview. Waite reported that it took abstractors a mean of 8.9 min per set of notes to abstract data to calculate a KFI score. This compared with the Charlson Index (5.9 min) and the Index of Coexistent Disease (ICED; 9.5 min) [90]. Several problems in interpreting the instructions for rating individuals using ICED have been reported [79].

Like the KFI (from which it was adapted), the ACE-27 requires special collection of comorbidity data. Registrars require training, which takes a full day to complete, to ensure the quality of the comorbidity data. Once training is completed, the authors report that the time required to obtain these data was minimal with the mean additional time for registrars to abstract comorbidity data estimated to be 2.1 min [69]. However, other studies have reported the time taken is longer, averaging 16.8 min per person in a cohort of patients with head and neck cancers [87]. Recent work involving the use of claims data to measure ACE-27 is promising [70].

2.12 Weighted Indices

Weighted indices score individuals based on the number of conditions that the individual has, with each condition weighted according to its severity.

The *Charlson Index* was the first example of this and is easily the most cited comorbidity index in the literature. It was developed in 1987 by Charlson et al. [16]. The comorbidity index was developed from a cohort of 604 general medical patients admitted during a one month period at a single New York hospital in 1984. At the time of admission, the number and severity of all comorbid conditions were recorded by the admitting doctor. Charlson et al. wanted to assess the combined effect of comorbid conditions. They first used a simple count of conditions, but were concerned about the assumption that all conditions had an equivalent impact on mortality. To account for this, they developed a weighted index with the weights being equivalent to the (rounded) adjusted relative risks for one-year mortality for each condition, with a maximum weight of six. Conditions with relative risks less than 1.2 were excluded from the index. The authors found this weighted index was superior in predicting one year survival to a simple count of conditions.

Algorithms have been developed by several authors to allow administrative data to be used to calculate individual Charlson scores [93–96]. Studies that have attempted to validate the Charlson index using administrative data have found that it performs reasonably well [27, 97–100]. More recently, questionnaires have been developed to allow the calculation of Charlson scores using patients' self-reports [101]. Other studies have used the Charlson approach, but re-weighted the index specifically for the outcome under study (for example [102–104]). The Charlson Index has been used as the basis for other comorbidity indices, most notably the NCI Comorbidity index, which uses the same conditions, but uses the beta coefficients (rather than the relative risk) of the association of each condition with one-year mortality to assign weights and does not exclude conditions with a RR less than 1.2 [27, 28].

The Charlson is the most widely used comorbidity index in cancer-related studies and has been used in just about every setting, with every cancer including breast [16, 105, 106], lung [107, 108], colorectal [42, 66, 109–112], urological cancers [113–115], cervical [116], head and neck [30, 64, 87] and haematological cancers [117].

Fleming et al. [118] first developed a 'Comprehensive Prognostic Index' which combined comorbidity, stage and age, to predict survival among a cohort of patients with breast cancer. Their aim was to produce a disease-specific index which outperformed more general indices such as the Charlson Index. Comorbidity data were collected for up to two years prior to diagnosis from Medicare claims data, and conditions were divided into 34 categories. Conditions with a prevalence of less than 1 % or greater than 50 % were excluded, leaving 28 categories. The association of each comorbid category with one year mortality was assessed, and those with a hazard ratio greater than 1.2 (n = 12) were included in a multivariable model which included two and three-way interaction terms for multiple comorbidities with (a combined) prevalence of at least 2 %. They calculated multiplicative indices for each of all-cause and breast cancer specific mortality by multiplying together the relative risk for each comorbidity category and by the interaction term of combinations of comorbidities if it was significant. In a later article, Fleming et al. [119] used a similar approach to develop a comorbidity index for prostate cancer patients'.

Both the *Washington University Head and Neck Comorbidity Index* (*WUHNCI*) [120] and the Simplified *Comorbidity Index* (SCI) [35] were developed for specific cancer sites (head and neck and lung cancer, respectively). Both assessed the impact of specified conditions on mortality and combined them by summing weights based on beta coefficients from multivariable models using mortality as the outcome of interest.

The *C3 index* was developed as a cancer specific comorbidity index for use with administratively collected data [37, 121]. It was developed using data from over 14,000 patients with a range of cancers. Comorbid conditions were identified using ICD-10 codes from administratively collected hospital discharge data, and included if they were were likely to have an impact on function or length of life. There were forty-two conditions in the final index and scores were calculated for each patient by adding together all parameter estimates (i.e. the log hazard ratios) for all comorbid conditions recorded for that patient. The index has been used for patients with colorectal, breast, urological, upper gastrointestinal and gynaecological cancers [37, 38, 122, 123].

The final group of weighted indices use pharmaceutical data to identify comorbid conditions. The first, the *Chronic Disease Score* was designed to measure the chronic disease status of a population [19]. The CDS was developed using data from a database held by a large Health Maintenance Organisation in the United States. A score was assigned on each pattern of medication use, based on the impact of the condition for which the medication was (likely to be) prescribed. For cardiac and respiratory disease, a higher score was assigned if more than one class of drug was used for its management. A CDS for each individual was calculated by summing the scores assigned for each class of medications using data over a one-year period. Subsequently, the CDS weights were refined [18] and later modified, and re-named the *RxRisk Model* [124]. The main purpose of this index was to predict health care costs in the managed care environment of the US [125, 126], although it has recently also been used in Australia [127]. The CDS and RxRisk scores have not been used extensively among cancer populations. CDS scores were used (with other measures of comorbidity) in studies relating to patients with head and neck, and prostate cancer [64, 65]. The CDS has also been used to adjust for comorbidity in a study of cancer outcomes among patients with diabetes [128, 129], and in a cost of illness study relating to cervical cancer [130].

A more recent pharmaceutical-based index, the *Pharmacy-based Comorbidity Index (PBCI)* was developed specifically as a measure of comorbidity for cancer populations [38]. Each medication identified in a pharmaceutical database was categorised according to its primary indication for use. Acute and self-limiting conditions were excluded, as were conditions with a prevalence of <1 % in the cancer populations studied. In the final index, 19 conditions were weighted according to their impact on non-cancer mortality and scores were assigned to individuals with cancer based on a sum of the weights for all conditions identified for that patient.

2.13 Content and Face Validity

The Charlson Index was not specifically developed for use among cancer patients, but was validated by its authors using a cohort of patients with breast cancer. While it is the most commonly used index, it is not without its problems. It includes some conditions that have not been shown to have an impact on survival among patients with cancer (e.g. peptic ulcer disease), it may exclude some that do have such an impact (e.g. non-cerebrovascular neurological conditions), and it assumes that the impact of multiple conditions is additive on a relative risk scale [95, 131–133]. The NCI index also used conditions identified by Charlson, although the weights for included conditions are cancer-specific.

The strengths of Fleming's indices are that the authors underwent a stringent process of comorbidity selection, and explicitly investigated the role of common combinations of comorbidity. Weights were empirically calculated, and combined. However these indices were designed for specific cancers, so it may not be easy to generalise this index to other populations with cancer. Similarly, for other site specific indices (WUHNCI and SCI), the process of identifying and combining conditions seems reasonable, but they have only been validated for those specific cancer sites.

The C3 index was designed specifically for cancer populations and included a large number of conditions that are likely to be relevant to cancer patients. Site specific and overall weights were provided and scores were calculated by adding the beta coefficients, which assumes that conditions have a multiplicative effect on each other.

Pharmaceutical-based indices (CDS, RxRisk and PBCI) are based only on conditions for which regular medications have been prescribed. This means that these indices may be subject to provider variation, due to prescribing habits, and utilisation bias, as only prescriptions that are filled will be identified. Medication-based indices may address some of the concerns about using administrative databases, such as inaccurate recording of diagnoses, and may be more likely to identify conditions managed in the outpatient system. They are based on the assumption that medications are being used for the purpose for which they are usually prescribed. The PBCI was specifically designed for cancer populations.

2.14 Criterion Validity

2.14.1 Concurrent

Charlson scores have been shown to be correlated with physician ratings of poor health and a range of other measures of comorbidity, including KFI, CIRS, ICED, Satariano, ACE-27, NCI combined index, Washington University Head and Neck Comorbidity Index, ASA score, C3 index and PBCI index, supporting the concurrent validity of both the Charlson index and these other measures of comorbidity [16, 29, 37, 38, 52, 64, 66, 67, 87]. The concurrent validity of the CDS was assessed by comparing CDS scores with physician-rated disease severity scores, and self-rated health status for individual patients, with moderate correlation with the former and poor correlation with the latter [19]. More recently, the Rx-Risk index was found to correlate poorly with the Charlson comorbidity index, whilst the correlation between the PBCI and the Charlson index was moderate [38, 127].

2.14.2 Predictive

Charlson et al. validated their new index using a cohort of 685 women with breast cancer, treated at a single hospital between 1962 and 1969. Age and comorbidity, as measured by the Charlson Comorbidity Score, were the only two independent predictors of comorbid death, with a relative risk of each increasing level of comorbidity index of 2.3 (1.9–2.8) compared to those with no noted comorbidity. Subsequently, the Charlson index has been found to predict cancer-specific and all-cause mortality in a large number of cancer-related settings [30, 42, 46, 54, 64–66, 108–110, 115, 116]. The predictive validity of the Charlson index appears to be somewhat less clear and consistent with shorter follow-up times, for example in studies that investigate in-hospital death, rather than 1-year mortality [40, 76, 104, 134].

The NCI outperformed the Charlson index in predicting two year non-cancer mortality, [27, 28] however the authors used a non-standard approach to calculating the Charlson index, meaning that several conditions were excluded from their Charlson score calculations (for example, for the prostate cancer cohort only eight conditions were included in the Charlson score).

The C3 index slightly outperformed both the Charlson and NCI indices, both overall and for some cancer sites, in terms of predicting non-cancer mortality [37]. All the site specific indices (Fleming, WUHNCI, SCI) were found to be predictive of mortality among the relevant cancer populations, with the SCI slightly outperforming Charlson in the lung cancer population studied [31, 75, 118, 119, 135].

The performance of pharmaceutical-based indices within cancer populations is mixed. In their study of 655 head and neck cancer patients, Hall et al. found that while CIRS, KFI and ICED scores were all strongly related to survival, CDS scores were not [64]. In contrast, Boulos et al. found that CDS was better than CIRS, ICED, KFI, or CCI, in distinguishing groups with different survival probabilities [65]. The PBCI was found to perform similarly to diagnostic-based comorbidity indices (Charlson and C3) in predicting non-cancer mortality among cancer populations [38].

2.15 Reliability

Many of the weighted indices are based on routinely collected administrative hospitalisation or pharmaceutical data. For these, reliability is not relevant, because data are extracted in a standardised way from electronically stored records. Generally, the reliability of the Charlson Index (using medical notes) has been found to be good, with ICCs or k statistics ranging from 0.67 to 0.93 [13, 46, 90, 91, 136]. The reliability of data collection for WUHNCI and SCI has not been formally reported.

2.16 Feasibility

Whilst measures based on administrative data do not require primary data collection, these databases are often large and unwieldy, and require expertise to manage them. Those that require data from notes review are more time consuming. Waite et al. found that collecting data for the Charlson index was considerably quicker than for either the KFI or ICED (5.9, 8.9, and 9.5 min, respectively) [90]. In contrast, Boulos et al. reported that data abstractors rated the Charlson Index as the least easy to use, when compared with ICED, KFI and CIRS in their study of 269 patients with prostate cancer [65].

2.17 Other Approaches to Measuring Comorbidity in Cancer Populations

Case mix approaches, such as the *ACG system*, described in the previous chapter, have been used as a proxy measure for comorbidity in some cancer studies [55, 137–139]. These systems categorise individuals into groups with similar health resource use expectations. The ACG system, for example, works by grouping ICD-9 diagnoses, identified from administrative data sources, on the basis of disease or condition characteristics, such as expected duration, severity and speciality care involvement of each condition into Ambulatory Diagnostic Groups (ADGs) [17, 140]. Patients can be included in multiple ADGs, which are then further divided into Adjusted Clinical Groups (ACGs), based on factors such as age, sex, the presence of specific ADGs, and the number of ADGs. Some are further subdivided, resulting in 102 final categories, each including individuals that would be expected to experience a similar pattern of resource use [17].

The *American Society of Anesthesiologists*' (*ASA*) classification was developed as a pre-operative summary measure of risk of perioperative complications [29]. The ASA classification is widely used clinically and is not commonly used as a general measure of comorbidity in the context of cancer. The ASA score ranges from 1 to 6 (1—healthy, 2—mild systemic disease, 3—severe systemic disease, 4—severe systemic disease that is a constant threat to life, 5—moribund and 6—brain dead). The ASA classification has been used as a method of measuring comorbidity in patients with head and neck, prostate, bladder and breast cancer [29, 141–145].

2.18 Content and Face Validity

The development of ACGs and similar case-mix approaches, is related to health resource consumption, rather than either cancer or comorbidity per se. Similarly, while ASA may be a useful measure of acute outcomes in the surgical setting, it was not developed for the purpose of measuring comorbidity in a cancer cohort [29].

2.19 Criterion Validity

2.19.1 Concurrent

The ASA class has been found to be moderately correlated with the Charlson index [146].

2.19.2 Predictive

The ACG system had similar predictive performance when compared to four other indices included in a study of treatment receipt and outcomes among patients with colon cancer [55].

The ASA class has been associated with all-cause mortality among patients with head and neck cancers in some [29, 147], but not all studies [142]. Similarly, higher ASA scores were associated with poorer all-cause and non-cancer mortality among men with early prostate cancer [141, 143].

2.20 Reliability

For case-mix approaches, reliability is not relevant, because data are extracted in a standardised way from electronically stored records. The reliability of the assignation of an ASA score has been questioned, but some evidence suggests that the reliability of this measure can be considerably improved with minimal training [29].

2.21 Feasibility

Specialised software is available to group patients into ACGs. The ASA classification is collected routinely for many surgical patients. It is simple and quick to do, but in administrative data will depend on the patient undergoing a surgical procedure.

2.22 So Which Index Is Best?

> Given the complexity and heterogeneity involved in comorbidity, however, no single definition or measure would serve all research or clinical purposes. Rather, definition and measurement of comorbidity approaches may vary depending on practice or research objectives (e.g. clinical, epidemiological, health service) and outcomes of interest (i.e. patient physical function, public health needs, mortality) (Yancik 2007).

There is no gold standard measure of comorbidity in the context of cancer [1]. In an ideal world, we would be able to perfectly measure the underlying construct of 'comorbidity' for every individual. However, because of the complexities of comorbidity, we are only ever going to be able to estimate a measure of this concept. All approaches that are designed to measure comorbidity are necessarily simplifications of this concept. In other words, there will always be some mis-measurement of comorbidity. The choice of measure depends on a number of factors and there is unlikely to be a single 'correct' choice in any context. Some of the key considerations in choosing a comorbidity measure are:

1. *The study question*: For example, if the question relates to a single cancer site, it may be reasonable to use an index developed specifically for that site. However, if comparability with other studies or other cancer sites is important, it may be more reasonable to use a more general index.
2. *The role of comorbidity in the study*: If comorbidity is being measured as a key exposure or outcome, it is likely to be important to optimise the measure to the extent possible. For example, if comorbidity is being considered as an exposure (for example, does comorbidity affect cancer survival), then mis-measurement of comorbidity will most commonly result in an underestimation of the association between comorbidity and the outcome of interest (although biases can occur in both directions). To minimise this bias, it would be reasonable to consider using the index with the highest possible validity for the particular study question. In contrast, if comorbidity is being considered as primarily a confounding (or mediating) variable, then the choice of measure may be less important. When different approaches to measure comorbidity have been compared in terms of their ability to adjust for confounding, there tends to be little difference, despite the fact that the measurement error inherent in the dissimilar approaches is likely to differ. For example, when indices derived from administrative data were compared with those derived from manual review of clinical notes, their ability to adjust a model was very similar, despite there being only moderate correlation between the indices themselves [99].
3. *Practical considerations*: If clinical data have been collected or if it is feasible to do so, indices which require this are available. However, if this is not the case, only indices based on routinely collected data can be considered. In this context, appropriate data and data management skills will be required to operationalise these indices.

Table 2.4 Qualitative criteria used to assess measures of comorbidity

Criteria	*	**	***	NR
Experience with cancer patients	Not generally used for cancer patients populations	Used in limited way with cancer patients. One or two sites only	Used extensively among cancer patient populations	
Content and face validity	Developed among non-cancer patients. Some relevant items likely to be excluded, and/or unreasonable scoring assumptions made	Most relevant items likely to be included. Some assumptions may not be reasonable	All relevant items likely to be included. Reasonable scoring assumptions made. Developed among cancer patient populations	
Concurrent validity	Evidence against concurrent validity	Some evidence to support concurrent validity	Strong evidence to support concurrent validity	No evidence relating to concurrent validity found
Predictive validity	Evidence against predictive validity	Some evidence to support predictive validity	Strong evidence to support predictive validity	No evidence relating to predictive validity found
Reliability	Evidence for poor reliability only	Evidence for moderate level of reliability	Evidence for high level of reliability	No evidence relating to reliability found
Feasibility	Requires substantial resource to implement	Moderate ease of implementation	Easy to implement. Does not require substantial resource	

Table reproduced and amended with permission from Sarfati et al. [1]

Table 2.4 provides some qualitative criteria to assess each measure of comorbidity in the context of cancer. While the criteria are highly simplified, they provide a basic framework to compare the various approaches. Table 2.5 provides the assessment for measures of comorbidity in the context of cancer, though it should be noted that the outcomes of this assessment may well differ if specific research questions or contexts were considered. For example, if clinical data have already been collected, the feasibility of clinical-notes based indices will be scored higher. Similarly, the score for cancer-site specific indices (e.g. WUHNC and SCI indices) are only relevant for studies of the site specified.

Table 2.5 Qualitative assessment of validity of indices in relation to cancer patient populations

Index name	Experience with cancer patients	Content/face validity	Concurrent validity	Predictive validity	Reliability[a]	Feasibility[b]
CIRS	***	**	***	***	**	*
KFI	**	**	***	**	**	*
Charlson	***	**	***	***	**	***
ACGs	*	*	NR	**	NA[c]	**
CDS/Rx-Risk	**	*	**	**	NA[c]	**
ICED	**	**	***	***	**	*
Satariano	**	**	**	**	***	***
TIBI/TIBI-CaP	**	*	***	**	NR	*
NIA/NCI collaborative study	***	**	NR	**	NR	*
Elixhauser (count)	***	**	NR	***	NA[c]	***
Comprehensive prognostic index	**	***	NR	***	NA[c]	**
NCI comorbidity index	***	**	**	***	NA[c]	***
ASA	**	*	**	**	**	**
Alcohol-Tobacco related comorbidities index	**	**	**	**	NA[c]	***
Washington University head and neck comorbidity index	**	***	NR	**	**	***
ACE-27	***	**	***	***	***	*
Tammemagi	**	***	**	**	NA[c]	**
SCI	**	**	**	**	NR	*
C3 index	***	***	***	***	NA[c]	***
PBCI	***	***	**	***	NA[c]	***

Table reproduced and amended with permission from Sarfati et al. [1]
[a]Reliability assessed when notes review or patient interview carried out
[b]The most simple approach is assessed e.g. if both notes review and administrative data are potential data sources, the latter will be assessed
[c]*NA* Not applicable

The content and face validity depends on the extent to which indices are likely to capture all elements of comorbidity important to cancer patients. All indices will do so to some extent. In general, those that are designed specifically for assessing outcomes among cancer patient populations may arguably have higher face validity than those that do not. For example, ACGs and Rx-Risk were developed as predictors of resource use, ASA was developed to predict acute perioperative risk and TIBI was primarily developed as a measure of case-mix. Some indices have not been used a lot in the context of cancer patients (e.g. ACG and ASA), so there is relatively little evidence on their validity in this particular context. These approaches also rate lower on content and face validity.

Another key consideration in relation to content and face validity relates to the process of assessing the severity of individual conditions and to combining them into a single metric. Simple counts of conditions make the implicit assumption that all conditions are equally important in relation to outcomes, regardless of their severity. Weighted indices use various approaches to combine conditions. For example, the Charlson index assumes that the impact of multiple conditions is additive, and that the prognostic impact of a condition is constant over time and regardless of the primary condition being investigated. Subsequent indices have used alternative approaches, including the use of beta coefficients as weights rather than relative risks, and the calculation of cancer specific weights. Few have explicitly explored the impact of specific combinations of conditions [118, 119]. Organ and systems-based approaches tend to use highly simplified scoring systems. For example, KFI and ACE-27 both assume that a 'severe' rating in any body system is equivalent to two 'moderate' ratings in different systems.

There is some evidence to support the predictive validity of all approaches. However, some indices have been used more extensively in the context of cancer than others, improving the evidence base for those indices (for example, CIRS, Charlson, ICED, Elixhauser, NCI combined, ACE-27, C3 index and PBCI). For all indices, where data could be found, there was also at least moderate evidence for concurrent validity. Studies that have compared the performance of various measures of comorbidity have had inconsistent results, depending on various factors, such as the size of the study, the cancer site studied, the way the comorbidity indices were categorised and the outcome measure used [1].

Reliability is most relevant for indices that are dependent on the manual collection of clinical data or from patients themselves. Reliability tends to depend on simplicity, clarity and ease of use of the index, as well as the quality of the training of the abstractors. For some indices, no specific data on reliability were found (e.g. for TIBI, NIA/NCI Collaborative Study Index or SCI). For CIRS, CCI and ICED and ACE-27, interrater reliability tended to be moderate to high in all studies reported [64, 65, 69, 77, 78, 91, 148–157]. Reliability is less of an issue for the other measures, because they are based on administrative data abstracted in a standard manner. However, there are inherent weaknesses with administrative data. Data may be missing or inaccurate, it can be difficult to differentiate complications of disease from pre-existing conditions, and there may be biases inherent in coding practices, for example in some jurisdictions there may be an over-emphasis on recording those conditions that attract higher funding [25, 99, 158].

The feasibility criterion for the indices relates the extent to which time and resource is likely to be required to use it. Those that require special collection of data, for example, may not be appropriate for population level cancer studies because of the resource required to collect the data. For this reason, some indices that scored well on all other criteria scored low on the feasibility criterion, for example, CIRS, ICED and ACE-27. The recent work underway to develop a claims-based version of ACE-27 will, if further validated, improve the feasibility of this measure [70].

In summary, many approaches to measuring comorbidity in cancer-related studies exist. They vary in terms of the purpose for which they were developed, the type of data required for their estimation and the methodological approaches they use. There is no approach that is clearly superior to the others, with the choice of measure being dependent on factors relating to the study questions, validity concerns and practical considerations.

2.23 Future Directions for Practice or Research

Whilst there are no gold standard measures of comorbidity, the assessment of the impact of comorbid conditions on cancers is important. Comorbidity is an important variable to consider as a moderator of cancer outcomes. Future work could focus on the impact of comorbidities in cancer care and outcomes from the perspective of those affected by cancer (such as the impact of comorbidity on survival, disability and individual costs of care) and from the perspective of the health system (such as overall cost of care and health care utilisation).

References

1. Sarfati D (2012) Review of methods to measure comorbidity in cancer populations: no gold standard exists. J Clin Epidemiol 65:924–933
2. de Groot V, Beckerman H, Lankhorst GJ, Bouter LM (2003) How to measure comorbidity. A critical review of available methods. J Clin Epidemiol 56(3):221–229
3. Grunau GL, Sheps S, Goldner EM, Ratner PA (2006) Specific comorbidity risk adjustment was a better predictor of 5-year acute myocardial infarction mortality than general methods. J Clin Epidemiol 59(3):274–280
4. van den Akker M, Buntinx F, Roos S, Knottnerus JA (2001) Problems in determining occurrence rates of multimorbidity. J Clin Epidemiol 54(7):675–679
5. Schneeweiss S, Maclure M (2000) Use of comorbidity scores for control of confounding in studies using administrative databases. Int J Epidemiol 29(5):891–898
6. Valderas JM, Starfield B, Sibbald B, Salisbury C, Roland M (2009) Defining comorbidity: implications for understanding health and health services. Ann Fam Med 7(4):357–363

7. Bonavita V, De Simone R (2008) Towards a definition of comorbidity in the light of clinical complexity. Neurol Sci 29(Suppl 1):S99–S102
8. Preen DB, Holman CD, Lawrence DM, Semmens JB, Spilsbury K (2004) Modelling comorbidity recency, duration and severity with risk adjustment for mortality and morbidity outcomes with administrative data. Aust Epidemiol 11(1):12–19
9. Gross CP, Guo Z, McAvay GJ, Allore HG, Young M, Tinetti ME (2006) Multimorbidity and survival in older persons with colorectal cancer. J Am Geriatr Soc 54(12):1898–1904
10. Byles JE, D'Este C, Parkinson L, O'Connell R, Treloar C (2005) Single index of multimorbidity did not predict multiple outcomes. J Clin Epidemiol 58(10):997–1005
11. Preen DB, Holman CD, Spilsbury K, Semmens JB, Brameld KJ (2006) Length of comorbidity lookback period affected regression model performance of administrative health data. J Clin Epidemiol 59(9):940–946
12. Streiner D, Norman G (2008) Health measurement scales. A practical guide to their development and use, 4th edn. Oxford University Press, Oxford
13. Hall SF, Groome PA, Streiner DL, Rochon PA (2006) Interrater reliability of measurements of comorbid illness should be reported. J Clin Epidemiol 59(9):926–933
14. Linn BS, Linn MW, Gurel L (1968) Cumulative illness rating scale. J Am Geriatr Soc 16 (5):622–626
15. Kaplan MH, Feinstein AR (1974) The importance of classifying initial co-morbidity in evaluating the outcome of diabetes mellitus. J Chronic Dis 27(7–8):387–404
16. Charlson M, Pompei P, Ales K, Mackenzie C (1987) A new method for classifying prognostic comorbidity in longitudinal studies: development and validation. J Chronic Dis 40:373–383
17. Weiner JP, Starfield BH, Steinwachs DM, Mumford LM (1991) Development and application of a population-oriented measure of ambulatory care case-mix. Med Care 29 (5):452–472
18. Clark DO, Von Korff M, Saunders K, Baluch WM, Simon GE (1995) A chronic disease score with empirically derived weights. Med Care 33(8):783–795
19. Von Korff M, Wagner EH, Saunders K (1992) A chronic disease score from automated pharmacy data. J Clin Epidemiol 45(2):197–203
20. Greenfield S, Apolone G, McNeil BJ, Cleary PD (1993) The importance of co-existent disease in the occurrence of postoperative complications and one-year recovery in patients undergoing total hip replacement. Comorbidity and outcomes after hip replacement. Med Care 31(2):141–154
21. Satariano WA, Ragland DR (1994) The effect of comorbidity on 3-year survival of women with primary breast cancer. Ann Intern Med 120(2):104–110
22. Greenfield S, Sullivan L, Dukes KA, Silliman R, D'Agostino R, Kaplan SH (1995) Development and testing of a new measure of case mix for use in office practice. Med Care 33(4 Suppl):AS47–AS55
23. Litwin MS, Greenfield S, Elkin EP, Lubeck DP, Broering JM, Kaplan SH (2007) Assessment of prognosis with the total illness burden index for prostate cancer: aiding clinicians in treatment choice. Cancer 109(9):1777–1783
24. Yancik R, Havlik RJ, Wesley MN et al (1996) Cancer and comorbidity in older patients: a descriptive profile. Ann Epidemiol 6(5):399–412
25. Elixhauser A, Steiner C, Harris DR, Coffey RM (1998) Comorbidity measures for use with administrative data. Med Care 36(1):8–27
26. Fleming LE, Bean JA, Rudolph M, Hamilton K (1999) Cancer incidence in a cohort of licensed pesticide applicators in Florida. J Occup Environ Med 41(4):279–288
27. Klabunde CN, Legler JM, Warren JL, Baldwin L-M, Schrag D (2007) A refined comorbidity measurement algorithm for claims-based studies of breast, prostate, colorectal, and lung cancer patients. Ann Epidemiol 17(8):584–590
28. Klabunde CN, Potosky AL, Legler J, Warren JL (2000) Development of a comorbidity index using physician claims data. J Clin Epidemiol 53:1258–1267

29. Reid BC, Alberg AJ, Klassen AC, Koch WM, Samet JM (2001) The American society of Anesthesiologists' class as a comorbidity index in a cohort of head and neck cancer surgical patients. Head Neck 23(11):985–994
30. Reid BC, Alberg AJ, Klassen AC et al (2002) A comparison of three comorbidity indexes in a head and neck cancer population. Oral Oncol 38(2):187–194
31. Piccirillo JF, Lacy PD, Basu A, Spitznagel EL (2002) Development of a new head and neck cancer-specific comorbidity index. Arch Otolaryngology Head Neck Surgery 128(10): 1172–1179
32. Piccirillo JF, Costas I, Claybour P, Borah A, Gorove L, Jeffe D (2003) The measurement of comorbidity by cancer registries. J Reg Mgmt 30(1):8–14
33. Tammemagi C, Nerenz D, Neslund-Dudas C, Feldkamp C, Nathanson D (2005) Comorbidity and survival disparities among black and white patients with breast cancer. JAMA 294 (14):1765–1772
34. Tammemagi CM, Neslund-Dudas C, Simoff M, Kvale P (2003) Impact of comorbidity on lung cancer survival. Int J Cancer 103(6):792–802
35. Colinet B, Jacot W, Bertrand D et al (2005) A new simplified comorbidity score as a prognostic factor in non-small-cell lung cancer patients: description and comparison with the Charlson's index. Br J Cancer 93(10):1098–1105
36. van Walraven C, Austin PC, Jennings A, Quan H, Forster AJ (2009) A modification of the Elixhauser comorbidity measures into a point system for hospital death using administrative data. Med Care 47(6):626–633
37. Sarfati D, Gurney J, Stanley J et al (2014) Cancer-specific administrative data-based comorbidity indices provided valid alternative to Charlson and NHI indices. J Clin Oncol 67 (5):586–595
38. Sarfati Lim B, Gurney J, McSherry C (2014) Development of a pharmacy-based comorbidity illness index for patients with cancer. Med Care 52(7):586–593
39. Mandelblatt JS, Bierman AS, Gold K et al (2001) Constructs of burden of illness in older patients with breast cancer: a comparison of measurement methods. [Erratum appears in Health Serv Res 2007 Oct; 42(5):2088 Note: Maserejan, N [corrected to Maserejian, N]]. Health Serv Res 36(6 Pt 1):1085–1107
40. Melfi C, Holleman E, Arthur D, Katz B (1995) Selecting a patient characteristics index for the prediction of medical outcomes using administrative claims data. J Clin Epidemiol 48 (7):917–926
41. Newschaffer CJ, Penberthy LT, Desch CE, Retchin SM, Whittemore M (1996) The effect of age and comorbidity in the treatment of elderly women with nonmetastatic breast cancer. Arch Intern Med 156(1):85–90
42. Sarfati D, Hill S, Blakely T et al (2009) The effect of comorbidity on the use of adjuvant chemotherapy and survival from colon cancer: a retrospective cohort study. BMC Cancer 9:116
43. Valery PC, Coory M, Stirling J, Green AC (2006) Cancer diagnosis, treatment, and survival in Indigenous and non-Indigenous Australians: a matched cohort study. Lancet 367(9525):1842–1848
44. Zeber JE, Copeland LA, Hosek BJ, Karnad AB, Lawrence VA, Sanchez-Reilly SE (2008) Cancer rates, medical comorbidities, and treatment modalities in the oldest patients. Crit Rev Oncol Hematol 67(3):237–242
45. Sarfati D, Tan L, Blakely T, Pearce N (2011) Comorbidity among patients with colon cancer. NZ Med J 124(1338):76–88
46. Newschaffer CJ, Bush TL, Penberthy LT (1997) Comorbidity measurement in elderly female breast cancer patients with administrative and medical records data. J Clin Epidemiol 50(6):725–733
47. Repetto L, Fratino L, Audisio RA et al (2002) Comprehensive geriatric assessment adds information to eastern cooperative oncology group performance status in elderly cancer patients: an Italian group for geriatric oncology study. J Clin Oncol 20(2):494–502

48. Yancik R, Wesley MN, Ries LA, Havlik RJ, Edwards BK, Yates JW (2001) Effect of age and comorbidity in postmenopausal breast cancer patients aged 55 years and older. JAMA 285(7):885–892
49. Martin JH, Coory MD, Valery PC, Green AC (2009) Association of diabetes with survival among cohorts of Indigenous and non-Indigenous Australians with cancer. Cancer Causes Control 20(3):355–360
50. Meyerhardt JA, Catalano PJ, Haller DG et al (2003) Impact of diabetes mellitus on outcomes in patients with colon cancer. J Clin Oncol 21(3):433–440
51. Polednak AP (2006) Comorbid diabetes mellitus and risk of death after diagnosis of colorectal cancer: a population-based study. Cancer Detect Prev 30(5):466–472
52. Silliman RA, Lash TL (1999) Comparison of interview-based and medical-record based indices of comorbidity among breast cancer patients. Med Care 37(4):339–349
53. Gross CP, McAvay GJ, Guo Z, Tinetti ME (2007) The impact of chronic illnesses on the use and effectiveness of adjuvant chemotherapy for colon cancer. Cancer 109(12):2410–2419
54. Hines RB, Chatla C, Bumpers HL et al (2009) Predictive capacity of three comorbidity indices in estimating mortality after surgery for colon cancer. J Clin Oncol 27(26):4339–4345
55. Baldwin L-M, Klabunde CN, Green P, Barlow W, Wright G (2006) In search of the perfect comorbidity measure for use with administrative claims data: does it exist? Med Care 44(8):745–753
56. Putt M, Long JA, Montagnet C et al (2009) Racial differences in the impact of comorbidities on survival among elderly men with prostate cancer. Med Care Res Rev 66(4):409–435
57. Brewer N, Borman B, Sarfati D et al (2011) Does comorbidity explain the ethnic inequalities in cervical cancer survival in New Zealand? A retrospective cohort study. BMC Cancer 11:132
58. Miller MD, Paradis CF, Houck PR et al (1992) Rating chronic medical illness burden in geropsychiatric practice and research: application of the cumulative illness rating scale. Psychiatry Res 41(3):237–248
59. Parmelee PA, Thuras PD, Katz IR, Lawton MP (1995) Validation of the cumulative illness rating scale in a geriatric residential population. J Am Geriatr Soc 43(2):130–137
60. Mistry R, Gokhman I, Bastani R et al (2004) Measuring medical burden using CIRS in older veterans enrolled in UPBEAT, a psychogeriatric treatment program: a pilot study. J Gerontol A Biol Sci Med Sci 59(10):1068–1075
61. Wedding U, Roehrig B, Klippstein A et al (2007) Comorbidity in patients with cancer: prevalence and severity measured by cumulative illness rating scale. Criti Rev Oncol Hematol 61(3):269–276
62. Wedding U, Rohrig B, Klippstein A, Pientka L, Hoffken K (2007) Age, severe comorbidity and functional impairment independently contribute to poor survival in cancer patients. J Cancer Res Clin Oncol 133(12):945–950
63. Castro MAF, Dedivitis RA, Ribeiro KCB (2007) Comorbidity measurement in patients with laryngeal squamous cell carcinoma. ORL J Otorhinolaryngol Relat Spec 69(3):146–152
64. Hall SF, Rochon PA, Streiner DL, Paszat LF, Groome PA, Rohland SL (2002) Measuring comorbidity in patients with head and neck cancer. Laryngoscope 112(11):1988–1996
65. Boulos DL, Groome PA, Brundage MD et al (2006) Predictive validity of five comorbidity indices in prostate carcinoma patients treated with curative intent. Cancer 106(8):1804–1814
66. Munro AJ, Bentley AH (2004) Deprivation, comorbidity and survival in a cohort of patients with colorectal cancer. Eur J Cancer Care 13(3):254–262
67. Piccirillo JF, Tierney RM, Costas I, Grove L, Spitznagel EL Jr (2004) Prognostic importance of comorbidity in a hospital-based cancer registry. JAMA 291(20):2441–2447
68. Piccirillo JF (2000) Importance of comorbidity in head and neck cancer. Laryngoscope 110(4):593–602
69. Johnston A, Piccirillo JF, Creech CM, Littenberg B, Jeffe D, Spitznagel EL (2001) Validation of a comorbidity education program. J Reg Mgmt 28:125–131

70. Fleming ST, Sabatino SA, Kimmick G et al (2011) Developing a claim-based version of the ACE-27 comorbidity index: a comparison with medical record review. Med Care 49(8): 752–760
71. Berger DA, Megwalu II, Vlahiotis A et al (2008) Impact of comorbidity on overall survival in patients surgically treated for renal cell carcinoma. Urology 72(2):359–363
72. Megwalu II, Vlahiotis A, Radwan M, Piccirillo JF, Kibel AS (2008) Prognostic impact of comorbidity in patients with bladder cancer. Eur Urol 53(3):581–589
73. Read WL, Tierney RM, Page NC et al (2004) Differential prognostic impact of comorbidity. J Clin Oncol 22(15):3099–3103
74. Yung KC, Piccirillo JF (2008) The incidence and impact of comorbidity diagnosed after the onset of head and neck cancer. Arch Otolaryngol Head Neck Surg 134(10):1045–1049
75. Sanabria A, Carvalho AL, Vartanian JG, Magrin J, Ikeda MK, Kowalski LP (2008) Validation of the Washington University Head and Neck Comorbidity Index in a cohort of older patients. Arch Otolaryngol Head Neck Surg 134(6):603–607
76. Soares M, Salluh JIF, Ferreira CG, Luiz RR, Spector N, Rocco JR (2005) Impact of two different comorbidity measures on the 6-month mortality of critically ill cancer patients. Intensive Care Med 31(3):408–415
77. Bennett CL, Greenfield S, Aronow H, Ganz P, Vogelzang NJ, Elashoff RM (1991) Patterns of care related to age of men with prostate cancer. Cancer 67(10):2633–2641
78. Greenfield S, Blanco DM, Elashoff RM, Ganz PA (1987) Patterns of care related to age of breast cancer patients. JAMA 257(20):2766–2770
79. Imamura K, McKinnon M, Middleton R, Black N (1997) Reliability of a comorbidity measure: the index of co-existent disease (ICED). J Clin Epidemiol 50(9):1011–1016
80. Krousel-Wood MA, Abdoh A, Re R (1996) Comparing comorbid-illness indices assessing outcome variation: the case of prostatectomy. J Gen Intern Med 11(1):32–38
81. Albertsen PC, Fryback DG, Storer BE, Kolon TF, Fine J (1996) The impact of co-morbidity on life expectancy among men with localized prostate cancer. J Urol 156(1):127–132
82. Stier DM, Greenfield S, Lubeck DP et al (1999) Quantifying comorbidity in a disease-specific cohort: adaptation of the total illness burden index to prostate cancer. Urology 54(3):424–429
83. Nagaratnam N, Gayagay G Jr (2007) Validation of the cumulative illness rating scale (CIRS) in hospitalized nonagenarians. Arch Gerontol Geriatr 44(1):29–36
84. Extermann M (2000) Measurement and impact of comorbidity in older cancer patients. Crit Rev Oncol Hematol 35(3):181–200
85. Lash TL, Mor V, Wieland D, Ferrucci L, Satariano W, Silliman RA (2007) Methodology, design, and analytic techniques to address measurement of comorbid disease. J Gerontol A Biol Sci Med Sci 62(3):281–285
86. Conwell Y, Forbes N, Cox C, Caine E (1993) Validation of a measure of physical illness burden at autopsy: the cumulative illness rating scale. J Am Geriatr Soc 41:38–41
87. Paleri V, Wight RG (2002) Applicability of the adult comorbidity evaluation—27 and the Charlson indexes to assess comorbidity by notes extraction in a cohort of United Kingdom patients with head and neck cancer: a retrospective study. J Laryngol Otol 116(3):200–205
88. Salvi F, Miller MD, Grilli A et al (2008) A manual of guidelines to score the modified cumulative illness rating scale and its validation in acute hospitalized elderly patients. J Am Geriatr Soc 56(10):1926–1931
89. Daskivich T, Sadetsky N, Kaplan SH, Greenfield S, Litwin MS (2010) Severity of comorbidity and non-prostate cancer mortality in men with early-stage prostate cancer. Arch Intern Med 170(15):1396–1397
90. Waite K, Oddone E, Weinberger M, Samsa G, Foy M, Henderson W (1994) Lack of association between patients' measured burden of disease and risk for hospital readmission. J Clin Epidemiol 47(11):1229–1236
91. Extermann M (2000) Measuring comorbidity in older cancer patients. Eur J Cancer 36 (4):453–471

92. Hudon C, Fortin M, Vanasse A (2005) Cumulative illness rating scale was a reliable and valid index in a family practice context. J Clin Epidemiol 58(6):603–608
93. Deyo RA, Cherkin DC, Ciol MA (1992) Adapting a clinical comorbidity index for use with ICD-9-CM administrative databases. J Clin Epidemiol 45(6):613–619
94. Quan H, Sundararajan V, Halfon P et al (2005) Coding algorithms for defining comorbidities in ICD-9-CM and ICD-10 administrative data. Med Care 43(11):1130–1139
95. Romano PS, Roos LL, Jollis JG (1993) Adapting a clinical comorbidity index for use with ICD-9-CM administrative data: differing perspectives. J Clin Epidemiol 46(10):1075–1079 Discussion 81–90
96. D'Hoore W, Bouckaert A, Tilquin C (1996) Practical considerations on the use of the Charlson comorbidity index with administrative data bases. J Clin Epidemiol 49(12): 1429–1433
97. Kieszak SM, Flanders WD, Kosinski AS, Shipp CC, Karp H (1999) A comparison of the Charlson comorbidity index derived from medical record data and administrative billing data. J Clin Epidemiol 52(2):137–142
98. Malenka DJ, McLerran D, Roos N, Fisher ES, Wennberg JE (1994) Using administrative data to describe casemix: a comparison with the medical record. J Clin Epidemiol 47 (9):1027–1032
99. Sarfati D, Hill S, Purdie G, Dennett E, Blakely T (2010) How well does routine hospitalisation data capture information on comorbidity in New Zealand? NZ Med J 123 (1310):50–61
100. Quan H, Li B, Couris C et al (2011) Updating and validating Charlson comorbidity index and score for risk adjustment in hospital discharge abstracts using data from 6 countries. Am J Epidemiol. doi:10.1093/aje/kwq433
101. Susser SR, McCusker J, Belzile E (2008) Comorbidity information in older patients at an emergency visit: self-report vs. administrative data had poor agreement but similar predictive validity. J Clin Epidemiol 61(5):511–515
102. Martins M, Blais R (2006) Evaluation of comorbidity indices for inpatient mortality prediction models. J Clin Epidemiol 59(7):665–669
103. van Doorn C, Bogardus ST, Williams CS, Concato J, Towle VR, Inouye SK (2001) Risk adjustment for older hospitalized persons: a comparison of two methods of data collection for the Charlson index. J Clin Epidemiol 54(7):694–701
104. Cleves MA, Sanchez N, Draheim M (1997) Evaluation of two competing methods for calculating Charlson's comorbidity index when analyzing short-term mortality using administrative data. J Clin Epidemiol 50(8):903–908
105. Ahern TP, Lash TL, Thwin SS, Silliman RA (2009) Impact of acquired comorbidities on all-cause mortality rates among older breast cancer survivors. Med Care 47(1):73–79
106. Newschaffer CJ, Bush TL, Penberthy LE, Bellantoni M, Helzlsour K, Diener-West M (1998) Does comorbid disease interact with cancer? An epidemiologic analysis of mortality in a cohort of elderly breast cancer patients. J Gerontol A Biol Sci Med Sci 53(5):M372–M378
107. Blanco JAG, Toste IS, Alvarez RF, Cuadrado GR, Gonzalvez AM, Martin IJG (2008) Age, comorbidity, treatment decision and prognosis in lung cancer. Age Ageing 37(6):715–718
108. Stevens W, Stevens G, Kolbe J, Cox B (2008) Ethnic differences in the management of lung cancer in New Zealand. J Thorac Oncol 3(3):237–244
109. Cronin DP, Harlan LC, Potosky AL, Clegg LX, Stevens JL, Mooney MM (2006) Patterns of care for adjuvant therapy in a random population-based sample of patients diagnosed with colorectal cancer. Am J Gastroenterol 101(10):2308–2318
110. Iversen LH, Norgaard M, Jacobsen J, Laurberg S, Sorensen HT (2009) The impact of comorbidity on survival of Danish colorectal cancer patients from 1995 to 2006—a population-based cohort study. Dis Colon Rectum 52(1):71–78
111. Lemmens VE, Janssen-Heijnen ML, Verheij CD, Houterman S, Repelaer van Driel OJ, Coebergh JW (2005) Co-morbidity leads to altered treatment and worse survival of elderly patients with colorectal cancer. Br J Surg 92(5):615–623

112. Rieker RJ, Hammer E, Eisele R, Schmid E, Hogel J (2002) The impact of comorbidity on the overall survival and the cause of death in patients after colorectal cancer resection. Langenbecks Arch Surg 387(2):72–76
113. Miller DC, Taub DA, Dunn RL, Montie JE, Wei JT (2003) The impact of co-morbid disease on cancer control and survival following radical cystectomy. J Urol 169(1):105–109
114. Nuttall M, van der Meulen J, Emberton M (2006) Charlson scores based on ICD-10 administrative data were valid in assessing comorbidity in patients undergoing urological cancer surgery. J Clin Epidemiol 59(3):265–273
115. Singh R, O'Brien TS (2004) Comorbidity assessment in localized prostate cancer: a review of currently available techniques. Eur Urol 46(1):28–41 Discussion
116. Brewer N, Borman B, Sarfati D et al (2011) Do comorbidities explain the ethnic inequalities in cervical cancer survival in New Zealand? BMC Cancer 11(1):1
117. Sorror ML, Maris MB, Sandmaier BM et al (2005) Hematopoietic cell transplantation after nonmyeloablative conditioning for advanced chronic lymphocytic leukemia. J Clin Oncol 23 (16):3819–3829
118. Fleming ST, Rastogi A, Dmitrienko A, Johnson KD (1999) A comprehensive prognostic index to predict survival based on multiple comorbidities: a focus on breast cancer. Med Care 37(6):601–614
119. Fleming ST, Pearce KA, McDavid K, Pavlov D (2003) The development and validation of a comorbidity index for prostate cancer among Black men. J Clin Epidemiol 56(11): 1064–1075
120. Piccirillo JF, Lacy PD, Basu A, Spitznagel EL (2002) Development of a new head and neck cancer-specific comorbidity index. Arch Otolaryngol Head Neck Surg 128(10):1172–1179
121. Sarfati D, Gurney J, Lim B et al (2013) Identifying important comorbidity among cancer populations using administrative data: prevalence and impact on survival. Asia Pac J Clin Oncol. doi:10.1111/ajco.12130
122. Gurney J, Sarfati D, Stanley J (2015) The impact of patient comorbidity on cancer stage at diagnosis. Br J Cancer 113:1375–1380
123. Sarfati D, Gurney J, Stanley J, Koea J (2014) A retrospective cohort study of patients with stomach and liver cancers: the impact of comorbidity and ethnicity on cancer care and outcomes. BMC Cancer 14:821
124. Fishman PA, Goodman MJ, Hornbrook MC, Meenan RT, Bachman DJ, O'Keeffe Rosetti MC (2003) Risk adjustment using automated ambulatory pharmacy data: the RxRisk model. Med Care 41(1):84–99
125. Sloan KL, Sales AE, Liu C-F et al (2003) Construction and characteristics of the RxRisk-V: a VA-adapted pharmacy-based case-mix instrument. Med Care 41(6):761–774
126. Johnson ML, El-Serag HB, Tran TT, Hartman C, Richardson P, Abraham NS (2006) Adapting the Rx-Risk-V for mortality prediction in outpatient populations. Med Care 44 (8):793–797
127. Lu CY, Barratt J, Vitry A, Roughead E (2011) Charlson and Rx-Risk comorbidity indices were predictive of mortality in the Australian health care setting. J Clin Epidemiol 64 (2):223–228
128. Bowker SL, Majumdar SR, Veugelers P, Johnson JA (2006) Increased cancer-related mortality for patients with type 2 diabetes who use sulfonylureas or insulin. Diabetes Care 29 (2):254–258
129. Bowker SL, Yasui Y, Veugelers P, Johnson JA (2010) Glucose-lowering agents and cancer mortality rates in type 2 diabetes: assessing effects of time-varying exposure. Diabetologia 53 (8):1631–1637
130. Helms LJ, Melnikow J (1999) Determining costs of health care services for cost-effectiveness analyses: the case of cervical cancer prevention and treatment. Med Care 37(7):652–661
131. Romano PS, Roos LL, Jollis JG (1993) Further evidence concerning the use of a clinical comorbidity index with ICD-9-CM administrative data. J Clin Epidemiol 46(10):1085–1090
132. Charlson M (1993) Adapting a clinical comorbidity index for use with ICD-9-CM administrative data: a response. J Clin Epidemiol 46(10):1083–1084

133. Deyo R (1993) Adapting a clinical comorbidity index for use with ICD-9-CM administrative data: a response. J Clin Epidemiol 46(10):1081–1082
134. Pompei P, Charlson ME, Ales K, MacKenzie CR, Norton M (1991) Relating patient characteristics at the time of admission to outcomes of hospitalization. J Clin Epidemiol 44(10):1063–1069
135. Jacot W, Colinet B, Bertrand D et al (2008) Quality of life and comorbidity score as prognostic determinants in non-small-cell lung cancer patients. Ann Oncol 19(8):1458–1464
136. Kiefe CI, Funkhouser E, Fouad MN, May DS (1998) Chronic disease as a barrier to breast and cervical cancer screening. J Gen Intern Med 13(6):357–365
137. Caldon LJM, Walters SJ, Reed JA, Murphy A, Worley A, Reed MWR (2005) Case-mix fails to explain variation in mastectomy rates: management of screen-detected breast cancer in a UK region 1997–2003. Br J Cancer 92(1):55–59
138. McArdle CS, Hole DJ (2002) Outcome following surgery for colorectal cancer: analysis by hospital after adjustment for case-mix and deprivation. Br J Cancer 86(3):331–335
139. Talsma AK, Reedijk AMJ, Damhuis RAM, Westenend PJ, Vles WJ (2011) Re-resection rates after breast-conserving surgery as a performance indicator: introduction of a case-mix model to allow comparison between Dutch hospitals. Eur J Surg Oncol 37(4):357–363
140. Starfield B, Weiner J, Mumford L, Steinwachs D (1991) Ambulatory care groups: a categorization of diagnoses for research and management. Health Serv Res 26(1):53–74
141. Froehner M, Koch R, Litz R, Heller A, Oehlschlaeger S, Wirth MP (2003) Comparison of the American society of anesthesiologists physical status classification with the Charlson score as predictors of survival after radical prostatectomy. Urology 62(4):698–701
142. Kanatas A, Gorton H, Smith AB, Mannion C, Ong TK, Mitchell D (2010) ASA grade and disease-free mortality in head and neck cancer patients: a prospective study. Br J Oral Maxillofac Surg 48(8):591–593
143. Froehner M, Koch R, Litz RJ et al (2005) Comparison of tumor- and comorbidity-related predictors of mortality after radical prostatectomy. Scand J Urol Nephrol 39(6):449–454
144. Lash TL, Thwin SS, Horton NJ, Guadagnoli E, Silliman RA (2003) Multiple informants: a new method to assess breast cancer patients' comorbidity. Am J Epidemiol 157(3):249–257
145. Prout GR Jr, Wesley MN, Yancik R, Ries LAG, Havlik RJ, Edwards BK (2005) Age and comorbidity impact surgical therapy in older bladder carcinoma patients: a population-based study. Cancer 104(8):1638–1647
146. Reid RJ, MacWilliam L, Verhulst L, Roos N, Atkinson M (2001) Performance of the ACG case-mix system in two Canadian provinces. Med Care 39(1):86–99
147. Nicolai P, Redaelli de Zinis LO, Tomenzoli D et al (1997) Prognostic determinants in supraglottic carcinoma: univariate and Cox regression analysis. Head Neck 19(4):323–334
148. Hall SF, Groome PA, Streiner DL, Rochon PA (2006) Interrater reliability of measurements of comorbid illness should be reported. J Clin Epidemiol 59(9):926–933
149. Hudon C, Fortin M, Vanasse A (2005) Cumulative illness rating scale was a reliable and valid index in a family practice context. J Clin Epidemiol 58(6):603–608
150. Melfi C, Holleman E, Arthur D, Katz B (1995) Selecting a patient characteristics index for the prediction of medical outcomes using administrative claims data. J Clin Epidemiol 48 (7):917–926
151. Miller MD, Paradis CF, Houck PR et al (1992) Rating chronic medical illness burden in geropsychiatric practice and research: application of the cumulative illness rating scale. Psychiatry Res 41(3):237–248
152. Salvi F, Miller MD, Grilli A et al (2008) A manual of guidelines to score the modified cumulative illness rating scale and its validation in acute hospitalized elderly patients. J Am Geriatr Soc 56(10):1926–1931
153. Newschaffer CJ, Bush TL, Penberthy LT (1997) Comorbidity measurement in elderly female breast cancer patients with administrative and medical records data. J Clin Epidemiol 50 (6):725–733

154. Waite K, Oddone E, Weinberger M, Samsa G, Foy M, Henderson W (1994) Lack of association between patients' measured burden of disease and risk for hospital readmission. J Clin Epidemiol 47(11):1229–1236
155. Kiefe CI, Funkhouser E, Fouad MN, May DS (1998) Chronic disease as a barrier to breast and cervical cancer screening. J Gen Intern Med 13(6):357–365
156. Imamura K, McKinnon M, Middleton R, Black N (1997) Reliability of a comorbidity measure: the index of co-existent disease (ICED). J Clin Epidemiol 50(9):1011–1016
157. Krousel-Wood MA, Abdoh A, Re R (1996) Comparing comorbid-illness indices assessing outcome variation: The case of prostatectomy. J Gen Intern Med 11(1):32–38
158. Mnatzaganian G, Ryan P, Norman PE, Hiller JE (2012) Accuracy of hospital morbidity data and the performance of comorbidity scores as predictors of mortality. J Clin Epidemiol 65 (1):107–115

Further reading

159. Streiner D, Norman G (2008) Health measurement scales. A practical guide to their development and use, 4th edn. Oxford University Press, Oxford
160. Devellis R (2012) Scale development: theory and applications. Sage Publications Inc., Los Angeles
161. Lash TL, Mor V, Wieland D, Ferrucci L, Satariano W, Silliman RA (2007) Methodology, design, and analytic techniques to address measurement of comorbid disease. J Gerontol A Biol Sci Med Sci 62(3):281–285
162. Hall SF (2006) A user's guide to selecting a comorbidity index for clinical research. J Clin Epidemiol 59(8):849–855
163. Sarfati D (2012) Review of methods to measure comorbidity in cancer populations: no gold standard exists. J Clin Epidemiol 65:924–933
164. de Groot V, Beckerman H, Lankhorst GJ, Bouter LM (2003) How to measure comorbidity. A critical review of available methods. J Clin Epidemiol 56(3):221–229

Chapter 3
Cancer, Chronic Conditions and Social Disadvantage—The Perfect Storm

Janelle V. Levesque, Afaf Girgis and Paul R. Ward

Abstract Socially disadvantaged, including low socio-economic groups, experience excess rates of cancer and other chronic conditions and worse outcomes for both. This chapter firstly provides a comprehensive conceptual framework for understanding 'social disadvantage' (social quality theory) and explores the equity of access to healthcare services for disadvantaged groups, highlighting that inequities in health care are complex and multi-faceted, including at the individual, health system and policy levels. The chapter then focuses on one particular socially disadvantaged group (people of culturally and linguistically diverse [CALD] backgrounds) as an example of interaction of disadvantage and disease, examining evidence on what works and what does not work in terms of creating equitable health services that address cancer and co-morbidity.

Keywords Social determinants of health · Socio-economic disadvantage · Marginalized groups · Culturally and linguistically diverse groups · Migrants · Culturally competent care

Key Points

- Disadvantaged and low socio-economic groups experience excess rates of and poorer outcomes from cancer and other chronic conditions
- Access to, quality of, and outcomes from healthcare are inequitable across a number of clinical areas, including screening for a variety of cancers, interventions and primary care services

---

J.V. Levesque (✉) · A. Girgis
Psycho-Oncology Research Group, Centre for Oncology Education and Research Translation (CONCERT), Ingham Institute for Applied Medical Research, South Western Sydney Clinical School, University of New South Wales, Sydney, Australia
e-mail: janelle.levesque@monash.edu

P.R. Ward
School of Health Sciences, Faculty of Medicine, Nursing and Health Sciences, Flinders University, Adelaide, Australia
e-mail: paul.ward@flinders.edu.au

B. Koczwara (ed.), *Cancer and Chronic Conditions*,
DOI 10.1007/978-981-10-1844-2_3

- A holistic conceptual umbrella (theory of social quality) is more useful for identifying the broader and cumulative forms of disadvantage and marginalization experienced by some population groups, rather than utilizing singular concepts such as social class, socio-economic status, or social capital
- By striving for a goal of 'equity in health', healthcare systems need to strive for the elimination of systematic differences in health status between groups on the basis of socio-economic status, ethnicity, age, gender and so on
- Despite growing multiculturalism and awareness of health-related disparities in cancer and other chronic conditions, there remains substantial work to be done to address the unequal outcomes
- Culturally and linguistically diverse patients face issues regarding communication with health care professionals, access to health systems and higher levels of unmet need
- A shift is required from viewing the patient as the agent responsible for changing their health outcomes to a broader view based on improving the system, so that it adequately addresses minority patient needs
- Creating a culturally competent health care system that is responsive to patients need is suggested as an avenue to address disparities in care for both cancer and the patient's comorbidities
- Policy reform at an organizational level, development, refinement and implementation of guidelines for minimum standards of care for disadvantaged patients and adoption of tested interventions may improve the equity of access to health care.

3.1 Introduction

It has been well established that more egalitarian societies have both better overall levels of health and reduced inequities in morbidity and mortality [1–4]. In addition, the concept of equity in health and health care has been shown to be important for health achievement [5]. The notion of equity is one of the most important and fundamental principles of health care systems in the developed world, whereby provision of healthcare services should be based solely on clinical need. However, there is a huge research literature demonstrating that access to, quality of, and outcomes from healthcare are inequitable across a number of clinical areas, including screening for a variety of cancers [6, 7], interventions for a variety of chronic conditions [8–10] and primary care [11–13]. These examples reflect or even fulfil Julian Tudor-Hart's notion of the 'inverse care law' [14], whereby the groups with the greatest levels of health care need receive the lowest levels of healthcare services.

In response to the 'inverse care law, it is widely recognized that public health policy and practice, needs to focus on addressing the social determinants of health, in order to increase the health of the most vulnerable and disadvantaged groups [4,

15, 16]. By focussing on developing relevant and appropriate health policy and practice responses for such groups, it is hoped that we can redress the current inequities in cancer and chronic conditions between the most and least advantaged groups within society. Building on seminal multi-national agreements such as the Ottawa Charter [17], the Alma Ata Declaration [18] and the Bangkok Declaration [19], the Commission on the Social Determinants of Health recognized the multiple forms of oppression and disadvantage experienced by the poorest members of society [4], calling for a 'joined up', multi-sectoral approach to addressing the problem of inequities in health. By focussing on the social determinants of health (e.g. poverty, inequitable access to healthcare services, social exclusion, discrimination), we can attempt to reduce the incidence of cancer and other major chronic conditions, such as heart disease, diabetes, mental health and musculoskeletal conditions, all of which are more prevalent in more disadvantaged populations. In this way, cancer and major chronic conditions represent comorbidities in disadvantaged groups, so focusing on the social determinants of health may improve both cancer and other chronic conditions.

3.2 The Theory of Social Quality as a Conceptual Framework for Understanding Socio-economic Status

We concur with the Commission on the Social Determinants of Health in terms of the need to focus on both the multiple forms of disadvantage and thus the development of complex and holistic policy responses. However, many conceptual frameworks currently used in public health research do not lend themselves easily to being useful for these purposes. For example, there is ample research evidence that certain population groups are more socially excluded [20], have lower levels of social capital [21], have poorer access to financial resources, health promoting or curative services [22] and that some groups are disempowered [23]. These factors are all social determinants of health as higher levels of social inclusion, social capital, access to finance and services and empowerment are all "good for your health". Taken on their own, studies highlighting these social determinants of health are useful only insofar as they paint part of the picture as to both the problems and potential solutions for improving the health of affected groups. However, they do not provide a conceptual and methodological framework for linking these various concepts for the same population groups, which would then highlight the potential for the multiple 'problems' that certain population groups can encounter or the particular 'problems' that other groups encounter.

Research studies may highlight the need to implement policy to increase the social capital for particular groups, or to facilitate more socially inclusive policies or systems, but rarely can such studies (due to their conceptual limitations) provide evidence for policies and systems which attend to the multiplicity of needs highlighted by the Commission on the Social Determinants of Health. Therefore, rather than utilizing singular concepts such as social class, socio-economic status, or social capital, in this chapter we outline a more holistic and hopefully more useful conceptual umbrella (theory of social quality) for identifying the broader and cumulative forms of disadvantage and marginalization experienced by some population groups.

The notion of social quality is gaining international recognition as an innovative theoretical and methodological tool for researchers and policy makers interested in understanding and responding to the multiple forms of disadvantage experienced by certain groups in society [24–34]. Social quality has been defined by Beck as: "*the extent to which people are able to participate in the social, economic life and development of their communities under conditions which enhance their wellbeing and individual potential*" [33] (p. 3). Social quality theory was originally developed as a response to the hegemony of individualized quality of life measures [35]. Walker argues that contemporary Western societies are preoccupied with measuring and increasing our well-being, quality of life, happiness and so on *as individuals*, rather than as individuals in groups, communities and other social relations [35] (p. 214). Social quality theory does not dismiss the individual quality of life approach, since it is useful for clinical situations and individualized solutions. However, the point is that it provides relatively little use for developing population-level social or public health policy. The individual quality of life approach can tell us a great deal about how to improve individual circumstances (e.g. functional well-being, psychological needs, cognitive impairments, etc.). However, it cannot tell us the reasons why some population groups fair worse than others in society, or more importantly, how we may be able to respond in terms of health policy and practice aimed at improving the health of the most vulnerable groups in society [29]. In addition, individual perspectives on quality of life tend to avoid consideration of the involvement of political and normative factors [29].

In terms of its underlying ideology, the social quality theory argues that there are four key *normative factors* that determine the 'quality of a society' [33]:

- Social justice
- Solidarity
- Equal value of all humans
- Human dignity

Any society can be judged according to these normative factors, both in a global sense (i.e. how good is the social quality of a particular society) but also in terms of the specific normative factors (i.e. which factors require policy response in a particular society). However, on their own, these normative factors are not easily operationalized and do not have a methodological framework. Therefore, within social quality theory, four *conditional factors* aim to render the normative factors 'researchable' (see Fig. 3.1):

- socio-economic security (linked to social justice)
- social cohesion (linked to solidarity)
- social inclusion (linked to equal value)
- social empowerment (linked to human dignity)

Socio-economic security **... based on ...** **Social Justice**	**Social cohesion** **... based on ...** **Solidarity**
Social inclusion **... based on ...** **Equal value of all humans**	**Empowerment** **... based on ...** **Human dignity**

Fig. 3.1 Architecture of social quality theory [34]

Socio-economic securityis concerned with the extent to which people or groups have access to, utilization of and successful outcomes related to a variety of resources over time. These resources may be related to, among other things, finance, housing, healthcare, employment and education. This domain has great historical credence in public health policy and practice, in terms of the importance of such factors in shaping inequalities in health and inequities in healthcare. Huge effort has been put into both public health policy [4, 36–39] and research around understanding the causes and mechanisms of inequalities in health, particularly in relation to education, housing and unemployment [4].

Social cohesion relates to the extent to which people and groups share social relations. Such relations may refer to shared identities, values and norms. This domain relates closely to issues of solidarity and trust, which are particularly important in terms of public health [40–42]. In many ways, this domain relates to the concept of social capital, which is now commonplace in public health policy [43] and research [43–46], although has its roots in sociological theory [47–51].

Social inclusion is, in many ways, similar to social cohesion, but differs as social inclusion is related to the extent to which people and groups have access to and are integrated into the different institutions and social relations of everyday life. This domain relates to the extent to which people and groups feel that they are part of, or are included in, society at an everyday level. The domain attempts to integrate processes at the level of systems (i.e. institutions and social systems) and the 'lifeworld' and, in so doing, it extends Parsons' notions of social systems by seeing their interconnectedness with individual lifeworlds. In this way, the domain of social inclusion fits neatly with theories expounded by Habermas [52–55], in addition to both public health policy and research [54, 55].

Social empowerment relates to the extent to which social relations enhance the personal capabilities of individuals. This domain takes concepts of social inclusion and cohesion, and explores the enabling factors which empower people to act as social agents. This domain builds on, and empirically develops, notions of reflexivity, outlined by Beck [56, 57] and Giddens [58, 59].

As can be seen in this brief overview, the multi-dimensional and multi-level approach represents an advancement of public health policy and practice, which is not solely aimed at either individuals or systems, but instead realises the intimate links between systems and life-world and aims at understanding both within the same theoretical framework. The long-term aim of developing and implementing the theory of social quality is to enhance the social quality of people's lives (especially vulnerable groups). This will imply the elaboration of the four conditional factors of social quality:

1. To increase socio-economic security, especially for the most vulnerable
2. To strengthen social cohesion in order to address the challenges regarding health and social care as a community
3. To increase social inclusion for the accessibility of the health and social care systems
4. To underpin social empowerment in order to take initiative in addressing problems on a community level as well as to find innovative ways for stimulating health, preventing diseases and new ways of coping with the consequences of diseases, illnesses and sicknesses.

3.3 The Role of Healthcare Services in Addressing Social Quality for Vulnerable Groups

It is important to argue that healthcare services can impact social quality and thus have a part to play as a social determinant of health. The most basic definitions of 'social' are that it involves communication or interaction [53, 60] and that it is not a 'natural' or 'given' state [60], which therefore makes it amenable to change through policy and practice. By these conceptualizations, we can immediately see how healthcare services are social and can thus impact social quality:

(a) They involve communication between patients and practitioners
(b) A person's social status may (and often does) have an impact on their experience of healthcare
(c) The outcomes of healthcare interventions may have an impact on social relationships
(d) Healthcare services are historically, geographically and culturally contingent, and therefore cannot be viewed as 'natural' entities, rather as 'social constructs' which are determined by both individuals and social systems

Talcott Parsons, an early functionalist sociologist, saw a central role for healthcare services in the smooth running of society by maintaining/increasing population-level health and reducing population-level illness [61, 62]. The importance of health services in promoting health and preventing illness is reflected in Parsons' quote, "*...by almost any definition health is included in the functional needs of the individual member of society.... From the point of view of the social system, too low a general level of health, too high an incidence of illness, is dysfunctional: this is in the first instance because illness incapacitates the effective performance of social roles*" [61]. This view provides particular roles:

(a) The health system—to turn 'illness' into 'health' (or to maintain health) in order to maintain social order
(b) The healthcare practitioners—to 'make people better' in order to make them 'functional' again
(c) The patients—to follow doctors' advice and to 'get better'

This was the central argument within Parsons' notion of 'the sick role', which is highly contentious and is not dealt with here (a useful critique can be found elsewhere [63]). Nevertheless, Parsons' functionalist theory set up healthcare services as central to the smooth running of society.

Similar to Parsons, Sen regards health as one of the most important conditions of human life, and central to the development of what have been called 'human capabilities' [64, 65]. This is similar to the widely held belief of 'health as a basic human right' [66, 67], which then enables each person to function as an agent—to pursue the various goals in life that he/she has reason to value. Whilst this is not a contentious issue, the role of healthcare services in 'creating' or maintaining health has been. For example, Sen minimises the role of healthcare services in the 'achievement of health' by stating that "*health equity cannot be understood in terms of the distribution of health care*" [68]. Taken as a singular argument, most people would tend to agree, although taken alongside other social determinants of health, the widely held view is that healthcare services can be understood as having a role in promoting health and preventing illness, and thereby have a role to play in promoting health equity [69].

A review of the international literatures for the Commission on Social Determinants of Health by the Knowledge Network on Health Systems [15] makes clear that health systems are a site for action to promote greater equity in health. The report goes on to show how the development of more equitable healthcare systems will lead to more equitable health, as long as this is done alongside action on other social determinants of health. This picks up on an earlier, but nonetheless important model of social determinants of health [69, 70] in which healthcare services are firmly located as one of the social determinants of health, all of which need to be addressed if we hope to have a sustained effort in reducing the current levels of inequity in cancer and chronic conditions.

3.4 The Need for More Equitable Access to Healthcare Services for Vulnerable Groups

By striving for a goal of 'equity in health', healthcare systems need to strive for the elimination of all systematic differences in health status between groups on the basis of socio-economic status, ethnicity, age, gender and so on. Therefore, the goal of equity in healthcare is to closely match services to levels of need within communities. Obviously, this may result in large differences in access and use between different socio-economic groups, favouring those groups in greatest need. This is the concept of 'vertical equity', which is outlined later in the chapter.

Numerous epidemiological studies and policy documents point to the effectiveness of investing in illness prevention programs across a whole range of cancers [71], highlighting the positive impact of investing in primary care on avoidable hospitalizations, and also the equitable impact that primary care has on vulnerable groups. A number of US studies have found that increasing access to primary care is associated with decreasing (avoidable) hospitalizations and more equitable health outcomes [72–74]. Compelling evidence is also provided on the specific role and impact of primary care on population health. First, population health is better in areas with more primary care general practitioners. Second, individuals who receive care from primary care general practitioners are healthier than those who do not. Third, there is an association between preventive care and improved health. Fourth, countries with stronger primary level care services have populations with better health, especially when health policy is supportive of primary care [73, 75, 76]. An Australian review of primary and community health services found positive and equitable impacts of a primary care approach on patient and community well-being, reduced mortality and morbidity and also on reduced health care expenditures [77]. Therefore, healthcare planners and providers now have the evidence to defend the planning and provision of equitable healthcare services and systems, on the basis of improving overall population health in addition to lowering the gap between those groups with the best and worst health outcomes.

3.5 Inequity, Inequality and Disparity: What Is the Difference and How Do We Measure 'Equity'?

Across the world, terms like 'inequalities', 'disparities' and 'inequities' are often used interchangeably in academic and policy literatures [16], and even when they are defined, there seems little consensus about their meaning or measurement [75, 78]. The terms 'inequality' and 'disparity' tend to be used in different geographical contexts, with 'inequality' being preferred in Western Europe whereas 'disparity' tends to predominate in the US [78]. Nevertheless, the two terms are very similar in meaning—essentially, they are defined by 'difference' with no reference to the context, nature or direction of the difference or who may be adversely affected by the difference. In this way, disparities or inequalities in healthcare may simply refer to differences in the use, access, availability or quality of healthcare by different groups.

The central ingredient missing from definitions of inequality or disparity is the idea of 'social justice' or 'fairness'. This is where 'equity' becomes particularly useful, since it focuses research, policy and practice on exploring, attending to and monitoring healthcare, which is deemed to be 'unfair'. There may be differences in healthcare use between groups, but are these fair? For example, we may find that older people use particular cancer services more than younger people, but that does not necessarily mean that access to those services is inequitable (i.e. unfair to younger people). Older people may just be in greater need for cancer services. Indeed, older people may in fact not be receiving high enough levels of those services, and therefore, the services may be inequitable in the opposite direction. Nevertheless, 'fairness' or 'social justice' is the key area of concern.

There is ample literature on defining, operationalizing and measuring equity in relation to primary healthcare services [75, 76, 78–80]. Equity has been generally conceptualized as either *horizontal equity* or *vertical equity*. Vertical equity works on the principle that individuals/groups that are 'different' should be treated differently, according to their levels of healthcare need. Whilst this is relatively uncontentious, it is not straightforward to operationalise and monitor in a public health context. Horizontal equity works on the principle of equal treatment for individuals or groups with the same (or similar) levels of healthcare need. For the example of cervical cancer screening, the major determinants of 'need' for population-based screening would be age and gender. Therefore, using the framework of horizontal equity, one may expect that the provision, access and uptake of cervical cancer screening services would be similar between a group of 50–60 year old women in one town and a similar group of women in another town. If there were systematic differences in uptake of cervical cancer screening services (i.e. differences in terms of social class, ethnicity etc.), then we could suggest an inequitable uptake.

Equity of healthcare has been divided into three domains: equal *access* to health care for people in equal need; equal *treatment* for people in equal need; and equal *outcomes* for people in equal need [79]. Whilst this is a simplification of the nature of equity, it is useful in delineating the various domains in which inequities may arise. For the purposes of this chapter, we briefly mention two of these concepts—access and need.

In a seminal paper, Aday and Anderson [81] outlined different mechanisms for understanding and defining access. They coined the terms "potential access" and "realized access" to differentiate between providing the mechanisms for people to access services (e.g. culturally appropriate information, adequately located services, appropriate staff mix etc.) and the actual utilization of those services. Goddard and Smith [79] have built on this definition of access, to provide the following: "*the ability to secure a* ***specified*** *range of services, at a* ***specified*** *level of quality, subject to a* ***specified*** *maximum level of personal inconvenience and cost, whilst in possession of a* ***specified*** *level of information*" (p. 1151, bold added). This definition

Table 3.1 Domains in the taxonomy of need [84, 85]

Domain 1: normative need This is a need defined by an 'expert', in the form of a local GP, school teacher or evidence-based guidelines for the treatment of a particular group of people (e.g. risk factors for lung cancer)	**Domain 2: felt need** This domain is determined by asking people what they feel they need (i.e. akin to 'wants'); and assumes perfect and equal information across groups in society about what services are available, which is obviously contestable [63, 86]
Domain 3: expressed need This may also be conceptualized as 'service utilization', measured through activity statistics, prescribing data or surgical statistics. Although not all 'felt need' gets turned into 'expressed need'—there will be groups of people who experience unmet need	**Domain 4: comparative need** This is akin to horizontal equity and is determined by studying the characteristics of differing populations in receipt of differing levels of a service (e.g. differing rates of cervical cancer screening)

begins to make 'access' amenable to policy makers, since the word 'specified' allows them to shape access in relation to local circumstances (i.e. allow for differences).

In terms of defining 'need', we can only scratch the surface here. There are huge literatures spanning philosophy, social policy, economics and public health, which cover everything from basic human needs [66, 67], human rights and capabilities [64, 65, 82], and health needs assessment [83]. For our purposes, a useful way of conceptualizing healthcare need is the 'Taxonomy of Need' [84, 85], which is widely used in healthcare needs assessment. This taxonomy has four domains of need (summarized in Table 3.1), which when taken together, Bradshaw argues that we can get somewhere close to understanding overall need.

Using the example of cervical cancer screening, a comparative approach to need (Domain 4) would assess the differences in screening rates between population A and population B, weighted to take account of the relevant risk factors in the patient populations. However, as this approach is purely comparative, if population A is deemed to be in need in comparison to population B, this does not necessarily mean that population B is not in need, as the screening rates in population B may not be at an adequate level. This approach merely attempts to assess comparative need (or equity), and makes no judgements about the appropriateness of screening rates.

In terms of understanding the role of healthcare systems in promoting 'inequities in health', a number of reasons have been put forward for the 'equity problems of health systems' [15]. Firstly, most health systems have weak population health and health equity orientation. With only limited and unsustained efforts being made at developing equitable health systems—the result is often the exclusion of socially and materially disadvantaged groups. Secondly, health care is rarely pro-poor, which means that services and systems are not necessarily offered on the basis of health care need, which is often highest in materially disadvantaged groups. There is a great deal of evidence that higher income groups make more use of services, get better access to services, receive higher quality services and get better health outcomes on the basis of these services. Finally, it has been suggested that socially marginalized groups often experience health care as demeaning and exclusionary, which results in poorer health outcomes, lower self-reported health status and a denial of dignity and basic human rights. These all point to lower levels of social quality.

Gilson et al. [15] argue that the driving forces behind the problems outlined above are macro in orientation: commercialization through a neo-liberal economic agenda; and public sector organizational culture and capacity. Health systems are obviously not immune to the globalized push towards a market-driven economy, whereby governments privilege privatization, consumerism, and commercialism. Both internally and externally, health systems that are funded by governments have to buy into these ideologies, and this can be seen internally by the increase in private health insurance, and increased competition between health care providers. Externally, the health system is in competition with other systems and organizations for scarce resources, which makes notions of 'intersectoral working' or 'whole-of-government' thinking more difficult. The increased impact of commercialization has been linked to worse and more inequitable access to health care services, and the greater reliance on private health care providers has been linked to increased inequities in treatment rates and outcomes between socio-economic groups [15]. There is also evidence that current levels of inequity in healthcare (and hence health) are compounded by organizational culture within public sector organizations internationally [15]. Such cultures are conceptualized as hierarchical, rule-bound and rigid, which impedes innovation such as inter-sectoral working and action. Also, such cultures often facilitate and maintain power and decision making with medically trained doctors. These doctors are trained to provide individuals (or their organs or diseases) with curative care; rather than providing preventive care for populations and the sub-groups of populations with the highest levels of need. This approach essentially limits the potential for health systems to focus on either population-based approaches or, more specifically, on an equity-based approach to policy and practice [15].

This chapter has broadly detailed the disadvantage or marginalization of particular groups. The following section examines one of these groups, people from culturally and linguistically diverse (CALD) backgrounds, providing evidence and possible solutions to improving equity of access to treatment. CALD patients are a particularly vulnerable group, facing not only potential economic difficulties, but also issues relating to communication, social inclusion and direct and indirect discrimination. Furthermore, worldwide migration is on the increase, and for some migrants the relocation to another country has a great impact on their social position, often through a decrease in status, therefore we may view this change as an acquired disadvantage. We also outline suggestions for meaningfully engaging with CALD groups, which may have applicability more broadly to other marginalized groups and within an international context.

3.6 Culturally Diverse Patients in the Context of Cancer Care and Chronic Disease

Migration is a world-wide phenomenon, with over 232 million, or 3 % of the world's population, being classified as migrants [87]. Over the past 20 years there has been an increase in net migration, from 2 million annually during the 1990s to 4.6 million annually between 2000 and 2010, with a current rate of approximately 3.6 million annually [87]. Approximately 50 % of all migrants take up residence in just 10 countries (listed from largest migrant intake to lowest): the United States of America (20 % of the global total), Russian Federation, Germany, Saudi Arabia, the United Arab Emirates, the United Kingdom, France, Canada, Australia and Spain [87]. Using the English speaking countries listed above as examples, the remainder of this chapter will examine the interaction between migration, cultural diversity, social disadvantage and health outcomes, with a specific focus on cancer care. It will also highlight current efforts to address disparities in cancer care for CALD patients, while also identifying factors that may contribute to service gaps, before future directions for research and practice are proposed.

3.6.1 Cultural Diversity and Its Challenges Within the USA, UK, Canada and Australia

Historically, the United States, Canada and Australia have British connections due to colonization efforts that underpinned the expansion of the British Empire [88]. While sharing this common element, the contemporary multicultural profiles of each country are distinctly different. According to the 2011 Census, 86 % of UK residents identify as white, with the remaining 14 % comprized of Asian (7.5 %, primarily Indian, Pakistani, and Bangladeshi), Black (3.3 %, from Africa or the Caribbean), and mixed or other ethnic backgrounds (3.2 %) [89]. In the United States, 62.1 % of the population identify as white, 17.4 % Hispanic or Latino, 13.2 % African-American, 5.4 % Asian American, and 1.4 % Native American/Alaska Native/Hawaiian Native [90]. In Canada, 20 % of the population were born overseas, with the most prominent migrant groups from the UK, France, Germany, Italy, China, Ukraine, East Indies, Netherlands and Poland [91]. Approximately one in four Australians were born overseas, with 28.1 % of the population being migrants [92]. The most common migrant groups within Australia are from the UK, New Zealand, China, India, Philippines, Vietnam, Italy, South Africa, Malaysia and Germany [92].

While the UK, USA, Canada and Australia have strong migration and multiculturalism policies, the reality is that culturally diverse individuals within each country face considerable social challenges and disadvantage. For example, in Australia the unemployment rate of migrants is higher than native born Australians (8.5 % compared to 4.6 %), many are under-employed (i.e. working in jobs that do not reflect their qualifications), with high numbers of migrants (including 38 % of skilled migrants) earning less than AUD$600 per week [93]. Other factors influencing employment for migrants in Australia include low English proficiency, barriers to integrating into a different culture, little recognition of foreign qualifications and race discrimination [94]. Consequently, it is suggested that migrants may take up to one generation of settlement in Australia to achieve the same professional level that they held in their home country [94]. A similar conclusion was reached in Canada, where migrants are at higher risk of poverty and are taking longer from the time of arrival to achieve professional parity with native-born Canadians [95]. The USA and UK both report poorer employment outcomes and higher unemployment rates for ethnic minorities [96–98]. As highlighted earlier in the chapter, employment issues influence socio-economic security and the associated conditional factor of social justice, and consequently significant attention has been paid to the relationship between employment and health outcomes [99–102].

3.7 Ethnicity and Cancer Care

The past 30 years have seen a steady increase in the volume of research investigating differential outcomes in cancer that may be due to variables such as age, sex, ethnicity and socio-economic status. As summarized by Halpern [103], this research is largely descriptive in nature, but it has shone the spotlight on important inequalities. Specifically, there is evidence that culturally diverse patients engage in cancer screening at lower levels than their mainstream peers [104–113]; that such patients are often diagnosed with more advanced disease [114, 115], have a higher number of co-morbid conditions [116–120], may not receive the same quality of care (e.g. most appropriate treatment, timely access to care, poorer communication with care providers) [114, 121–127]; and have poorer psychological and physical outcomes, including survival [114, 115, 128–130].

As presented in the earlier sections of this chapter, the disadvantage experienced by culturally diverse patients is complex and will involve more than residing in a low socio-economic area or barriers to employment success. Inequitable health outcomes may reflect differing cultural expectations of cancer screening [131–134] and preventive healthcare [135–137] and different cultural meanings about cancer [136, 138, 139]. There is also increasing argument that both socio-economic deprivation and persistent racial bias interact with personal (e.g. patient and health care professional) and systemic (e.g. organizational and governmental) factors to create a situation in which ethnically diverse patients are truly disadvantaged [140, 141]. When CALD patients engage with health care systems they may be reminded how their personal health values lie outside the norm of the mainstream culture, they may not be provided with the same level of service or care, and they may feel quite powerless to change their situation or address their health concern. Using Social Quality Theory as the explanatory framework, we can therefore conclude that CALD patients face challenges pertaining to all elements of social quality. The remainder of this section highlights communication challenges faced by culturally diverse patients in receiving adequate cancer care, an issue selected as it potentially differentiates culturally diverse patients from other disadvantaged groups.

3.7.1 Communication with Culturally Diverse Patients in Cancer Care Settings

Communication is a fundamental skill in medical care with the potential to influence the extent to which the patient understands their conditions while also impacting on psychological and physical outcomes [142, 143]. Communicating with individuals from different cultural groups has been identified by health care professionals as challenging and stressful [144, 145]. Patients also face challenges, as sensitive topics may be discussed and unfamiliar terminology may be used. Additional challenges arise when there are discrepancies between patients' and doctors' values and beliefs pertaining to health, illness, the role of the doctor, and communication expectations [146, 147]. Linguistic and cultural differences are often nominated as barriers to establishing and maintaining a suitable relationship between health care professionals and patients and are noted as having an impact on compliance, level of understanding, and patient, engagement during the consultation [147–151]. For example, Gordon et al. [148] highlighted that African American patients with pulmonary nodules or lung cancer received less information from doctors and were less active in consultations compared to white patients. This difference was exacerbated in consultations when there was racial discordance between doctors and patients (i.e. white doctor with black patients) [148]. Similarly, in their review of cultural difference in medical communication, Schouten and Meeuwesen [147] concluded that ethnically diverse patients were less expressive, affective and assertive compared to white patients; and that doctors demonstrated less affective interactions during consultations with CALD patients.

Involving interpreters in cancer care consultations is often perceived as one way to mitigate the problem of a lack of understanding when there is racial discordance between patients and clinicians. Unfortunately, current research suggests that this may not be the case, due to a relative lack of appropriately trained interpreters, an over-reliance on family and friends for interpretation, the impact of interpreter presence on consultation flow, and interpretation inaccuracies [150, 152–155]. Additionally, Gargan and Chianese [155] highlight the ethical issues regarding the use of both formal and informal interpreters, arguing that many CALD patients are unable to give informed consent to treatment, are excluded from potentially beneficial clinical trials, and face confidentiality violations, especially when using a family or friend to translate.

In Australia, Butow et al. [152, 153] have examined audio recordings of consultations with cancer patients (Anglo-Australian, Chinese, Greek and Arabic) to examine the content and process of doctor-patient communication in cancer care, particularly when a poor prognosis was going to be communicated to the patient. Findings revealed significant differences in how doctors communicated with immigrant patients with interpreters, including less overall verbal interaction, less discussion of cancer related issues, less information provision and summarizing of consultation content, and more time on other medical issues and providing direct advice [153]. In these consultations, despite migrant patients giving more cues indicating a need for information or emotional support, one in five cues were not interpreted, and when they were, doctors tended to delay responding to or ignore such cues [153]. In consultations involving the delivery of poor prognostic information, doctors communicated less messages of hope to CALD patients, and the presence of an interpreter actually increased the use of medical jargon, in comparison to consultations involving non-CALD patients [152].

While the use of interpreters may alter the style and content of consultations, there are also issues pertaining to the accuracy of translation and the suitability of using family and friends in comparison to professional interpreters. A review conducted by Flores [156] concluded that the quality of care is markedly reduced when a translator is not available or when ad hoc translators (e.g. family, friends, bilingual medical staff or strangers) took on the interpreter role. While concluding that there were differences in the quality of care, Flores [156] did note that many CALD patients report that they are more comfortable with using family members or bilingual staff, and are therefore more likely to raise sensitive topics in such situations when compared to using professional translators.

The level of accuracy reported in translated consultations varies across studies [153, 155–158]. For example, Simon et al. [157] found that overall accuracy was high (74 % of content), however accuracy decreased as the complexity of the consultation increased. The rate of inaccuracy especially increased when research related concepts such as clinical trials and randomization were introduced, especially if medical staff spoke for extended periods and used jargon [157]. Flores et al. [158] found that in 57 consultations almost 1900 interpretation errors were made, of which 18 % (or on average six errors per consultation) had potential clinical consequences. When examining these serious errors, Flores et al. [158] found that professional translators made a significantly lower proportion of clinically relevant errors compared to ad hoc translators (12 % vs. 22 % respectively), concluding that the use of ad hoc interpreters doubled the risk of a clinically relevant error being made. Omission of consultation content is the most frequent source of error; with Flores et al. [158] finding 47 % of errors were omissions, with the rate higher when ad hoc translators were used. Butow et al. [152] found that 23 % of prognostic statements made by doctors were never interpreted for patients and an additional 27 % were interpreted inaccurately. Additionally, patient statements or requests relating to prognosis were not interpreted 59 % of the time. Butow et al. [152] found comparable omissions and inaccuracies for both professional and family translators, suggesting that prognostic information is deeply embedded in cultural beliefs, and therefore may be altered by interpreters to reduce patient distress or to hide a poor prognosis.

3.8 Addressing the Needs of Culturally Diverse Patients

While the above evidence highlights the challenges and disparities experienced by culturally diverse patients, these issues and barriers have been recognized by key stakeholders, including governments, health care administrators, health care providers, support organizations and researchers. Consequently, there is growing awareness of the disparities experienced by CALD patients and efforts are being undertaken to address these.

Possibly the most commonly mentioned method to address the disparities in care and health outcomes for CALD patients is the concept of "culturally competent care". To achieve this goal, change is required at all levels of the health care system, not just at the patient-provider level. While an agreed upon definition of culturally competent care is difficult to find, Renzaho et al. [159] proposed that cultural competence is "a set of congruent behaviours, attitudes and policies that come together in a system, agency or among professionals, and enable that system, agency or those professionals to work effectively in cross-cultural situations" (p. 262). It is crucial to recognise that culturally competent care does not happen at an individual level, but rather encompasses the organizations and systems that underpin health care [160, 161]. Betancourt et al. [161] argue that cultural competence requires:

(a) An understanding of the socio-cultural influences that shape CALD patients' health beliefs and behaviours
(b) Consideration of how those factors influence engagement with heath care, from the organizational and structural processes through to clinical care
(c) The development of interventions to address these issues to ensure delivery of high quality care for all

While there are various models, interventions and training packages designed to enhance cultural competence [162–164] the framework proposed by Betancourt et al. [161] acknowledges the levels at which intervention is required while also identifying common barriers and interventions needed at each level. This framework is summarized in Table 3.2.

Crucially, it has been acknowledged that culturally competent interactions between patients and healthcare providers occurs with all staff in health care centers, and requires more than just awareness of typical cultural beliefs [164, 165]. Campinha-Bacote [164] proposes that culturally competent care is comprized of five, interwoven constructs:

(a) Cultural awareness
(b) Cultural knowledge
(c) Cultural skill
(d) Cultural encounters
(e) Cultural desire

Table 3.2 Culturally competent care framework [161]

Level	Barriers	Interventions
Organizational How the processes of health care are shaped by managers and politicians, and the staff who carry out their visions of care	• Lack of cultural minority representation in the workforce and in leadership roles • Culturally insensitive policies and procedures • Inappropriately designed delivery systems	• Increase minority representation at a leadership level • Ensure workforce reflects cultural diversity of the population it is servicing • Increased minority representation in health care training institutes and core professional organizations
Structural How the rules and economic forces that underpin health care increase the complexity of the system with which the patient must engage	• Lack of interpreter services • Lack of culturally appropriate information material • Arduous intake processes • Long waiting times for appointments • Need for health insurance • Difficulties in referrals to specialists • Lack of continuity of care	• Development of health care materials that are available in home languages and culturally sensitive • Community consultation and conduct of a socio-cultural assessment of local population and service provision barriers • Review of policies and procedures to address issues with intake, continuity of care and transfer of care to specialists • Development of specific quality care measures for evaluating care delivered to CALD patients • Linguistically suitable signage • Community engagement in the delivery of health promotion and prevention efforts
Clinical The sociocultural differences between patient and provider	• Attitudes to health care • Misaligned health beliefs • Reduced trust in care and lower patient satisfaction • Stereotyping of patients • Reduced patient involvement in decision making • Bias and discrimination	• Cultural awareness training for staff • Integration of cultural competence skills in undergraduate training programs for health care workers • Communication skills training

While the lay person may consider *cultural awareness* as being knowledge of other cultures, it actually refers to the health-care providers' self-awareness and reflection upon their cultural and professional background to identify biases and consider how they may influence practice. *Cultural knowledge* involves deliberately seeking information about cultural groups, specifically focusing on cultural values related to health, variation in disease incidence and prevalence among cultural groups, and treatment efficacy. *Cultural skill* comprises two elements—the ability to conduct a cultural assessment of the client and their underlying condition, and secondly, to perform a culturally based physical examination that takes into consideration physical and biological differences between ethnic groups. Directly interacting with culturally diverse clients to enhance cultural understanding is the essence of *cultural encounters,* while the motivation to engage in activities to enhance cultural awareness, knowledge and skill underpins the construct of *cultural desire*. While each of these elements is important in its own right, Campinha-Bacote [164] argues that it is when all five intersect that culturally competent care is achieved, and therefore the greater the area of intersection, the more culturally competent the service.

Nested within the concept of culturally competent care are opportunities to adapt or develop interventions specifically designed to meet the needs of minority patients. While often conducted as pilot projects with limited samples sizes, the research evidence is encouraging that interventions designed and tailored to address specific needs or concerns can be effective in improving CALD patients' outcomes in numerous areas of health, including cancer care [166–170]. A recent review by Harun et al. [167] examined interventions designed to enhance participation in decision making, communication with health care providers and treatment compliance for CALD patients with cancer. While findings were mixed, the evidence suggested that decision aids and patient navigators improved communication between minority patients and health care providers, with decision aids also effective in increasing shared decision making and patient perceived adherence [167].

Interventions using a patient navigator have been developed to specifically address barriers pertaining to CALD patients entering and successfully engaging with the health care system. Patient navigation is defined as "support and guidance offered to persons with abnormal cancer screening or a new cancer diagnosis in accessing the cancer care system; overcoming barriers; and facilitating timely, quality care provided in a culturally sensitive manner" (p. 3392) [171]. Patient navigators assist patients in a variety of ways, including providing informational and emotional support, assist with scheduling appointments, assist with forms, provide appointment reminders, meet patients for their appointments and assist with communication with health care professionals [172–174]. Evidence to date suggests that such interventions are effective, with reports of increased screening rates [175, 176] reduced time between testing and diagnostic resolution, reduced anxiety, increased patient satisfaction [177], increased adherence to diagnostic testing [172, 174] and more timely diagnostic testing in comparison to patients engaging in usual care [174]. It is however noted that there is a lack of evidence pertaining to the value of patient navigation in addressing issues that arise related to treatment adherence and cancer survivorship [176, 178].

In earlier sections of this chapter, we presented findings that culturally diverse patients tend to engage in cancer screening at lower levels than their Anglo peers. There is encouraging evidence to suggest that interventions designed to improve screening rates in cultural minority group patients are effective [179–182]. For example, Walsh et al. [182] developed an intervention to enhance colon cancer screening for members of the Latino and Vietnamese communities in the USA. The intervention included brochures with culturally tailored content and design features, individualized telephone counseling in their preferred language to discuss identified barriers to screening; and customized fecal occult blood test (FOBT) kit with simplified bilingual instructions. Involving a rigorous randomized controlled trial methodology and adequately powered sample size (n = 1358), Walsh et al. [182] found that screening rates increased by 12 % in the brochure/FOBT kit group and 21 % in the brochure/counselling/FOBT group, compared to 4 % in the usual care group. Other studies have utilized different awareness approaches targeting different cancer diagnoses, including education sessions with culturally congruent lay health workers for breast cancer screening in Korean-American women [181], brochure, flipchart and video delivery targeting couples for breast cancer screening in Hmong communities [180]; and home visits by lay health workers to enhance cervical cancer screening in Vietnamese American women [179].

From the field of mental health, there is evidence to suggest that empirically based interventions can be successfully adapted for use with cultural minority patients [183–185]. Griner and Smith [183] reviewed 76 studies, and concluded that there was a moderately strong benefit for culturally modified interventions, and that this benefit was increased if they were conducted in the client's preferred language and/or in groups of patients with the same cultural heritage. To increase the likelihood that interventions will be culturally acceptable and therapeutically effective, practitioners and researchers considering developing or adapting interventions for culturally diverse patients are strongly advized to consider the underpinning theoretical framework for the intervention while also following a specific model for intervention design and adaptation. There are numerous possible models to consider for developing culturally appropriate intervention content including intervention mapping [186], ecological validity model [187–189], community engagement [190], cultural targeting and tailoring [191], and the cultural adaptation process [192]. Utilizing such models will ensure that relevant engagement with the community is undertaken, cultural values and health beliefs are incorporated, consideration is given to the language and style of the intervention content, and potential barriers and risks can be identified and addressed in the planning phases.

3.9 Barriers to Supporting Culturally Diverse Patients

Despite growing acknowledgement of the need to address socio-cultural disparities in health care and outcomes for culturally diverse patients, numerous issues exist which pose barriers to progress. Sheikh [193] argues that there is systemic lack of investment in health needs of minority patients. In a social environment driven by the economic bottom line, the costs of developing interventions and resources for CALD patients are considerably higher than equivalent programs for English-speaking patients [193]. This is due to the additional costs of translation and interpreter services, engagement of bi-lingual staff (often at a higher base salary due to their additional skills), extended periods of community consultation and specialized services required to produce information resources (e.g. DVDs) in languages other than English. While these may present as barriers for development, it is important that we consider how proactive engagement with CALD patients may be more cost effective in the long-term if such programs can enhance the health outcomes of this vulnerable group.

An additional barrier is the perception of ethnic minority patients as hard to reach and therefore difficult to recruit and retain in research, which in turn limits the knowledge base upon which researchers and practitioners can draw to develop appropriate interventions and supportive care services [194]. Numerous barriers to the recruitment and retention of CALD patients in research have been identified including distrust, lack of community involvement, sampling approach, timing of contact with potential participants, housing instability, psychosocial distress, lack of knowledge about research/clinical trials, perceived harm arising from research, provider-related factors, culture, and logistical issues such as transportation, time, and costs [194–198].

However, Wendler et al. [199] challenge the conclusion that ethnic minority patients are reluctant to participate in research, finding that there were non-significant differences in willingness to participate in intervention, surgical and non-intervention health research between white, Hispanic and African American patients. Furthermore, there is evidence to suggest that minority patients perceive participation in research as beneficial, both to themselves and others [196]. Sheikh argues that we must acknowledge that the current trend to label CALD patients as hard to reach implies that they are to blame for their lack of participation due to poor health literacy, lack of research understanding and distrust and cultural beliefs that would make them decline research invitations [193]. Such an explanation fails to acknowledge the broader issues that may limit participation in research, for example that many mainstream research projects specifically exclude CALD patients on the grounds of limited English proficiency [200]. Strategies to enhance involvement of ethnic minority patients in research include community engagement, use of culturally congruent research staff, utilizing a targeted recruitment strategy with follow-up procedures, recruitment through word of mouth, cultural adaptations with personalized communications to participants, and flexible consenting procedures that allow auditory information presentations and verbal consent that is more appropriate to oral cultures and patients with limited literacy [194, 196, 198, 200–202].

Barriers to engagement in research are not exclusive to culturally diverse members of the community. Several other groups are considered hard to reach including (but not limited to) the elderly, the disabled, Indigenous, rural residents, gay, lesbian, bisexual and transgender, the homeless and mentally ill [177]. It is notable that such groups are often part of the most disadvantaged in our society, and therefore highlights that much of our contemporary medical knowledge is based upon the white, middle and upper classes, highly educated members of society. Barriers to recruitment in hard-to-reach groups were similar to ethnic minority patients and included mistrust, particularly from populations with a history of mistreatment, fear of authority, risk of harm, stigma, fear of exposure, possible exploitation, ill health, time commitment to take part, and a lack of perceived benefit to self or community [177, 203, 204]. Strategies to enhance recruitment of under-represented members of the community included community partnerships, use of media and social marketing, ensuring confidentiality, developing adequate rapport with participants, reducing the impact of gatekeepers in accessing populations, greater recruitment of and through caregivers, use of technology to gather data, broadening eligibility criteria and addressing logistical barriers in the study design, such as eliminating problems with transport and providing childcare for participants to attend research sessions [177, 204–208].

3.10 Future Directions for Research and Practice

Despite growing multiculturalism and awareness of health-related disparities in cancer and other chronic conditions, substantial work remains to be done in order to address the unequal outcomes. Clarke et al. [209] advocate for a shift from viewing the patient as the agent responsible for changing their health outcomes to a broader view based on improving the system so that it adequately addressed minority patient needs. This can be achieved through:

(a) policy reform, which is implemented at an organizational level
(b) development/refinement and implementation of guidelines for minimum standards of care for CALD patients
(c) educational interventions (e.g. communication skills training, interpreter training)
(d) interventions that engage with culturally diverse sectors of the community across the spectrum of health care from prevention and health promotion through to palliative care

While culturally competent care is viewed as a way to address this issue, the evidence base is not conclusive. Research examining organizational level interventions is scant and structural level changes may be implemented without adequate evaluation. Stronger evidence employing rigorous study designs is required and greater emphasis on interventions at the organizational and structural level may be encouraged if the economic feasibility can be demonstrated [210].

While studies of interventions designed to improve doctor-patient communication yield positive results [211, 212], there is very little evidence that it improves patient outcomes [159, 213]. Furthermore, the existing evidence base contains lower quality research with insufficient published information regarding the intervention/training, inadequate control of confounding variables, an almost exclusive focus on how interventions improve clinician knowledge rather than outcomes, and an absence of randomized controlled trials [159, 211, 213].

To increase the efficacy of clinical level interventions, two crucial elements are proposed. Firstly, Betancourt et al. [161] advocate that a categorical approach to cross-cultural education that highlights attitudes, beliefs and values of specific cultural groups may be inadequate and unsustainable considering the expanding cultural diversity within the USA, UK, Canada and Australia. Instead, they propose that training should focus on social issues and health beliefs that cut across cultures, while developing attitudes and skills that will encourage clinicians to handle different communication styles, navigate patient preferences for decision making, appreciate the role of family and gender issues, and how mistrust and discrimination may influence their patients' engagement with care [161]. Such training may reduce the current perception that cultural competence is a distinct skill rather than an integral element to clinical competence [214]. Secondly, several researchers and practitioners argue that culturally competent care requires practitioner reflexivity and consideration of personal factors that can interact with patient socio-cultural factors to influence the experience of care [215]. This poses a challenge for managers of health care settings in creating an environment that encourages such practice and allocates time for practitioners to talk and share their experiences and critically evaluate the cultural needs of each patient.

Finally, while the evidence for interventions designed specifically for CALD patients is encouraging, there are questions regarding their long-term sustainability and application to other cultural groups. Much of the published research reports on pilot studies or initial studies, but there are very few studies that have examined the long-term impact of such interventions and whether they have been integrated into usual care, or discontinued after the end of the funding period. Furthermore, Miranda et al. [185] argue that while there is evidence regarding the effectiveness of adapted psychosocial interventions, direct comparisons of adapted versus standard interventions have not been conducted. These matters are earmarked as areas requiring urgent attention to allow demonstration of the superiority of culture-specific interventions and the long-term value of such interventions, especially considering that they can be costly to develop.

3.11 Conclusions

In this chapter, we presented a comprehensive conceptual framework for understanding social disadvantage and highlighted the abundance of evidence on inequities in incidence of various cancers and most major chronic conditions, revealing the cumulative effects of socio-economic status on the likelihood of getting both cancer and other chronic conditions. It is clear that the reasons that underpin the inequities in health care are complex and multi-faceted, including at the individual, health system and policy levels. However, more in-depth examination of the social determinants of health for one disadvantaged sub-group, people of culturally and linguistically diverse backgrounds, suggests that whilst there are clear interactions between migration, cultural diversity, social disadvantage and health outcomes, there are also promising avenues for addressing some of the current disparities in health care. For example, evidence suggests that decision aids and patient navigators improves communication between minority patients and health care providers, with decision aids also effective in increasing shared decision making and patient perceived adherence. Also, whilst culturally diverse patients tend to engage in cancer screening at lower levels than their Anglo peers, there is encouraging evidence to suggest that interventions designed to improve screening rates specifically in cultural minority group patients are effective. Evidence from CALD groups might inform strategies to support more equitable care for other marginalized groups.

References

1. Marmot M, Wilkinson R (2006) Social determinants of health. Oxford University Press, Oxford
2. Wilkinson RG, Pickett KE (2007) The problems of relative deprivation: why some societies do better than others. Soc Sci Med 65:1965–1978
3. Wilkinson RG, Pickett KE (2006) Income inequality and population health: a review and explanation of the evidence. Soc Sci Med 62:1768–1784
4. Commission on Social Determinants of Health (2008) Closing the gap in a generation: health equity through action on the social determinants of health. Final report of the CSDH. World Health Organisation, Geneva
5. Anand S, Peter F, Sen A (2006) Public health, ethics, and equity. Oxford University Press, Oxford
6. Ward PR, Kelly B, Tucker G, Luke C (2006) Theoretical and conceptual issues around equity in health care: application to cervical cancer screening in South Australia. Public Health Bull 5:9–14
7. McCaffery K, Wardle J, Nadel M, Atkin W (2002) Socioeconomic variation in participation in colorectal cancer screening. J Med Screen 9:104–108
8. Battersby J, Flowers J, Harvey I (2004) An alternative approach to quantifying and addressing inequity in healthcare provision: access to surgery for lung cancer in the east of England. J Epidemiol Commun Health 58:623–625
9. Hippisley-Cox J, Pringle M (2000) Inequalities in access to coronary angiography and revascularisation: the association of deprivation and location of primary care services. Br J Gen Pract 50:449–454
10. Majeed A, Eliahoo J, Bardsley M, Morgan D, Bindman AB (2002) Variation in coronary artery bypass grafting, angioplasty, cataract surgery, and hip replacement rates among primary care groups in London: association with population and practice characteristics. J Public Health Med 24:21–26
11. Hull SA, Cornwell J, Harvey C, Eldridge S, Bare PO (2001) Prescribing rates for psychotropic medication amongst east London general practices: low rates where Asian populations are greatest. Fam Pract 18:167–173

12. Ward PR, Noyce PR, St Leger AS (2005) Multivariate regression analysis of associations between general practitioner prescribing rates for coronary heart disease drugs and healthcare needs indicators. J Epidemiol Commun Health 59:86–87
13. Ward PR, Noyce PR, St Leger AS (2007) How equitable are GP practice prescribing rates for statins? An ecological study in four primary care trusts in the North West of England. Int J Equity Health. doi:10.1186/1475-9276-6-2
14. Tudor Hart J (1971) The inverse care law. Lancet 297(6):405–412
15. Gilson L, Doherty J, Loewenson R, Francis V (2007) Challenging inequity through health systems. World Health Organisation Commission on Social Determinants of Health
16. Pittman PM (2006) Beyond the sound of one hand clapping: experiences in six countries using health equity research in policy. J Health Polit Polic 31:33–49
17. Ottawa Charter for Health Promotion (1986) First international conference on health promotion, Canada
18. International Conference on Primary Health Care (1978) Declaration of alma-ata. Association of South East Asian Nations, Kazakhstan
19. World Conference on Human Rights (1993) Bangkok declaration, Bangkok
20. Giddens A (1994) Beyond left and right. Polity Press, Cambridge
21. Ahern MM, Hendryx MS (2003) Social capital and trust in providers. Soc Sci Med 57: 1195–1203
22. Spicer N (2009) Places of exclusion and inclusion: asylum-seeker and refugee experiences of neighbourhoods in the UK. J Ethn Migr Stud 34:491–510
23. Ward PR, Coates A (2006) "We shed tears, but there is no one there to wipe them up for us": narratives of (mis)trust in a materially deprived community. Health 10:283–301
24. Ward PR, Redgrave P, Read C (2006) Operationalizing the theory of social quality: theoretical and experiential reflections from the development and implementation of a public health programme in the UK. Eur J Soc Qual 6:9–18
25. Ward PR, Meyer SB (2009) Trust, social quality and wellbeing: a sociological exegesis. Dev Soc 38:339–363
26. Ward PR (2006) Social quality and modern public health: developing a framework for the twenty-first century. Eur J Soc Qual 6:1–7
27. Ward PR (2006) Trust, reflexivity and dependence: a 'social systems theory' analysis in/of medicine. Eur J Soc Qual 6:121–133
28. Walker A, van der Maesen L (2004) Social quality and quality of life. In: Glatzer W, Von Below S, Stoffregen M (eds) Challenges for quality of life in the contemporary world: advances in quality-of-life studies, theory and research. Kluwer Academic Publishers, Dordrecht, pp 13–31
29. van der Maesen LJG, Walker A (2005) Indicators of social quality: outcomes of the European Scientific Network. Eur J Soc Qual 5:8–24
30. Taylor-Gooby P (2006) The rational actor reform paradigm: delivering the goods but destroying public trust? Eur J Soc Qual 6:121–141
31. Meyer SB, Luong CN, Tsourtos G, Ward PR (2010) Operationalising the theory of social quality: analysis of the reliability of an instrument to measure social quality. Dev Soc 39:327–356
32. Beck W, van der Maesen L, Thomese F, Walker A (2001) Introduction: who and what is the European Union for? In: Beck W (ed) Social quality: a vision for Europe. Kluwer Law International, The Hague, pp 1–17
33. Beck W, van der Maesen L, Thomese F, Walker A (eds) (1998) The social quality of Europe. Policy Press, Bristol
34. Ward P, Mamerow L, Meyer S (2013) Identifying vulnerable populations using a social determinants of health framework: analysis of national survey data across six Asia-Pacific countries. PLoS ONE 8:e83000. doi:10.1371/journal.pone.0083000
35. Walker A (2009) The social quality approach: bridging Asia and Europe. Dev Soc 38: 209–235

36. WHO Task Force on Research Priorities for Equity in Health (2005) Priorities for research to take forward the health equity policy agenda. B World Health Org 83:948–953
37. Commission on Social Determinants of Health (2005) Action on the social determinants of health: learning from previous experiences. World Health Organisation, Geneva
38. Commission on Social Determinants of Health (2007) Achieving health equity: from root causes to fair outcomes. World Health Organisation, Geneva
39. Graham H, Kelly M (2004) Health inequalities: concepts, frameworks and policy. Health Development Agency, London
40. Ward P, Coffey C, Javanparst S, Wilson C, Meyer S (2015) Institutional (mis)trust in colorectal cancer screening: a qualitative study with Greek, Iranian, Anglo-Australian and Indigenous groups. Health Expect 18:2915–2927
41. Ward P, Coffey C, Meyer S (2015) Trust, choice and obligation: a qualitative study of enablers to colorectal cancer screening in South Australia. Sociol Health Illn 37:988–1006
42. Ward P, Mamerow L, Meyer S (2014) Interpersonal trust across six Asia-Pacific countries: testing and extending the 'high trust society' and 'low trust society' theory. PLoS ONE 9: e95555
43. Health Development Agency (2004) Social capital for health: issues of definition, measurement and links to health. Health Development Agency, London
44. Kim D, Subramanian SV, Kawachi I (2006) Bonding versus bridging social capital and their associations with self rated health: a multilevel analysis if 40 US communities. J Epidemiol Commun Health 60:116–122
45. Skrabski A, Kopp M, Kawachi I (2003) Social capital in a changing society: cross sectional associations with middle aged female and male mortality rates. J Epidemiol Commun Health 57:114–119
46. Subramanian SV, Lochner KA, Kawachi I (2003) Neighbourhood differences in social capital: a compositional artifact or a contextual construct? Health & Place 9:33–44
47. Yip W, Subramanian SV, Mitchell AD, Lee DT, Wang J, Kawachi I (2007) Does social capital enhance health and well-being? Evidence from rural China. Soc Sci Med 64:35–49
48. Durkheim E (1951) Suicide: a study in sociology. Free Press, Glencoe
49. Bourdieu P (1984) Distinction: a social critique of the judgement of taste. Routledge, London
50. Poortinga W (2006) Social relations or social capital? Individual and community health effects if bonding social capital. Soc Sci Med 63:255–270
51. Poortinga W (2006) Social capital: an individual or collective resource for health? Soc Sci Med 62:292–302
52. Habermas J (1997) The theory of communicative action: vol 1 reason and rationalization of society. Polity Press, Cambridge
53. Habermas J (2001) On the pragmatics of social interaction: preliminary studies in the theory of communicative action. Polity Press, Cambridge
54. Scrambler G (2001) Habermas, critical theory and health. Routledge, London
55. Scrambler G, Britten N (2001) System, lifeworld and doctor-patient interaction: issues of trust in a changing world. In: Scrambler G (ed) Habermas, critical theory and health. Routledge, London, pp 45–67
56. Beck U (2005) World risk society. Polity Press, Cambridge
57. Beck U, Giddens A, Lash S (1994) Reflexive modernization: politics, tradition and aesthetics in the modern social order. Polity Press, Cambridge
58. Giddens A (1990) The consequences of modernity. Polity Press, Cambridge
59. Giddens A (1991) Modernity and self identity. Polity Press, Cambridge
60. Luhmann N (1995) Social systems. Stanford University Press, Stanford
61. Parsons T (1951) The social system. Free Press, Glencoe
62. Parsons T, Norfolk C (1971) The system of modern societies. Prentice-Hall, Englewood Cliffs, NJ
63. Shilling C (2002) Culture, the "sick role" and the consumption of health. Brit J Sociol 53:621–638
64. Sen A (1999) Development as freedom. Oxford University Press, Oxford

65. Nussabaum M (2000) Women and human development: the capabilities approach. Cambridge University Press, Cambridge
66. Doyal L (1993) Thinking about human need. New Left Rev 201:113–128
67. Doyal L, Gough I (1991) A theory of social need. Macmillan, London
68. Sen A (2006) Why health equity? In: Anand S, Fabienne P, Sen A (eds) Public health, ethics, and equity. Oxford University Press, Oxford
69. Whitehead M, Dahlgren G (1991) What can be done about inequalities in health? Lancet 338:1059–1063
70. Whitehead M (1992) The concepts and principles of equity and health. Int J Health Services 22:429–445
71. Department of Health (2000) The NHS cancer plan. Department of Health, London
72. Kozak LJ, Hall MJ, Owings MF (2001) Trends in avoidable hospitalizations, 1980–1998. Health Aff 20:225–232
73. Starfield B, Shi L, Macinko JA (2005) Contribution of primary care to health systems and health. Milbank Q 83:457–502
74. Parchman ML, Culler SD (1999) Preventable hospitalizations in primary care shortage areas. Arch Fam Med 8:487–491
75. Macinko JA, Starfield B (2002) Annotated bibliography on equity in health, 1980–2001. Int J Equity Health 1:1
76. Starfield B (2006) State of the art in research on equity in health. J Health Polit Polic Law 31:11–32
77. McDonald J, Hare L (2004) The contribution of primary and community health services. The Centre for Health Equity, Training, Research and Evaluation, University of New South Wales, Sydney
78. Braveman P (2006) Health disparities and health equity: concepts and measurement. Ann Rev Public Health 27:167–194
79. Goddard M, Smith P (2001) Equity of access to health care services: theory and evidence from the UK. Soc Sci Med 53:1149–1162
80. Oliver A, Mossialos E (2004) Equity of access to health care: outlining the foundations for action. J Epidemiol Commun Health 58:655–658
81. Aday LA, Andersen RM (1981) Equity of access to medical care: a conceptual and empirical overview. Med Care 19:4–27
82. Sen A (2003) Inequity reexamined. Oxford University Press, Oxford
83. Stevens A, Rafferty J, Mant J, Simpson S (2004) Health care needs assessment: the epidemiologically based needs assessment reviews. Radcliffe Publishers, Oxford
84. Bradshaw J (1972) A taxonomy of social need. In: McLachlan G (ed) Problems and progress in medical care. Nuffield Provincial Hospital Trust, Oxford
85. Bradshaw J (1994) The conceptualisation and measurement of need. In: Popay J, Williams G (eds) Researching the people's health. Routledge, London, pp 45–57
86. Fuller S (2000) The governance of science. Open University Press, Buckingham
87. United Nations and OECD (2013) World migration in figures 2013. http://www.oecd.org/els/mig/World-Migration-in-Figures.pdf. Accessed 14 Jan 2016
88. Ashkanasy NM, Trevor-Roberts E, Earnshaw L (2003) The Anglo cluster: legacy of the British Empire. J World Bus 37:28–39
89. Office of National Statistics (2012) Ethnicity and national identity in England and Wales 2011. http://www.ons.gov.uk/ons/dcp171776_290558.pdf. Accessed 14 Jan 2016
90. United States Census Bureau (2015) Quick facts 2015. http://www.census.gov/quickfacts/table/PST045215/00. Accessed 14 Jan 2016
91. Statistics Canada (2011) Immigration and ethnocultural diversity in Canada http://www.12.statcan.gc.ca/nhs-enm/2011/as-sa/99-010-x/99-010-x2011001-eng.pdf. Accessed 14 Jan 2016
92. Australian Bureau of Statistics (2015) 3412.0 Migration, Australia, 2013–2014 http://www.abs.gov.au/ausstats/abs@.nsf/Latestproducts/3412.0Main%20Features32013-14?opendocument&tabname=Summary&prodno=3412.0&issue=2013-14&num=&view=. Accessed 14 Jan 2016

93. Human Rights Law Centre (2015) Australia's 2015 UPR: culturally and linguistically diverse people and communities. http://hrlc.org.au/wp-content/uploads/2015/07/13+Final+CALD+Fact+Sheet.pdf. Accessed 14 Jan 2016
94. Department of the Attorney General (2009) Equality before the law bench book. www.supremecourt.wa.gov.au/_files/equity_before_the_law_benchbook.pdf. Accessed 14 Jan 2016
95. Canadian Department of Immigration (2010) The current state of multiculturalism in Canada and research themes on Canadian multiculturalism 2008–2010. http://www.cic.gc.ca/english/pdf/pub/multi-state.pdf. Accessed 14 Jan 2016
96. Bureau of Labor Statistics (2015) Foreign-born workers: Labor force characteristics http://www.bls.gov/news.release/pdf/forbrn.pdf. Accessed 14 Jan 2016
97. Bureau of Labor Statistics (2014) Labor force characteristics by race and ethnicity, 2013. http://www.bls.gov/cps/cpsrace2013.pdf. Accessed 14 Jan 2016
98. Dustmann C, Frattini T (2011) The socio-economic integration of migrants. http://www.ucl.au.uk/~uctpb21/reports/Final_report_CLG_06_2011.pdf. Accessed 14 Jan 2016
99. Hergenrather KC, Zeglin RJ, McGuire-Kuletz M, Rhodes SD (2015) Employment as a social determinant of health: a systematic review of longitudinal studies exploring the relationship between employment status and physical health. Rehab Res Polic Educ 29:2–26
100. Jin RL, Shah CP, Svoboda TJ (1995) The impact of unemployment on health: a review of the evidence. Can Med Assoc J 153:529–540
101. Mathers CD, Schofield DJ (1998) The health consequences of unemployment: the evidence. Med J Aust 168:178–182
102. Clougherty JE, Souza K, Cullen MR (2010) Work and its role in shaping the social gradient in health. Ann NY Acad Sci 1186:102–124
103. Halpern MT (2014) Cancer disparities research: it is time to come of age. Cancer 121: 1158–1159
104. Bansal N, Bhopal RS, Brewster DH (2012) Major ethnic group difference in breast cancer screening uptake in Scotland are not extinguished by adjustment for indicies of geographical residence, area deprivation, long-term illness and education. Brit J Cancer 106:1361–1366
105. Wain G, Morrell ST, Taylor RS, Momoon H, Bodkin N (2001) Variation in cervical cancer screening by region, socio-economic, migrant and Indigenous status in women in New South Wales. Gynaecol Oncol 41:320–325
106. Robb K, Wardle J, Stubbings S, Ramirez A, Austoker J, Macleod U et al (2010) Ethnic disparities in knowledge of cancer screening programmes in the UK. J Med Screen 17:125–131
107. Renshaw C, KJack RH, Dixon S, Moller H, Davies EA (2010) Estimating attendance for breast cancer screening in ethnic groups in London. BMC Public Health 10:157
108. Robb KA, Solarin I, Power E, Atkin W, Wardle J (2008) Attitudes to colorectal cancer screening among ethnic minority groups in the UK. BMC Public Health 8:34
109. Quan H, Fong A, De Coster C, Wang J, Musto R, Noseworthy TW et al (2006) Variation in health services utilization among ethnic populations. Can Med Assoc J 174:787–791
110. McDonald JT, Kennedy S (2007) Cervical cancer screening by immigrant and minority women in Canada. J Immigr Minor Health 9:323–334
111. Amankwah E, Ngwakongnwi E, Quan H (2009) Why many visible minority women in Canada do not participate in cervical cancer screening. Ethn Health 14:337–349
112. Friedemann-Sanchez G, Griffin J, Partin M (2007) Gender differences in colorectal cancer screening barriers and information needs. Health Expect 10:148–160
113. Beeker C, Kraft JM, Southwell BG, Jorgensen CM (2000) Colorectal cancer screening in older men and women: qualitative research findings and implications for intervention. J Epidemiol Commun Health 25:263–278
114. Chornokur G, Dalton K, Borysova M, Kumar N (2011) Disparities at presentation, diagnosis, treatment and survival in African American men affected by prostate cancer. Prostate 71:985–997
115. Yang R, Cheung MC, Byrne MM, Huang Y, Nguyen D, Koniaris G (2010) Do racial or socioeconomic disparities exist in lung cancer treatment? Cancer 116:2437–2447

116. Braithwaite D, Tammemagi CM, Moore DH, Ozanne EM, Hiatt RA, Esserman L (2009) Hypertension is an independent predictor of survival disparity between African American and white breast cancer patients. Int J Cancer 124:1213–1219
117. Cook LS, Nelson HE, Cockburn M, Olson SH, Muller CY, Wiggins CL (2013) Comorbidities and endometrial cancer survival in Hispanics and non-Hispanic whites. Cancer Cause Control 24:61–69
118. Sarfati D, Gurney J, Stanley J, Koea J (2014) A retrospective cohort study of patients with stomach and liver cancers: the impact of comorbidity and ethnicity on cancer care and outcomes. BMC Cancer 14:821
119. Tammemagi CM, Nerenz D, Neslund-Dudas C, Feldkamp C, Nathanson D (2005) Comorbidity and survival disparities among black and white patients with breast cancer. JAMA 294:1765–1772
120. Holmes L Jr, Chan W, Jiang Z, Ward D, Essien EJ, Du XL (2009) Impact of andogren deprivation therapy on racial/ethnic disparities in survival of older men treated for locoregional prostate cancer. Cancer Control 16:176–185
121. Hamilton AS, Fleming ST, Wang D, Goodman M, Wu X-C, Owen JB et al (2016) Clinical and demographic factors associated with receipt of non guideline-concordant initial therapy for nonmetastatic prostate cancer. Am J Clin Oncol 39:55–63
122. Siminoff LA, Graham GC, Gordon NH (2006) Cancer communication patterns and the influence of patient characteristics: disparities in information-giving and affective behaviors. Pat Educ Couns 62:355–360
123. Redman J, Higginbottom GMA, Massey MT (2008) Critical review of literature on ethnicity and health in relation to cancer and palliative care in the United Kingdom. Divers Health Social Care 5:137–150
124. Elkan R, Avis M, Cox K, Wilson E, Patel S, Miller S et al (2007) The reported views and experiences of cancer service users from minority ethnic groups: a critical review of the literature. Eur J Cancer Care 16:109–121
125. Fazil Q, Aujla N, Hale C, Kai J (2015) Unequal treatment: health care experiences and needs of patients with cancer from minority ethnic communities. Divers Equal Health Care 12:95–103
126. Magai C, Consedine NS, Adjei BA, Hershman D, Neugut A (2008) Psychosocial influences on suboptimal adjuvant breast cancer treatment adherence among African American women: implications for education and intervention. Health Educ Behav 35:835–854
127. Purificacion SJ, French JG, d'Agincourt-Canning L (2015) Inequities in access to cancer care in Canada: an ethical perspective. Healthc Manage Forum 28:265–269
128. Butow PN, Aldridge L, Bell ML, Sze M, Eisenbruch M, Jefford M et al (2013) Inferior health-related quality of life and psychological well-being in immigrant cancer survivors: a population-based study. Eur J Cancer 49:1948–1956
129. Hislop TG, Bajdik CD, Regier MD, Barroetavena MC (2007) Ethnic differences in survival for female cancers of the breast, cervix and colorectum in British Columbia, Canada. Asian Pac J Cancer Preven 8:209–214
130. Macmillan (2013) The rich picture: people with cancer from BME groups. http://www.macmillan.org.uk/Documents/AboutUs/Research/Richpictures/2013updates/BMERichPicture2013-FINAL.pdf. Accessed 14 Jan 2016
131. Holroyd E, Twinn S, Adab P (2004) Socio-cultural influences on Chinese women's attendance for cervical screening. J Adv Nurs 46:42–52
132. Rajaram S, Rashidi A (1999) Asian-Islamic women and breast cancer screening: a socio-cultural analysis. Women Health 28:45–58
133. Rajaram S, Rashidi A (1998) Minority women and breast cancer screening: the role of cultural explanatory models. Prevent Med 27:757–764
134. Christie J, Jandorf L, Itzkowitz S (2003) Attitudes and practices of colon cancer screening compared to breast cancer screening in women in East Harlem, NY. Am J Gastroent 98:S125

135. Jenkins C, Le T, McPhee S, Stewart S, Ha N (1996) Health care access and preventative care among Vietnamese immigrants: do traditional beliefs and practices pose barriers? Soc Sci Med 43:1049–1056
136. Jenkins C, McPhee S, Bird J, Bonilla N (1990) Cancer risks and prevention practices among Vietnamese refugees. West J Med 153:34–39
137. Gannotti M, Kaplan L, Handwerker W, Groce N (2004) Cultural influences on health care use: differences in perceived unmet needs and expectations of providers by Latino and Euro-American parents of children with special health care needs. J Dev Behav Paed 25:156–165
138. Chattoo S, Ahmad W (2004) The meaning of cancer: illness, biography and social identity. In: Kelleher D, Leavey G (eds) Identity and health. Routledge, London, pp 19–36
139. Gordon D, Eugenio P (1997) Disclosure practices and cultural narratives: understanding concealment and silence around cancer in Tuscany, Italy. Socl Sci Med 44:1433–1452
140. Nazroo JY, Karlsen S (2001) Ethnic inequalities in health: social class, racism and identity. Available from: http://www.lancaster.ac.uk/fass/projects/hvp/pdf/fd10.pdf. Accessed 14 Jan 2016
141. Robert Wood Johnson Foundation (2009) Issue brief 5: race and socioeconomic factors 2009 Available from: https://www.comissiononhealth.org. Accessed 14 Jan 2016
142. Schofield PE, Butow PN, Thompson JF, Tattersall MHN, Beeney LJ, Dunn SM (2003) Psychological responses of patients receiving a diagnosis of cancer. Ann Oncol 14:48–56
143. Fallowfield L, Jenkins V, Farewell V, Saul J, Duffy A, Eves R (2002) Efficacy of a cancer research UK communication skills training model for oncologists: a randomised controlled trial. Lancet 359:650–655
144. Fallowfield L, Lipkin M, Hall A (1998) Teaching senior oncologists communication skills: results from Phase I of a comprehensive longitudinal program in the United Kingdom. J Clin Oncol 16:1961–1968
145. Richardson A, Thomas VN, Richardson A (2006) "Reduced to nods and smiles": experiences of professionals caring for people with cancer from black and ethnic minority groups. Eur J Oncol Nurs 10:93–101
146. Gudykunst WB (1997) Cultural variability in communication. Commun Res 24:327–348
147. Schouten BC, Meeuwesen L (2006) Cultural differences in medical communication: a review of the literature. Patient Educ Couns 64:21–34
148. Gordon HS, Street RL Jr, Sharf BF, Souchek J (2006) Racial differences in doctors' information giving and patients participation. Cancer 107:1313–1320
149. Harmsen H, Meeuwesen L, van Wieringen J, Bersen R, Bruijnzeels M (2003) When cultures meet in general practice: intercultural differences between GPs and parents of child patients. Patient Educ Couns 51:99–106
150. Ramirez AG (2003) Consumer-provider communication research with special populations. Patient Educ Couns 50:51–54
151. Suurmond J, Seeleman C (2006) Shared decision-making in an intercultural context: barriers in the interaction between physicians and immigrant patients. Patient Educ Couns 60: 253–259
152. Butow PN, Sze M, Eisenbruch M, Bell ML, Aldridge LJ, Abdo S et al (2013) Should culture affect practice? A comparison of prognostic discussions in consultations with immigrant versus native-born cancer patients. Patient Educ Couns 92:246–252
153. Butow PN, Goldstein D, Bell ML, Sze M, Aldridge LJ, Abdo S et al (2011) Interpretation in consultations with immigrant patients with cancer: How accurate is it? J Clin Oncol 29: 2801–2807
154. Butow P, Bell M, Goldstein D, Sze M et al (2011) Grappling with cultural differences: communication between oncologists and immigrant cancer patients with and without interpreters. Patient Educ Couns 84:398–405
155. Gargan N, Chianese J (2007) A review of the literature surrounding the provision of interpreters in health care, focusing on their role in translating information for

non-English-speaking cancer patients and issues relating to informed consent. J Radiother Pract 6:201–209
156. Flores G (2005) The impact of medical interpreter services on the quality of health care: a systematic review. Med Care Res Rev 62:255–299
157. Simon CM, Zyzanski SJ, Durand E, Jimenez X, Kodish ED (2006) Interpreter accuracy and informed consent among Spanish-speaking families with cancer. J Health Commun 11: 509–522
158. Flores G, Abreu M, Barone CP, Bachur R, Lin H (2012) Errors of medical interpretation and their potential clinical consequences: a comparison of professional versus ad hoc versus no interpreters. Ann Emerg Med 60:545–553
159. Renzaho AMN, Romios P, Crock C, Sonderlund AL (2013) The effectiveness of cultural competence programs in ethnic minority patients-centred health care—A systematic review of the literature. Int J Qual Health Care 25:261–269
160. Surbone A (2008) Cultural aspects of communication in cancer care. Support Care Cancer 16:235–240
161. Betancourt JR, Green AR, Carrillo JE, Ananeh-Firempong O (2003) Defining cultural competence: a practical framework for addressing racial/ethnic disparities in health and health care. Public Health Rep 118:293–302
162. Beach MC, Price EG, Gary TL, Robinson KA, Gozu A, Palacio A et al (2005) Cultural competency: a systematic review of health care provider educational interventions. Med Care 43:356–373
163. Betancourt JR, Green AR, Carrillo JE (2002) Cultural competence in health care: emerging frameworks and practical approaches. http://www.commonwealthfund.org/usr_doc/betancourt_culturalcompetence_576.pdf. Accessed 14 Jan 2016
164. Campinha-Bacote J (2002) The process of cultural competence in the delivery of healthcare services: a model of care. J Transcult Nurs 13:181–184
165. Kagawa-Singer M, Kassim-Lakha S (2003) A strategy to reduce cross-cultural miscommunication and increase the likelihood of improving health outcomes. Acad Med 78:577–587
166. Eakin EG, Bull SS, Riley KM, Reeves MM, McLaughlin P, Gutierrez S (2007) Resources for health: a primary-care based diet and physical activity intervention targeting urban latinos with multiple chronic conditions. Health Psychol 26:392–400
167. Harun A, Harrison JD, Young JM (2013) Interventions to improve patient participation in the treatment process for culturally and linguistically diverse people with cancer: a systematic review. Asia-Pac J Clin Oncol 9:99–109
168. Pendo FJ, Traeger L, Dahn J, Molton I, Gonzalez JS, Schneiderman N et al (2007) Cognitive behavioral stress management intervention improves quality of life in Spanish monolingual Hispanic men treated for localized prostate cancer: results of a randomised controlled trial. Int J Behav Med 14:164–172
169. Tsoh JY, Burke NJ, Gildengorin G, Wong C, Le K, Nguyen A et al (2015) A social network family-focused intervention to promote smoking cessation in Chinese and Vietnamese American male smokers: a feasibility study. Nicotine Tob Res 17:1029–1038
170. Ward EC, Brown RL (2015) A culturally adapted depression intervention for African American adults experiencing depression: Oh happy day. Am J Orthopsychiatry 85:11–22
171. Freund KM, Battaglia TA, Calhoun E, Dudley DJ, Fiscella K, Paskett E et al (2008) National Cancer Institute patient navigation research program: methods, protocol, and measures. Cancer 113:3391–3399
172. Maxwell AE, Jo AM, Crespi CM, Sudan M, Bastani R (2010) Peer navigation improves diagnostic follow-up after breast cancer screening among Korean American women: results of a randomised trial. Cancer Cause Control 21:1931–1940
173. Ferrante JM, Chen P-H, Kim S (2007) The effect of patient navigation on time to diagnosis, anxiety, and satisfaction in urban minority women with abnormal mammograms: a randomised controlled trial. J Urban Health 85:114–124

174. Ell K, Vourlekis B, Lee P-J, Xie B (2007) Patient navigation and case management following an abnormal mammogram: a randomised clinical trial. Prevent Med 44:26–33
175. Christie J, Itzkowitz S, Lihau-Nkanza I, Castillo A, Redd W, Jandorf L (2008) A randomised controlled trial using patient navigation to increase colonoscopy screening among low-income minorities. J Natl Med Assoc 100:278–284
176. Paskett ED, Harrop JP, Wells KJ (2011) Patient navigation: an update on the state of the science. CA-Cancer J Clin 61:237–249
177. Bonevski B, Randell M, Paul C, Chapman K, Twyman L, Bryant J et al (2014) Reaching the hard-to-reach: a systematic review of strategies for improving health and medical research with socially disadvantaged groups. BMC Med Res Methodol 14:42
178. Robinson-White S, Conroy B, Slavish KH, Rosenzweig M (2010) Patient navigation in breast cancer: a systematic review. Cancer Nurs 33:127–140
179. Taylor VM, Jackson JC, Yasul Y, Nguyen TT, Woodall E, Acorda E et al (2010) Evaluation of a cervical cancer control intervention using lay health workers for Vietnamese American Women. Am J Public Health 100:1924–1929
180. Tanjasiri SP, Kagawa-Singer M, Foo MA, Chao M, Linayao-Putman I, Nguyen J et al (2007) Designing culturally and linguistically appropriate health interventions: the "life is precious" Hmong breast cancer study. Health Educ Behav 34:140–153
181. Han-H-R, Lee H, LKim MT, Kim KB (2009) Tailored lay health worker intervention improves breast cancer screening outcomes in non-adherent Korean-American women. Health Educ Res 24:318–329
182. Walsh JME, Salazar R, Nguyen TT, Kaplan C, Nguyen L, Hwang J et al (2010) Healthy colon, healthy life: a novel colorectal cancer screening intervention. Am J Prev Med 39:1–14
183. Griner D, Smith TB (2006) Culturally adapted mental health interventions: a meta-analytic review. Psychother Theor Res 43:531–548
184. Huey SJ, Polo AJ (2008) Evidence-based psychosocial treatments for ethnic minority youth: a review and meta-analysis. J Clin Child Adolesc 37:262–301
185. Miranda J, Bernal G, Lau A, Kohn L, Hwang W-C, LaFromboise T (2005) State of the science on psychosocial interventions for ethnic minorities. Ann Rev Clin Psychol 1: 113–142
186. Bartholomew LK, Parcel GS, Kok G, Gottlieb NH (2006) Planning health promotion programs: an intervention mapping approach. Jossey-Bass, San Francisco
187. Bernal G, Bonilla J, Bellido C (1995) Ecological validity and cultural sensitivity for outcome research: issues for the cultural adaptation and development of psychosocial treatments with Hispanics. J Abnorm Child Psychol 23:67–82
188. Bernal G, Jimenez-Chafey MI, Rodriguez MMD (2009) Cultural adaptation of treatments: a resource for considering culture in evidence-based practice. Prof Psychol-Res Pract 40: 361–368
189. Bernal G, Saez-Santiago E (2006) Culturally centered psychosocial interventions. J Commun Psychol 34:121–132
190. Bender MS, Clark MJ, Gahagan S (2014) Community engagement approach: developing a culturally appropriate intervention for Hispanic mother-child dyads. J Transcult Nurs 25:373–382
191. Kreuter MW, Lukwago SN, Bucholtz DC, Clark EM, Sanders-Thompson V (2002) Achieving cultural appropriateness in health promotion programs: targeted and tailored approaches. Health Educ Behav 30:133–146
192. Rodriguez MMD, Baumann AA, Schwartz AL (2011) Cultural adaptation of an evidence based intervention: from theory to practice in a Latino/a community context. Am J Commun Psychol 14:170–186
193. Sheikh A (2005) Why are ethnic minorities under-represented in US research studies? PLoS Med 3:e49
194. Wallengren S, Mellgren C (2015) The other way around: the Roma minority's view on doing research on sensitive topics. Int J Soc Sci Stud 3:14

195. Ford JG, Howerton MW, Lai GY, Gary TL, Bolen S, Gibbons MC et al (2008) Barriers to recruiting underrepresented populations to cancer clinical trials: a systematic review. Cancer 112:228–242
196. Roberson NL (1994) Clinical trial participation: Viewpoints from racial/ethnic groups. Cancer 74:2687–2691
197. Shavers VL, Lynch CF, Burmeister LF (2002) Racial differences in factors that influence the willingness to participate in medical research studies. Ann Epidemiol 12:248–256
198. Yancey AK, Ortega AN, Kumanyika SK (2006) Effective recruitment and retention of minority research participants. Ann Rev Public Health 27:1–28
199. Wendler D, Kington R, Madans J, Van Wye G, Christ-Schmidt H, Pratt LA et al (2006) Are racial and ethnic minorities less willing to participate in health research? PLoS Med 3:e19
200. Hussain-Gambles M, Atkin K, Leese B (2004) Why ethnic minority groups are under-represented in clinical trials: a review of the literature. Health Soc Care Commun 12:382–388
201. Knobf MT, Juarez G, Lee S-YK, Sun V, Sun Y, Haozous E (2007) Challenges and strategies in recruitment of ethnically diverse populations for cancer nursing research. Oncol Nurs Forum 34:1187–1194
202. Symonds RP, Lord K, Mitchell AJ, Raghavan D (2012) Recruitment of ethnic minorities into cancer clinical trials: experience from the front line. Brit J Cancer 107:1017–1021
203. Fudge N, Wolfe CDA, McKevitt C (2007) Involving older people in health research. Age Ageing 36:492–500
204. Glover M, Kira A, Johnston V, Walker N, Thomas D, Chang AB et al (2014) A systematic review of barriers and facilitators to participation in randomized controlled trials by Indigenous people from New Zealand, Australia, Canada and the United States. Glob Health Promot 22:21–31
205. Ellard-Gray A, Jeffrey NK, Choubak M, Crann SE (2015) Finding the hidden participant: solutions for recruiting hidden, hard-to-reach and vulnerable populations. Int J Qual Res 5:1–10
206. Fox S, Arnold A-L, Dunn R, Keeffe J, Taylor H (2010) Sampling and recruitment methodology for a national eye health survey of Indigenous Australians. Aust NZ J Public Health 34:554–562
207. Lennox N, Taylor M, Rey-Conde T, Bain C, Purdie DM, Boyle F (2005) Beating the barriers: recruitment of people with intellectual disability to participate in research. J Intellect Disabil Res 49:296–305
208. McMurdo ME, Roberts H, Parker S, Wyatt N, May H, Goodman C et al (2011) Improving recruitment of older people to research through good practice. Age Ageing 40:659–665
209. Clarke AR, Goddu AP, Nocon RS, Stock NW, Chyr LC, Akuoko JAS et al (2013) Thirty years of disparities intervention research: what are we doing to close racial and ethnic gaps in health care? Med Care 51:1020–1026
210. Beach MC, Gary TL, Price EG, Robinson K, Gozu A, Palacio A et al (2006) Improving health care quality for racial/ethnic minorities: a systematic review of the best evidence regarding provider and organizational interventions. BMC Public Health 6(104)
211. Griffin SJ, Kinmonth A-L, Veltman MWM, Gillard S, Grant J, Stewart M (2004) Effect on health-related outcomes of interventions to alter the interaction between patients and practitioners: a systematic review of trials. Ann Fam Med 2:595–608
212. Schouten BC, Meeuwesen L, Harmsen HAM (2005) The impact of an intervention in intercultural communication on doctor-patient interaction in The Netherlands. Patient Educ Couns 58:288–295
213. Lie DA, Lee-Ray E, Gomez A, Bereknyel S, Braddock CH (2010) Does cultural competency training of health professionals improve patient outcomes? A systematic review and proposed algorithm for future research. J Gen Int Med 26:317–325
214. Vega WA (2005) Higher stakes ahead for cultural competence. Gen Hosp Psychiatry 27:446–450

215. Chenowethm L, Jeon Y-H, Goff M, Burke C (2006) Cultural competency and nursing care: an Australian perspective. Int Nurs Rev 53:34–40

Further Reading

216. Wilkinson R, Pickett K (2009) The spirit level: what greater equality makes stronger societies. Bloomsbury Press, New York
217. Marmot M, Wilkinson R (2006) Social determinants of health. Oxford University Press, Oxford
218. Anand S, Peter F, Sen A (2006) Public health, ethics, and equity. Oxford University Press, Oxford
219. Campinha-Bacote J (2002) The process of cultural competence in the delivery of healthcare services: a model of care. J Transcult Nurs 13:181–184
220. Elkan R, Avis M, Cox K, Wilson E, Patel S, Miller S et al (2007) The reported views and experiences of cancer service users from minority ethnic groups: a critical review of the literature. Eur J Cancer Care 16:109–121
221. Flores G (2005) The impact of medical interpreter services on the quality of health care: a systematic review. Med Care Res Rev 62:255–299
222. Betancourt JR, Green AR, Carrillo JE, Ananeh-Firempong O (2003) Defining cultural competence: a practical framework for addressing racial/ethnic disparities in health and health care. Public Health Rep 118:293–302

Chapter 4
Impact of Comorbidity on Cancer Screening and Diagnosis

Steven T. Fleming, Diana Sarfati, Gretchen Kimmick, Nancy Schoenberg and Ruth Cunningham

Abstract The presence of coexistent chronic disease or comorbid illness has been shown to have an impact on the pathogenesis of cancer and on the frequency of screening, the stage at diagnosis, the intensity of treatment, and, therefore, on cancer outcomes. This chapter will focus on how comorbid illness affects cancer screening and diagnosis. There is some disagreement in the literature regarding how the comorbidity burden affects the screening and stage of cancer, particularly when specific comorbidities and the overall burden of comorbidity, measured by some aggregate index, are examined. Moreover, the extent of the relationship between comorbidity and cancer may be affected by the method by which the comorbidity burden is measured, with regard to breadth (number of comorbidities) and depth (severity of comorbidities). We consider some of these factors in this chapter as we examine the literature in view of four hypotheses: (1) The surveillance hypothesis, which suggests that patients with comorbid illnesses are screened more regularly or are more likely to be diagnosed earlier because they have more frequent contact with the medical care system. (2) The competing demand hypothesis, which posits that patients with comorbidities are screened less or diagnosed later because other chronic conditions represent a competing demand upon physician time and focus. (3) The physiological hypothesis, which argues that comorbid illness actually affects the pathogenesis, progression, and/or severity of cancer. (4) The death from other causes hypothesis, which suggests that patients or their physicians choose not to screen, because of the risk of death from a cause of other than cancer.

Keywords Comorbidity · Comorbid illness · Chronic disease · Multimorbidity

S.T. Fleming (✉) · N. Schoenberg
University of Kentucky, Lexington, USA
e-mail: steven.fleming@uky.edu

D. Sarfati · R. Cunningham
University of Otago Wellington, Wellington, New Zealand
e-mail: diana.sarfati@otago.ac.nz

G. Kimmick
Duke University School of Medicine, Durham, USA

B. Koczwara (ed.), *Cancer and Chronic Conditions*,
DOI 10.1007/978-981-10-1844-2_4

Key Points

1. Patients with comorbidities have more contact with their clinicians providing an opportunity for cancer screening recommendations to be provided
2. Comorbid illness may distract physicians from or complicate the important task of recommending regular cancer screening
3. For some patients with comorbid illness that results in a limited life expectancy, screening may not be appropriate
4. Some comorbidities such as diabetes, may influence the biology of cancer, such that there is increased risk for the disease, greater risk of cancer progression, and higher stage and tumor aggressiveness
5. Physicians and patients may avoid cancer screening because the prognosis or estimated risk of death from other causes is deemed to outweigh the benefits of screening. Such patients may still be good candidates for both screening and cancer treatment to improve quality of life and to prevent morbidity
6. The impact of comorbidity burden on cancer depends upon the number and severity of comorbidities
7. The link between cancer screening and stage of illness is presumed, but only well established for some screening modalities and cancers.

4.1 Introduction

The aging of the population is a global phenomenon that will affect economies across the world. For example, the PEW Research Center [1] estimates that 16.5 % of the population in the United States or 56 million people will be 65 years or older by 2020. This percentage is expected to rise to 20 % or 73 million people by 2030 [1]. In Europe, by 2030, about 25 % of the population will be 65 and older [2]. This unprecedented growth of the older population portends huge increases in patients with multiple chronic conditions or comorbidities (multiple morbidity), forcing providers and patients to face increasingly complex clinical and lifestyle decisions. We currently lack sufficient evidence-based guidelines on the management of cancer patients with multiple chronic conditions. Even less is known about the relationship between multiple morbidity and its impact on diagnosis and screening [3, 4]. It is unclear whether multiple morbidity, or even one comorbidity, for that matter, increases the odds that a patient will be diagnosed with late rather than early stage cancer. This chapter will focus on the impact of one or more chronic conditions, hereinafter referred to as "comorbidity burden," on the screening and diagnosis of cancer. We will develop a conceptual model of the relationship between comorbidity burden and cancer screening, diagnosis, treatment, and outcome. We will also describe several hypotheses that seek to explain the variability in the effects of comorbidities on screening and diagnosis. We will focus on diabetes and obesity as examples of comorbid conditions that have an impact on cancer screening and diagnosis.

4.2 Conceptual Model of Cancer and Comorbid Illness

A conceptual model of the relationship between cancer and comorbid illness is illustrated in Fig. 4.1. Cancer progresses through a preclinical or asymptomatic stage, to a clinical or symptomatic stage. Valanis has defined the "clinical horizon" as the point when the disease has detectable signs and symptoms [5]. We posit another point in the natural history of disease, let's call it the "sub-clinical horizon," when the disease is detectable only though imaging, laboratory or other technologies, and not by clinical symptoms. Further, Valanis defines the "critical point" as the point in the natural history of disease beyond which serious consequences, such as the metastasis of cancer, occur. Cancer screening is useful at either the clinical (e.g., clinical breast exam for breast cancer) or sub-clinical (e.g., fecal occult blood test for colorectal cancer) horizons, if they occur before the critical point of disease. In such cases, cancer screening can increase the likelihood of an early-stage diagnosis, when the disease is curable. If the critical point occurs before the clinical horizon(s), then metastases are subclinical and will eventually become apparent later. Certainly, as illustrated in Fig. 4.1, additional key factors, such as age or ethnicity/race, may affect the likelihood of cancer (i.e., cancer risk increases with age), the likelihood of being screened, and even the kinds of treatment that are received for cancer. Comorbid illness also can directly affect the incidence of cancer (e.g., colorectal cancer is more common among those with diabetes), the likelihood of being screened, and the kinds of treatment received. Treatment for cancer may

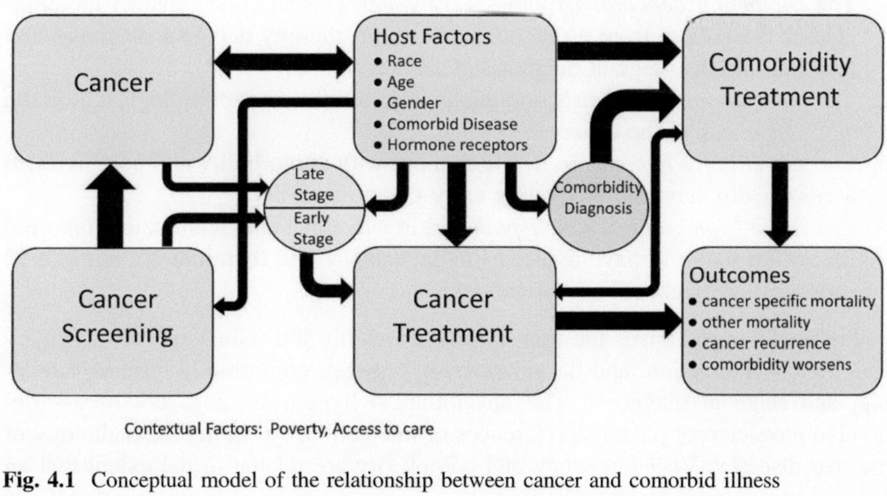

Fig. 4.1 Conceptual model of the relationship between cancer and comorbid illness

also impact the management of another comorbid illness. For example, hormone therapies for breast and prostate cancer can destabilize and exacerbate diabetes, and the cancer treatment may become a competing demand for the ongoing management of coexisting chronic diseases. Of course, the converse is also true, when the treatment for comorbidity may impact on the cancer treatment. For example, chemotherapy toxicity is more likely among patients on multiple medications because of drug to drug interactions. Treatment for both cancer and the coexisting disease affects the outcomes of care for both.

4.3 Impact of Comorbidity on Screening for Cancer

There are contrasting and not necessarily mutually exclusive possibilities regarding the impact of comorbidity on the detection and diagnosis of cancer [6–8]. On one hand, patients with comorbidity may be diagnosed earlier and/or be more likely to be offered screening for cancer, because they tend to be accessing health services more regularly and to be under a higher level of medical scrutiny than people without chronic conditions. Alternatively, the concomitant existence of chronic disease may mask early symptoms of cancer, and may distract either or both the patient and clinician from considering a diagnosis of cancer. It is also reasonable to assume that in some cases, a rational decision is made for patients with severe chronic disease not to undergo screening or investigations for cancer, because of their reduced life expectancy.

A review of the evidence to date, suggests that a lack of screening may be multifactorial, and the balance among the various mechanisms may vary depending on health system and patient factors. Consistent with these ideas, Fleming et al. [7] proposed four separate hypotheses to explain the varying associations among comorbidity and stage of cancer at diagnosis. These are four possible explanations:

1. The *competing demands* hypothesis, in which comorbidities distract the clinician or the patient from a diagnosis of cancer, thereby delaying diagnosis and resulting in later stage at diagnosis
2. The *pathological hypothesis*, in which comorbidities impact biologically on the aggressiveness of the cancer
3. The *surveillance hypothesis*, in which those with comorbidity are more likely to access health services, facilitating early diagnosis
4. The *death from other causes hypothesis*, in which patients with major comorbid illness are likely to have reduced life expectancy and therefore are not offered screening or diagnostic investigations.

Figure 4.2 summarizes the four hypothesis within the framework of the physician patient interaction, and the relationship between comorbidity burden, screening, and stage at diagnosis. The physiological hypothesis does not necessarily involve physician or patients preferences or interaction, but rather the pathology of the two diseases. Visit frequency and complexity are related to the extent that an

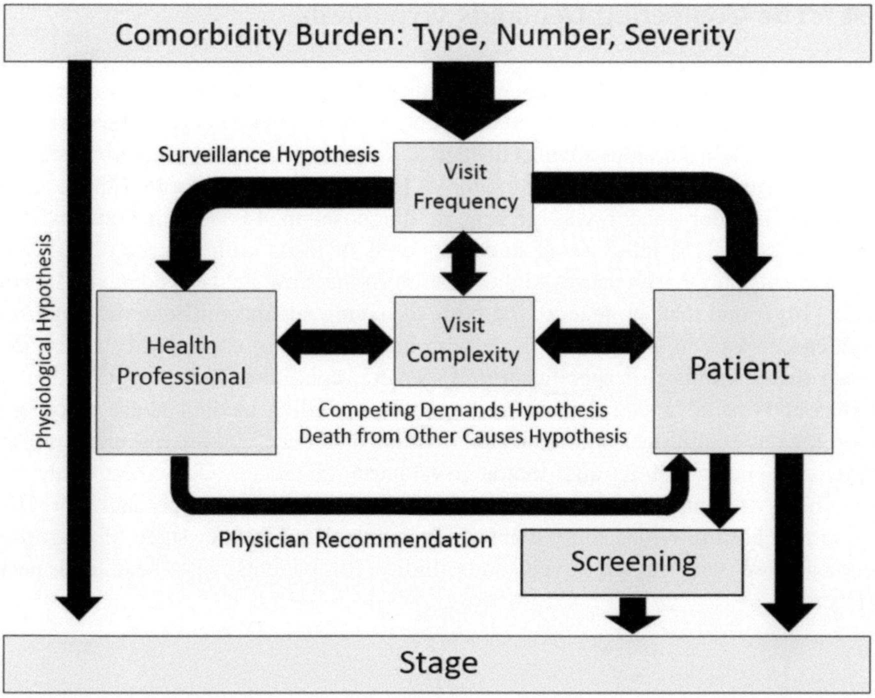

Fig. 4.2 The framework of the physician patient interaction, and the relationship between comorbidity burden, screening, and stage at diagnosis

increase in the former may decrease the complexity of the latter. More contact with the medical care system provides increased opportunity for screening recommendations through the surveillance hypothesis. The competing demands hypothesis could work through either or both the health professional and the patient, to the extent that visit complexity distracts from a focus on health screening. The death from other causes hypothesis would also relate to visit complexity, the focus on one or more comorbid conditions, and the presumption that cancer screening is not an immediate priority as the patient may die from other causes instead. We will discuss each of the four hypotheses, how more than one hypothesis may be needed to explain the evidence, and how the number, type, and severity of comorbidities that constitute the "comorbidity burden" are critical. We will then focus on the importance of physician recommendation, particularly with regards to the surveillance and death from other causes hypothesis, the relationship between comorbidity burden and stage at diagnosis, and the impact of multiple comorbidities, in terms of breadth (number) and depth (severity), and the impact of mental illness. Finally, we will illustrate the application of most of these hypotheses to explain the impact of diabetes mellitus on breast and colorectal cancer.

4.4 The Competing Demands Hypothesis

If health professionals and/or patients are distracted from the possibility of cancer, because of other health-related demands, one would expect a delay in the diagnosis of cancer, and thus a more advanced stage at diagnosis. There are numerous studies reporting this pattern [9–14]. For example, Koppie et al. [10] reported that locally extensive bladder cancer was present at diagnosis in 43 % of patients with a Charlson et al. [15] index score under 3, 49 % of those with a score of 3–5 and 56 % among those with scores higher than 5. In the New Zealand context, Gurney et al. [14] found that, in general, the odds of having advanced disease at diagnosis with cancer were higher among those with higher levels of comorbidity. They also found that a number of specific, usually severe, conditions were associated with higher odds of advanced disease at diagnosis, including alcohol abuse disorders, neurological conditions, pulmonary circulation disorders, cerebrovascular disease, congestive heart failure and major psychiatric disorders. Consistent with the hypothesis of competing demands on clinicians and patients, Teppo and Alho [12] found that both provider and patient delay were related to later stage of diagnosis among those with higher levels comorbidity for patients with head and neck cancers.

4.5 The Physiological Hypothesis

The general findings of later stage at diagnosis for those with chronic disease are also consistent with the theoretical possibility that cancer is somehow more aggressive among those with comorbidity [7]. Aksoy et al. [16] suggested that some comorbidities may be related to higher levels of proangiogenic growth factors which may encourage cancer growth. Similarly, insulin resistance, as seen in type II diabetes, is associated with high levels of blood insulin, growth factors and the activation of pathways that may also promote cancer growth [17]. In contrast, it is plausible that some conditions or their treatment are associated with slower cancer growth. For example, non-steroidal anti-inflammatory drugs (NSAIDs) used in arthritis may slow the growth of colorectal and other cancers [17, 18].

4.6 The Surveillance Hypothesis

The surveillance hypothesis suggests that those with comorbidity are more likely to access health services because of their increased healthcare needs, and are therefore more likely to be offered screening and/or have symptoms noticed and investigated, when compared to those who are less exposed to health services. Consistent with this hypothesis, some authors have reported either no difference in stage distribution according to comorbidity, or a pattern of earlier stage at diagnosis with higher comorbidity levels [8, 19, 20, 21, 22, 23]. Walter et al. [24] found that a greater number of visits to health clinics was related to higher rates of screening, supporting the contention that those with high levels of medical surveillance, due to chronic disease, may be more likely to be offered screening. Vaeth et al. [8] found that women with one or more of five functionally limiting comorbid conditions were less likely to present with late stage breast cancer. They concluded that these conditions are likely to be associated with higher levels of medical surveillance, which resulted in more opportunity for referral to screening. Furthermore, there may also be an element of 'reverse causality', where patients who tend to access health care services frequently are more likely to be diagnosed with minor comorbidity and may also be more likely to undergo screening.

4.7 The Death from Other Causes Hypothesis

This hypothesis relates to the possibility that those with comorbidity might be less likely to be offered screening (or diagnostic investigations) due to an explicit decision on the part of the health professional or patient that there is little point to such investigations due to their risk of death from other causes. The evidence to support this hypothesis is difficult to disentangle from that of the competing demands hypothesis. Patients may be less likely to be referred for screening either because of competing demands of care for their comorbidity or because of a rational decision on the part of the health professional and patient that screening may not be worthwhile, given that the mortality reduction benefits of screening for cancer tend not to accrue until many years after the initial screening test [25–29].

4.8 Multiple Mechanism Hypotheses

The net impact of comorbidity burden on cancer screening and diagnoses likely involves multiple mechanisms, represented by the four hypotheses, particularly where that burden involves a complexity of considerations and care needs. This complexity derives from more than one chronic disease at more than one level of severity, involving more than one management plan or strategy of care. Moreover, some barriers to screening that are erected as a result of the overall comorbidity burden may be explained by more than one hypothesis. For example, consider patients with multiple chronic diseases and complex patterns of care for all these conditions. These patients may feel that the management of these diseases represents a "competing demand" from their perspective. In other words, they have enough to worry about keeping up with the management of their conditions, so screening would take a secondary priority. They may also worry that one or more of their conditions pose challenges for screening. For example, diabetic patients may worry about blood sugar level changes during a colonoscopy preparation, whilst heart disease patients may worry about sedation.

4.9 How to Make Sense of the Evidence?

The summary of evidence relating to the impact of comorbidity on diagnosis above, suggests that there are different mechanisms at play that vary depending on specific circumstances. Key characteristics that are likely to be important are:

- *Type of cancer*: the impact of comorbidity may vary by type of cancer, availability of screening, and recognition of presenting symptoms, as distinct from the comorbid illness. For example, a patient with chronic respiratory disease may report increasing shortness of breath or cough to their health professional, who may assume this is an exacerbation of their underlying disease, rather than investigating the possibility of lung cancer.
- *Type of comorbidity*: Patients with unstable and/or life threatening comorbidities may be more likely to have symptoms overlooked and less likely to undergo screening, because of diversion of resources to manage the active condition(s), rather than considering new ones. In contrast, patients with stable or less severe comorbidities may be more likely to access health services, and therefore have greater opportunity to undergo screening or to have early symptoms of cancer investigated. There is some evidence to support this contention. Yasmeen et al. [22] studied a cohort of 118,742 women with breast cancer. They identified comorbid conditions and divided them into those that could be classified as stable (those that affect daily activities) and unstable (those that may be life-threatening or difficult to control). They found that the presence and number of stable conditions were associated with higher screening mammography rates and earlier stage at diagnosis, while the converse was true for unstable conditions. Similarly, Fleming and colleagues examined the impact of comorbidity on stage at diagnosis of prostate [30] and breast [7] cancers and found that those comorbidities that tended to be associated with earlier stage of cancer diagnosis, were often more mild conditions or conditions that might more accurately be considered risk factors for future ill-health (such as benign hypertension, dyslidipaemia, musculoskeletal conditions, and non-malignant breast disease). Those comorbidities associated with later stage of cancer diagnosis, tended to be those that were likely to have a greater negative impact on life expectancy, or those associated with poorer mental health (such as peripheral vascular disease, severe renal and psychiatric disorders).
- *Health service structure, funding and organisation*. Health services with a strong focus on screening, or where funding is attached to screening coverage may minimize differences in screening rates by comorbidity level. A number of studies have investigated the uptake of CRC screening within the equal access Veterans Administration (VA) health system in the US [24, 31, 32]. All found

that there was little or no difference in the rates of screening for men with life-limiting comorbidity, concluding that physicians may not be taking shortened life expectancy into account when they offer screening. This finding may be explained by colorectal cancer screening rates' use as a performance measure in the VA health system. Such a protocol may have had the unforeseen consequence of encouraging inappropriate screening [33].

4.10 Screening and Comorbidity: The Important Role of Physician Recommendation

In some settings, there is evidence that those with comorbidity are less likely to be offered screening, and as a result have later stage at diagnosis of screen-detectable cancers. For example, Gonzalez et al. [34] studied the association of higher levels of comorbidity with late stage at diagnosis among patients with potentially screen-detectable cancers (breast, colorectal, prostate and melanoma). They found that for all four sites, comorbidity was a significant predictor of late stage at diagnosis cancers ('any' comorbidity compared with none was associated with a 17 % greater risk for late stage diagnosis for CRC, 24 % for breast, 30 % for prostate and 62 % for melanoma). To assess whether chronic disease reduced breast and cervical cancer screening uptake, Kiefe et al. [3] carried out a review of medical records amongst a cohort of primary care patients. They found that higher Charlson index scores were associated with a reduced rate of screening for these cancers (each unit increase in Charlson score resulted in a 17 % lower likelihood of mammography and a 20 % lower rate of Pap test after adjustment for demographics, clinic use and insurance status). In other contexts, screening rates among those with comorbidity have been found to be similar to those without multiple chronic disease [24, 33]. This finding may be particularly evident where screening coverage rates are related to health service funding or quality indicators, which may encourage the screening of those with high levels of comorbidity, e.g., by offering higher reimbursement. Of note is that reduced screening among those with limited life expectancy is entirely consistent with best practice relating to screening, because finding early stage cancers that would take years, perhaps longer than the patient's lifetime, to cause symptoms, is unnecessary and does not improve quality or quantity of life [27, 28].

Extensive evidence demonstrates that recommendations by physicians are a key determinant of cancer screening, particularly for colorectal cancer (CRC) screening [4, 26, 33]. Although, in a national survey of primary care physicians, 95 % indicated that they recommend CRC screening [35], some evidence suggests that comorbidity burden may place colorectal and other cancer screenings lower on a list of priorities for both patients and their providers [26, 36]. Fontana et al. [37] also found that women with diabetes were less likely to have a mammogram and those with both heart disease and diabetes were more likely to forego screening for uterine cervical cancer with a Pap test. The authors speculate that because primary care providers emphasize "disease-centered care in an encounter-based system" (p. 1195), prevention services tend to be neglected. Patients with multiple morbidities are challenged to maintain complex, costly, and time consuming regimens, and represent a competing demand for the provider's limited office time [38]. Both patients and physicians frequently focus on the most disabling, threatening, and painful comorbidities. This focus is reasonable, as failure to manage these conditions may push the patient into a trajectory of more severe decompensation, disability, complications, and death. Prevention, including the highly effective CRC screening tests, loses its priority to other preexisting conditions, most particularly, acute and serious chronic conditions [38, 39]. Indeed, Yarnell et al. [40] have estimated that if a physician attempted to administer the health care prevention and maintenance recommended by the US Preventive Services Taskforce [41], he or she would spend 8 h on these responsibilities alone, forsaking acute and chronic disease complaints.

Physicians may also feel disinclined to provide a screening recommendation to patients they consider physically unable to endure screening or whose life expectancy may be compromised by multiple comorbidities [39]. This may be considered a variant of the death from other causes hypothesis (let us call it the "complications from other causes" hypothesis) in which the chronic disease itself is a barrier to the more invasive forms of screening, such as colonoscopy. Kiefe et al. [3] found that patients in a primary care setting were screened significantly less frequently for breast or cervical cancer as their chronic disease burden increased. Each increase in the Charlson index decreased a woman's likelihood of having a mammogram, clinical breast exam, or Pap test by 15, 13, and 19 %, respectively. These results were consistent with other clinically-based studies that showed an inverse dose response relationship between illness burden and likelihood of mammogram [39, 42]. May et al. [43] found that women with a higher index of comorbidity were significantly less likely to receive a mammogram recommendation from their physician and, not surprisingly, less likely to obtain a mammogram. Lipscombe et al. [44] corroborated these findings. They found that, after adjusting for age and other covariates, the odds of women with diabetes having a mammogram was 0.68 of that of women without diabetes. Obesity, another chronic condition, is associated with a lower likelihood of CRC screening [45].

It is important to emphasize that not offering screening to individuals with substantial comorbidity and shortened life expectancy is entirely consistent with clinical guidelines [24, 33]. There are harms associated with screening, and the potential benefits (in terms of reduced mortality) generally accrue several years after the test. Thus, there is a tension for health professionals to appropriately offer screening to some patients with comorbidity who have a life expectancy that is long enough to realize the benefits of screening, but also to not offer screening to others, for whom the harms will outweigh the benefits. There are now tools to assist health professionals and individuals themselves to make these decisions, such as ePrognosis [46] (http://eprognosis.ucsf.edu), which provides estimates of life expectancy, based on readily available clinical information in older patients.

These varying and inconclusive results with regards to the impact of comorbidity burden on screening may be due to several factors. First, methodological differences pervade these studies, including differing data collection techniques (chart reviews, claims data, interview data), the measurement of comorbidity burden (Charlson index, a single index condition, a tally of conditions), different populations (older people, general population) and different health care systems. Kiefe et al. [3] has offered another plausible explanation—that the association between comorbidity burden and cancer screening rates is skewed. It was suggested that those with only one or two co-morbidities or with less severe comorbidity, may be more likely to receiving screening due to greater physician contact, while those with multiple morbidities (>2) or more severe comorbidity are less likely to receive screening because of competing demands or physicians' perceptions of limited life expectancy, reduced quality of life, or patient lack of acceptance [36]. In addition, other factors, most especially older age, have been conflated with comorbidity burden. For example, Bynum et al. [47] found that screening decisions were significantly related to health status and to chronological age (and race).

4.11 Relationship Between Comorbidity and Stage at Diagnosis

The lack of congruence among the four hypotheses described earlier, surveillance, competing demand, physiological, and death from other causes, suggests that the relationship between comorbidity burden and either screening or stage at diagnosis, and the link between screening and stage at diagnosis is complex. Screening does not necessarily result in earlier stage diagnosis, for example, interval cancers and aggressive tumors are quite common, and late stage disease may occur even with regular screening. Gurney et al. [14] conducted a study with 14,096 patients with nine different cancers in New Zealand using cancer registry linked to hospitalization data and the C3 comorbidity index of 42 chronic conditions. They concluded that the presence of comorbid illness increased the odds of distant metastases (supporting the physiological and competing demand hypotheses), but that it did not lead to an earlier diagnosis (refuting the surveillance hypothesis). Compared to patients with no comorbidity burden, patients with moderate and high burden had 29 and 49 % higher odds, respectively, of distant stage disease. Furthermore, of the 42 investigated comorbid conditions, 27 increased the odds that the cancer was unstaged, possibly due to clinicians being unwilling to put patients with severe comorbidity through the rigors of diagnostic investigation, perhaps consistent with the death from other causes hypothesis. The implications of this study are that comorbidity burden may, in fact, be a barrier to regular screening or early diagnosis, possibly leading to more late stage disease.

The difficulty with examining the effect of comorbidities and other variables on mammography screening and stage at diagnosis has been recently examined by

Lipscomb et al. [48]. They analysed 7620 women diagnosed with breast cancer in 2004 from 7 states in the United States, who participated in the CDC sponsored "Breast and Prostate Patterns of Care Study". They addressed the question of whether covariates such as method of detection (mammography or other) are subject to bias in the studies that seek to estimate the determinants of late stage breast cancer, particularly in studies that use cancer registry data. Important confounders, such as breast density and family history, are usually missing and are predictors of both method of detection and stage of cancer. They used a two-stage regression with the mammography capacity in the county of residence as an instrumental variable to correct for this possible selection bias. With regards to mammography, the model confirmed selection bias and demonstrated a strong inverse relationship between mammography screening and late stage disease (OR = 0.037, $p < 0.001$), mammography screening was associated with a drastic reduction in the odds of late stage disease. The impact of comorbidities on late-stage disease was, however, less clear. Comorbidity burden was classified as none, mild, moderate, or severe based on the ACE-27 comorbidity index, which examines 26 different comorbid conditions [49]. In the single equation models that did not correct for the bias associated with missing confounders, patients who had a severe comorbidity burden were nearly half as likely to indicate a method of detection by mammography (OR = 0.60, $p < 0.08$) and more likely to be diagnosed at an advanced stage (OR = 1.46, $p < 0.04$). With the two stage models, however, the elevated risk of late stage cancer associated with severe comorbidity was statistically attenuated. This result likely does not mean that comorbidity burden is unrelated to screening, but rather that proportionately fewer women with severe comorbidity are screened, that most of the late stage disease is mediated by screening uptake, and that important confounders such as breast density and family history probably bias the impact of screening on stage. Moreover, any single comorbidity metric that consolidates the impact of multiple diseases probably hides the individual (and perhaps antagonistic) effects of these comorbidities on the risk of screening or late stage disease.

We mentioned earlier that the "type" of comorbidity really matters. The relationship between comorbidity burden, screening, and diagnosis is developed further by Sarfati and colleagues [50], who argue that the impact of comorbidity burden on cancer diagnosis through screening may depend on the type and severity of comorbidity. In other words, the surveillance hypothesis—that more frequent physician visits leads to a greater opportunity for physician screening recommendations—may only be valid for some comorbidities and not others. Sarfati suggests that surveillance is useful to promote screening for mild or stable comorbidities but detrimental, as competing demands predominate, for the more severe or unstable comorbid conditions. Moreover, health service factors, such as insurance coverage or widespread screening, that strengthen the link between screening and diagnosis, or even interactions between the cancer and comorbidity, may have an impact on screening and diagnosis. For example, end stage renal dialysis patients are diagnosed earlier for colorectal cancer [51], because they had higher rates of lower endoscopy, due to high rates of gastrointestinal symptoms in this group. A comorbidity metric that consolidates the effects of different conditions, such as the Charlson comorbidity index [15] or the ACE-27, discussed above, may hide these important differences. In an effort to expose the complex interaction between comorbid illness and cancer, we will show how the hypotheses explain the impact of comorbid illness on breast or colorectal cancer.

4.12 Competing Demands, Surveillance, and Multiple Morbidities

The increased burden of multiple comorbidities complicates the decision-making process of both clinicians and patients. More than one hypothesis may be needed to explain the empirical results. Fleming, Schoenberg and others, for example, conducted a study in Appalachian Kentucky, dealing with the impact of multiple comorbidities on colorectal cancer screening. The study had both a quantitative and qualitative design components. The quantitative component [52] included a cross-sectional study of 1153 subjects aged 50–76 from Appalachia Kentucky. The qualitative component [53] was comprised of two in-depth interviews with open-ended semi-structured and structured questionnaires, with each of forty-one subjects followed up by nine focus groups (six with providers, three with patients). The cross-sectional study showed a trend where a greater number of comorbidities was associated with higher rates of any guideline concordant colorectal cancer screening. Among subjects with none, 1, 2–3, 4–5, and 6+ morbidities, the rates of screening were 56.6, 59.1, 65.6, 70.8, and 79.6 %, respectively. In the multivariate analysis that controlled for demographic variables, such as age, gender, race, and socioeconomic status, only the highest level of comorbidity burden (6+) was associated with increased odds of screening by 2.2 times.

This curious and unexpected result is supportive of the surveillance hypothesis, since subjects with multiple chronic conditions are likely to see the physician more often. The results also illustrate the difference between the "depth" and "breadth" of comorbidity burden. Earlier we mentioned that the work of Corkum et al. [23] suggested that the more stable comorbidities were associated with higher screening rates, but the unstable or more severe comorbidities were associated with lower screening rates, the former governed by the surveillance hypothesis and the latter by the competing demands hypothesis. Thus, stability or severity might be considered the "depth" of comorbidity burden, the deeper the burden, the more likely that competing demands will prevail over surveillance. The "breadth" of comorbidity burden would simply be the number of different conditions which the physician(s) must manage. The results of Fleming and colleagues would suggest, at first glance, that a wider breadth of comorbidity burden is associated with higher screening rates, at least in the context in which the study was done.

In an effort to understand the apparent direct relationship between comorbidity "breath" and colorectal cancer screening, Tarasenko et al. [53] examined a subset of the Appalachian respondents (n = 1012) who had a least one (16 %) or more than one (84 %) morbidities and investigated whether there was a link between the perceived burden of multiple morbidities and colorectal screening. Respondents answered a number of survey questions regarding the perceived burden of their morbidities. Whereas more morbidities were associated with higher rates of colonoscopy overall, those who perceived that their morbidities were barriers to screening had lower rates of screening. For example, respondents who affirmed that "with all my health conditions, I worry about being put to sleep before a colonoscopy" had a 33 % lower prevalence of colonoscopy than those who did not agree with that statement. Individuals who affirmed that "with all my health conditions, I am not physically up for CRC screening" had a 25 % lower prevalence of colonoscopy. In fact for each of the perceived burden questions dealing with fears, worry, time, cost, and physician discussion of screening, both crude and adjusted prevalence rates were consistently lower for those who perceived that their morbidities represented a burden. This research clarifies the impact of the breadth of comorbidity burden on screening, at least from the patient's perspective. The surveillance hypothesis trumps competing demands only for those patients who do not perceive that their comorbidities are a barrier to screening. Alternatively, one could argue that those patients who were worried about their multiple morbidities, were indeed those who had the most severe disease and therefore were appropriately not being screening.

The qualitative aspect of the study involved two in-depth interviews of 41 white, mostly female (71 %), aged 51–77 subjects [54]. In terms of barriers to screening, they indicated that provider availability in rural settings was an issue, as was lack of finances or insurance. They felt that prevention was a secondary priority over the management of multiple morbidities, that the disease management of multiple chronic conditions was exhausting, leaving little time or energy for screening, and that multiple morbidities may make the preparation for colonoscopy challenging or increase worries about sedation, all of which is consistent with the competing demands hypothesis.

Jensen et al. [55] completed a historical cohort study in Demark, involving 149,234 women who were invited to the first breast cancer screening in 2008–2009. They investigated the link between 11 chronic disease groups and several measures of multimorbidity, with the likelihood of non-participation in the screening program, using prevalence ratios as the measure of association. Chronic disease was measured within two time periods (≤2 years and 2–10 years) prior to the screening invitation, based on an emergency, outpatient, or admission to a Danish hospital during that time period. Within the ≤2 year window, the prevalence of non-compliance was higher for patients with cancer, chronic mental illness, chronic obstructive pulmonary disease, chronic neurological disorders, and chronic kidney disease (50, 51, 51, 24, and 70 % higher, respectively). In most cases, the prevalence of non-compliance with the 2–10 year window was still elevated, but somewhat lower than the shorter time window, indicating that the proximity of chronic disease care represents a higher barrier to screening. Multimorbidity demonstrated a dose-response relationship with non-compliance for patients, with one, two, and three or more chronic disease groups having a 20, 47 and 58 % higher prevalence of non-compliance with screening, respectively. This study was incongruous with the Fleming et al. [52] work discussed earlier, since multimorbidity was associated with decreased rather than increased screening. The study showed that comorbidity burden, at least in Denmark, was more likely to be a barrier rather than a facilitator of screening.

4.13 Competing Demands and Surveillance in the Context of Mental Illness

The presence of coexisting mental illness has been found to have an influence on cancer screening uptake and cancer diagnosis. The competing demands and surveillance hypotheses may explain the apparently contradictory findings of studies in this area. Three recent systematic reviews have found that a history of mental illness is associated with lower uptake of cancer screening [56–58]. In a pooled meta-analysis of 24 studies, Lord et al. [56] found that mental illness was associated with significantly reduced rates of mammography screening (OR 0.71, 95 % CI 0.66–0.77), while women with severe mental illness (including schizophrenia, bipolar disorder and other non-organic psychosis) had a further reduced rate of screening compared to women without mental illness (pooled OR 0.54, 95 % CI 0.45–0.65). Women with psychological distress, but not meeting the criteria for mental illness, had the same rate of mammography as women without any mental health problems. In a systematic review of studies of breast and cervical screening receipt in women with mental illness, Aggarwal et al. [58] reported that more severe mental illness tended to be associated with lower screening receipt. For example, in a study of mammography receipt using insurance claims data from the United States, Carney and Jones [59] found that women with low severity mood disorders were 7 % less likely to have had a mammogram, while women with high severity mood disorders were 66 % less likely to have had one. Women with psychotic and substance use disorders had low screening rates regardless of severity. These findings of lower screening uptake with more severe comorbid mental illness may reflect competing demands, with more severe illness more readily overshadowing or distracting from screening recommendation by practitioners or screening attendance.

There are, however, studies which link mental illness with higher rates of cancer screening. For example, a number of studies have found that depression is associated with being more likely to have had a mammogram [60], a colonoscopy [61], or a cervical smear [62]. This suggests that surveillance has an impact on screening uptake, as depression is associated with higher rates of health service utilisation, particularly in older people [63].

The association of mental illness with cancer stage at diagnosis is unclear, with some studies finding that mental illness is associated with an earlier diagnosis [64], some with later diagnosis [65], and some with no association [66]. Variation in the type and severity of mental illness, other patient factors, such as age and physical health, and the health system within which mental health care and cancer diagnosis are occurring, are all likely to be important in understanding the variation among these findings. For example, a study of people using mental health services in London, England, did not find any difference in cancer stage at diagnosis (all cancers combined), between people with schizophrenia or bipolar disorder and people not known to mental health services [66]. A similar study of adults using mental health services in New Zealand found that those with schizophrenia or bipolar disorder had their breast and colorectal cancers diagnosed later than people without a history of mental illness [65]. This difference, however, may relate to the cost barriers to primary care in New Zealand [67].

4.14 The Physiological Hypothesis and Diabetes

Diabetes mellitus (DM) has reached epidemic proportions in many parts of the world, and deserves special consideration when discussing the confluence of multiple chronic conditions and cancer screening and diagnosis. In the United States, for example, the 1.7 million new cases each year (2012) adds to the pool of 29.1 million cases or 9.3 % of the population [68]. Globally, there are about 382 million cases (2013) or 8.3 % of the population, with significant differences in prevalence across countries, e.g., 23.9 % prevalence in Saudi Arabia but 3.2 % prevalence in Iceland [69, 70].

The physiological hypothesis provides a reasonable explanation for why diabetes has been associated with an increased risk of a cancer [71–75], including both breast and colorectal cancer, possibly due to hyperinsulinemia [76], "disturbed glucose/insulin homeostasis", which is associated with an increased production of factors contributing to DNA mutations, a compromised immune response [77], or adipocytokines and inflammatory mediators [78]. Data suggest an important role for the insulin pathway in the pathogenesis of breast cancer. Three mechanisms have been proposed to explain the association between diabetes and breast cancer [79]:

- Activation of the insulin pathway
- Activation of the insulin-like-growth-factor pathway
- Impaired regulation of endogenous sex hormones.

As an example, we know that insulin is able to directly affect proliferation of breast cancer cells [80], insulin receptor levels are high on human breast cancer cells [81], and insulin receptor expression is associated with a worse prognosis among breast cancer patients [82]. While high insulin receptor levels were found to be associated with expression of ER, most ER-negative tumors also show high levels [81]. In support of this theory, Goodwin et al. [83] confirmed that serum insulin levels were correlated with BMI and both were associated with worse outcome in 512 women with early-staged breast cancer [84]. Thus, high insulin levels may be the major link between type 2 diabetes and breast cancer and may explain the association between diabetes and low expression of hormone receptors.

In addition, DM itself may affect the aggressiveness or progression of the disease. Lipscombe et al. [85] recently completed a population-based study using databases from Ontario, Canada, on 38,407 women with breast cancer, including 6115 individuals with diabetes (which was also stratified by duration). They reported that women with diabetes had a 14, 21, and 16 % increased odds of stage II, III, or IV cancer, respectively, versus stage I. As importantly, diabetes was associated with a 16 % higher odds of increased tumor size (>2 cm) and a 16 % higher odds of positive lymph nodes, and longer duration diabetes (>2 years) was associated with an elevated and statistically significant risk. Since the authors controlled for mammography screening, and both increased tumor size and lymph node involvement are indicators of aggressiveness, they conclude that the study "supports a biological mechanism for the association between diabetes and breast cancer. Indolent tumors may progress more rapidly in patients with diabetes, or diabetes may lead to a higher metastatic potential" [85, p. 619]. The authors argue that disease progression is more advanced in diabetes patients, because of a more rapid growth of tumors due to hyperglycemia, hyperinsulinemia, insulin resistance [86–88], the mitogenic effect of insulin on breast cells [89], the overexpression of insulin receptors on breast cells [90], and the up-regulation of the insulin mitogenic pathway [91].

Diabetes is also a risk factor for more aggressive colorectal cancer, through some of the same mechanisms discussed above. Hu et al. [92] reported that DM was associated with a higher risk of colorectal cancer (OR = 1.43), a higher risk of advanced colorectal cancer (OR = 1.56), and a higher risk of fatal colorectal cancer (OR = 2.39). They reported that even after adjusting for age, body mass index, physical activity, and other covariates, diabetic women had a 56 % increased odds of advanced colorectal cancer, compared to non-diabetics. Siddiqui et al. [93] conducted a case control study of 155 patients with type 2 diabetes and colorectal cancer and 144 patients with colorectal cancer, but without type 2 diabetes. The authors found that subjects with poorly controlled diabetes (HbA1C > 7.5 %) had nearly twice the odds of right-sided colorectal cancer, and a 36 % higher odds of more advanced stage colorectal cancer, both related to poorer prognosis. Sharma et al. [94] studied the histopathologic differences in tumor characteristics among 534 patients with colorectal cancer, which included 282 individuals with diabetes. They found that subjects with (versus without) diabetes had a higher depth of tumor invasion, greater lymphovascular invasion, and higher staging. The multivariate analysis showed 11.4 times the log odds of signet cell histology, 1.74 times the log odds of transverse tumor location as well as an association with increased depth of tumor and lymphovascular invasion. The authors concluded that "the study found more adverse histopathologic features in patients with CRC who had diabetes as compared to those without diabetes" [94, p. 60]. With regards to colorectal cancer, hyperinsulinemia may result in elevated fecal bile acid [95], increased iron overload [96], a lower than normal level of antioxidant activity [97], or delayed stool transit and other gastrointestinal abnormalities [95], each of which might create a "cancer-promoting gastrointestinal milieu" [98]. To complicate matters further, metformin, the medication used to treat type II diabetes, is known to have an anti-cancer effect, which may to some degree counter balance the proliferative effects of diabetes itself [99].

To summarize, the physiological hypothesis can be brought to bear upon our understanding of why some comorbidities, in this case diabetes, seem to be related to an increased incidence of cancer, through various physiological and pathological mechanisms. It should be pointed out, however, that the same mechanisms that lead to an increased incidence of disease can also affect the aggressiveness with which cancer presents, thus a higher stage of diagnosis and/or more difficult to treat receptor negative tumor biology.

4.15 The Competing Demands Hypothesis, Diabetes, and Obesity

Despite the higher risk of breast cancer among those with diabetes, a number of studies have shown that diabetes itself is a potential barrier to regular mammography screening, the increased surveillance to the contrary notwithstanding. The relationship between diabetes and screening can be explained by the competing demands hypothesis, wherein this comorbidity represents a competing demand on the physician's time, energy and focus. McBean and Yu [100] used SEER-Medicare data to show that older women with diabetes were less likely to have a mammogram in the next 2–4 years, compared to women without the disease. In a retrospective cohort study, Lipscombe et al. [44] reported that women with diabetes were less likely to have had a mammogram during a two-year follow up period compared to those without diabetes, even though they had more health care visits. Beckman et al. [101] also found that women with diabetes were significantly less likely to get mammography screening compared to the controls. In a study based on a survey of 1030 Kentucky residents (695 women), Fleming et al. [102] found that those with diabetes who were 42 and older were significantly less likely to report regular mammography (68.5 %), compared to those without the disease (81.6 %). Similar results were found for women with and without diabetes in Appalachian Kentucky. In each of these studies it would seem that the competing demands hypothesis prevails over the surveillance hypothesis.

Obesity, an established risk factor for diabetes, may also be a significant barrier to mammography screening. According to Fontaine et al. [103], both the underweight and obese were more likely to delay mammography screening. Compared to normal weight women, white women with higher BMI were less likely to have breast cancer screening [104] and severely obese women were not as likely to comply with physician recommendations for breast cancer screening [105].

The combination of the physiological impact of diabetes on cellular proliferation, in addition to delays or avoidance of mammography screening among those with either diabetes or obesity, may lead to advanced stage of breast cancer at presentation. A small study by Wolf et al. [106] found that women with diabetes were more likely to present with more advanced stage of disease, larger tumor size, and hormone receptor negative status, compared to women without diabetes, even after adjusting for BMI, which was higher among diabetic patients. Fleming et al. [7] found that diabetes increased the odds of late (versus early) stage breast cancer by 19 %, controlling for age, race, twenty-three other comorbidities, mammography use two years prior to cancer diagnosis, and the number of physician and specialist visits. In separate analyses, both older (>74) and younger (≤74) women with DM, who had a mammography within 2 years of breast cancer diagnosis, were at higher risk (27 % increased odds and 28 % increased odds, respectively) of a late-stage breast cancer diagnosis compared to those without [7]. In an analysis of 6912 patients with stage I-III breast cancer from five different states, Sabatino et al. [107] found that 19.1 % of those patients with moderate to severe diabetes had stage III breast cancer compared to only 12.6 % of patients with mild diabetes ($P = 0.0565$). An exploratory, but unpublished, multivariate analysis of a larger subset of the Sabatino data source included stage IV cases (n = 6157) and both in situ and stage IV cases (n = 7539). Controlling for age and obesity, women with severe (vs. no) diabetes had 2.5 times the odds of late (vs. early) stage breast cancer ($p = 0.037$). Inclusion of in situ cases decreased the odds to 2.3. Inclusion of race/ethnicity decreased the odds even more (OR = 2.2, $p = 0.057$) as the African American cases had a higher odds of late stage disease (OR = 2.0) and nearly twice the rate of severe diabetes, when compared with the Caucasian cases.

4.16 Future Direction for Research and Practice

More research is needed, which looks at the impact of comorbidity burden and at the depth and breadth of such burden, to differentiate between the impact of multiple comorbidities and the severity of such comorbidities. We must also determine if comorbidity burden has a threshold, such that a low burden would increase the probability of screening and presumably decrease the risk of late stage illness and a high burden would decrease screening and increase late stage disease through competing demands. More qualitative research could focus specifically on the decision making process of the physician, to determine exactly how comorbid illness becomes a competing demand in patient care. Do comorbidities compete with physician time or focus? Do they conflict with perceived appropriate recommendations? Research on specific comorbidities like diabetes or heart disease would be useful to determine if there are distinct differences in the way that physicians deal with these additional morbidities. We also need research that attempts to disentangle the competing demands from the death from other causes hypothesis. In other words, we need to know why physicians are not recommending screening, i.e. whether it relates to a lack of time or focus or a conscious decision on the part of the physician, the patient, or both.

Primary care providers and specialists need to be aware that comorbid illness may not only increase the risk of cancer, but that it also represents a competing demand upon their time, so that cancer screening has a lower priority. Patients highly value the recommendations of physicians, particularly with regards to cancer screening. Some patients may require repeated recommendations for the more invasive and uncomfortable procedures, such as colonoscopy. Physicians need to be vigilant, proactive and insistent with regards to cancer screening among patients with comorbid illness. Finally, physicians need to be cognizant of the screening guidelines for their comorbid patients, so as not to either over-screen those with a limited life expectancy or to under-screen those for whom screening may be beneficial, because of their additional illnesses.

4.17 Conclusions

We have described a model showing that comorbidities have an impact on screening, stage at diagnosis, treatment, and outcome and that cancer treatment may have an impact on the management and outcome of comorbid conditions. We have suggested that there are inconsistencies in the literature regarding whether comorbidities increase or decrease the rates of cancer screening, increase or decrease the rate of late stage disease, and the degree to which there is a link between screening and stage at diagnosis as moderated by comorbidity burden. We have posited four distinct hypotheses, all of which are plausible to explain the association between comorbidities and screening, with the positive associations explained by the 'surveillance' hypothesis and the negative associations explained by the 'competing demands', 'physiological', or the 'death from other causes' hypothesis. We suggested that not all comorbidities are the same, and that the depth and breadth of comorbidity burden may dictate how many of the four hypothesis are valid and which hypothesis will prevail. Finally, we specifically focused on the comorbidity diabetes, and demonstrated how diabetes could impact not only the risk of developing either colorectal or breast cancer, but could also have an impact on both the likelihood of cancer screening and the stage of disease at diagnosis. The take away message for providers is that comorbid illness may complicate clinical decision making, particularly with regards to screening advocacy. Some, but not all, patients with comorbidities may need motivational messages. Clinicians must carefully balance the risks and benefits of screening, especially for their comorbid patients.

References

1. PEW. http://www.pewglobal.org/2014/01/30/global-population. Accessed 29 Oct 15
2. Population Reference Bureau. http://www.prb.org/Publications/Datasheets/2006/EuropesPopulationAgingWillAccelerateSaysDataSheet.aspx. Accessed 29 Oct 15
3. Kiefe CI, Funkhouser E, Fouad MN, May DS (1998) Chronic disease as a barrier to breast and cervical cancer screening. JGIM 13:357–365
4. Brawarsky P, Brooks DR, Mucci LA, Woods PA (2004) Effect of physician recommendation and patient adherence on rates of colorectal cancer testing. Cancer Detect Prev 28:260–268
5. Valanis B (1999) Epidemiology in healthcare, 3rd edn. Stamford, Appleton and Lange
6. Ogle KS, Swanson GM et al (2000) Cancer and comorbidity: redefining chronic diseases. Cancer 88:653–663
7. Fleming ST, Pursley HG, Newman B, Pavlov D, Chen K (2005) Comorbidity as a predictor of stage of illness for patients with breast cancer. Med Care 43:132–140
8. Vaeth PA, Satariano WA et al (2000) Limiting comorbid conditions and breast cancer stage at diagnosis. J Gerontol Ser A Biol Sci Med Sci 55:M593–M600
9. Miller MD, Paradis CF et al (1992) Rating chronic medical illness burden in geropsychiatric practice and research: application of the cumulative illness rating scale. Psychiatry Res 41:237–248
10. Koppie TM, Serio AM, Vickers AJ et al (2008) Age-adjusted Charlson comorbidity score is associated with treatment decisions and clinical outcomes for patients undergoing radical cystectomy for bladder cancer. Cancer 112:2384–2392
11. Tetsche MS, Dethlefsen C et al (2008) The impact of comorbidity and stage on ovarian cancer mortality: a nationwide Danish cohort study. BMC Cancer 8:31
12. Teppo H, Alho O-P (2009) Comorbidity and diagnostic delay in cancer of the larynx, tongue and pharynx. Oral Oncol 45:692–695
13. Grann A, Froslev T, Olesen AB et al (2013) The impact of comorbidity and stage on prognosis of Danish melanoma patients, 1987–2009: a registry-based cohort study. Br J Cancer 109:265–271
14. Gurney J, Sarfati D, Standley J (2015) The impact of patient comorbidity on cancer stage at diagnosis. Br J Cancer 2015(113):1375–1380
15. Charlson ME, Pompei P, Ales KL, MacKenzie CR (1987) A new method of classifying prognostic comorbidity in longitudinal studies: development and validation. J Chron Dis 40:373–383
16. Aksoy S, Aksoy H, Harputluoglu H et al (2006) Treatment of comorbidities besides the treatment of primary tumor may further increase effective management of cancer. Med Hypotheses 67:744–746
17. Extermann M (2007) Interaction between comorbidity and cancer. Cancer Control 14:13–22
18. Gonzalez-Perez A, Garcia Rodriguez LA, López-Ridaura R (2003) Effects of non-steroidal anti-inflammatory drugs on cancer sites other than the colon and rectum: a meta-analysis. BMC Cancer 3:28
19. Satariano WA, Ragland DR (1994) The effect of comorbidity on 3-year survival of women with primary breast cancer. Ann Intern Med 120:104–110
20. Yancik R, Wesley MN et al (2001) Effect of age and comorbidity in postmenopausal breast cancer patients aged 55 years and older. JAMA 285:885–892
21. Zafar SY, Abernethy AP et al (2008) Comorbidity, age, race, and stage at diagnosis in colorectal cancer: a retrospective, parallel analysis of two health systems. BMC Cancer 8:345. doi:10.1186/1471-2407-8-345
22. Yasmeen S, Xing G, Morris C et al (2011) Comorbidities and mammography use interact to explain racial/ethnic disparities in breast cancer stage at diagnosis. Cancer 117:3252–3261
23. Corkum M, Urquhart R, Kendell C et al (2012) Impact of comorbidity and healthcare utilization on colorectal cancer stage at diagnosis: literature review. Cancer Causes Control 23:213–220

24. Walter LC, Lindquist K et al (2009) Impact of age and comorbidity on colorectal cancer screening among older veterans. Ann Intern Med 150:465–473 [Summary for patients in Ann Intern Med. 2009 Apr 7;150(7):I-42; PMID: 19349627]
25. Zappa M, Visiolli CB et al (2003) Mammography screening in elderly women efficacy and cost-effectiveness. Crit Rev Oncol Hematol 46:235–239
26. Schonberg MA, McCarthy EP et al (2004) Breast cancer screening in women aged 80 and older: results from a national survey. J Am Geriatr Soc 52:1688–1695
27. Gross CP, McAvay GJ, Krumholz HM et al (2006) The effect of age and chronic illness on life expectancy after a diagnosis of colorectal cancer: implications for screening. Ann Intern Med 145:646–653 [Summary for patients in Ann Intern Med. 2006 Nov 7;145(9):I20; PMID: 17088573]
28. Walter LC, Bertenthal D et al (2006) PSA screening among elderly men with limited life expectancies. JAMA 296:2336–2342
29. Wolf AMD, Wender RC et al (2010) American Cancer Society guideline for the early detection of prostate cancer: update 2010. CA Cancer J Clin 60:70–98
30. Fleming ST, McDavid K, Pearce K, Pavlov D (2006) Comorbidities and the risk of late-stage prostate cancer. TSW Urol 1:163–173. doi:10.1100/tswurol.2006.142
31. Sultan S, Conway J et al (2006) Colorectal cancer screening in young patients with poor health and severe comorbidity. Arch Intern Med 166:2209–2214
32. Fisher DA, Galanko J, Shaheen NJ et al (2007) Impact of comorbidity on colorectal cancer screening in the veterans healthcare system. Clin Gastroenterol Hepatol 5:991–996
33. Fisher DA, Judd L, Sanford NS (2005) Inappropriate colorectal cancer screening: findings and implications. Am J Gastroenterol 100:2526–2530
34. Gonzalez EC, Ferrante JM, Van Durme DJ et al (2001) Comorbid illness and the early detection of cancer. South Med J 94:913–920
35. Klabunde CN, Frame PS, Meadow A et al (2003) A national survey of primary care physicians' colorectal cancer screening recommendations and practices. Prev Med 26:352–362
36. Grady KE, Lemkau JP, McVay JM et al (1996) Clinical decision-making and mammogram referral. Prev Med 25:327–338
37. Fontana SA, Baumann LC, Helberg C, Love RR (1997) The delivery of preventive services in primary care practices according to chronic disease status. AJPH 87:1190–1196
38. Fenton JJ, Von Korff M, Lin EHB et al (2006) Quality of preventive care for diabetes: effects of visit frequency and competing demands. Ann Fam Med 4:32–39
39. Shoen RE, Marcus M, Braham RL (1994) Factors associated with the use of screening mammography in a primary care setting. J Community Health 19:239–252
40. Yarnell KS, Pollak K, Ostbye T, Krause KM, Michener JL (2003) Primary care: is there enough time for prevention. Am J Pub Health 93:635–641
41. http://www.uspreventiveservicestaskforce.org/
42. Burack RC, Liang J (1989) The acceptance and completion of mammography by older black women. Am J Public Health 79:721–726
43. May DS, Kiefe CI, Funkhouser E, Fouad MN (1999) Compliance with mammography guidelines: physician recommendation and patient adherence. Prev Med 28:386–394
44. Lipscombe LL, Hux JE, Booth GL (2005) Reduced screening mammography among women with diabetes. Arch Intern Med 165:2090–2095
45. Rosen AB, Schneider EC (2004) Colorectal cancer screening disparities related to obesity and gender. J Gen Intern Med 19:332–338
46. http://eprognosis.ucsf.edu
47. Bynum JPW, Braunstein JB, Sharkey P et al (2005) The influence of health status, age, and race on screening mammography in elderly women. Arch Intern Med 165:2083–2088
48. Lipscomb J, Fleming ST, Trentham-Dietz A et al (2015) What predicts an advanced-stage diagnosis of breast cancer? Sorting out the influence of method of detection, access to care and biological factors. Cancer Epidemiol Biomark Prev

49. Piccirillo JF, Creech C, Zequeira R et al (1999) Inclusion of comorbidity into oncology data registries. J Reg Manag 26:66–70
50. Sarfati D, Koczwara B, Jackson C. The impact of comorbidity on cancer and its treatment. CA Cancer J Clin 2016 66(4): 337–350
51. Taneha S, Mandayam S, Kayani ZZ, Yong-Fang K, Shahinian VB (2007) Comparision of stage at diagnosis of cancer in patients on dialysis versus the general population. Clin J Am Soc Nephrol 2:1008–1013
52. Fleming ST, Schoenberg NE, Tarasenko YN, Pearce KA (2011) The prevalence of colorectal cancer screening among a multi-morbid rural Appalachian population. South Med J 104:811–818
53. Tarasenko Y, Fleming ST, Schoenberg NS (2013) The relationship between perceived burden of chronic conditions and colorectal cancer screening among Appalachian residents. J Rural Health 30:40–49
54. Bardach SH, Schoenberg NE, Fleming ST, Tarasenko YN (2010) Rural residents' perspectives on multiple morbidity management and disease prevention. J Appl Gerontol 30:671–699
55. Jensen LF, Pedersen AF, Andersen B, Vestergaard M, Vedsted P (2015) Non-participation in breast cancer screening for women with chronic diseases and multimorbidity: a population-based cohort study. BMC Cancer 15:798. doi:10.1186/s12885-015-1829-1
56. Lord O, Malone D, Mitchell AJ (2010) Receipt of preventive medical care and medical screening for patients with mental illness: a comparative analysis. Gen Hosp Psychiatry 32:519–543
57. Mitchell AJ, Pereira IES, Yadegarfar M et al (2014) Breast cancer screening in women with mental illness: comparative meta-analysis of mammography uptake. Br J Psychiatry 205:428–435
58. Aggarwal A, Pandurangi A, Smith W (2013) Disparities in breast and cervical cancer screening in women with mental illness. Am J Prev Med 44:392–398
59. Carney CP, Jones LE (2006) The influence of type and severity of mental illness on receipt of screening mammography. J Gen Intern Med 21:1097–1104
60. Green CA, Polen MR, Brody KK (2003) Depression, functional status, treatment for psychiatric problems, and the health-related practices of elderly HMO members. Am J Health Promot 17:269–275
61. Peytremann-Bridevaux I, Voellinger R, Santos-Eggimann B (2008) Healthcare and preventive services utilization of elderly Europeans with depressive symptoms. J Affect Disord 105:247–252
62. Stecker T, Fortney JC, Prajapati S (2007) How depression influences the receipt of primary care services among women: a propensity score analysis. J Women's Health
63. Luppa M, Sikorski C, Motzek T et al (2012) Health service utilization and costs of depressive symptoms in late life—a systematic review. Curr Pharm Des 18:5936–5957
64. Bergamo C, Sigel K, Mhango G et al (2014) Inequalities in lung cancer care of elderly patients with schizophrenia: an observational cohort study. Psychosom Med 76(215–220):2. doi:10.1097/PSY.0000000000000050
65. Cunningham R, Sarfati D, Stanley J et al (2015) Cancer survival in the context of mental illness: a national cohort study. Gen Hosp Psychiatry 37:501–506
66. Chang C-K, Hayes RD, Broadbent MTM et al (2014) A cohort study on mental disorders, stage of cancer at diagnosis and subsequent survival. BMJ Open 4:e004295
67. Jatrana S, Crampton P (2009) Primary health care in New Zealand: who has access? Health Policy 93:1–10
68. American Diabetes Association (ADA). http://www.diabetes.org/diabetes-basics/statistics/. Accessed 23 Oct 15
69. Index Mundi. http://www.indexmundi.com/facts/indicators/SH.STA.DIAB.ZS/rankings. Accessed 23 Oct 15
70. Health Intelligence. http://healthintelligence.drupalgardens.com/content/prevalence-diabetes-world-2013. Accessed 23 Oct 15

71. Hjartaker A, Langseth H, Weiderpass E (2008) Obesity and diabetes epidemics: cancer repercussions. Adv Exp Med Biol 630:72–93
72. Gupta S, Vittinghoff E, Bertenthal D et al (2006) New-onset diabetes and pancreatic cancer. Clin Gastroenterol Hepatol 4:1366–1372
73. Larsson SC, Orsini N, Brismar K, Wolk A (2006) Diabetes mellitus and risk of bladder cancer: a meta- analysis. Diabetologia 49:2819–2823
74. Friberg E, Orsini N, Mantzoros CS, Wolk A (2007) Diabetes mellitus and risk of endometrial cancer: a meta-analysis. Diabetologia 50:1365–1374
75. Huxley RR, Ansary-Moghaddam A, Clifton P et al (2009) The impact of dietary and lifestyle risk factors on risk of colorectal cancer: a quantitative overview of the epidemiological evidence. Int J Cancer 125:171–180
76. Lipscombe LL, Goodwin PJ, Zinman B et al (2006) Increased prevalence of prior breast cancer in women with newly diagnosed diabetes. Breast Cancer Res Treat 98:303–309
77. Gunter MJ, Hoover DR, Yu H et al (2009) Insulin, insulin-like growth factor-I, and risk of breast cancer in postmenopausal women. J Natl Cancer Inst 101:48–60
78. Cebioglu M, Schild HH, Golubnitschaja O (2008) Diabetes mellitus as a risk factor for cancer: stress or viral etiology? Infect Disord Drug Targets 8:76–87
79. Alokail MS, Al-Daghri NM, Al-Attas OS, Hussain T (2009) Combined effects of obesity and type 2 diabetes contribute to increased cancer risk in premenopausal women. Cardiovasc Diabetol 8(33). doi:10.1186/1475-2840-8-33
80. Wolf I, Sadetzki S, Catane R, Karasik A, Kaufman B (2005) Diabetes mellitus and breast cancer. Lancet Oncol 6:103–111
81. Chappell J, Leitner JW, Solomon S et al (2001) Effect of insulin on cell cycle progression in MCF-7 breast cancer cells. Direct and potentiating influence. J Biol Chem 276:38023–38028
82. Papa V, Pezzino V, Costantino A, Belfiore A, Giuffrida D, Frittitta L et al (1990) Elevated insulin receptor content in human breast cancer. J Clin Invest 86:1503–1510
83. Goodwin PJ, Ennis M, Pritchard KI, Trudeau ME, Koo J, Madarnas Y et al (2002) Fasting insulin and outcome in early-stage breast cancer: results of a prospective cohort study. J Clin Oncol 20:42–51
84. Belfiore A, Frittitta L, Costantino A et al (1996) Insulin receptors in breast cancer. Ann N Y Acad Sci 784:173–188
85. Lipscomb LL, Fischer HD, Austin PC et al (2015) The Association between diabetes and breast cancer stage at diagnosis: a population based study. Breast Cancer Res Treat 150:613–620
86. Hernandez AV et al (2014) Association between insulin resistance and breast carcinoma: a systematic review and meta-analysis. PLoS ONE 9(6):e99317
87. Godsland IF (2010) Insulin resistance and hyperinsulinaemia in the development and progression of cancer. Clin Sci 118(5):315–332
88. Lawlor DA, Smith GD, Ebrahim S (2004) Hyperinsulinaemia and increased risk of breast cancer: findings from the British Women's Heart and Health Study. Cancer Causes Control 15(3):267–275
89. Belfiore A et al (2009) Insulin receptor isoforms and insulin receptor/insulin-like growth factor receptor hybrids in physiology and disease. Endocr Rev 30(6):586–623
90. Milazzo G et al (1992) Insulin receptor expression and function in human breast cancer cell lines. Cancer Res 52(14):3924–3930
91. De Meyts P et al (1995) Role of the time factor in signaling specificity: application to mitogenic and metabolic signaling by the insulin and insulin-like growth factor-I receptor tyrosine kinases. Metabolism 44(10 Suppl 4):2–11
92. Hu FB, Manson JE, Liu S et al (1999) Prospective study of adult onset diabetes mellitus (type 2) and risk of colorectal cancer in women. J Natl Cancer Inst 91:542–547
93. Siddiqui AA, Spechler SJ, Huerta S et al (2008) Elevated HbA1c is an independent predictor of aggressive clinical behavior in patients with colorectal cancer: a case-control study. Dig Dis Sci 53:2486–2494

94. Sharma A, Ng H, Kumar A, Teli K, Randhawa J, Record J, Maroules M (2014) Colorectal cancer: histopathologic differences in tumor characteristics between patients with and without diabetes. Clin Colorectal Cancer 13(1):54–61. doi:10.1016/j.clcc.2013.10.002
95. Will JC, Galuska DA, Vinicor F, Calle EE (1998) Colorectal cancer: another complication of diabetes mellitus? Am J Epidemiol 147(9):816–825
96. Nelson R, Persky V, Davis F (1997) Re: Diabetes mellitus and risk of large bowel cancer. J Nat Canc Inst 89:1232. doi:10.1093/jnci/89.16.1232
97. Ross CM (1999) Re: prospective study of adult onset diabetes mellitus (Type 2) and risk of colorectal cancer in women. J Nat Canc Inst 91:1334
98. Chang CK, Ulrich CM (2003) Hyperinsulinaemia and hyperglycaemia: possible risk factors of colorectal cancer among diabetic patients. Diabetologia 46:595–607
99. Kasznicki J, Sliwinska A, Drzewoski J (2014) Metformin in cancer prevention and therapy. Ann Transl Med 2:57. doi:10.3978/j.issn.2305-5839.2014.06.01
100. McBean AM, Yu X (2007) The underuse of screening services among elderly women with diabetes. Diabetes Care 30:1466–1472
101. Beckman TJ, Cuddihy RM, Scheitel SM et al (2001) Screening mammogram utilization in women with diabetes. Diabetes Care 24:2049–2053
102. Fleming ST, Love MM, Bennett K (2011) Diabetes and cancer screening rates among Appalachian and non-Appalachian residents of Kentucky. J Am Board Fam Pract 24:682–692
103. Fontaine KR, Heo M, Allison DB (2001) Body weight and caner screening among women. J Women's Health Gend Med 10:463–470
104. Wee CC, McCarthy EP, Davis RB, Phillips RS (2004) Obesity and breast cancer screening. J Gen Intern Med 19:324–331
105. Ferrante JM, Chen PH, Crabtree BF, Wartenberg D (2007) Cancer screening in women: body mass index and adherence to physician recommendations. Am J Prev Med 32:525–531
106. Wolf I, Sadetzki S, Gluck I, Oberman B, Ben-David M, Papa MZ, Catane R, Kaufman B (2006) Association between diabetes mellitus and adverse characteristics of breast cancer at presentation. Eur J Cancer 42):1077–1082
107. Sabatino SA, Thompson TD, Wu X, Fleming ST, Kimmick GG, Trentham-Dietz A, Cress R, Anderson RT (2014) The influence of diabetes severity on receipt of guideline concordant treatment for breast cancer. Breast Cancer Res Treat 146:199–209. doi:10.1007/s10549-014-2998-3
108. Bauer KR, Brown M, Cress RD et al (2007) Descriptive analysis of estrogen receptor (ER)-negative, progesterone receptor (PR), and HER2-negative invasive breast cancer, the so-called triple-negative phenotype: a population—based study from the California Cancer Registry. Cancer 109:1721–1728
109. Landman GW, Ubink-Veltmaat LJ, Kleefstra N et al (2008) Increased cancer mortality in type 2 diabetes (ZODIAC-3). Anticancer Res 28:1373–1375

Further Reading

110. Fleming ST, Pursley HG, Newman B, Pavlov D, Chen K (2005) Comorbidity as a predictor of stage of illness for patients with breast cancer. Med Care 43:132–140
111. Satariano WA, Ragland DR (1994) The effect of comorbidity on 3-year survival of women with primary breast cancer. Ann Intern Med 120:104–110
112. Gurney J, Sarfati D, Standley J (2015) The impact of patient comorbidity on cancer stage at diagnosis. Br J Cancer 2015(113):1375–1380

Chapter 5
Impact of Comorbidity on Treatment Decision Making and Outcomes

Jae Jin Lee and Martine Extermann

Abstract Cancer, like many chronic conditions, is a disease of aging, and more than half of cancer patients in developed countries are 65 years or older. Therefore, many cancer patients have comorbidities, high use of medications, altered body composition, pharmacokinetics, and pharmacodynamics. Therefore, the treatment plans need to be individually tailored to achieve optimal outcomes. This chapter on comorbidity in cancer decision making gives some general principles and then will review some specific comorbidities with their incidence, considerations for decision making and treatment outcome. Scores to assess the risk of toxicity from chemotherapy will also be reviewed. Comorbidity burden is a major influencer of life expectancy and should be integrated in life expectancy estimates. The most assessed comorbidities are renal insufficiency and hepatic diseases. Creatinine clearance should be systematically calculated, and for several types of treatment, the Child-Pugh classification can be used. We also review the treatment of patients with cardiovascular diseases, auto-immune/inflammatory diseases, and diabetes. All risk factors of comorbidity should be comprehensively evaluated before cancer treatment, in order to reduce treatment-related toxicity and improve patient outcomes. Future research should address how to integrate the impact of multiple concomitant comorbidities, and more specifically which subgroups most affect various cancer outcomes.

Keywords Comorbidity · Elderly · Cancer · Clinical decision making · CRASH score · Life expectancy · Renal function · Hepatic function · Geriatric oncology

Key Points

- Many cancer patients have concomitant comorbidity. More than 90 % of cancer patients aged 70 and above have at least one comorbidity
- Comorbidity is a major influencer of life expectancy, and an individualized estimation of life expectancy should be conducted

J.J. Lee · M. Extermann (✉)
Moffitt Cancer Center, 12902 Magnolia Drive, Tampa, FL 33612, USA
e-mail: martine.extermann@moffitt.org

B. Koczwara (ed.), *Cancer and Chronic Conditions*,
DOI 10.1007/978-981-10-1844-2_5

- Comorbidity influences the behavior and outcomes of cancer and its treatment
- Creatinine clearance should always be calculated, as older patients can have serious limitations of renal function with normal creatinine levels
- Many of the new targeted therapies have a cardiovascular impact and should be used with caution in patients with cardiovascular disorders
- In diabetic patients receiving short-duration steroids, as given in many chemotherapy regimens, a combination of insulin detemir and aspart leads to better glycemic control than sliding scale insulin
- Risk indexes, such as the Chemotherapy Risk Assessment Score for High-age patients (CRASH) score and the Cancer and Aging Research Group (CARG score), exist to help assess the individual patient risk of toxicity from chemotherapy
- More research work in patients with multimorbidity needs to be done to assess which subgroup most influences outcome.

5.1 Introduction

Cancer, like many chronic conditions, is a disease associated with aging, and more than half of the cancer patients in the USA are 65 years or older [1]. Therefore many cancer patients have comorbidities [2–4], a high use of medications [5, 6], altered body composition, pharmacokinetics, and pharmacodynamics [7–9]. In such patients the treatment plans need to be individually tailored.

Many clinical trials have reported benefits for the inclusion of older cancer patients compared to younger patients with adequate cancer treatment in many solid tumors and hematologic malignancies, sometimes at the cost of some increased toxicity. However, these selected older patients typically have a low level of comorbidity. How then, can we transfer the evidence to patients with comorbidities? Is there direct evidence generated in patients with comorbidities? This chapter on comorbidity in cancer decision making will address two aspects: how the comorbidity burden of a patient affects life expectancy and fitness; and highlights of specific comorbidities with their incidence, considerations for decision making and treatment outcomes. Moreover, the MAX2 index and CRASH score for predicting chemotherapy-induced toxicity will be introduced.

5.2 General Considerations

The comorbidity burden of cancer patients can considerably influence their life expectancy. Walter et al. [10] demonstrated large variations in life expectancy between the top and the bottom quartile of the US population for similarly aged patients. A more detailed analysis of the impact of comorbidity using the Charlson Comorbidity Index in the SEER/Medicare registry is also available [11]. Validated geriatric tools are available online to help us estimate a patient's 1-year, 5-year, or 10-year risk of death if they are aged 65 or more. www.ePrognosis.org. This can be particularly helpful when deciding what adjuvant treatment to choose for patients in their late seventies or eighties. When deciding adjuvant treatment, it is also very important to know the time dynamic of the risk of relapse. For example, the risk of relapse of an estrogen-receptor positive breast cancer is fairly constant over a long period of time, whereas the risk of relapse from colon cancer is mostly in the first 5 years [12]. Although more research still needs to be done to quantify this effect, comorbidity does contribute to a decrease of functional reserve that is linked to frailty. Several frailty indexes integrating comorbidity have been studied in cancer patients [13–15].

As comorbidity is a multidimensional construct, quantifying it in order to assess its impact is a challenge. Most validated indices have used either mortality risk as an endpoint (e.g. Charlson Comorbidity Index [16], Kaplan-Feinstein Index [17]), or an expert assessment of the functional and mortality impact of the diseases (Cumulative Illness Rating Scale-Geriatric (CIRS-G) [18, 19], Index of Coexistent Diseases (ICED) [20]). Every comorbidity has a more detailed specific severity rating, but in this review we chose to address to overall comparison ratings in the context of oncology.

Another issue related to comorbidity is polypharmacy. Older American cancer patients take an average of six medications, two of them interacting with the CYP450 cytochrome system [21]. As an increasing number of chemotherapies and targeted agents are liver metabolized, careful attention should be paid to a review of the patient's medications and to eliminating superfluous prescriptions, or replacing some medications with others less likely to interact with the intended cancer treatment drug. The presence of high level drug interactions significantly increases the risk of severe toxicity from chemotherapy [22].

5.3 Individual Comorbidities

5.3.1 Renal Function

5.3.1.1 Renal Insufficiency and Its Incidence

According to Cumulative Illness Rating Scale-Geriatrics (CIRS-G) [18], kidney as comorbidity is considered as one category (Table 5.1). There are five rating scores which range from 0—no problem to 4—with dialysis. Their severity is determined by serum creatinine levels and depends on the treatment. In the Kaplan-Feinstein Index (KFI) [17], renal dysfunction is considered as a cogent comorbidity and its severity is defined to have proteinuria, azotemia, and renal decompensation. Adult

Table 5.1 Assessment of renal insufficiency in several comorbidity indexes

Measurement	Grade 1	Grade 2	Grade 3	Grade 4
CIRS-G	History of kidney stone passage within 10 years or asymptomatic kidney stone; pyelonephritis within five years	Serum creatinine >1.5 but <3.0 without diuretic or antihypertensive medication	Serum creatinine >3.0 or serum creatinine >1.5 in conjunction with diuretic, antihypertensive, or bicarbonate therapy' current pyelonephritis	Requires dialysis; renal carcinoma
Kaplan-Feinstein index	Proteinuria (tests of 3+ or 4+ on two or more urinalyses, or excretion of 1 g on 24-h urine collection); recurrent lower urinary infections or renal stones	Azotemia, manifested by elevated BUN (>25 mg%) and/or creatinine (>3.0 mg%) without secondary effects; nephrotic syndrome; recurrent infections; hydronephrosis	Uremia, renal decompensation with secondary anemia, edema, hypertension	–
AEC-27	Creatinine 2–3 mg/dl; stable transplant >6 months ago	Creatinine >3 mg/dl; stable transplant ≤6 months; chronic dialysis	Creatinine >3 mg/dl with multiple organ failure, shock, or sepsis; acute transplant rejection, acute dialysis	–
NCI/NIA Life-Threat Model	–	–	–	Renal failure
Charlson comorbidity index	–	Moderate or severe renal disease; serum creatinine >3 mg/dL; dialysis; transplantation; uremic syndrome	–	–

Comorbidity Evaluation-27 (ACE-27) [23] includes renal disease as comorbidity with four levels of severity of none to severe and the Index of Coexistent Disease (ICED) scales [20] with four levels of severity.

In the National Cancer Institute/National Institute on Aging (NCI/NIA) Life-Threat Model [24], renal failure is considered a high impact comorbidity, even without active management. In the Charlson comorbidity index (CCI) [25], renal disease including elevated creatinine, dialysis, and transplantation rates '2 points' (Table 5.1).

Among cancer patients, the incidence of renal insufficiency remains unclear. High prevalence of renal insufficiency in cancer patients has been observed by French investigators of the Renal Insufficiency and Cancer Medicine (IRMA) Study Group [26]. It was somewhat different depending on the methods used to calculate the renal function. The prevalence was 57.5 % using Cockcroft-Gault or 52.9 % with the abbreviated Modification of Diet in Renal Disease (aMDRD). Renal insufficiency was defined to be less than 90 mL/min of GFR by the Working Group of the National Kidney Foundation [27]. Stage 3 (GFR of 30–59 mL/min) or higher (GFR of less than 30 mL/min) renal insufficiency made up about 20 % by both of methods. According to the IRMA study group, a high prevalence of renal insufficiency of 60.3 % was observed in cancer patients who had normal serum creatinine, when this was calculated according to the Cockcroft-Gault formula. Furthermore, the prevalence of renal insufficiency in cancer patients aged 75 years and older was 74.1 %, as calculated by the MDRD formula.

5.3.1.2 Treatment Decision Making with Renal Insufficiency

Estimating Renal Function

Renal function should be assessed by calculation of GFR or creatinine clearance (CrCl) in all patients, even if serum creatinine levels are within normal range [28]. For assessment of renal function, we should consider sex, age, and weight of the patient for parameters of representing the muscle mass of the patient. There are various formulae to estimate GFR or CrCl. The SIOG renal insufficiency task force recommends the abbreviated MDRD (aMDRD) formula or the Cockcroft-Gault formula for older cancer patients [29].

Dose Adjustment Recommendation

Kintzel and Dorr [30] provided recommendation for 17 drugs which had a renal clearance equal to or exceeding 30 % of the administered dose out of 48 anticancer drugs reviewed. Recommendations for the adjustment of dosing in elderly cancer patients with renal insufficiency were developed by the International Society of Geriatric Oncology (SIOG) taskforce on the basis of the Kintzel and Dorr study [31]. In those studies, the alkylating agents included carmustine, ifosfamide, melphalan, dacarbazine, and temozolomide. The platinum agents were carboplatin, cisplatin, and oxaliplatin. The antimetabolites fludarabine, methotrexate, capecitabine, cytarabine, hydroxyurea, raltitrexed, and pemetrexed were also reviewed. As topoisomerase inhibitors, etoposide and topotecan were included. Beside anticancer drugs, they suggested guidelines for bisphosphonates, including zoledronic acid, pamidronate, and ibandronate.

Furthermore, the guidelines for anticancer drugs with limited renal excretion were suggested. They were chlorambucil in alkylating agents, gemcitabine and fluorouracil in antimetabolites, vincristine, vinblastine, and vinorelbine in vinca alkaloids, paclitaxel, ABI 007, and docetaxel in taxanes, irinotecan in topoisomerase inhibitors, doxorubicin, liposomal doxorubicine, epirubicin, daunorubicine, mitoxantrone, mitomycin, and idarubicin in antitumor antibiotics, tamoxifen and-bicalutamide in hormonal therapy, and thalidomide, bortezomib, and anti-VEGF antibiodies in other drugs.

Other Considerations for Patients with Renal Insufficiency

Beside estimating renal function, an assessment and optimization of hydration status should be performed per SIOG recommendation for renal insufficiency in older cancer patients, as renal insufficiency affects the ability of the body to control the fluid balance [32]. They also recommended that co-administration of known nephrotoxic drugs such as NSAIDs or Cox-2 inhibitors should be avoided or minimized.

5.3.1.3 Life Expectancy and Outcomes

In a study of the effects of unidentified renal insufficiency in metastatic colorectal cancer patients treated with capecitabine in combination with oxaliplatin, all the patients had normal values of serum creatinine and the ranges of GFR were very broad, from <30 to >90 mL/min [33]. The patients with GFR of 60 mL/min or less experienced more severe toxicities with cytopenia (76 % vs. 61 %, OR = 1.86, $p < 0.001$), diarrhea (34 % vs. 29 %, OR = 3.76, $p = 0.007$), stomatitis (10 % vs. 6 %, OR = 2.81, $p = 0.002$), and hand-foot syndrome (18 % vs. 11 %, OR = 2.56, $p = 0.045$) than those with GFR of 60 mL/min or more. The response rate and time to progression (4.5 vs. 5.5 months, HR = 1.57, $p = 0.015$) were significantly lower in renal insufficiency patients. Unidentified renal insufficiency patients received more dose modification (34 % vs. 14 %, OR = 1.98, $p < 0.001$) and dose interruption (52 % vs. 26 %, OR = 1.72, $p < 0.001$). The authors of this study suggested that estimating renal function with GFR should be required for all metastatic colorectal cancer patients before initial chemotherapy.

A retrospective Japanese study of advanced urothelial cancer, reported that 3-year overall survival for patients having GFR ≥60 mL/min/1.73 m^2 was better than that for those with GFR of <60 mL/min/1.73 m^2, when treated with a gemcitabine and cisplatin combination therapy (31.4 % vs. 14.1 %) [34]. The reason was a high dose reduction rate of gemcitabine and cisplatin (43.9 %). The 1-year survival of patients with a reduced dose of the two drugs was significantly lower than that for those treated with standard-dose among the patients with an estimated GFR of <60 mL/min/1.73 m^2 (26.2 % vs 60.3 %, $p = 0.01$).

An advanced non-small cell lung cancer study by Langer et al. demonstrated that patients with mild (GFR of 51–80 mL/min) or moderate (GFR of 50 mL/min or less) renal insufficiency had response rates and toxicity similar to patients with normal renal function, when treated with weekly nab-paclitaxel (100 mg/m^2) or paclitaxel 200 mg/m2 every three weeks, in combination with carboplatin (AUC = 6 every three weeks) [35]. The median dose intensity and cumulative exposure was better for nab-paclitaxel weekly across all levels of renal function. Other outcomes were comparable as well.

An ancillary study of CALGB 49907, which randomized older breast cancer patients to capecitabine vs. AC or CMF analyzed the impact of renal function on outcomes [36]. Patients with an estimated creatinine clearance (Cockroft-Gault) ≥30 ml/min were enrolled. Methotrexate and capecitabine were dose-adapted to renal function. With this dose-adaptation, renal function did not predict whether a patient would receive a dose modification, complete treatment per protocol, or experience hematologic toxicity for any regimen. It was however associated with non-hematologic toxicity in a heterogeneous fashion: increased creatinine clearance was associated with a decreased risk of toxicity in patients receiving AC, and an increased risk of toxicity in patients receiving capecitabine. It was not predictive of RFS or OS.

5.3.2 Hepatic Function

5.3.2.1 Hepatic Dysfunction and Its Incidence

According to Cumulative Illness Rating Scale-Geriatrics, liver diseases as comorbidity are considered as one category (Table 5.2). There are five rating scores which range from 0 with no problem to 4 with active hepatitis. Their severity is determined by a liver function test, including bilirubin and depending on their activity. The Kaplan-Feinstein Index considers hepatic dysfunction as a cogent comorbidity and its severity is defined by laboratory findings and clinical manifestation. Adult Comorbidity Evaluation-27 includes liver disease as comorbidity with four levels of severity of none to severe. The index of Coexistent Disease scales includes hepatobiliary disease with four levels of severity.

In the National Cancer Institute/National Institute on Aging Life-Threat Model, liver dysfunction is considered as a low to moderate impact comorbidity depending on active management. The Charlson comorbidity index takes liver disease into account, including liver cirrhosis without portal hypertension or with portal hypertension and rates ‘1 or 3 of points’ (Table 5.2).

Unfortunately, most clinical trials have excluded patients with hepatic dysfunction. So, the prevalence of hepatic dysfunction is poorly known in cancer patients. Besides comorbidities, hepatic dysfunction also results from the

Table 5.2 Assessment of hepatic dysfunction in several comorbidity indexes

Measurement	Grade 1	Grade 2	Grade 3	Grade 4
CIRS-G	History of hepatitis >five years ago	Mildly elevated LFT (up to 150 % of normal); hepatitis within five years; daily or heavy alcohol use within five years	Elevated bilirubin (total >2); marked elevation of LFT (>150 % of normal)	Active hepatitis
Kaplan-Feinstein index	Chronic liver disease manifested on biopsy or by persistently elevated BSP (>15 % retention) or bilirubin (>3 mg%)	Compensated hepatic failure (cutaneous spiders, palmar erythema, hepatomegaly or other clinical evidence of chronic liver disease)	Hepatic failure (ascites, icterus, encephalopathy); or esophageal varices	–
AEC-27	Chronic hepatitis or cirrhosis w/o PHT; chronic liver on biopsy or with bilirubin >3 mg/dl	Chronic hepatitis, cirrhosis, PHT with moderate symptoms "compensated hepaticfailure"	PHT and or esophageal bleeding ≤6 months (encephalopathy, ascites, jaundice with bilirubin >2; h/o transplant ≤6 months or acute rejection	–
NCI/NIA Life-Threat Model		No current management/history only	Under active management	–
Charlson comorbidity index	Mild liver disease; cirrhosis without PHT; chronic hepatitis	–	Moderate or severe liver disease; cirrhosis with PHT± variceal bleeding	–

LFT liver function test; *PHT* portal hypertension

metastases of solid tumors, including breast cancer, lung cancer, and colorectal cancer to the liver. A retrospective study of the association of comorbidity with survival and treatment-related toxicities reported that the incidence of liver disease as comorbidity was 30.8 %, which included biliary disease and pancreatic disease as assessed by CIRS-G [37]. Grade 3 or 4 of hepatic dysfunction made up 7.3 % in this study. According to annual report by the NIH, incidence of hepatic dysfunction, including liver cirrhosis, chronic hepatitis, and moderate to severe liver disease, was

0.8 % in breast cancer, colorectal cancer, lung cancer, and prostate cancer patients of 65 years and older [38]. A retrospective study of nonhepatic cancer in patients with liver cirrhosis reported 19.8 % of the incidence of nonhepatic cancer [39].

5.3.2.2 Treatment Decision Making with Hepatic Dysfunction

Similar to estimating renal function with creatinine or creatinine clearance, hepatic dysfunction has been estimated with laboratory findings including the level of bilirubin, albumin, and prothrombin time and clinical manifestation including ascites, encephalopathy, nutritional status, peripheral edema, and complications of portal hypertension. Hepatic dysfunction affects the hepatic clearance of drugs, low albumin increases the fraction of free drug, and portal hypertension affects drug absorption.

Estimating Hepatic Dysfunction

There are several classifications for estimating hepatic function, but no single test has been developed for clinical use to adjust drugs in patients with hepatic dysfunction. The Child-Pugh classification (Table 5.3) is one of the best known assessments for hepatic dysfunction. Assessment of the Child-Pugh classification results in (A) mild degree with 5 or 6 points, (B) moderate degree with 7–9 points, or (C) severe degree with 10–15 points.

The model for end-stage liver disease (MELD) is based on serum bilirubin, serum creatinine, the internationalized ratio (INR) of prothrombin time, and the underlying liver disease. The MELD score accurately predicts 3-month mortality for patients on a liver transplant waiting list.

The Maddrey discriminant function (df) is for patients with acute alcoholic hepatitis, the disease is not severe if df < 54, is severe when the score is between 55

Table 5.3 Child-Pugh classification

Variables	1 point	2 points	3 points
Encephalopathy grade[a]	None	1 or 2	3 or 4
Ascites	Absent	Slight	Moderate
Serum bilirubin, mg/dL	<2	2–3	>3
Serum albumin, g/L	>3.5	2.8–3.5	<2.8
Prothrombin time, s prolonged	<4	4–6	>6

[a]Grade 0: Normal consciousness, personality, neurological examination, electroencephalogram
Grade 1: Restless, sleep disturbed, irritable/agitated, tremor, impaired handwriting, 5 cps (cycles per second) waves
Grade 2: Lethargic, time-disoriented, hyperactive reflexes, rigidity, slower waves
Grade 4: Unrousable coma, no personality/behavior, decerebrate, slow 2–3 cps delta activity

and 92, and probably lethal when 93 or more and left untreated. The df is calculated as follows:

$$\mathrm{df} = 4.6 \times (\text{prothrombin time, in seconds}) + \text{serum total bilirubin, mg/dL}$$

As another markers of hepatic function, Indocyanine Green clearance correlated significantly with Child-Pugh's classification (r = 0.86, p = 0.0001) and antipyrine clearance correlated significantly with Child-Pugh's classification (r = 0.67, p = 0.0003).

Dose Adjustment Recommendation

There are three classifications for the hepatic contribution to the elimination of the drug which are: no hepatic contribution, limited (<20 %) hepatic elimination, and extensive (>20 %) hepatic elimination.

Taxanes, vinca alkaloids, irinotecan, and anthracyclines may generate unacceptable toxicity in patients with poor hepatic function. Continuous infusion of 5-fluorouracil, capecitabine, mechlorethamine, cyclophosphamide, topotecan, and oxaliplatin are relatively well tolerated in patients with hepatic dysfunction [40].

Both the Food and Drug Administration (FDA) and the European medicines Agency (EMEA) have published an industry guideline about pharmacokinetics of medical products in patients with impaired hepatic function. These guidelines recommend that the Child-Pugh classification could categorize patients according to their degree of hepatic dysfunction and exogenous markers might be used to assess the elimination capacity by different mechanisms.

Some general considerations were recommended by Verbeeck for patients with hepatic dysfunction [41] and can apply to anticancer agents as well:

1. Drugs with a relatively high hepatic extraction ratio: the oral bioavailability of these drugs can be drastically increased in patients with chronic liver disease, and the dosage should be reduced accordingly. Following systemic administration (iv, im, sc, etc.), the plasma clearance may be reduced if hepatic blood flow is decreased.
2. Drugs with a low hepatic extraction and high plasma protein binding (>90 %): the oral and intravenous clearance of these drugs is determined by the intrinsic capacity of the hepatic elimination mechanisms and the unbound drug fraction in blood or plasma. The intrinsic clearance will be reduced to a degree determined by the fractional status of the liver and the specific metabolic pathways involved in the elimination of the drug. Because the unbound fraction of drug in blood or plasma may be significantly increased in patients with chronic liver disease, pharmacokinetic evaluation should be based on the unbound blood/plasma concentrations and dosage adjustment may be necessary even though total blood/plasma concentrations are within the normal range.

3. Drugs with a low hepatic extraction ratio and low plasma protein binding (<90 %): the oral and intravenous clearance of these drugs is determined by the intrinsic capacity of the hepatic elimination mechanisms and unbound drug fraction in blood or plasma. The intrinsic clearance will be reduced to a degree determined by the functional status of the liver and the specific metabolic pathways involved in the elimination of the drug. Fluctuations in the unbound drug fraction in blood or plasma are rather small and will not significantly affect blood/plasma clearance of the drug. Dosage adjustment may be necessary and should be aimed at maintaining normal total (bound and unbound) plasma concentrations.
4. The elimination of drugs that are partly excreted in unchanged form by the kidneys will be impaired in patients with the hepato-renal syndrome. It should be taken into account that creatinine clearance significantly overestimates glomerular filtration rate in these patients.
5. The volume of distribution of hydrophilic drugs may be increased in patients with chronic liver disease who have edema or ascites. As a consequence, the loading dose may have to be increased in these patients if a rapid and complete effect of the drug is required. Since many hydrophilic drugs are eliminated primarily in unchanged form by the kidneys, renal function should be taken into consideration.
6. Extreme caution is recommended when using drugs with a narrow therapeutic index in patients with liver disease and when administering any drug to patients with severe liver dysfunction (Child-Pugh class C).

5.3.2.3 Life Expectancy and Outcomes

In a prospective study of the impact of liver cirrhosis on the outcome of ovarian cancer, compensated liver cirrhosis (Child-Pugh class A) affected neither disease-free survival (95 % CI, 19.9–26.7 months vs. 19.4–26.1 months, $p = 0.719$) nor overall survival (95 % CI, 21.6–25.7 months vs. 21.1–25.1 months $p = 0.524$) in ovarian cancer patients treated with debulking surgery followed by adjuvant chemotherapy with paclitaxel (175 mg/m^2) and carboplatin (AUC, 5) compared those without liver disease [42].

An Italian study of established cirrhosis and hepatocellular carcinoma treated with sorafenib demonstrated that treatment duration or incidence of adverse event between Child-Pugh class A and class B were not significantly different [43]. A retrospective study of sorafenib for advanced hepatocellular carcinoma patients with Child-Pugh class B liver cirrhosis observed that overall survival was significantly different among class A, class B score 7, and class B score 8–9 (6.1 vs. 5.4 vs. 2.7 months, $p = 0.002$) but progression-free survival was similar among them (3.2 vs. 3.2 vs. 2.3 months, $p = 0.26$) [44]. Among them, most of adverse events had a similar incidence except anemia, gastrointestinal bleeding and hepatic encephalopathy, which developed in class B score 8–9.

A retrospective study investigated prevalence, complication after oncologic treatment, and prognostic predictors of nonhepatic cancer in patients with liver cirrhosis [39]. The prevalence of nonhepatic cancer was 19.8 % and was mainly colorectal cancer, prostate cancer, and tobacco-related cancers. Low bilirubin ($p = 0.01$), normal albumin ($p = 0.005$), and absence of ascites ($p < 0.0001$) were related significantly to longer survival. In that study, Child-Pugh classification and MELD score were suitable parameters to predict mortality. The rate of post-interventional death after specific treatment was high although all patients with long-term survival received specific oncologic treatment.

5.3.3 Immunologic Disorders

5.3.3.1 Immunologic Disorders and Their Incidence

Examples of autoimmune diseases are rheumatic arthritis, systemic lupus erythematosus, antiphospholipid syndrome, multiple sclerosis, scleroderma, primary biliary cirrhosis, autoimmune hepatitis, Graves' disease, Hashimoto's thyroiditis, and Sjogren's disease. Immunologic disorders usually involve joint organs and most of the assessments of comorbidity classify immunologic diseases in the musculoskeletal category.

According to Cumulative Illness Rating Scale-Geriatrics, autoimmune disease is considered to be in the musculoskeletal/integument category (Table 5.4). There are five rating scores which range from 0 with no problem to 4 with severe joint deformity. Their severity is determined by their function of activity in daily life. In the Kaplan-Feinstein Index, locomotive impairment is considered as a cogent comorbidity and its severity is defined by the level of limitation of activity. The Adult Comorbidity Evaluation-27 includes rheumatologic disease as comorbidity with four levels of severity of none to severe. The Index of Coexistent Disease scale includes arthritis with four levels of severity.

In the National Cancer Institute/National Institute on Aging Life-Threat Model, arthritis is considered as a negligible to low impact comorbidity, depending on active management. In the Charlson comorbidity index, connective tissue disease, including systemic lupus erythematosus (SLE), polymyositis, mixed connective tissue disease (CTD), polymyalgia rheumatica, and moderate to severe rheumatoid arthritis (RA) rate 1 point.

In this chapter, we will focus on rheumatoid arthritis as an example of autoimmune diseases (Table 5.4).

According to a cancer registry study by Piccirillo et al. [23], the prevalence of reported rheumatologic disease was 1.8 % in cancer patients. By annual report including four solid tumors patients of 65 years and older diagnosed between 1992 and 2005, the incidence of rheumatologic disease was 2.0 % [38]. A study of

Table 5.4 Assessment of immunologic disorder in several comorbidity indexes

Measurement	Grade 1	Grade 2	Grade 3	Grade 4
CIRS-G	Uses prn meds for arthritis; mild limited ADL's from joint pathology	Daily antiarthritic meds; use of assistive devices; moderate limitation in ADL's	Severely impaired ADL's secondary to arthritis; requires steroids for arthritic condition	Wheelchair bound' severe joint deformity or severe impaired usage
Kaplan-Feinstein Index	Slightly impaired (some limitation of activity)	Moderate impaired (confined to home, nursing home, or convalescent setting)	Bed-to-chair existence	–
AEC-27	CTD on NSAIDS or no treatment	CTD on steroids or immunosuppressant medications	CTD with secondary end-organ failure (renal, cardiac, CNS)	–
NCI/NIA Life-Threat Model	No current management/history only: arthritis	Under active management: arthritis	–	–
Charlson comorbidity index	SLE; polymyositis; mixed CTD; polymyalgia rheumatic; moderate to severe RA	–	–	–

ADL activity of daily livings; *CTD* connective tissue disorder

Hodgkin's lymphoma with pre-existing autoimmune disease reported an incidence of autoimmune diseases to be 2.7 % among [45]. On the other hand, cancer incidence among patients with rheumatoid arthritis has been reported as high, especially lymphoid malignancies (standardized incidence ratios, SIR = 2.0, 95 % CI, 1.5–2.6) [46].

5.3.3.2 Treatment Decision Making with Immunologic Disorders

Cancer patients may develop rheumatic manifestations after chemotherapy [47]. Patients receiving adjuvant chemotherapy with cyclophosphamide combined with either methotrexate and fluorouracil or doxorubicin and fluorouracil experienced myalgia, arthralgia, and tenosynovitis [48]. Tamoxifen has been known to be associated with occasional rheumatic symptoms [49]. Aromatase inhibitors can be associated with arthralgias and tenosynovitis [50] Bleomycin, vinblastine, cisplatin,

5-fluorouracil have been associated with Raynaud's phenomenon [51, 52]. Interferon-α and -γ have been associated with the generation of auto-antibodies and the induction of autoimmune disorders [53–55]. Recently developed checkpoint inhibitors, for example, ipilimumab, pembrolizumab, nivolumab and lambrolizumab, have toxic immune-mediated effects such as pneumonitis, colitis, and hepatitis [56–58], linked to their mechanism of breaking immune tolerance. Patients with preexisting autoimmune disorders were excluded from clinical trials, and therefore no information is available about the potential of these drugs for flare ups of an underlying autoimmune disease.

5.3.3.3 Life Expectancy and Outcomes

In a prospective study of survival outcomes in non-Hodgkin's lymphoma patients with rheumatoid arthritis, RA patients with NHL had similar overall survival compared with non-RA controls (HR = 0.95, 95 % CI, 0.70–1.30) [59]. In the study, RA with HNL had low risk of lymphoma progression or relapse (HR = 0.41, 95 % CI, 0.25–0.68) and of lymphoma or treatment-related death (HR = 0.60, 95 % CI, 0.37–0.98), but had a more than double the risk of death from causes unrelated to lymphoma, compared with non-RA controls (HR = 2.16, 95 % CI, 1.33–3.50). The median duration of RA disease was 14 years and 95 % of RA patients had prior Disease-Modifying Anti-Rheumatic Drug (DMARD) use, including methotrexate, hydroxychloroquine, gold salt, sulfasalazine, azathioprine, and others.

A study of survival patterns in patients with Hodgkin's lymphoma with a pre-existing autoimmune disease observed that Hodgkin's lymphoma patients with autoimmune disease had a high risk for death compared with those without autoimmune disease (HR = 1.8, 95 % CI, 1.3–2.4 for women, and HR = 1.7, 95 % CI, 1.3–2.2 for men) [45]. The most common causes of death were lymphoma and treatment-related complications (76 % of women and 68 % of men) in the study.

5.3.4 Cardiovascular Disorders

5.3.4.1 Cardiovascular Disorders and Their Incidence

Cardiovascular diseases are coronary artery disease, congestive heart failure, arrhythmia, valvular disease, pericardial disease, hypertension, and peripheral atherosclerotic disease.

According to Cumulative Illness Rating Scale-Geriatrics, heart and vascular comorbidity are separate categories (Table 5.5). There are five rating scores which range from 0—no problem to 4—intractable congestive heart failure for heart category or previous surgery for vascular category. The Kaplan-Feinstein Index considers cardiovascular disorder as a cogent comorbidity and its ailments are

Table 5.5 Assessment of cardiovascular disorders in several comorbidity indexes

Measurement	Grade 1	Grade 2	Grade 3	Grade 4
CIRS-G Heart category	Remote MI (>5 years ago); occasional angina treated with prn meds	CHF compensated with meds; daily anti-angina meds; left ventricular hypertrophy; atrial fibrillation; bundle branch block; daily antiarrhythmic drugs	Previous MI < 5 years; abnormal stress test; s/p PCA or CABG; bifasicular block; pacemaker for cardiogenic syncope	Marked activity restriction secondary to cardiac status (i.e., unstable angina or intractable congestive heart failure)
CIRS-G Vascular category	Hypertension compensated with salt restriction and weight loss; serum cholesterol with normal range	Daily antihypertensive meds; one symptom of atherosclerotic disease (angina, claudication, bruit, amaurosis fugax, absent pedal pulses); aortic aneurysm <4 cm	Two or more symptoms of atherosclerosis; two or more antihypertensive drugs for control; evidence of left ventricular hypertrophy	Previous surgery for vascular problem; aortic aneurysm >4 cm
Kaplan-Feinstein Index Cardiac ailment	MI more than 6 months ago; ECG evidence of coronary disease; or atrial fibrillation	CHF more than 6 months ago; or angina pectoris not requiring hospitalization	Within past 6 months; CHF, MI, significant arrhythmias, or hospitalization required for angina pectoris or angina-like chest pain	–
Kaplan-Feinstein Index Hypertension	DBP 90-114 mmHg, without secondary effects or symptoms	DBP 115-129 mmHg; or at any level below 130, with secondary cardiovascular or symptomatic effects such as headaches, vertigo, epistaxis	Severe or malignant; papilledema; encephalopathy; or DBP 130 mm Hg or higher	–
Kaplan-Feinstein Index Peripheral vascular ailment	Old amputation; intermittent claudication	Recent amputation or gangrene of extremity	–	–
AEC-27 MI	Old MI on ECG only, age undetermined	MI >6 months ago	MI ≤6 months	–

(continued)

Table 5.5 (continued)

Measurement	Grade 1	Grade 2	Grade 3	Grade 4
CAD	ECG/stress/angio evidence of CAD without symptoms; angina not requiring hosp.; CABG, PCA, stent >6 months prior	Chronic exertional angina; CABG, PCA, stent ≤6 months	Unstable angina	
CHF	CHF with dyspnea that responded to TX; exertional dyspnea, paroxysmal mocturnal dyspnea	Hosp for CHF >6 months prior; CHF w/dyspnea limiting ADLs	Hosp for CHF < 6 months; EF <20 %	
Arrhythmias	Sick sinus syndrome	Ventricular arrhythmia >6 months ago; chronic AFib/flutter; pacemaker	Ventricular arrhythmia ≤ 6 months ago	
Hypertension	DBP 90–114; DBP <90 on medication	DBP 115–129; Secondary CV symptoms: vertico, epistaxis, HA	DBP >130; severe malignant papilledema/eye changes; encephalopathy	
Venous disease	Old DVT no longer treated	DVT controlled with Coumadin or heparin; old PE >6 months	Recent PE ≤6 months; venous filter for PE	
PAD	Intermittent claudication; untreated thoracic or abdominal aneuvrysm (<6 cm); s/p abdominal or thoracic aortic repair	Bypass or amputation for gangrene or arterial insufficiency >6 months ago; chronic insufficiency	Bypass or amputation for gangrene or arterial insufficiency ≤ 6 months ago; untreated thoracic or abdominal aneurysm >6 cm	

(continued)

Table 5.5 (continued)

Measurement	Grade 1	Grade 2	Grade 3	Grade 4
NCI/NIA Life-Threat Model		No current management/history only; arrhythmias, hypertension	No current management/history only; angina, MI, valvular disease: Under active management; DVT, hypertension	No current management/history only; cardiac arrest, congestive heart failure Under active management; angina, arrhythmias, cardiac arrest, CHF, MI, valve disease
Charlson comorbidity index	History of MI, symptomatic CHF with response to specific treatment; intermittent claudication, peripheral arterial bypass for insufficiency, gangrene, acute arterial insufficiency, untreated aneurysm (≥6 cm)	–	–	–

AFib atrial fibrillation, *CABG* coronary artery bypass graft; *CAD* coronary artery disease, *CHF* congestive heart failure; *DBP* diastolic blood pressure; *DVT* deep vein thrombosis; *HA* headaches; *hosp*. hospitalization; *MI* myocardial infarct; *PAD* peripheral arterial disease, *PCA* percutaneous angioplasty divided into cardiac, hypertension, and peripheral vascular disease. Adult Comorbidity Evaluation-27 includes 7 categories of cardiovascular diseases, which are hypertension, angina, myocardial infarction, arrhythmias, congestive heart failure, peripheral vascular disease, and venous disease as comorbidity with four levels of severity from none to severe. The Index of Coexistent Disease scales includes five categories of cardiovascular diseases, which are organic heart disease, ischemic heart disease, primary arrhythmias and conduction problems, congestive heart failure, and hypertension with four levels of severity.

In the National Cancer Institute/National Institute on Aging Life-Threat Model, cardiovascular disorder is considered as low to high impact comorbidity, depending on disease severity and active management. By the Charlson comorbidity index, cardiovascular disease, including myocardial infarct, congestive heart failure, and peripheral vascular disease, rates 1 point.

The prevalence of cardiovascular disease has been reported ranging from 12 % to 60 % in cancer patients [60]. According to a cancer registry study by Piccirillo et al., the prevalence of hypertension was 40.2 %, and the most common comorbidity in cancer patients [23] and a 71.9 % prevalence of cardiovascular disorders was observed. By annual report, including four solid tumors patients with 65 years and older diagnosed between 1992 and 2005, the incidence of cardiovascular disease was 17.3 %, including 9.7 % of congestive heart failure, 4.3 % of peripheral vascular disease, and 3.3 % of myocardial infarction [38]. The prevalence of the CIRS-G heart category in a secondary analysis of clinical trials including six solid tumors, was 36.3 % and that of the vascular category was 78.4 % [37].

5.3.4.2 Treatment Decision Making in Patients with Cardiovascular Disorder

Numerous chemotherapies, targeted therapies, and hormonal therapies are associated with cardiovascular toxicity, and have been reviewed by others [61–64]. The literature is sparser concerning the management of patients with pre-existing cardiovascular disease.

Congestive Heart Failure (CHF)

CHF is mostly an issue with anthracycline-based regimens. Older patients are at higher cumulative risk of CHF with anthracyclines. A study by [65] showed that while the risk of CHF was low up to 400 mg/m^2 for all patients, patients aged over 65 had a HR of 3.28 of developing CHF beyond that cumulative threshold, compared to younger patients. Whereas for some diseases, such as breast cancer, some good alternatives exist, for other diseases, such as diffuse large B-cell lymphoma (DLBCL), no first line regimen has demonstrated the same curative potential as CHOP-R. In a recent review of 859 DLBCL patients, about 5 % had a preexisting heart failure, half systolic, half diastolic. Patients with diastolic heart failure received CHOP-like regimens more frequently than the others. 24 % of cardiac events were observed, defined as hospitalization for CHF, for cerebrovascular insult, for chest pain, for ischemic or non-ischemic cardiac events or cardiac-related deaths, in the group treated with R-CHOP, vs. 16.7 % in the non-R-CHOP group, but this was not statistically significant (*p* value 0.7), given low patient numbers. Overall, 90.9 % of the patients treated with a non-R-CHOP chemotherapy completed the planned treatment versus 58.3 % in the R-CHOP group (*p* value 0.09). Although patients treated with a R-CHOP regimen tended to have higher complete remission rates compared to non R-CHOP regimens (73.7 % vs. 55.5 % respectively), this result was not statistically significant ($p = 0.37$), and there was no significant difference in overall survival or 2-year relapse free survival, but the numbers were small [66]. Regimens needing intense hydration can be a challenge, especially in patients with decreased diastolic relaxation.

To minimize the anthracycline cardiotoxicity, one can use less cardiotoxic therapies, for example continuous infusion, use of epirubicin, desrazoxane, liposomal anthracycline formulation, or sequential administration of conventional anthracyclines and trastuzumab in HER2-positive breast cancer [67].

Coronary Artery Disease

A large SEER registry study identified coronary artery disease as a risk factor for chemotherapy-induced CHF in older women (HR, 1.58; 95 % CI, 1.39–1.79), independent of age, race, diabetes, and hypertension. However, that series did not report the ejection fraction of patients with coronary artery disease (CAD), or the proportion of patients that had an actual myocardial infarction [68]. A recent study assessed the risk of CHF after anthracycline therapy and found a significant association of CAD with CHF (11.8 % early CHF, 17.4 % late CHF, vs. 3.1 % in the control group ($p < 0.01$) [69]. There is to our knowledge no study that assessed whether pre-existing CAD with a normal cardiac muscle function led to a higher incidence of anthracycline-induced CHF. In the absence of decreased ejection fraction, most oncologists would give anthracyclines if essential to the treatment plan, but there might be an increased risk of CHF. On the other hand, fluoropyrimidines, such as 5-FU and capecitabine, can induce coronary vasospasm, which are most frequently asymptomatic and should be used with caution in patients with preexisting CAD [70].

Arrhythmia Management

In clinical experience, patients with a well-compensated arrhythmia typically fare well with chemotherapy. Although some arrhythmias, such as atrial fibrillation, are very frequent in the elderly, we couldn't find literature exploring their impact on chemotherapy tolerance. For patients on full anticoagulation, it might be wise to choose chemotherapy agents that minimize anemia and platelets toxicity to prevent bleeding. Caution should be exercised with many new agents, notably kinase inhibitors, which can lead to QT prolongation. A careful review of potential drug interactions is warranted. In patients receiving arsenic trioxide, potassium levels should be maintained at 4.0 mg/dl or above, and magnesium levels should also be maintained at 1.8 mg/dl or above.

5.3.4.3 Life Expectancy and Outcomes

A retrospective study of treatment of DLBCL patients with preexisting congestive heart failure, including either systolic or diastolic heart failure, observed that elderly patients with DLBCL and baseline systolic CHF were more likely to receive non R-CHOP (rituximab, cyclophosphamide, doxorubicin, vincristine, and prednisolone) based regimens, compared to patients with diastolic dysfunction and non R-CHOP treatments seemed to be better tolerated, without any obvious differences in outcome (the numbers were small) [66]. A study of lung cancer and comorbid illness [71] demonstrated that 18 % of patients with CHF received chemotherapy in comparison with 36 % of those without comorbid illness. In this study, patients with CHF had a significantly decreased survival rate (HR = 1.38, 95 % CI, 1.18–1.62) in multivariate analysis. A study of colon cancer patients reported that the use of adjuvant chemotherapy was 36.2 % in patients with heart failure compared to 64.9 % of those without heart failure [72]. Among patients with heart failure, the 5-year survival was significantly higher in patients treated with adjuvant chemotherapy (43, 95 % CI, 40–47 % vs. 30, 95 % CI, 27–34 %). A study of breast cancer patients showed that patients with early stage disease and CHF had significantly poorer survival (HR = 1.89, 95 % CI, 1.44–2.48) [73].

5.3.5 Diabetes

5.3.5.1 Diabetes and Its Incidence

With the rise in obesity in the US, the prevalence of metabolic syndrome is 40 % in patients above the age of 65 (NHANES). The prevalence of diabetes is also rapidly increasing and was 20 % for patients above the age of 65 in 2014 (CDC, accessed 1/18/2016 http://www.cdc.gov/diabetes/statistics/prev/national/figbyage.htm).

In the CIRS-G and ACE 27, diabetes is rated by level of control. The Kaplan-Feinstein index was designed for diabetic patients, so diabetes is not included in the comorbidity rating. In the NIA/NCI index, the impact of diabetes is considered negligible if untreated; low if treated (medication unknown in SEER registry); and high if insulin-treated. The Charlson score attributes 1 point to diabetes without complications, and 2 points to diabetes with end-organ complications (Table 5.6).

Table 5.6 Assessment of diabetes in several comorbidity indexes

Measurement	Grade 1	Grade 2	Grade 3	Grade 4
CIRS-G	DM controlled with diet	Insulin or oral agents required	Intermediate level of severity between 2 and 4	Brittle or poorly controlled diabetes. Hx of diabetic coma in past year
Kaplan-Feinstein Index	N/A (the index was developed for diabetic patients)			
AEC-27	NIDDM controlled by oral agents	IDDM without complications; poorly controlled NIDDM	Hosp ≤6 months for keto-acidosis; diabetes with end-organ failure	–
NCI/NIA Life-Threat Model	untreated	On active management (meds unknown)	–	On insulin
Charlson comorbidity index	Diabetes without complication	Diabetes with end organ damage	–	–

(N)IDDM (non) insulin-dependent diabetes mellitus

5.3.5.2 Treatment Decision Making with Diabetes

Toxicity Issues

Many chemotherapy regimens contain high-dose steroids. Since they are given for one day only (most of the time), there is little literature on acute effects. Other regimens give it for five days. Temporary insulin regimens to control steroid-induced hyperglycemia have been proposed. In a study of 40 diabetic patients with hematologic malignancies receiving dexamethasone, intravenous or oral, for three days, a baseline and bolus regimen with insulin detemir and aspart produced better glycemic control than a sliding scale insulin regimen. Three keto-acidoses developed in the sliding scale insulin group versus 0 in the baseline/bolus group [74].

Diabetic patients have increased toxicity from chemotherapy. In a study, diabetic patients were shown to have an increased severity and a delayed recovery of paclitaxel-induced peripheral neuropathy [75] (Morena-Barrio 15). In another study, older patients treated with CHOP for NHL or docetaxel for prostate cancer were assessed for the impact of diabetes and hyperglycemia on toxicity. In both populations, hyperglycemia during chemotherapy was associated with the occurrence of severe toxicity. For prostate cancer patients, a known diagnosis of diabetes was also associated with the occurrence of severe toxicity [76].

5.3.5.3 Life Expectancy and Outcomes

A secondary analysis of a large randomized trial showed that diabetic patients treated with a 5-FU based adjuvant chemotherapy had a shorter PFS, EFS and OS than patients without diabetes [77]. In the study on NHL and prostate cancer patients mentioned above, neither a known diagnosis of diabetes nor hyperglycemia during treatment were associated with PFS or OS [76]. Among diabetic patients, the type of treatment they receive might influence the prognosis of their cancer. Diabetic prostate cancer patients who take metformin seem to have a lesser risk of recurrence [78]. Similar results have been found in colorectal and pancreatic cancer patients [79, 80]. Diabetic breast cancer patients on metformin have a better CR rate on chemotherapy than other diabetic patients or non-diabetic patients [81]. Prospective studies are ongoing.

5.3.6 Prediction of Chemotherapy-Induced Toxicity in the Elderly

5.3.6.1 MAX2 Index

The MAX2 index [82–84] was evaluated to assess the average per patient risk for chemotherapy toxicity. Severe toxicity is defined as grade 4 hematologic toxicity and/or grade 3 and 4 non-hematologic toxicity by common terminology criteria for adverse events version 3.0.

The MAX2 index is defined as follows:

$$\frac{\text{Most frequent grade 4 hematologic toxicity} + \text{most frequent grade 3 and 4 non-hematologic toxicity}}{2}$$

The MAX 2 value for a regimen should be derived from three published studies which had at least 20 patients with a reliable reporting of toxicity. The most useful studies are the ones that provide a separate reporting of grade 4 absolute neutrophil count. Among non-hematologic toxicities, alopecia is excluded. Febrile neutropenia counts as a non-hematologic toxicity.

If ANC was not reported, ANC is extracted as follows:

$0.6 \times (\text{G3} + 4 \text{ leucopenia})$ if G4 leukopenia $< 30\,\%$
$0.8 \times (\text{G3} + 4 \text{ leucopenia})$ if G4 leukopenia is $30\,\%$ or higher

When the MAX2 index was evaluated for validation with ECOG trials, the association of the MAX2 index with the patient incidence of grade 4 hematologic and/or grade 3 and 4 non-hematologic toxicity was highly significant for the overall group and for the elderly subgroup.

5.3.6.2 CRASH (Chemotherapy Risk Assessment Scale for High-Age Patients) Score

The CRASH score [85] was constructed in a prospective multicentric study in patients aged 70 years and older. Severe chemotherapy toxicity was defined as grade 4 hematologic toxicity or grade 3 and 4 non-hematologic toxicity according to Common Terminology Criteria for Adverse Events version 3.0. In the study, 64 % of patients experienced severe toxicity. Hematologic and non-hematologic toxicities had different predictors, and therefore the CRASH score consists of two sub-scales, which are hematologic toxicity and non-hematologic toxicity. The best predictive model for hematologic toxicity includes diastolic blood pressure (>72 mmHg; 1 point), instrumental activities of daily living (<26; 1 point), the level of LDH (equal or more than 0.75 × upper normal limit; 2 points), and toxicity of regimen. The best predictive model for non-hematologic toxicity included ECOG performance status (PS 1-2; 1 point: PS 3-4; 2 points), mini-mental status score (<30; 2 points), mini-nutritional assessment score (<28; 2 points), and toxicity of regimen. Toxicity of regimen is based on the MAX2 index. According to the level of MAX2 index, the risk of toxicity of a regimen is divided into three categories from 0 to 2.

The CRASH *score and MAX2 index are available on-line at the following website:*

https://moffitt.org/tests-treatments/treatments/senior-adult-oncology-program/senior adult-oncology-program-tools/.

5.3.6.3 The CARG (Cancer and Aging Research Group) Score

Another toxicity risk predictive score is the CARG score [86]. This score defines severe toxicity as grade 3–5 by CTCAE. The adjustment for toxicity of chemotherapy was made by classifying it as single agents vs. combination, standard vs. reduced dose, and by tumor type. The predictors of toxicity are: creatinine clearance <34 ml/min, one or more falls in the past 6 months (3 points), age ≥72 years, GI or GU cancer, standard dose chemotherapy, polychemotherapy, hearing fair or worse, somewhat or a lot limited in walking a block (2 points), taking medications with some help/unable, limited at least some time in social activity because of physical/emotional health (1 point). A score of 0–5 is low-risk, 6–9 represents a medium risk, and a score of between 10 and 19 represents a high risk. Validation is ongoing in a CALGB trial. The score can be found online at http://www.mycarg.org/Chemo_Toxicity_Calculator.

5.4 Summary and future direction for research and practice

In conclusion, we have provided some elements to address the impact of comorbidity on survival, as well as the management of individual comorbidities in cancer treatment. More research work needs to be done, notably on the impact of multimorbidity and on other outcomes, such as relapse, progression, tolerance to chemotherapy and functional recovery or maintenance. New tools need to be developed to identify clusters of diseases with the highest impact on these outcomes.

References

1. Howlader N NA, Krapcho M, Garshell J, Miller D, Altekruse SF, Kosary CL, Yu M, Ruhl J, Tatalovich Z, Mariotto A, Lewis DR, Chen HS, Feuer EJ, Cronin KA (eds) SEER cancer statistics review, 1975–2012. National Cancer Institute, Bethesda, MD. http://seer.cancer.gov/csr/1975_2012/, Apr 2015
2. Extermann M, Overcash J, Lyman GH et al (1998) Comorbidity and functional status are independent in older cancer patients. J Clin Oncol 16:1582–1587
3. Extermann M (2000) Measuring comorbidity in older cancer patients. Eur J Cancer 36:453–471
4. Extermann M (2000) Measurement and impact of comorbidity in older cancer patients. Crit Rev Oncol Hematol 35:181–200
5. Anderson G, Kerluke K (1996) Distribution of prescription drug exposures in the elderly: description and implications. J Clin Epidemiol 49:929–935
6. Kennerfalk A, Ruigomez A, Wallander MA et al (2002) Geriatric drug therapy and healthcare utilization in the United kingdom. Ann Pharmacother 36:797–803
7. Beaufrere B, Morio B (2000) Fat and protein redistribution with aging: metabolic considerations. Eur J Clin Nutr 54(Suppl 3):S48–53
8. McLean AJ, Le Couteur DG (2004) Aging biology and geriatric clinical pharmacology. Pharmacol Rev 56:163–184
9. Balducci L, Extermann M (1997) Cancer chemotherapy in the older patient: what the medical oncologist needs to know. Cancer 80:1317–1322
10. Walter LC, Schonberg MA (2014) Screening mammography in older women: a review. JAMA 311:1336–1347
11. Cho H, Klabunde CN, Yabroff KR et al (2013) Comorbidity-adjusted life expectancy: a new tool to inform recommendations for optimal screening strategies. Ann Intern Med 159:667–676
12. Jatoi I, Chen BE, Anderson WF, Rosenberg PS (2007) Breast cancer mortality trends in the United States according to estrogen receptor status and age at diagnosis. J Clin Oncol 25:1683–1690
13. Kristjansson SR, Rønning B, Hurria A et al (2012) A comparison of two pre-operative frailty measures in older surgical cancer patients. J Geriatr Oncol 3:1–7
14. Tucci A, Ferrari S, Bottelli C et al (2009) A comprehensive geriatric assessment is more effective than clinical judgment to identify elderly diffuse large cell lymphoma patients who benefit from aggressive therapy. Cancer 115:4547–4553
15. Extermann M, Wedding U (2012) Comorbidity and geriatric assessment for older patients with hematologic malignancies: a review of the evidence. J Geriatr Oncol 3:49–57

16. Charlson ME, Pompei P, Ales KL, MacKenzie CR (1987) A new method of classifying prognostic comorbidity in longitudinal studies: development and validation. J Chronic Dis 40:373–383
17. Kaplan MH, Feinstein AR (1974) The importance of classifying initial co-morbidity in evaluating the outcome of diabetes mellitus. J Chronic Dis 27:387–404
18. Miller MD, Paradis CF, Houck PR et al (1992) Rating chronic medical illness burden in geropsychiatric practice and research: application of the Cumulative Illness Rating Scale. Psychiatry Res 41:237–248
19. Miller M, Tower A (1991) A manual of guidelines for scoring the cumulative illness rating scale for geriatrics (CIRS-G). University of Pittsburgh, Pittsburgh, PA
20. Greenfield S, Blanco DM, Elashoff RM, Ganz PA (1987) Patterns of care related to age of breast cancer patients. JAMA 257:2766–2770
21. Wallace K, Overcash J, Yoder J, Vranas P, Extermann M (2005) Influence of concomitant medications on toxicity from chemotherapy in elderly patients. Focus on cytochrome P-450 inhibition and protein binding effects. Proc Am Soc Clin Oncol 23:735s
22. Popa MA, Wallace KJ, Brunello A et al (2014) Potential drug interactions and chemotoxicity in older patients with cancer receiving chemotherapy. J Geriatr Oncol 5:307–314
23. Piccirillo JF, Costas I, Claybour P et al (2003) The measurement of comorbidity by Cancer Registries
24. Yancik R, Wesley MN, Ries LA et al (1998) Comorbidity and age as predictors of risk for early mortality of male and female colon carcinoma patients: a population-based study. Cancer 82:2123–2134
25. Charlson ME, Sax FL, MacKenzie CR et al (1986) Assessing illness severity: does clinical judgment work? J Chronic Dis 39:439–452
26. Launay-Vacher V, Oudard S, Janus N et al (2007) Prevalence of renal insufficiency in cancer patients and implications for anticancer drug management: the renal insufficiency and anticancer medications (IRMA) study. Cancer 110:1376–1384
27. Foundation NK (2002) K/DOQI clinical practice guidelines for chronic kidney disease: evaluation, classification, and stratification. Am J Kidney Dis 39:S1–266
28. Giannelli SV, Patel KV, Windham BG et al (2007) Magnitude of underascertainment of impaired kidney function in older adults with normal serum creatinine. J Am Geriatr Soc 55:816–823
29. Launay-Vacher V, Chatelut E, Lichtman SM et al (2007) Renal insufficiency in elderly cancer patients: International Society of Geriatric Oncology clinical practice recommendations. Ann Oncol Off J Eur Soc Med Oncol/ESMO 18:1314–1321
30. Kintzel PE, Dorr RT (1995) Anticancer drug renal toxicity and elimination: dosing guidelines for altered renal function. Cancer Treat Rev 21:33–64
31. Lichtman SM, Wildiers H, Launay-Vacher V et al (2007) International Society of Geriatric Oncology (SIOG) recommendations for the adjustment of dosing in elderly cancer patients with renal insufficiency. Eur J Cancer 43:14–34
32. Launay-Vacher V, Chatelut E, Lichtman SM et al (2007) Renal insufficiency in elderly cancer patients: International Society of Geriatric Oncology clinical practice recommendations. Ann Oncol 18:1314–1321
33. Chen J, Wang XT, Luo PH, He QJ (2015) Effects of unidentified renal insufficiency on the safety and efficacy of chemotherapy for metastatic colorectal cancer patients: a prospective, observational study. Support Care Cancer 23:1043–1048
34. Ichioka D, Miyazaki J, Inoue T et al (2015) Impact of renal function of patients with advanced urothelial cancer on eligibility for first-line chemotherapy and treatment outcomes. Jpn J Clin Oncol 45:867–873
35. Langer CJ, Hirsh V, Ko A et al (2015) Weekly nab-paclitaxel in combination with carboplatin as first-line therapy in patients with advanced non-small-cell lung cancer: analysis of safety and efficacy in patients with renal impairment. Clin Lung Cancer 16:112–120

36. Lichtman SM, Cirrincione CT, Hurria A et al. (2016) Effect of pretreatment renal function on treatment and clinical outcomes in the adjuvant treatment of older women with breast cancer: alliance A171201, an Ancillary Study of CALGB/CTSU 49907. J Clin Oncol
37. Lee JJ, Kim J, Sehovic M, Extermann M (2015) The association of comorbidity with toxicities and clinical outcomes in elderly cancer patients treated with chemotherapy using heat maps: preliminary results. SIOG
38. Edwards BK, Noone AM, Mariotto AB et al (2014) Annual Report to the Nation on the status of cancer, 1975–2010, featuring prevalence of comorbidity and impact on survival among persons with lung, colorectal, breast, or prostate cancer. Cancer 120:1290–1314
39. Gundling F, Seidl H, Schmidtler F et al (2011) Nonhepatic cancer in liver cirrhosis: a retrospective study of prevalence, complication rate after specific oncological treatment, follow-up and prognostic predictors of outcome in 354 patients with cirrhosis. Anticancer Res 31:2931–2938
40. Eklund JW, Trifilio S, Mulcahy MF (2005) Chemotherapy dosing in the setting of liver dysfunction. Oncology (Williston Park) 19:1057–1063; discussion 1063–1064, 1069
41. Verbeeck RK (2008) Pharmacokinetics and dosage adjustment in patients with hepatic dysfunction. Eur J Clin Pharmacol 64:1147–1161
42. Refky B, Kotb S, Fady T et al (2015) Impact of liver cirrhosis due to chronic hepatitis C viral infection on the outcome of ovarian cancer: a prospective study. BMC Cancer 15:754
43. Inghilesi AL, Gallori D, Antonuzzo L et al (2014) Predictors of survival in patients with established cirrhosis and hepatocellular carcinoma treated with sorafenib. World J Gastroenterol 20:786–794
44. Chiu J, Tang YF, Yao TJ et al (2012) The use of single-agent sorafenib in the treatment of advanced hepatocellular carcinoma patients with underlying Child-Pugh B liver cirrhosis: a retrospective analysis of efficacy, safety, and survival benefits. Cancer 118:5293–5301
45. Landgren O, Pfeiffer RM, Kristinsson SY, Bjorkholm M (2010) Survival patterns in patients with Hodgkin's lymphoma with a pre-existing hospital discharge diagnosis of autoimmune disease. J Clin Oncol 28:5081–5087
46. Gridley G, McLaughlin JK, Ekbom A et al (1993) Incidence of cancer among patients with rheumatoid arthritis. J Natl Cancer Inst 85:307–311
47. Abu-Shakra M, Buskila D, Ehrenfeld M et al (2001) Cancer and autoimmunity: autoimmune and rheumatic features in patients with malignancies. Ann Rheum Dis 60:433–441
48. Loprinzi CL, Duffy J, Ingle JN (1993) Postchemotherapy rheumatism. J Clin Oncol 11:768–770
49. Warner E, Keshavjee al N, Shupak R, Bellini A (1997) Rheumatic symptoms following adjuvant therapy for breast cancer. Am J Clin Oncol 20:322–326
50. Morales L, Pans S, Verschueren K et al (2008) Prospective study to assess short-term intra-articular and tenosynovial changes in the aromatase inhibitor-associated arthralgia syndrome. J Clin Oncol 26:3147–3152
51. Vogelzang NJ, Bosl GJ, Johnson K, Kennedy BJ (1981) Raynaud's phenomenon: a common toxicity after combination chemotherapy for testicular cancer. Ann Intern Med 95:288–292
52. Papamichael D, Amft N, Slevin ML, D'Cruz D (1998) 5-Fluorouracil-induced Raynaud's phenomenon. Eur J Cancer 34:1983
53. Dumoulin FL, Leifeld L, Sauerbruch T, Spengler U (1999) Autoimmunity induced by interferon-alpha therapy for chronic viral hepatitis. Biomed Pharmacother 53:242–254
54. Ronnblom LE, Alm GV, Oberg K (1991) Autoimmune phenomena in patients with malignant carcinoid tumors during interferon-alpha treatment. Acta Oncol 30:537–540
55. Ronnblom LE, Alm GV, Oberg KE (1991) Autoimmunity after alpha-interferon therapy for malignant carcinoid tumors. Ann Intern Med 115:178–183
56. Topalian SL, Hodi FS, Brahmer JR et al (2012) Safety, activity, and immune correlates of anti-PD-1 antibody in cancer. N Engl J Med 366:2443–2454
57. Hamid O, Robert C, Daud A et al (2013) Safety and tumor responses with lambrolizumab (anti-PD-1) in melanoma. N Engl J Med 369:134–144

58. Nishino M, Sholl LM, Hodi FS et al (2015) Anti-PD-1-related pneumonitis during cancer immunotherapy. N Engl J Med 373:288–290
59. Mikuls TR, Endo JO, Puumala SE et al (2006) Prospective study of survival outcomes in Non-Hodgkin's lymphoma patients with rheumatoid arthritis. J Clin Oncol 24:1597–1602
60. Ogle KS, Swanson GM, Woods N, Azzouz F (2000) Cancer and comorbidity: redefining chronic diseases. Cancer 88:653–663
61. Hamo CE, Bloom MW (2015) Getting to the heart of the matter: an overview of cardiac toxicity related to cancer therapy. Clin Med Insights Cardiol 9:47–51
62. Ades F, Zardavas D, Pinto AC et al (2014) Cardiotoxicity of systemic agents used in breast cancer. Breast 23:317–328
63. Suter TM, Ewer MS (2013) Cancer drugs and the heart: importance and management. Eur Heart J 34:1102–1111
64. Aapro M, Bernard-Marty C, Brain EG et al (2011) Anthracycline cardiotoxicity in the elderly cancer patient: a SIOG expert position paper. Ann Oncol Off J Eur Soc Med Oncol/ESMO 22:257–267
65. Swain SM, Whaley FS, Ewer MS (2003) Congestive heart failure in patients treated with doxorubicin. Cancer 97(11):2869–2879
66. Dougoud-Chauvin V, Fradley MG, Chen L, Kim J, Walko CM, Sehovic M, Extermann M (2015) Treatment of diffuse large B-cell lymphoma and preexisting congestive heart failure: a retrospective analysis from Moffitt Cancer Center TCC database. Blood 126 (abstr 3957)
67. Aapro M, Bernard-Marty C, Brain EG et al (2011) Anthracycline cardiotoxicity in the elderly cancer patient: a SIOG expert position paper. Ann Oncol 22:257–267
68. Pinder MC, Duan Z, Goodwin JS et al (2007) Congestive heart failure in older women treated with adjuvant anthracycline chemotherapy for breast cancer. J Clin Oncol 25:3808–3815
69. Qin A, Thompson CL, Silverman P (2015) Predictors of late-onset heart failure in breast cancer patients treated with doxorubicin. J Cancer Surviv 9:252–259
70. Stewart T, Pavlakis N, Ward M (2010) Cardiotoxicity with 5-fluorouracil and capecitabine: more than just vasospastic angina. Intern Med J 40:303–307
71. Dy SM, Sharkey P, Herbert R et al (2006) Comorbid illnesses and health care utilization among Medicare beneficiaries with lung cancer. Crit Rev Oncol Hematol 59:218–225
72. Gross CP, McAvay GJ, Guo Z, Tinetti ME (2007) The impact of chronic illnesses on the use and effectiveness of adjuvant chemotherapy for colon cancer. Cancer 109:2410–2419
73. Siegelmann-Danieli N, Khandelwal V, Wood GC et al (2006) Breast cancer in elderly women: outcome as affected by age, tumor features, comorbidities, and treatment approach. Clin Breast Cancer 7:59–66
74. Gosmanov AR, Goorha S, Stelts S et al (2013) Management of hyperglycemia in diabetic patients with hematologic malignancies during dexamethasone therapy. Endocr Pract 19:231–235
75. de la Morena Barrio P, Conesa MA, Gonzalez-Billalabeitia E et al (2015) Delayed recovery and increased severity of Paclitaxel-induced peripheral neuropathy in patients with diabetes. J Natl Compr Canc Netw 13:417–423
76. Brunello A, Kapoor R, Extermann M (2011) Hyperglycemia during chemotherapy for hematologic and solid tumors is correlated with increased toxicity. Am J Clin Oncol 34:292–296
77. Meyerhardt JA, Catalano PJ, Haller DG et al (2003) Impact of diabetes mellitus on outcomes in patients with colon cancer. J Clin Oncol Off J Am Soc Clin Oncol 21:433–440
78. Hwang IC, Park SM, Shin D et al (2015) Metformin association with lower prostate cancer recurrence in type 2 diabetes: a systematic review and meta-analysis. Asian Pac J Cancer Prev 16:595–600
79. Hassabo H, Hassan M, George B, Wen S, Baladandayuthapani V, Kopetz S, Fogelman DR, Kee BK, Eng C, Garrett CR (2011) Survival advantage associated with metformin usage in patients with colorectal cancer (CRC) and type II noninsulin-dependent diabetes (NIDDM). J Clin Oncol 29 (abstr 3618)

80. Sadeghi N, Abbruzzese JL, Yeung SJ, Hassan M, Li D (2011) Effect of metformin on survival of diabetic patients with pancreatic adenocarcinoma. J Clin Oncol 29 (abstr 4063)
81. Jiralerspong S, Palla SL, Giordano SH et al (2009) Metformin and pathologic complete responses to neoadjuvant chemotherapy in diabetic patients with breast cancer. J Clin Oncol 27:3297–3302
82. Extermann M, Bonetti M, Sledge GW et al (2004) MAX2–a convenient index to estimate the average per patient risk for chemotherapy toxicity; validation in ECOG trials. Eur J Cancer 40:1193–1198
83. Extermann M, Chen H, Cantor AB et al (2002) Predictors of tolerance to chemotherapy in older cancer patients: a prospective pilot study. Eur J Cancer 38:1466–1473
84. Extermann M, Reich RR, Sehovic M (2015) Chemotoxicity recurrence in older patients: risk factors and effectiveness of preventive strategies-a prospective study. Cancer
85. Extermann M, Boler I, Reich RR et al (2012) Predicting the risk of chemotherapy toxicity in older patients: the chemotherapy risk assessment scale for high-age patients (CRASH) score. Cancer 118:3377–3386
86. Hurria A, Togawa K, Mohile SG et al (2011) Predicting chemotherapy toxicity in older adults with cancer: a prospective multicenter study. J Clin Oncol Off J Am Soc Clin Oncol 29:3457–3465

Further Reading

87. References 2–4, 14, 29, 61, 73, 84 and 85 provide a good starting point for the reader wanting to deepen further their knowledge.

Chapter 6
The Impact of Cancer and Chronic Conditions on Caregivers and Family Members

Sylvie D. Lambert, Janelle V. Levesque and Afaf Girgis

Abstract Caregiving by a family member or a friend is critical in maintaining and improving the health and well-being of individuals living with cancer, and in reducing demands on the health care system. The increased prevalence of cancer and co-morbidities is applying pressure on already stretched cancer care resources and high-quality cancer care now relies on caregivers taking on more and more complex illness management roles (once performed by health care professionals). Caregivers provide about 70–80 % of patients' cancer care, the economic value of which is estimated to be at least in the millions. Although caregiving is a valued societal and financial resource, caregivers remain largely a hidden workforce. Caregivers often take on their roles and responsibilities with little to no formal training, leading to high levels of burden and lower quality of life for both the caregivers and the person they are caring for. Cancer caregivers are a particularly vulnerable sub-group, as they report higher burden than caregivers for individuals with diabetes or frail elders. Although across caregiver studies it might be assumed that many of the patients cared for have co-morbidities, this information is not always explicit and there are no studies specifically examining the burden endured by caregivers of patients with cancer and co-morbidities. Therefore, the purpose of this chapter is to summarize what is known about cancer caregiving and note how these findings might be extrapolated to begin to understand the issues faced by caregivers of patients with cancer and co-morbidities. The chapter provides an overview of caregivers' roles in cancer care and the impact of this involvement on caregivers' health and functioning; their patterns of health care services utilization; a description of the type of support caregivers require more of (unmet needs); and the effectiveness of interventions that can support caregivers throughout the cancer trajectory. A discussion of future directions for research and practice concludes this chapter.

S.D. Lambert (✉)
McGill University, St. Mary's Research Centre, Montreal, Canada
e-mail: sylvie.lambert@mcgill.ca

J.V. Levesque · A. Girgis
Psycho-Oncology Research Group Centre for Oncology Education and Research Translation (CONCERT), Ingham Institute for Applied Medical Research South Western Sydney Clinical School, University of New South Wales, Sydney, Australia

B. Koczwara (ed.), *Cancer and Chronic Conditions*,
DOI 10.1007/978-981-10-1844-2_6

Keywords Cancer · Caregiver · Family members · Quality of life · Psychosocial interventions

Key Points

- With the expected growth in the number of caregivers due to the aging of the population and changes in the health care system as well as the substantial burden endured, caregiving is now a public health priority.
- Caregivers fulfill a wide range of roles and responsibilities and often feel unprepared to meet the multiple demands of caregiving.
- An extensive reliance on caregivers adversely impacts on their own physical health, immune function, health behaviors and lifestyle, mental health, social functioning, and financial status, which may limit the extent to which they can sustain their involvement.
- Despite significant challenges, caregiving can also be a positive experience, whereby between 42 and 98 % of caregivers identify at least one positive element in or change arising from their caregiving experience.
- Caregivers report unmet needs in the following domains: comprehensive cancer care, emotional and psychological, partner or caregiver impact and daily activities, relationship, information, and spiritual.
- Although caregivers seem to engage with health care services in regards to cancer screening and primary care visits, there is evidence to suggest that caregivers under-utilize available services, particularly in relation to their mental health needs.
- The ultimate goal of caregiver interventions is to identify the most effective ways of supporting caregivers and meeting their most pressing needs. Significant effects of caregiver interventions are particularly noted for improving knowledge, appraisal, self-efficacy, coping, relationship communication, psychological well-being, sexual functioning and intimacy, and relationship functioning.

6.1 Introduction

Cancer is among the most common conditions worldwide requiring help from informal caregivers, such as a friend, partner, family member, or neighbor. The cost-containment health care context and the increased reliance on outpatient cancer treatment is shifting cancer care from the hospital to the community and is leading to an unprecedented dependence on caregivers' support for high-quality care [1]. Also, with the aging of the population and the concurrent increase in life expectancy, there is a rise in the incidence of cancer, and co-existing chronic diseases, which is leading to an ever increasing cohort of caregivers needing assistance to sustain their role.

Caregivers are patients' primary source of support, with the informal care provided often involving a considerable number of hours per week [2]. Although caregivers' support reduces the demands on the health care system [3], too often caregivers take on their novel roles and responsibilities with little to no formal training [1, 4]. Many caregivers assume their roles and responsibilities without being fully aware of the burden these might cause, and regardless of their readiness to do so. Despite caregivers' best efforts to manage the demands of their role, these might inadvertently exceed their capabilities and result in high levels of physical, emotional, social, and/or financial burden [5–9]. Of concern, caregivers often put aside their own needs to focus on supporting patients [6] and resist using health services to alleviate their burden, which might decrease their ability to sustain their caregiving role and increase caregivers' risk for long-term health complications [10].

With the expected growth in the number of caregivers due to the aging of the population and changes in the health care system, the increased complexity of their role due to the rise in multi-morbidities, and the substantial burden endured, caregiving is now a public health priority. The recognition of caregivers' personal, physical, social, and financial investments in patients' recovery by researchers, clinicians, and policy makers has been coupled with an exponential increase in the research on the psychosocial impact of a cancer diagnosis on caregivers [11]. However, this literature has mainly focused on cancer caregiving in isolation, ignoring the presence of co-morbidities for many patients. This, despite the fair assumption that as the complexity of care increases for patients with multi-morbidities, so does the complexity of informal caregiving. Although it can be supposed that in most cancer caregiver studies the patients had at least one other co-morbidity, these co-morbidities are rarely reported (mainly limited to cancer type, stage, and treatment) and it is therefore difficult to draw conclusions from these studies for this sub-group of caregivers. Given the scarcity of studies examining the issues specifically faced by caregivers of patients with cancer and co-morbidities, this chapter will summarize what is known about cancer caregiving to date and identify directions for future research. This chapter commences with a review of who the caregivers are and what their main roles and responsibilities in cancer care are. Then, the impact of these roles and responsibilities on caregivers' health, functioning, and well-being is presented. This is followed by an overview of caregivers' common supportive care needs and their patterns of health care service utilization. The last section of this chapter provides in-depth evidence about the effectiveness of caregiver interventions. A discussion about the implications of these findings for caregivers of patients with co-morbidities and priorities for future directions for research and practice concludes this chapter.

The definition of caregiver used in this chapter is: family member, partner, friend or neighbor assisting with health care activities for someone with cancer who is unable to independently care for him or herself or needs assistance to manage his/her cancer care or cancer treatment [12].

6.2 The Roles of Caregivers in Cancer Care

6.2.1 How Many Caregivers Provide Care?

Caregivers are a diverse group representing a significant proportion of the population [3, 13, 14]. Whilst the assessment of caregiving responsibilities differs across countries, the proportion of the population defined as caregivers ranges from 10 to 50 %. For example, in a survey conducted by the National Alliance for Caregiving (NAC) in the US, 18.2 % of respondents were caregivers in the previous year, with top conditions requiring caregivers' assistance including "old age," Alzheimer's disease or dementia, surgery or wounds, and cancer [13]. This translates to cancer alone accounting for 7 % of all informal caregivers in the US [13]. In Canada, 28 % of Canadians aged 15 years or older report providing care in the previous 12 months to a family member or friend experiencing a health or age related condition [3]. This rate increases to 46 % when considering whether similar care was provided at some point in their lives [3]. Top conditions requiring assistance from caregivers include: age-related needs, cancer, cardiovascular disease, mental illness, and Alzheimer's disease or dementia [3]. Hence, in Canada, 11 % of caregivers provide care for someone with cancer [3]. In Australia, 12 % of the population were caregivers in 2012 [14], with cancer also representing 1 of the 10 most common health conditions for which people received informal care [14, 15].

6.2.2 Who Provides Care?

Although caregivers across all health conditions are overwhelmingly family members, cancer caregivers are more likely to be the spouses of the care recipient. This is in contrast to those caring for someone with mental health-related needs or age-related needs who are more commonly a parent or adult child, respectively [3, 13]. An estimated 54–60 % of caregivers are women [3, 13, 14], although the number of men taking on caregiving responsibilities has markedly increased [13, 16, 17] and is expected to continue to increase due to the aging population and changing conceptualizations of family and gender roles [18, 19].

Caregivers are predominantly between the ages of 45 and 64 [3, 13]. It is noteworthy that currently nearly one in 10 American caregivers is over the age of

75 [13]. Similarly, Canadian seniors aged 65 years or older represent 12 % of all caregivers. Although a relatively small proportion of the caregiver population, these individuals are the most likely to spend the longest hours providing care [3]. Another particularly vulnerable group are those "sandwiched" between raising children and taking on additional caregiving responsibilities, a growing group because of the overall aging of the population [3].

Information about the race and ethnicity of caregivers is scant, though it is estimated that in US, 62 % of caregivers are White, 17 % are Hispanic, 13 % are African American, and 6 % are Asian American [13].

In the US, The American Cancer Society's (ACS) *Quality of Life Survey* for Caregivers (N = 739 caregivers) is the most complete source of information on cancer caregivers [20, 21]. Overall, the findings of this survey have been consistent with those of studies examining caregivers as a whole: cancer caregivers are predominantly Caucasian, middle-aged women who were the spouses of the care recipient [22, 23]. One notable difference is that nearly 90 % of the participants are Caucasian. This might be related to particular patient populations being more likely to participate in research and subsequently nominating their caregivers [20]. In Australia, a 5-year longitudinal *Partners and Caregivers Well-Being Study* (N = 547) reported similar demographics [5, 8, 9].

6.2.3 How Much Care Is Provided?

Most patients with cancer identify an informal caregiver, who fulfills essential roles and responsibilities that contributes to their illness adjustment [24]. In the US, Kim and Schulz [2] found that cancer caregivers provided on average 31 h of informal caregiving per week, with the burden of cancer caregiving among the highest compared to other caregivers. A report by Statistics Canada found that cancer caregivers were among the top three caregiver sub-groups providing more than 10 h of care per week [3]. In another study, Yabroff and Kim [24] found that on average cancer caregivers dedicated 8.3 h per day (in a range from 4.2 to 12.0 h) to providing care over approximately 13.7 months (in a range from 11.4 to 16.7 months). Medical characteristics, such as the type of cancer and the stage at diagnosis, further increased caregiving intensity, with ovarian and lung cancers requiring the greatest time commitment (>10 h), compared to kidney and bladder cancers (<7 h), which required the least time input. Also, caregivers' socioeconomic status was inversely related to the number of hours per day spent providing care. Finally, Hayman et al. [25] reported that individuals treated for cancer received on average 10 h of informal caregiving per week, compared to about seven hours for those who were diagnosed with cancer, but did not receive treatment in the last year ($p < 0.05$).

6.2.4 *What Kind of Care Is Provided?*

The transition to the caregiving role is life changing [26], with many caregivers perceiving their responsibilities as unknown and demanding [27]. Caregiver roles and responsibilities typically include: practical care, emotional support, household tasks, financial management, and advocacy/decision-making. In Australia's *Partners and Caregivers Well-Being Study,* caregivers reported being mostly involved in: household tasks (daily 68.5 %), emotional support (daily 39.9 %), and managing money (daily 22.7 %) [6]. Interestingly, providing emotional support, liaising with doctors, making appointments and assessing needs for and managing medication were more associated with caregiver anxiety than other tasks [6].

6.2.4.1 Practical Care

Practical care involves the home-based provision of specialized medical care, planning and coordinating care, monitoring the patient's health status and anticipating health needs, and meeting the day-to-day needs (e.g., activities of daily living, personal care) of the person with cancer [28–30]. Ussher et al. [30] reported that medical tasks typically assumed by caregivers include administering injections, dispensing medications, maintaining a colostomy bag, and wound care. In a study by Kim and Schulz [2], activities of daily living most often performed by cancer caregivers included helping patients transfer into and out of a bed, chair, or toilet; providing assistance with bathing; showering and dressing; and feeding the care recipient. Transportation of the patient to and from medical appointments can also constitute a significant task for caregivers, particularly for those who rely on public transport [31].

6.2.4.2 Emotional Support

Emotional support involves providing accompaniment, encouragement, and distraction throughout the cancer experience [32]. It involves tasks such as talking, engaging in pleasurable activities together, being present during medical consultations, encouraging questions during appointments with healthcare providers, and openly discussing worries [24]. Many caregivers experience least confidence and greatest uncertainty in performing these emotional tasks [29, 33], and acting as an emotional buffer and dealing with the psychological responses to cancer are among the most difficult tasks for caregivers [29]. Nonetheless, caregivers recognize the benefits of providing emotional accompaniment for both themselves and the patient [27].

6.2.4.3 Household Tasks

Many caregivers are challenged by the additional responsibilities in the household tasks previously performed by the ill person [30], such as shopping, housework, meal preparation, garden maintenance, and being the family designated driver [8, 30]. Men and women caregivers report assuming different household tasks, primarily those previously performed by their spouse of the opposite gender; this is especially prevalent in the older adult age group [30]. Additionally, those with children have the added pressure of maintaining daily routines and providing childcare [27, 28]. The assumption of these household tasks is especially cumbersome during times in which the patient is perceived to be in poorer health [28].

6.2.4.4 Financial Management

Managing money is another daily task that has long-term implications for caregivers, including mitigating the loss of savings for retirement, altered educational plans for family members, and loss and/or change of housing [2, 8, 15]. Financial management includes distribution of family income to cover illness-related costs, paying household bills, and supporting lifestyle activities [34]. In support of this, Parker et al. [35] identified three main financial concerns among caregivers of patients with terminal cancer: (a) expenses directly related to patient care, (b) costs associated with caregiver lifestyles (e.g., mortgage); and (c) managing financial assistance from insurance companies and government aid.

6.2.4.5 Advocacy/Decision Making

Caregivers often adopt the role of decision-maker [30]. Although patients are encouraged to make their own care decisions, cognitive changes or communication difficulties may result in the caregiver confronting the decisions about treatment and care provision [28, 30], end-of-life care, and household matters [26]. Caregivers also often advocate for the patient by obtaining the necessary support, information, and resources [27]. McIlfatrick et al. [36] found that caregivers assumed the role of advocate through first identifying the knowledge gaps of the patient, and then helping him/her acquire the necessary information to make informed decisions. Likewise, Bowman et al. [37] found that caregivers played a key role in health maintenance advocacy, which mainly encompassed encouraging health-promoting activities (e.g., exercise, healthy eating) among patients.

6.2.5 *What Kind of Skills Do Caregivers Need?*

To engage effectively in caregiving processes, caregivers must first have knowledge of the illness, the possible treatment, the patient's care plan, and the short- and long-term implications of the illness [38]. Once this foundational knowledge is in place, caregiver skills can be developed, i.e. the "ability to engage effectively and smoothly" in various care-related processes [39]. Given et al. [38] identified three categories of caregiver skills: psychomotor, cognitive, and psychological skills. Psychomotor skills involve the coordinated activity required to perform medical tasks. Cognitive skills involve higher-order thinking related to illness management such as symptom monitoring, decision-making, and problem-solving. Finally, psychological skills allow the caregiver to provide emotional support and manage the emotional burden associated with caregiving. Schumacher et al. [39] identified nine key caregiver skills: monitoring, interpreting, decision-making, taking action, adjusting to changing needs, comforting with hands-on care (direct care), accessing resources, working with the ill person, and negotiating the health care system.

Research suggests that cancer caregivers score relatively low on measures of self-efficacy or their confidence in their ability to provide the required care [40]. However caregivers' self-efficacy varies greatly across studies [38], and some factors contribute to enhanced self-efficacy. For example, the following factors positively influenced self-efficacy in caring for lung cancer patients: (a) being older, (b) caring for a patient who has never undergone chemotherapy or radiation, and (c) reduced symptoms and distress among patients [40]. Improved self-efficacy has positive implications for both the patient and the caregiver [40, 41]. Among caregivers, higher self-efficacy has been associated with a reduced risk of mood disturbances and role strain [41] and improved energy levels, reduced time in bed, and improved symptoms among patients [41].

6.3 The Impact of Cancer Caregiving

For many, caregiving can become an enduring and exhausting experience. The following section summarizes the impact of cancer caregiving on their physical health, immune function, health behaviors, mental health, social activities, and finance. An overview of the positive impact of caregiving is also provided.

6.3.1 *Physical Health*

As many caregivers are elderly themselves, they are not only managing patients' illness(es), but they are also coping with their own chronic illness(es), which affects and is affected by the caring role [42]. Caregivers often prioritize patients' health needs over their own, and they might consequently lose control of the management of their illness(es) [12]. Common physical chronic illnesses among caregivers include hypertension, high cholesterol, chronic back pain, heart disease, and arthritis, with the majority of caregivers reporting more than one chronic illness [42]. Although Shaffer [43] found that cancer caregivers had comparable cardiovascular health to the general population, Ji et al. [44] found that spouses of patients with cancer had greater risk for coronary heart disease and stroke after their spouse was diagnosed compared to those without a spouse with cancer. Possible reasons explaining these different findings include: timing of measurements, caregivers' age, type of caregivers included, and methods used to determine disease status [43].

A recent review reported that caregivers' main physical health problems included sleep disturbance, fatigue, pain, loss of physical strength, loss of appetite, and weight loss [7]. Dhruva et al. [45] found that approximately 40–60 % of caregivers experience sleep disturbances, with a similar proportion reporting moderate levels of fatigue. A study of caregivers of individuals with advanced cancer found that 69 % reported fatigue at baseline, which increased as the patients' disease progressed over time [46]. Other factors that contribute to caregiver fatigue and sleep disturbance include emotional distress [47, 48], financial problems [47, 48], an inadequate support system [47, 48], and high level of patient fatigue [47]. Caregivers' physical health problems can extend for years. For example, a study by Asgeirsdóttir et al. [49] examined the impact of spousal loss among widowers on chronic pain 4–5 years later and suggested that low-preparedness prior to a wife's death may contribute to an increased risk of chronic pain among younger widowers and comorbid anxiety, depression, and sleep disorder.

Although a number of quality of life studies have found that caregivers' physical health is comparable to population norm (commonly determined by the SF-12 or SF-36 health surveys) [12, 22, 42, 50–52], others have emphasized the strain of caregivers' roles on their physical health [52–55]. The longitudinal study by Lambert et al. [54] found that caregivers' physical health was comparable to the population norm at 6 months following the diagnosis of cancer in the patient. However, a steady decrease in physical health over time meant that by 2 years post-diagnosis, their physical health fell below population norm. This decline was noted until the last data collection time point of 5 years post-diagnosis. Caregivers' physical health has also been found to be lower than what patients report [56, 57]. Key risk factors associated with low caregiver physical functioning include: being a women [52, 56] or older [22, 50, 51, 53, 56]; reporting lower education [22, 52, 53], unemployment [22, 52, 53], or lower socioeconomic status [50, 52]; not having all the support needed [51]; experiencing symptoms [53]; reporting high psychological distress [56], caregiver stress [53], or depression [54, 55]; caring for someone who also report high distress [56] or lower physical functioning [22, 52]; and caregiving for other family members [22].

6.3.2 Immune Function

Recently studies have documented that caring for a patient with cancer has an adverse impact on caregivers' immune function [58, 59], providing evidence of biological mechanisms that might underpin caregivers' poorer health in comparison to non-caregivers. For instance, Wells-Di Gregario et al. [60] examined the impact of breast cancer recurrence and cancer-specific stress on spousal health and immune function. The results indicated that only the cancer-specific stress was associated with increased physical symptoms and lower T-cell blastogenesis in caregivers, whilst patient recurrence status did not significantly predict caregivers' physical health or immune function. Mortimer et al. [61] added that living for a longer time with an ill spouse, reporting depression symptoms, and having more intrusive thoughts were associated with suppressed cell-mediated immunity. Of note, Rohleder et al. [59] found that the C-reactive protein level of caregivers of patients with brain cancer in the year following the diagnosis was in the range associated with a higher risk of coronary heart disease.

6.3.3 Health Behaviors

Caregivers report multiple unhealthy behaviors, including low fruit and vegetable intake, increased use of tobacco and alcohol, low physical activity, and being overweight [62–67]. Beesley et al. [62] found that after three years, 54 % of caregivers of women with ovarian cancer did not meet the Australian guidelines for physical activity, 71 % were overweight/obese, 40 % ate less than two servings of fruits per day, 80 % ate less than five servings of vegetables per day, 37 % consumed more than two alcoholic beverages per occasion, and 10 % were smokers. In this study, slightly more than half of caregivers reported more than one negative health behavior change since they took on their role. However, some positive changes were also noted, including 14 % of caregivers increased their physical activity, 7 % increased their fruit, and 13 % their vegetable intake, 20 % purposefully lost weight, and 3 out of 13 quit smoking. Of concern, Kershaw et al. [67] found that caregivers tended to use alcohol and drugs as a coping strategy more so than patients (although this strategy was the least used avoidant coping strategy for both patients and caregivers).

Few studies have examined risk factors for caregivers' unhealthy behaviors, but those that have, draw attention to: being a woman [64]; low caregiver health [64, 66], social support [64], and education [62]; and high interference in daily activities due to caregiving [62, 68] and distress [62]. Humpel et al. [69] found that family and friends of cancer survivors who perceive a greater risk of developing cancer were more likely to increase their physical activity and sun-prevention behavior than those family members who did not perceive a greater risk. Stage along the cancer trajectory, and associated variations in caregiver burden, also seem to have an impact, with active caregivers more likely to report higher levels of unhealthy behaviors than those in the survivorship phase [65]. Despite caregivers being prone to unhealthy behaviors, some studies underscore caregivers' motivation and perceived benefits to improve their health behaviors [63, 64]. Cooley et al. [63] found that family members of patients with lung cancer had high rates of unhealthy behaviors; however, between 42 and 56 % expressed readiness to change one unhealthy behavior in the next 30 days. In this study, most (92 %) were interested to participate in a health promotion program.

6.3.4 Mental Health

The most common mental health issues experienced by cancer caregivers are psychological distress, anxiety, and/or depression [70–72]. A quarter (26 %) of caregivers report depression (range = 18.4–35.0 %), and 40.1 % report anxiety (range = 25.4–55.9 %) [73]. The prevalence of caregivers' psychological distress, anxiety, and depression is often reported as being greater than that of the general population [9, 72, 74–76], and in some cases, rates exceed those reported by the patients' [70–72]. For instance, among a mixed group of caregivers of cancer survivors, Lambert et al. [9] noted that 35.8 % of caregivers reported clinically significant levels of anxiety 6 months post patient diagnosis. This prevalence exceeded the anxiety rate reported by the patients themselves [77] and population norm [9]. However, at 12 months, 30.5 % of caregivers reported anxiety, a rate comparable to population norm. The proportion of caregivers reporting clinically significant depression exceeded population norm at both 6 and 12 months post patient diagnosis (15.1 and 15.9 % respectively) [9]. Although caregivers' anxiety and depression tend to decrease over time [78–81], Lambert et al. [5] further reported that caregivers reporting clinically significant anxiety or depression at 6 months continued to do so throughout the first 2 years post-diagnosis.

Predictors for increased risk of psychological distress, anxiety, and/or depression in caregivers include:

- *Gender*: Females experience in general poorer mental health than their male counterparts, regardless of their role in the illness (i.e., caregiver versus patient) [70, 82–87].
- *Marital status*: Spouses experience more anxiety than other caregivers (i.e., relatives, friends) [84, 86, 88, 89], and caregivers living with the patient tend to be more depressed [89].
- *Age*: Young to middle-aged caregivers tend to be more anxious than older caregivers [74, 85].
- *Physical/mental functioning*: Caregivers who are in poor health and are unable to function normally are more likely to experience depression [86].

- *Role in family*: Caregivers who are adult children of patients with cancer and/or those who have children at home tend to experience high anxiety and depression [85, 88, 90].
- *Employment status*: Caregivers who are employed report higher levels of depression [90].
- *Quality of life*: Caregivers with lower quality of life are more anxious and depressed [74, 75, 87].
- *Social support*: Caregivers with lower social support tend to be more anxious and depressed [5, 9, 72, 91–95].
- *Care burden*: Burden appears to be a key predictor of depression in caregivers [86].
- *Unmet needs*: Higher unmet needs tend to be associated with greater levels of anxiety [9, 87].
- *Coping*: Avoidant coping is a recurrent predictor of high caregiver anxiety or depression [9, 91]. Also, higher use of problem-focused coping by patients has been associated with higher fatigue among caregivers [82].
- *Interference with regular activities*: Interference with caregivers' schedule is associated with anxiety and depression [9].
- *Phase along the illness trajectory*: Caregivers tend to report the most anxiety or depression around the time of diagnosis [96, 97].
- *Type of cancer*: Caregivers of patients diagnosed with lung, hematological or head and neck cancers have been found to experience high anxiety and depression [9].
- *Type of treatment*: Caregivers of patients who have surgery and chemotherapy or surgery and radiation therapy tend to be more anxious and depressed than caregivers of patients who undergo surgery alone [97, 98]. Increases in patients' symptoms and severity have also been linked to more distress, anxiety, and/or depression in caregivers [99].

In addition to these variables, a meta-analysis by Hagedoorn [100] has found a moderate, positive association between patients' and caregivers' levels of distress ($r = 0.29$, $p < 0.001$); which implies mutuality in response. That is, if one member of the dyad is distressed, the other is also more likely to be distressed, suggesting that patients and their caregivers react to the cancer diagnosis as an interdependent, emotional system. Of note, increases in caregivers' levels of distress tend to be higher at time of diagnosis and treatment, whereas patients' distress tend to be higher once treatment is completed; however, these differences disappear over time where both patients and caregivers experience similar levels of distress [96].

6.3.5 Social Activities and Relationships

Social changes associated with caregiving include disrupted household routines, reductions in time for family or social activities, and changes in family functioning and relationship quality with family, friends, and the patient [52, 101]. Although caregivers may want to participate in various social activities to help them cope with the stress of their role, they often worry or feel guilty if time is spent away from the person they are caring for [8]. Litzelman et al. [101] found that, among caregivers of patients with lung or colorectal cancer, social stressors (e.g., others making too many demands on them, being critical of them) were more often reported than disruptions in family functioning and relationship quality. In this study, older caregivers, with higher education, who were the patients' primary caregiver and involved in more caregiving tasks, were at risk of experiencing more social stress. Similarly, Mosher et al. [52] found that social changes most frequently reported by caregivers of patients with lung cancer were reductions in time for social activities with friends (57 %) and for family activities (47 %), whereby relationships with the patient and family were least negatively affected. This is consistent with reports that 42 % of patients and spouse caregivers find cancer brought them closer [102]. Although many couples identify remaining strong during the turmoil of cancer, those experiencing troubles pre-diagnosis often find their relationship further deteriorates with the added stress of cancer [103]. Relationship vulnerabilities for couples include interruptions in intimate relationships [104, 105], incorporating the prospect of death and separation [105], managing differential preferences for communicating about cancer [105], negotiating what is helpful or not to the other person [105], accommodating changes (e.g., change in personality, goals for the future, behaviors) in the other person [105], and coping with each other's emotional reactions [104, 105]. Despite these challenges, the claim that cancer leads to higher rates of divorce in comparison to the general population is not supported [106, 107].

In some instances, caregivers report lower social support and higher loneliness than both the patients and matched controls [108]. Although lower social support can adversely impact on their mental health [5, 9, 72, 91–95], it is important to note that not all types of support equally buffer caregivers' burden [5, 109]. For example, Lambert et al. [5] examined the impact of four different types of support—emotional/informational, practical, positive social interaction, and tangible support—on caregivers' anxiety and depression, and found that only low emotional/informational support was significantly associated with high anxiety and depression. In addition, the stress buffering effect of social support seems to depend on the extent to which patients and caregivers are willing to provide or engage in a particular type of support. Incongruence in the type of support patients and caregivers prefer to receive or engage in might actually lead to poorer outcomes (even if that support is considered inherently positive) [95]. Regan et al. [94] further documented that among wives of men with prostate cancer, wives' support behaviors had no impact on their own anxiety and depression, but an increase in men's supportive behaviors predicted an increase (not a decrease) in wives' anxiety and depression. This might reflect wives' discomfort in eliciting support from their partner whom she recognizes is also under significant stress, or it is possible that engaging in open discussions with a partner about serious and sensitive issues might initially increase their salience, resulting in greater distress [94]. In this study, wives' perceptions of men's negative support behaviors were also associated with an increase in their anxiety and depression, which further highlights that the perception of whether the support behavior is positive or negative might be as important (if not more) than the actual behavior itself in determining effects [94].

6.3.6 Finance and Work

As patients and caregivers are preoccupied with the diagnosis, treatment, and recovery, they are often unaware of the impact of cancer on their finances [34]. However, both the direct out-of-pocket and indirect expenses incurred by patients and their caregivers can be substantial and contribute to financial strain [34, 110–112]. Sources of costs include travel to and accommodation during treatments, treatments and medication, taking time off work, reorganization of daily and home life (e.g., help with housework), and coping with the disease (e.g., long distance calls to other family members) [34, 110–113]. Hanly et al. [110] estimated that the cost of the first year of informal care was €29,842 per caregiver, with time lost from other activities accounting for 85 % of the total economic burden, out-of-pocket costs 13 % (e.g., medicine, household expenses), and travel costs 2 %. Others have corroborated that time costs for caregivers contributed the most to the economic burden endured, with caregivers' direct care effort accounting for the majority of the total time costs followed by time lost related to work and leisure [114]. In a study by Carey et al. [113], half of the caregivers reported personal expenses related to their role, with common expenses including parking (36 %), travel to cancer appointments (33 %), and drugs or treatments (25 %). Longo et al. [115] found that 35.6 % of patients required others to take time from work, with these caregivers loosing a mean of 7 work days in the previous 30 days. In addition to missing work, other effects of caregiving on work include: leaving work for appointments, receiving interrupting phone calls, using holidays or special leave, and decreasing work hours [116]. This not only results in loss of income, but could lead to concerns about job loss, employability, lack of promotion, and inadequate pension build-up [34, 113]. To manage financial burden, caregivers might have to sell their assets, use their and other family members' savings, take out loans, or take on an extra job [112]. Further consequences might include house repossession, bankruptcy, loss of independence, and relationship breakdown [34]. Two sub-groups of caregivers appear to be at high-risk for financial strain: those caring for someone in active treatment [110, 111, 113] and caregivers of patients diagnosed with a later stage cancer [24].

6.3.7 Positive Impact of Caregiving

Despite the challenges faced by cancer caregivers, caregiving can also be a positive experience; with between 42 and 98 % of caregivers identifying at least one positive element in or change arising from their cancer caregiving experience [102,

117–119]. A recent review by Li and Loke [120] concluded that positive aspects of caregiving included: (a) improvement in the quality of the relationship between caregiver, care recipient, and the broader family unit; (b) feeling of accomplishment incorporating awareness of their knowledge and capabilities to help the patient and receiving a sense of respect and appreciation from the patient; and (c) meaning derived from caregiving, including elements of reprioritization, altered values, and efforts to maintain normality for the patient and the family unit.

Recognition of the potential benefits that can be derived from the caregiving experience has led to increased research into the concepts of post-traumatic growth and benefit finding, both of which are possible in both spouses [119, 121, 122], adult children and other family caregivers [121–124], in the short- [122, 125] and long-term [122–124] and throughout the cancer trajectory [125, 126]. Weiss [119] found that 88 % of husbands with a wife with breast cancer reported post-traumatic growth in the areas of connection with partner, life priorities, personal strength, and spirituality. Kim et al. [121] found six domains of benefit finding: acceptance, empathy, appreciation, family, positive self-view and reprioritization. Similar results were found in the qualitative study by Levesque and Maybery [124], whereby adult children of patients with cancer reported benefit finding in their relationship with their sick parent, increased emphasis on family, altered life priorities, and personal development. Levesque and Maybery [123] also reported that the level of benefit finding is likely to be higher in caregivers who also report high levels of caregiver satisfaction, suggesting that the two concepts are related and reflect the caregivers' cognitive efforts to positively appraise stressful situations, potentially as a coping mechanism.

The link between post-traumatic growth or benefit finding and the psychological outcomes of cancer caregiving is not yet definitively known. Although the review by Li and Loke [120] concluded that benefit finding contributed to overall caregiver well-being, other research suggests the situation is equivocal. Kim et al. [121] found that different domains of benefit finding had different patterns of association with psychological adjustment. Specifically, higher levels of acceptance and appreciation and lower levels of reprioritization were positively associated with positive adjustment, whereas high levels of empathy and reprioritization and low levels of acceptance and positive self-view were predictive of higher levels of depression. In a study examining the psychological outcomes of the adult children of cancer patients, Levesque [118] found that benefit finding was unrelated to anxiety and well-being, but was a protective factor for depression, whereas Teixeira and Pereira [125] found that positive growth moderated the association between distress and the presence of post-traumatic stress disorder symptoms. Another beneficial outcome is that for some caregivers, the caregiving experience provides an avenue for emotional expression, eliminating feelings of guilt [127], saying goodbye, spiritual development, and gaining a sense of closure [128], which in turn has been shown to assist with grief and adjustment post-bereavement.

Although not denying the negative impact of caregiving, it is equally important to acknowledge the positive aspects of this experience. If attention is not paid to benefit finding and post-traumatic growth, the perception of caregiving will be biased, limiting the extent to which comprehensive theories of caregiver adjustment can be generated [129, 130]. Cohen et al. [117] proposed that screening caregivers for positive elements of the experience may be a way to identify caregivers at heightened risk of poor outcomes. Whilst some have proposed that interventions designed to assist caregivers in acknowledging positive changes brought about by their caregiving role can be beneficial [121, 122], others have expressed concern about the suitability of such interventions, primarily due to disagreement and ambiguity regarding the origins of post-traumatic growth or benefit finding, its measurement, and its relations to psychological health [131–133].

6.4 Common Unmet Supportive Care Needs

Supportive care needs assessment can facilitate the appropriation of services and support for caregivers by optimizing intervention development and allocation of limited economic resources for addressing those needs that remain unmet [71, 134]. A need is labelled as 'unmet' when the services required to deal with a particular issue are not received [135]. Caregivers' most prominent supportive care needs often remain unmet [136], compromising their quality of life [137–140] and adversely impacting on patients' distress [139]. Hence, both patients' and caregivers' illness adjustment may be optimized if caregivers' unmet needs are addressed [140].

6.4.1 Prevalence of Unmet Needs Reported by Caregivers

A recent systematic review identified that caregivers report between 1.3 and 16 unmet needs on average (in a range from 17 to 67), suggesting that 5–47 % of caregivers' needs remain unmet [136]. In some studies, caregivers' needs often exceed the levels reported by patients [136, 141]. Caregivers of individuals in the acute post-diagnosis phase [140], or advanced or palliative care phase [142, 143] and those diagnosed with a brain tumor [138] report considerably high unmet needs. To date, as there has been no attempt to quantify the clinical significance of a given unmet need, it is difficult to determine the significance of experiencing one unmet need [144]. However, many of the top ranking unmet needs reviewed below pertain to key aspects of the caregiving process and it is foreseeable that experiencing any one (even only one) of these would adversely impact clinical outcomes.

6.4.2 Types of Unmet Needs Reported by Caregivers

Caregivers report unmet needs in the following six domains: comprehensive cancer care (prevalence = 1.1–96 %), emotional and psychological (prevalence = 2–93 %), caregiver impact and daily activities (prevalence = 3–79 %), relationship (prevalence = 3.7 and 58 %), information (prevalence = 2.2–86 %), and spiritual (prevalence = 6.7–43 %) [136]. Below are examples of prominent unmet needs across each domain.

6.4.2.1 Comprehensive Cancer Care Unmet Needs

Prevalent unmet needs within this domain include: to be told about the help health care professionals can offer, have a supportive relationship with health care professionals, access to health services, and have possibilities to participate or help in patients' care [136]. Eriksson and Lauri [145] reported that although 63 % of caregivers felt accepted by health care professionals, 96 % felt that health care professionals rarely asked them whether they wanted to talk about their experiences and 86 % were not provided sufficient information about ways they can partake in the patient's care. Overall, fewer caregivers of patients with head and neck cancer [146] or cancer survivors [147] identified needing help with this domain, but higher caregiver unmet needs in this domain were found in studies where the care recipients were hospitalized patients [145], in the acute diagnostic and treatment phases [148, 149], or in the palliative care phase [87, 142, 150, 151].

6.4.2.2 Emotional and Psychological Unmet Needs

Top emotional and psychological unmet needs include: help dealing with own emotional distress, get emotional support for self/have someone to talk to, know how to provide emotional support to patient or others, and manage fears about the situation getting worse [136]. Overall, lower prevalence of emotional unmet needs was reported by caregivers of cancer survivors [139, 147, 152]. Conversely, Buscemi et al. [142] reported that 86 and 83.1 % of caregivers of patients diagnosed with terminal cancer identified needing more help to deal with feeling of loss and getting emotional support for self, respectively; and two studies of wives of men with prostate cancer reported a high prevalence of unmet needs for help to emotionally support the patients (53–59 %) [148, 149].

6.4.2.3 Caregiver Impact and Daily Activities Unmet Needs

Finding out about financial support, knowing how to maintain sense of control, dealing with uncertainty and life after cancer, and curtailing impact on lifestyle and schedule are common unmet needs in this domain [136]. Similar to the previous domains, a lower prevalence of unmet needs was reported in survivorship studies [139, 140, 147, 152]; with a higher prevalence in caregivers of patients in the palliative care phase [142, 151]. For instance, in a study by Eriksson et al. [151] examining the support caregivers received from health care professionals before and after the patient's death, 79 % did not receive much information regarding financial support available. Caregivers of patients diagnosed with terminal cancer who participated in the Buscemi et al. [142] study identified the following impact and daily activities unmet needs: know how to maintain self-control (66.1 %), have more time for myself (59.3 %), and deal with uncertainty and life after cancer (44.1 %).

6.4.2.4 Relationship Unmet Needs

Two unmet needs are particularly prominent in this domain: help communicating with patient about illness and his/her concerns and have an intimate relationship with the patient and consideration for sexual needs [136]. Overall, the pattern of prevalence is consistent with the other domains: studies of caregivers of cancer survivors reported lower unmet needs [139, 147, 152, 153] than caregivers either in the early phases of the illness [149] or in the palliative care phase [142].

6.4.2.5 Information Unmet Needs

Overall patterns of unmet needs previously noted according to illness trajectory were further corroborated for this domain, with the most common information unmet needs including: knowing what to expect, the illness and treatment, death and dying, and providing care to the patient [136].

6.4.2.6 Spirituality Unmet Needs

Spirituality needs are less often documented than the other domains, but a common unmet need in this domain related to feeling there is hope for the future [136].

6.4.3 Comparison Between Patients' and Caregivers' Unmet Needs

Although patients and caregivers share a number of common unmet needs, some needs are unique to the challenges faced by caregivers. Soothill et al. [154] noted the following overlapping unmet needs among patients diagnosed with breast, colorectal, lymphoma, or lung cancer and their caregivers: help with financial matters, help in filling out forms, help with anger, opportunities for meeting others who are in a similar situation, and advice about food and diet. The following top three unmet needs were unique to caregivers: help in considering sexual needs, help with feeling of guilt, and help in dealing with tiredness. Hodgkinson et al. [139] found that patients' and their caregivers' highest unmet needs domains were different, with caregivers needing help in the areas of relationships and partner impact and patients' highest needs pertained to the existential survivorship and comprehensive cancer domains. However, when comparing individual unmet needs items, patients and caregivers identified the same top three unmet needs: managing concerns about the cancer coming back, more accessible hospital parking, and reducing stress in survivors' life. Similarly, a survivorship study by Turner et al. [155] noted that within-dyad agreement was the highest ($\geq$50 %) for help for managing fears of recurrence, coordinated care, and having complaints dealt with properly.

6.4.4 Change in Caregivers' Unmet Needs Over Time

A longitudinal by Girgis et al. [147] found that 50 % of caregivers reported at least one unmet need at 6 months post-diagnosis, with a significant decrease to 35.9 % at 12 months and 30.7 % at 24 months, with the average number of unmet needs also decreasing across these time points (from 4.6 at 6 months to 2.1 at 24 months). Interestingly, ranking of unmet needs revealed some core unmet needs across time, including managing concerns about cancer coming back, reducing stress in the person with cancer's life, understanding the experience of the person with cancer, and more accessible hospital parking. However, at 12 and 24 months, a shift in unmet needs was apparent, with needs related to caregivers' well-being and relationships (e.g., impact that cancer has had on your relationship with the person with cancer, looking after own health) taking priority over patient-focused needs. This might reflect a change in focus for caregivers from prioritizing the patient's recovery within the first year post-diagnosis to processing and managing the impact cancer has had on themselves in survivorship. Conversely, Butow et al. [143] identified increasing unmet needs among caregivers of women with ovarian cancer in the last year of life, with 58 % of caregivers reported at least one unmet need 10–12 months before the patient's death, 70 % 7–9 months, 83 % 4–6 months, and 88 % 0–3 months. Butow et al. [143] also noted that reducing the patient's stress was the only unmet need consistently prevalent across time. A shift in top unmet needs was also noted, with the initial focus on obtaining support for the wider family, discussing cancer in social situations, and issues around sexuality being replaced with needing help with disappointment and fear and making decision within the context of uncertainty.

6.4.5 *Variables Associated with Caregivers' Unmet Needs*

6.4.5.1 Caregiver Demographics

Several studies have not supported a relationship between demographics and level of unmet needs [136]. However, those that have, note that caregivers who are not the patient's spouse (or partner) experienced higher unmet needs [31, 87, 145, 150, 151].

6.4.5.2 Psychosocial Variables

Generally, studies have found that partner or caregiver distress [71, 139], anxiety [71, 134, 138, 142, 147, 152, 153, 155], and/or depression [138, 142, 147, 152, 153] are associated with higher unmet needs. Some studies have also noted that patients reporting higher distress [134, 139] and higher unmet needs [71, 134, 139] have caregivers reporting higher unmet needs of their own. Low social support [31, 147], low relationship satisfaction [139], and having caring responsibilities [31, 142, 147] have all been associated with higher unmet needs.

6.4.5.3 Health/Illness Variables

Although trends have been noted whereby caregivers of individuals with advanced cancer reported higher unmet need, a number of studies do not support a significant relationship between caregiver or patient health/illness variables and unmet needs [31, 134, 138, 139, 152, 153, 155].

6.4.5.4 Health Care Context and Care Variables

Some studies have suggested a relationship between some cancer care variables and unmet needs [137, 150, 156]. For example, Nikoletti et al. [156] found that caregivers who received information from the breast nurse counselor and medical staff had fewer unmet needs than those receiving their information from any other source.

6.4.6 *Implications for Service Delivery*

A review of caregivers' unmet needs provides a strong evidence-base to guide the design and implementation of supportive care services, especially as many caregivers' unmet needs are amenable to change. In addition, caregivers' range of unmet needs highlight that a multidisciplinary approach to supportive care is most appropriate. Although a multidisciplinary approach is the preferred model of care for patient, it is unknown whether this approach has reached caregivers in the same way [31]. However, as caregivers often do not access services, even when these are available [10], this suggests that health care professionals might first need to reassure caregivers that by taking time to meet their own needs they are not only contributing to their own well-being, but to patients' quality of life.

6.5 Health Care Service Utilization by Caregivers

Overall, very little is known about the way that caregivers engage with the health care system to meet their supportive care needs. There is evidence to suggest that caregivers under-utilize available services, particularly in relation to their mental health needs [10, 157–159]. Specifically, in a study of caregivers providing care to patients with advanced cancer, Vanderwerker et al. [10] found that despite 13 % of their sample meeting the diagnostic criteria for a psychiatric disorder; only 46 % of this group accessed mental health services. Studies of bereaved caregivers with a diagnosed mental disorder have also found low numbers of mental health service utilization, ranging from 27 to 47 % [158, 159]. Negative perceptions of mental health professionals, guilt about accessing services for their own needs rather than patient needs, and wanting to self-manage emotional concerns are core barriers to obtaining professional help [160].

However, caregivers do engage with other types of health care services, especially cancer screening and primary care visits. For example, Son et al. [161] found that spousal caregivers undertook screening behaviors for gastric, colorectal, cervical and breast cancer at a significantly higher rate, often more than double the rate, than matched controls. Reeves et al. [162] found that there was no overall difference in screening behaviors between caregivers and non-caregivers; however, they did find that caregivers were more likely to have had a pap test and clinical breast exam within the past 12 months. Finally, a longitudinal study of Australian female caregivers found that caregivers reported a higher number of GP visits compared to women who had never undertaken the caregiving role or who had stopped caregiving [163]. This study futher documented that caregivers were more likely to be taking medication for sleep, nervous conditions, or depression [163].

Caregivers also access some supportive care and psychosocial services. For example, Mosher et al. [164] found that lung cancer caregivers who were currently not receiving services expressed an interest in complementary and alternative medicine (40 %), mental health services (29 %) and practical support (29 %), with a smaller proportion considering couples or family counselling (15 and 19 % respectively). Applebaum et al. [165] found that 92 % of caregivers currently not receiving support were interested in counselling services; however, 48 % of these caregivers identified barriers to accessing this care, including time, guilt at leaving patient, finances and scheduling conflicts. In both of these studies caregivers expressed a preference for phone interventions, potentially as they are more flexible, less costly, and would allow caregivers to receive support in their home without having to be away from their care recipient [164, 165].

6.6 Caregiver Interventions

Without the help of informal caregivers, the costs of cancer to the formal healthcare system would be considerably higher. However, caregivers' own supportive care needs must be addressed to enable them to confront the complexities of their caregiver roles in a way that leads to the best possible patient outcomes [4, 166]. Therefore, over the past decade there has been a rapid increase in the number of interventions developed to: (a) improve caregivers' ability to provide care; (b) reduce the adverse impacts of caregiving on caregivers' health and functioning; (c) enhance patients' reported outcomes; and (d) reduce the cost to society and the health care of caring for patients with cancer. None of these interventions have explicitly targeted caregivers of patients with multi-morbidities. A challenge particular to cancer caregivers (in comparison to, for instance, caregivers of individuals with dementia or the elderly) is that they are given a short timeline to learn all that is required and apply these new skills to the situation to have an impact on clinical outcomes [166]. This section will provide an overview of the caregiver interventions published to date and of their effectiveness.

6.6.1 Types

Caregiver interventions typically employ cognitive, physical, emotional, and/or social mechanisms of action or strategies to have an impact on caregivers' outcomes, and can be categorized in five major types:

1. *Psycho-educational*: Educate caregivers regarding the patient's disease process and other aspects of care, and provide information on available services. Attention is also given to meeting the supportive care needs of patients, caregivers, and/or marital or family relationships [4].
2. *Skills training*: Develop coping and self-management skills (e.g., coping, communication, and problem-solving skills), including increase caregivers' motivation and confidence to apply these to their situation [4, 167].
3. *Counseling*: Opportunity to address problems, concerns, and/or feelings related to caregiving with health care professionals [4].

4. *Palliative care/hospice interventions*: Relieve suffering and improve the quality of life of those living with or dying from advanced illness as well as their caregivers [166].
5. *Respite*: Designed to give the caregiver time off [166].

Most caregiver interventions are psycho-educational or include a combination of psycho-education and skills training [4, 167–169]. The literature reviewed below pertains mainly to these types of interventions.

6.6.2 Format

Caregiver interventions are commonly delivered jointly to the patient and his/her caregiver (also referred to as dyadic interventions) [168–171], by a nurse or a combination of health professionals, and face-to-face, either in the clinical or home setting [4, 168, 172–174]. However, the health care professional delivering the intervention varies according to the type of intervention, with couple-based interventions more often delivered by psychologists, therapists, or counselors [167, 169, 173, 174]. Another popular option is to use the telephone [4, 167, 168, 172, 173], which matches previous reports of caregivers' preferences for supportive cancer care [164, 165]. Although group interventions are less often used [4, 167, 171], this format appears most used for caregivers of patients in the palliative phase [166]. Groups have the advantage of providing opportunities for individuals in a similar situation to interact; however, it might be too difficult for caregivers to attend these [175]. When a combination of formats is used, typically this includes face-to-face sessions with telephone-based follow-ups [167, 172, 173]. Although dose and duration vary widely, caregiver interventions appear to include on average 6–7 sessions [4, 167, 170]. This is in contrast with the literature that longer psychosocial interventions (8–12 sessions) are more efficacious than shorter interventions [176].

6.6.3 Focus

Caregiver interventions can be grouped as: caregiver self-care, marital/family care, and/or patient caregiving [4]. Intervention foci are not mutually exclusive, and many interventions will include some content to address all three [4, 167]. The intervention by Carter [177], which included self-assessment of maladaptive habits affecting caregivers' sleep quality, stimulus control, relaxation techniques, cognitive therapy, and sleep hygiene to maximize caregivers' ability to improve their sleep quality is an example of a caregives self-care intervention. One example of a marital/family care intervention is the counselling intervention by Kuijer et al. [178], which is focused on patient and caregiver mutual support to reduce feelings of inequity and enhance relationship quality. The psycho-educational and skills training intervention developed by Northouse et al. [179] is an example of patient caregiving intervention. This intervention included home visits and telephone follow-ups to provide caregivers with the information, skills, and support needed to manage patient's care and assist patients with managing uncertainty and maintaining an optimistic attitude. This intervention also had a marital/family care component (e.g., improving family functioning) and caregiver self-care content.

Similarly, a review by Badr et al. [172] emphasized that interventions delivered jointly to patients and caregivers involve caregivers in one of two ways. In the first approach, the focus is on promoting individual change in the patient and the role of the caregiver is mainly to facilitate learning and coping skills in the patient [180]. In the second one, the focus is on both patients' and caregivers' needs, both member of the dyad are treated together [172].

6.6.4 Efficacy

Overall, meta-analyses [4, 170] and reviews [167, 173, 174, 181] have supported the efficacy of caregiver interventions on a range of caregiver-reported outcomes. To contextualize the effect sizes presented below, those for psychological and behavioral intervention typically range from 0.35 to 0.50 [182], and the effect sizes for psychosocial interventions for patients with cancer are generally small to moderate: range = 0.17–0.42 [176, 183, 184] (although some types of interventions have been found to result in large effect sizes on selected outcomes [176, 184]).

6.6.4.1 Proximal Outcomes

Proximal outcomes are conceptualized to be more directly affected by an intervention and can be clearly identified from the content and goals of the intervention. The psycho-education and skills training focus of most caregiver interventions means that key proximal outcomes include monitoring caregivers' acquisition of the required knowledge, coping skills, and self-efficacy. Most often the selection of proximal outcomes is based on Lazarus and Folkman's [185] Stress and Coping Framework. Despite the focus of interventions on changing proximal outcomes, these typically receive less attention than more distal outcomes (e.g., anxiety, depression, quality of life).

- *Information needs and knowledge* (*positive findings*): Only the meta-analysis by Northouse et al. [4] has reported on the overall significant effect of interventions on this outcome (effect size = 1.36).
- *Caregiving benefit* (*mixed findings*): Post-intervention findings tend to be non-significant (effect size = 0.17); however, significant findings have been found at follow-ups (effect size = 0.31) [4]. A review by Brandão et al. [174]

noted that significant benefits of couple-based interventions among women with breast cancer and their spouse included reporting more post-traumatic growth.

- *Caregiving burden* (*mixed findings*): Small but significant effect sizes noted post-intervention (effect size = 0.22 [4]). However, effects do not seem to be sustained [4].
- *Self-efficacy* (*positive findings*): The hypothesis that the main underlying mechanism by which caregiver interventions are expected to have an impact is through increased self-efficacy has been confirmed [4].
- *Coping* (*positive findings*): Intervention studies have also reported significant improvements in caregivers' ability to cope (i.e., promoting active coping, and reducing ineffective coping) [173], with a moderate effect size (effect size = 0.47) and enduring effects noted [4]. In recent years, a growing literature is going beyond individual caregiver coping to consider how patients and caregivers engage in the coping process together (termed dyadic coping) [94, 95, 186]. Few studies have reported on the effect of caregiver interventions on dyadic coping. However, those that do have found that caregivers participating in an intervention report higher dyadic coping in comparison to those who do not [186, 187].
- *Communication* (*positive findings*): The few interventions that measure changes in communication have generally noted improvements [167, 173]. For instance, Kayser's [186] Partners in Coping Program for women with breast cancer and their partners resulted in partners being more willing to communicate their stress to patients as well as more positive individual and dyadic coping.

6.6.4.2 Distal Outcomes

Whereas proximal outcomes are directly affected by the content of an intervention, distal outcomes depend on factors that are not directly influenced by the intervention [188]. The challenge of focusing on such distal outcomes, is that change might not be a reasonable expectation given the short periods of time [181].

- *Quality of life* (*positive findings*): Weak to moderate effect sizes (effect sizes = 0.05–0.54) have been noted, not only immediately after the intervention, but also at follow-ups [167, 168, 173].
- *Psychological outcomes* (*mixed findings*): The Badr and Krebs [170] meta-analysis of couple-based interventions reported a small, but significant effect on psychological outcomes (effect size = 0.18). The Northouse et al. [4] meta-analysis reported encouraging effect sizes for distress and anxiety, both post-intervention and at follow-up. However, caregiver interventions have not been found to be as effective in reducing depression [4, 173]. This finding might be partially explained by low levels of baseline caregiver depression and the high rate of attrition of depressed caregivers [4, 181].

- *Physical functioning* (*non-significant findings*): Caregiver interventions do not seem efficacious post-intervention on this outcome (effect size = 0.11 [4]); however, they might be at follow-up (effect size = 0.22–0.26 [4]).
- *Social functioning* (*mixed findings*): Mixed results have been noted regarding improving caregivers' ability to maintain family, vocational, and social roles [173], with minimal effect noted post-intervention (effect size = 0.11 [4]). However, a positive effect has been noted at follow-up (effect size = 0.39 [4]).
- *Sexual functioning* (*positive findings*): Few studies have focused on sexual functioning and intimacy of the caregiver, but those that have, have shown some positive impact [169].
- *Relationship functioning and satisfaction* (*mixed findings*): Marital satisfaction and relationship functioning have generally been found to improve following caregiver interventions [4, 167, 170, 173]. However, improvements in relationship functioning obtained following a caregiver intervention do not seem to be sustained over time [4], which might emphasize the need for booster sessions to improve long-term outcomes.

6.6.4.3 Impact on Patient-Reported Outcomes

There is increasing evidence that when interventions engage both the caregiver and patient as a dyad, important synergies are achieved that significantly enhances each person's outcomes [170, 171, 173]. The meta-analysis by Badr and Krebs [170] emphasized that interventions jointly delivered to patients and caregivers had a significant impact on the patients' psychological (effect size = 0.18), physical (effect size = 0.31) and relationship (effect size = 0.25) functioning. The Regan et al. [173] review of couple-based interventions documented that the benefits of these interventions for patients paralleled those noted for their spouse caregivers, including improved psychological and physical distress, sexuality and relationship functioning, communication, and coping. These findings were echoed by the Brandão et al. [174] review of couple-based interventions for women with breast cancer and their spouse, whereby many of the benefits for the spouse were noted for the patient as well.

There is also evidence that dyadic interventions are potentially more efficacious than patient-only interventions in enhancing patients' well-being outcomes [189, 190]. For instance, Nezu et al. [190] examined the efficacy of a problem-solving therapy (PST) among a mixed sample of patients diagnosed with cancer and included two treatment groups: one in which patients attended the PST alone and a second one where PST was attended with a significant other. Post-PST positive effects on quality of life and distress were similar in the two treatment groups. However, at 6- and 12-month follow-ups, patients participating in PST with their significant other reported lower distress than patients who attended the PST alone. The support and shared learning that occurs in dyadic interventions might increase the likelihood of improvements [173].

6.6.5 Moderators of Intervention Effects

Northouse et al. [4] examined the potential impact of four study characteristics on intervention effects: (a) participants (caregiver alone vs. caregiver-patient dyad), (b) mode of delivery (face-to-face vs. phone vs. group vs. mixed), (c) type of intervention, and (d) duration and dose. For many outcomes, none of these characteristics had a significant effect. Inconsistent findings were noted for intervention length, whereby caregivers receiving longer interventions reported significantly more burden and depression and lower relationship functioning than those in shorter interventions. However, the opposite was noted for coping. Coping was also more favorable for interventions delivered face-to-face or using a group format than those using mixed modes of delivery. Caregiver-only interventions reported more positive outcomes in terms of appraisal of caregiving benefit than dyadic interventions. This might be because these interventions focused more on caregivers' own needs. Overall these findings emphasize that decisions about intervention design need to take into consideration the desired outcomes.

A systematic review by Regan et al. [173] also did not note any differences in efficacy based on mode of delivery. However, interventions targeting early-stage cancer were suggested to result in greater improvement in comparison to interventions targeting late-stage or advanced cancers. Also, interventions with patient-caregiver dyads or couples in less supportive relationships or in a shorter relationship were found to be more efficacious. This suggests that tailoring interventions to key risk factors might increase the likelihood of positive outcomes.

A review by Baik and Adams [171] concluded that couple-based interventions focused on improving communication, reciprocal understanding, and intimacy in the couple appeared to be most promising in reducing illness-related distress for caregivers and improving dyadic adjustment. Similarly, Waldron et al. [168] also emphasized that interventions targeting communications pose to make the greatest impact on caregivers, as well if these integrate problem-solving skills training.

Of note, the review by Wootten et al. [169] found that cognitive behavioral-based interventions appeared to be more effective than psycho-educational interventions in improving sexual intimacy and satisfaction for partners of men with prostate cancer. However, psycho-educational interventions were as effective as cognitive behavioral based interventions in reducing distress. This might indicate that the lack of information is a significant contributor to psychological distress for caregivers. This review also emphasized that face-to-face interventions produced more beneficial outcomes than those delivered solely over the telephone.

6.6.6 Attrition and Retention

Caregiver interventions are typically acceptable to caregivers, with high satisfaction reported [181, 191], but uptake rates across studies vary widely. In a review by

Regan et al. [192] of interventions targeting both the patients and their spouse caregivers, uptake rates varied from 13.6 to 94.2 % (overall rate = 48.8 %). Specifically for caregivers, uptake rates for dyadic interventions (46.3 %) was slightly lower than for individual-based interventions (48 %), and both were lower than coaching interventions (59.2 %), possibly reflecting logistical issues if patients and caregivers are unable to participate in an intervention simultaneously or feel they need different levels of support [192, 193]. Caregivers' uptake rates were higher for psycho-educational or coping skills training interventions (51, 51.8 %) than for those focusing on communication (43.1 %). Finally, face-to-face intervention had a higher uptake (49.8 %) than telephone interventions (45 %).

Regan et al. [192] also found that caregivers' attrition rates post-intervention ranged from 0 to 38.7 % (overall rate = 17.6 %). Attrition rates for dyadic interventions (22.5 %) were higher than for individual-based (18.5 %) and coaching (attrition rate = 15.8 %) interventions. Attrition rates were higher for psycho-educational and coping skills interventions (22.4, 22.7 %) than communication-focused interventions (13.8 %), suggesting that although communication interventions might not initially be attractive to patients and caregivers, their benefits might become more apparent as they engage with the intervention [193]. This, in turn, raise a critical issue regarding marketing the benefits of these interventions to participants. In addition to a higher uptake rate, face-to-face interventions had a lower attrition rate (16.7 %) than telephone interventions (19.9 %).

One of the most common barriers to intervention uptake and completion includes distance to the intervention being too great [170, 173, 192]. Although delivering interventions via other means is increasingly popular to overcome this barrier, caregivers usually desire some level of face-to-face [173]. Other frequent barriers include timing or scheduling issues (e.g., too busy) [168, 170, 173, 192, 194], high patient symptom severity [173], compromised caregiver health [168, 194], high caregiver burden and strain [168, 169] and perception that interventions do not meet caregivers' needs [171, 173]. Consumer involvement in the process of developing the interventions through participatory research strategies might address this last limitation [175].

6.6.7 Under-Researched, but Potentially Promising Caregiver Interventions

6.6.7.1 Orientation Programs

A Cochrane review [195] of information interventions to orient patients and their caregivers to a cancer care facility and the services available within a centre supported their efficacy in reducing distress but not anxiety.

6.6.7.2 Physical Activity Interventions for Caregivers

The health benefits of physical activity (PA) for the general population are well-recognized [196], with evidence that these benefits extend to individuals diagnosed with cancer [197]. A recent systematic review of the impact of PA Interventions on caregivers by Lambert et al. [198] found one among cancer caregivers, with benefits of decreasing distress and increasing aspects of quality of life noted. The remaining 13 trials were mostly conducted among caregivers of individuals with dementia or Alzheimer's, with benefits including increased PA, reduced burden, increased physical outcomes, and improved sleep quality.

6.6.7.3 Self-directed Intervention

Most caregiver interventions raise access barriers related to travel and sustainability due to their high cost and reliance on health care professionals' availability. An increased interest in a self-directed (or self-administered) format is evident as an alternate approach to provide ongoing instruction and support to caregivers in a cost-effective manner. A self-directed format offers caregivers the flexibility to choose when and where to engage in the program and requires less direct input from clinicians. As caregivers are often less likely than patients to access conventional services, self-directed interventions might play a particularly prominent role in supporting them in their coping efforts [10]. Lambert et al. [57, 193] developed *Coping-Together*, a manual-based, self-directed coping skills intervention for couples facing cancer, with initial feasibility testing highly endorsing its dyadic focus and self-directed format.

6.6.7.4 Online Interventions

Web-based interventions are increasingly recognized as a convenient, cost-effective, and efficacious approach for delivering support to large numbers of individuals [199]. The few interventions developed to date show promise in enhancing caregivers' health and well-being [200]. Given the popularity of the internet for delivering psychosocial interventions and the potential effectiveness of this mode of delivery, it is an encouraging platform to deliver caregiver interventions and overcome barriers of conventional caregiver interventions.

6.6.7.5 GP Supported Interventions

In recognition that general practice (GP) consultations provide an opportunity to address caregivers needs, Mitchell et al. [201, 202] have examined the efficacy of a GP-based intervention incorporating a caregiver-reported needs checklist (The Needs Assessment Tool—Carers [203]) and a supporting GP compendium of resources to address caregivers' identified needs. In a randomized controlled trial with caregivers of people with advanced cancer, this novel approach improved mental well-being among caregivers who were clinically anxious at baseline. For caregivers whose baseline anxiety was within the normal range, the intervention led to a significant improvement in their physical functioning. Although the intervention did not reduce the number of unmet needs, drawing caregivers' attention to their needs may prompt them and/or the GP to put in place extra resources to address these. Additional studies are needed to further examine the potential benefits of systematically using a needs assessment tool to improve caregivers' outcomes.

6.6.8 Potential Implications for Caregivers of Patients with Multi-morbidities

As patients with multi-morbidities often have greater self-care needs, an increased reliance on informal caregivers to meet these needs might lead to these caregivers spending more time providing care per week, being involved in more tasks, with potentially lower self-efficacy than caregivers of patients without co-morbidities. These caregivers may also engage in a greater frequency of tasks and more care co-ordination and communicating with health care teams. Since greater caregiving intensity or higher interference in caregivers' daily activities due to their caring role are recurrent risk factors for a number of adverse health and well-being outcomes, caregivers of patients with multi-morbidities may report worse outcomes than those caring for someone with cancer alone. The impact of caregiving for someone with multi-morbidities might be comparable to those caring for someone in the palliative phase. However, more intense caregiving might also mean that these caregivers report higher levels of benefit finding, with Levesque and Maybery [124] noting that adult children who reported greater impact of caring and higher emotional reactions to their parents' illness also noted a higher number of positive outcomes.

As reviewed in this chapter, caregiver education and skill building are key to supporting caregivers. However, caregiver interventions are often disease-specific, and do not take into consideration the multiple demands that might arise across illnesses. Although this approach reflects the disease-specific model used to provide health services [204], it may actually further isolate caregivers of patients with cancer and co-morbidities. The staggering increase in prevalence of multi-morbidities can no longer be ignored and further urges the identification of caregiver interventions and approaches that are effective across illnesses. An integrated approach to caregiver interventions is also justified by findings that caregiver burden is comparable across illnesses [204–206], and is mainly predicted by caregivers' similar needs and approach to coping (not patients' diagnosis) [205, 206]. However, one challenge in the planning and implementation of interventions for caregivers of patients with multi-morbidities is that although they might benefit more from the interventions due to the additional burden and needs, attrition rates might be even higher in this sub-group as key barriers might be enhanced (e.g., too busy, higher patient symptom severity).

6.7 Conclusion and Future Directions

6.7.1 Conclusion

For many, the caregiving role is equivalent to a full-time job, resulting in significant burden in their health, economic and social outcomes. Caregivers also report unmet needs in relation to comprehensive cancer care, emotional and psychological support, partner or caregiver impact and daily activities, relationship, information, and spiritual issues. However, many caregivers also report deep levels of satisfaction from their caregiving role.

Patients and their caregiver react to cancer (and potentially other diagnoses) as a unit, and as a result, both have legitimate needs for help from health professionals; hence, comprehensive care plans should ideally focus on the patient-caregiver dyad [4]. It is imperative that health care professionals identify caregivers who are at most risk and support them through direct care or by referrals to community resources to help meet the needs of this vulnerable population. Utilizing tools such as screening checklists can provide a more systematic approach to needs assessment to ensure the highest priority needs are addressed. Despite the promise of caregiver interventions to achieve clinically significant outcomes, few interventions (if any) have been translated for or implemented in clinical practice [4]. Hence, health care professionals can also become aware of caregiver interventions, detailed in this chapter, which are most effective for supporting caregivers and meeting their most pressing needs and consider some alternate approaches and format that might favor translational in routine cancer care.

6.7.2 Future Directions

Our understanding of the impact of caregiving is limited to the populations and outcomes that have been studied to date. It is difficult to draw inferences to other caregiver populations, including those caring for patients with multi-morbidities, with a high degree of confidence. Hence, extending the research to include under-studies caregiver populations is of high priority. As previously mentioned, the chronic disease profile that comes with the aging of the population is creating an urgency to increase our understanding of the experiences of caregiving of patients with cancer and co-existing chronic diseases. In addition, most studies to date have focused on the patients' spouse or partner as their primary caregiver [168], and more studies are needed to examine the impact of caregiving potentially on other caregiver sub-group, who have been found to be more at risk of adverse outcomes (e.g., daughters higher burden than spouse) [85, 88, 90]; and on same-sex couples [173]. Our understanding of the impact of caregiving on people of different racial, cultural, and socio-economic backgrounds is also limited by the lack of research in these populations. Northouse et al. [4] noted that less than 16 % of participants across 29 intervention studies reviewed were self-identified as members of a minority; and only two studies were identified which tailored interventions for a particular cultural or racial group [207, 208]. Most caregiver intervention studies have focused on breast or prostate cancer populations [167, 170], with only a handful of studies focusing on caregivers sub-group actually at highest risk of anxiety and depression (e.g., caregiver of patients with hematological, head and neck, or lung cancer [9]). Further research into more "accessible" interventions such as using e-Health technology is required, as well as assessing the cost-effectiveness of different intervention approaches [4, 170].

Finally, with significant challenges encountered by many studies in low recruitment and high attrition rates, the challenge to achieve required sample sizes to reach statistical significance calls for more research to clarify the definition of clinically meaningful changes in the outcomes examined, as even small effect sizes can still be clinically significant and important [170].

References

1. Northouse LL, McCorkle R (2010) Spouse caregivers of cancer patients. In: Holland JC, Breitbart WS, Jacobsen PB, Lederberg MS, Loscalzo MJ, McCorkle R (eds) Psycho-Oncology. Oxford University Press, New York, pp 516–521
2. Kim Y, Schulz R (2008) Family caregivers' strains - Comparative analysis of cancer caregiving with dementia, diabetes, and frail elderly caregiving. J Aging Health 20(5):483–503. doi:10.1177/0898264308317533
3. Sinha M (2013) Spotlight on Canadians: results from the general social survey. Portrait of caregivers, 2012
4. Northouse LL, Katapodi MC, Song L, Zhang L, Mood DW (2010) Interventions with family caregivers of cancer patients: meta-analysis of randomized trials. CA Cancer J Clin 60 (5):317–339. doi:10.3322/caac.20081
5. Lambert SD, Jones B, Girgis A, Lecathelinais C (2012) Distressed partners and caregivers do not recover easily: adjustment trajectories among partners and caregivers of cancer survivors. Ann Behav Med 44(2):225–235. doi:10.1007/s12160-012-9385-2
6. Girgis A, Lambert SD (2009) Caregivers of cancer survivors: the state of the field. Cancer Forum 33(3):167–171
7. Stenberg U, Ruland CM, Miaskowski C (2010) Review of the literature on the effects of caring for a patient with cancer. Psycho-Oncology 19(10):1013–1025. doi:10.1002/pon.1670
8. Girgis A, Lambert S, Johnson C, Waller A, Currow D (2013) Physical, psychosocial, relationship, and economic burden of caring for people with cancer: a review. J Oncol Pract 9 (4):197–202. doi:10.1200/JOP.2012.000690
9. Lambert SD, Girgis A, Lecathelinais C, Stacey F (2013) Walking a mile in their shoes: anxiety and depression among partners and caregivers of cancer survivors at 6 and

12 months post-diagnosis. Support Care Cancer 21(1):75–85. doi:10.1007/s00520-012-1495-7
10. Vanderwerker L, Laff R, Kadan-Lottick N, McColl S, Pigerson H (2005) Psychiatric Disorders and mental health service use among caregivers of advanced cancer patients. J Clin Oncol 23(28):6899–6907
11. Rankin N, Butow P, Price M, Evans A (2011) Views of psycho-oncology health professionals on priority psycho-oncology research questions. Support Care Cancer 19 (8):1133–1141. doi:10.1007/s00520-010-0922-x
12. Given BA, Given CW, Sherwood P (2012) The challenge of quality cancer care for family caregivers. Semin Oncol Nurs 28(4):205–212. doi:10.1016/j.soncn.2012.09.002
13. National Alliance for Caregiving (NAC), American Association of Retired Persons (AARP) (2015) Caregiving in the U.S. Public Policy Institute, Washington, DC
14. Australian Bureau of Statistics (ABS) (2012) Disability, ageing and carers, Australia: summary of findings. Australian Bureau of Statistics, Canberra, Australia
15. Aoun S (2004) The hardest thing we have ever done full report of the National Inquiry into the Social Impact of Caring for Terminally Ill People: incorporating a literature review and analysis of public submissions. Accessed from http://nla.gov.au/nla.cat-vn3255721. Palliative Care Australia, Deakin West, A.C.T
16. Ducharme F, Lévesque L, Lachance L, Zarit S, Vézina J, Gangbè M, Caron CD (2006) Older husbands as caregivers of their wives: a descriptive study of the context and relational aspects of care. Int J Nurs Stud 43(5):567–579
17. Baker KL, Robertson N, Connelly D (2010) Men caring for wives or partners with dementia: masculinity, strain and gain. Aging Ment Health 14(3):319–327
18. Kramer BJ, Thompson EH (2002) Men as caregivers: theory, research, and service implications. Springer Series: Focus on Men. Springer Publishing Company
19. Russell R (2007) The work of elderly men caregivers from public careers to an unseen world. Men Masculinities 9(3):298–314
20. Romito F, Goldzweig G, Cormio C, Hagedoorn M, Andersen BL (2013) Informal caregiving for cancer patients. Cancer 119(Suppl 11):2160–2169. doi:10.1002/cncr.28057
21. Kim Y, Shaffer KM, Carver CS, Cannady RS (2015) Quality of life of family caregivers 8 years after a relative's cancer diagnosis: follow-up of the National Quality of Life Survey for Caregivers. Psycho-Oncology. doi:10.1002/pon.3843
22. Kim Y, Spillers RL (2010) Quality of life of family caregivers at 2 years after a relative's cancer diagnosis. Psycho-Oncology 19(4):431–440. doi:10.1002/pon.1576
23. Kim Y, Kashy DA, Kaw CK, Smith T, Spillers RL (2009) Sampling in population-based cancer caregivers research. Qual Life Res 18(8):981–989
24. Yabroff KR, Kim Y (2009) Time costs associated with informal caregiving for cancer survivors. Cancer 115(S18):4362–4373. doi:10.1002/cncr.24588
25. Hayman JA, Langa KM, Kabeto MU, Katz SJ, DeMonner SM, Chernew ME, Slavin MB, Fendrick AM (2001) Estimating the cost of informal caregiving for elderly patients with cancer. J Clin Oncol Official J Am Soc Clin Oncol 19(13):3219–3225
26. McConigley R, Halkett G, Lobb E, Nowak A (2010) Caring for someone with high-grade glioma: a time of rapid change for caregivers. Palliat Med 24(5):473–479. doi:10.1177/0269216309360118
27. Blindheim K, Thorsnes SL, Brataas HV, Dahl BM (2013) The role of next of kin of patients with cancer: learning to navigate unpredictable caregiving situations. J Clin Nurs 22 (5/6):681–689. doi:10.1111/j.1365-2702.2012.04349.x
28. Clemmer SJ, Ward-Griffin C, Forbes D, Clemmer SJ, Ward-Griffin C, Forbes D (2008) Family members providing home-based palliative care to older adults: the enactment of multiple roles. Can J Aging 27(3):267–283
29. Adams E, Boulton M, Rose P, Lund S, Richardson A, Wilson S, Watson E (2012) A qualitative study exploring the experience of the partners of cancer survivors and their views on the role of primary care. Support Care Cancer 20(11):2785–2794. doi:10.1007/s00520-012-1400-4

30. Ussher JM, Tim Wong WK, Perz J (2011) A qualitative analysis of changes in relationship dynamics and roles between people with cancer and their primary informal carer. Health: 15 (6):650–667. doi:10.1177/1363459310367440
31. Soothill K, Morris SM, Harman JC, Francis B, Thomas C, Illmurray MB (2001) Informal carers of cancer patients: what are their unmet psychosocial needs? Health Soc Care Community 9(6):464–475
32. Nicholls W, Hulbert-Williams N, Bramwell R (2014) The role of relationship attachment in psychological adjustment to cancer in patients and caregivers: a systematic review of the literature. Psycho-Oncology 23(10):1083–1095
33. Bakas T, Lewis RR, Parsons JE (2001) Caregiving tasks among family caregivers of patients with lung cancer. Oncol Nurs Forum 28(5):847–854
34. Amir Z, Wilson K, Hennings J, Young A (2012) The meaning of cancer: implications for family finances and consequent impact on lifestyle, activities, roles and relationships. Psycho-Oncology 21(11):1167–1174. doi:10.1002/pon.2021
35. Parker D, Grbich C, Maddocks I (2001) Financial issues in caring for someone with terminal cancer at home. Aust J Primary Health 7(2):37–42
36. McIlfatrick S, Sullivan K, McKenna H (2006) What about the carers?: exploring the experience of caregivers in a chemotherapy day hospital setting. Eur J Oncol Nurs 10 (4):294–303. doi:10.1016/j.ejon.2005.12.003
37. Bowman KF, Rose JH, Deimling GT (2005) Families of long-term cancer survivors: health maintenance advocacy and practice. Psycho-Oncology 14(12):1008–1017
38. Given B, Sherwood PR, Given CW (2008) What knowledge and skills do caregivers need? AJN Am J Nurs 108(9):28–34
39. Schumacher KL, Stewart BJ, Archbold PG, Dodd MJ, Dibble SL (2000) Family caregiving skill: development of the concept. Res Nurs Health 23(3):191–203
40. Porter LS, Keefe FJ, Garst J, McBride CM, Baucom D (2008) Self-efficacy for managing pain, symptoms, and function in patients with lung cancer and their informal caregivers: associations with symptoms and distress. Pain (03043959) 137(2):306–315. doi:10.1016/j.pain.2007.09.010
41. Keefe FJ, Ahles TA, Porter LS, Sutton LM, McBride CM, Pope MS, McKinstry ET, Furstenberg CP, Dalton J, Baucom DH (2003) The self-efficacy of family caregivers for helping cancer patients manage pain at end-of-life. Pain 103(1–2):157–162. doi:10.1016/S0304-3959(02)00448-7
42. Kim Y, Carver CS, Cannady RS, Shaffer KM (2013) Self-reported medical morbidity among informal caregivers of chronic illness: the case of cancer. Qual Life Res 22(6):1265–1272. doi:10.1007/s11136-012-0255-y
43. Shaffer KM (2013) Risk and manifestation of cardiovascular disease among cancer caregivers: effects of stress, depression, and gender. University of Miami
44. Ji J, Zoller B, Sundquist K, Sundquist J (2012) Increased risks of coronary heart disease and stroke among spousal caregivers of cancer patients. Circulation 125(14):1742–1747. doi:10.1161/CIRCULATIONAHA.111.057018
45. Dhruva A, Lee K, Paul SM, West C, Dunn L, Dodd M, Aouizerat BE, Cooper B, Swift P, Miaskowski C (2012) Sleep-wake circadian activity rhythms and fatigue in family caregivers of oncology patients. Cancer Nurs 35(1):70–81
46. Aranda SK, Hayman-White K (2001) Home caregivers of the person with advanced cancer: an Australian perspective. Cancer Nurs 24(4):300–307
47. Fletcher BA, Schumacher KL, Dodd M, Paul SM, Cooper BA, Lee K, West C, Aouizerat BE, Swift PS, Wara W, Miaskowski C (2009) Trajectories of fatigue in family caregivers of patients undergoing radiation therapy for prostate cancer. Res Nurs Health 32 (2):125–139. doi:10.1002/nur.20312
48. Aslan O, Sanisoglu Y, Akyol M, Yetkin S (2009) Quality of sleep in Turkish family caregivers of cancer patients. Cancer Nurs 32(5):370–377. doi:10.1097/NCC.0b013e3181a87fb9

49. Asgeirsdóttir HG, Valdimarsdóttir U, Fürst CJ, Steineck G, Hauksdóttir A (2013) Low preparedness before the loss of a wife to cancer and the widower's chronic pain 4–5 years later-a population-based study. Psycho-Oncology 22(12):2763–2770. doi:10.1002/pon.3345
50. Kim Y, Spillers RL, Hall DL (2012) Quality of life of family caregivers 5 years after a relative's cancer diagnosis: follow-up of the national quality of life survey for caregivers. Psycho-Oncology 21(3):273–281. doi:10.1002/pon.1888
51. Bergelt C, Koch U, Petersen C (2007) The influence of disease and treatment-related variables on the quality of life of partners of cancer patients. Psycho-Oncology 16(9):S211–S212
52. Mosher CE, Bakas T, Champion VL (2013) Physical health, mental health, and life changes among family caregivers of patients with lung cancer. Oncol Nurs Forum 40(1):53–61. doi:10.1188/13.ONF.53-61
53. Kershaw TS, Mood DW, Newth G, Ronis DL, Sanda MG, Vaishampayan U, Northouse LL (2008) Longitudinal analysis of a model to predict quality of life in prostate cancer patients and their spouses. Ann Behav Med 36(2):117–128
54. Lambert SD, Girgis A, Descallar J, Levesque JV, Jones B (2014) Partners' and caregivers' psychological and physical adjustment to cancer within the first five years post survivor diagnosis. Psycho-Oncology 23(Suppl. 3):78
55. Janda M, Steginga S, Langbecker D, Dunn J, Walker D, Eakin E (2007) Quality of life among patients with a brain tumor and their carers. J Psychosom Res 63(6):617–623. doi:10.1016/j.jpsychores.2007.06.018
56. Kim Y, Kashy DA, Wellisch DK, Spillers RL, Kaw CK, Smith TG (2008) Quality of life in couples dealing with cancer: dyadic and individual adjustment among breast and prostate cancer survivors and their spousal caregivers. Ann Behav Med 35(2):230–238. doi:10.1007/s12160-008-9026-y
57. Lambert SD, McElduff P, Girgis A, Levesque JV, Regan TW, Turner J, Candler H, Mihalopoulos C, Shih STF, Kayser K, Chong P (2016) A pilot, multisite, randomized controlled trial of a self-directed coping skills training intervention for couples facing prostate cancer: Accrual, retention, and data collection issues. Support Care Cancer 24(2):711–722
58. Sherwood PR, Weimer J, Price T, Ren D, Lieberman F, Donovan H (2014) Stress induced immune dysfunction in neuro-oncology caregivers. Neuro-Oncology 16:ii110. doi:10.1093/neuonc/nou174
59. Rohleder N, Marin TJ, Ma R, Miller GE (2009) Biologic cost of caring for a cancer patient: dysregulation of pro- and anti-inflammatory signaling pathways. J Clin Oncol 27(18):2909–2915. doi:10.1200/JCO.2008.18.7435
60. Wells-Di Gregorio S, Carpenter KM, Dorfman CS, Yang HC, Simonelli LE, Carson WE (2012) Impact of breast cancer recurrence and cancer-specific stress on spouse health and immune function. Brain Behav Immun 26(2):228–233. doi:10.1016/j.bbi.2011.07.237
61. Mortimer JS, Sephton SE, Kimerling R, Butler L, Bernstein AS, Spiegel D (2005) Chronic stress, depression and immunity in spouses of metastatic breast cancer patients. Clin Psychol 9(2):59–63. doi:10.1080/13284200500221094
62. Beesley VL, Price MA, Webb PM (2011) Loss of lifestyle: health behaviour and weight changes after becoming a caregiver of a family member diagnosed with ovarian cancer. Support Care Cancer 19(12):1949–1956
63. Cooley ME, Finn KT, Wang Q, Roper K, Morones S, Shi L, Litrownik D, Marcoux J, Zaner K, Hayman LL (2013) Health behaviors, readiness to change, and interest in health promotion programs among smokers with lung cancer and their family members: a pilot study. Cancer Nurs 36(2):145–154. doi:10.1097/NCC.0b013e31825e4359
64. Mazanec SR, Flocke SA, Daly BJ (2015) Health behaviors in family members of patients completing cancer treatment. Oncol Nurs Forum 42(1):54–62. doi:10.1188/15.ONF.54-62
65. Ross A, Sundaramurthi T, Bevans M (2013) A labor of love: the influence of cancer caregiving on health behaviors. Cancer Nurs 36(6):474–483. doi:10.1097/NCC.0b013e3182747b75

66. Willette-Murphy K, Lee KA, Dodd M, West C, Aouizerat BE, Paul S, Swift P, Wara W, Miaskowski C (2009) Relationship between sleep and physical activity in female family caregivers at the initiation of patients' radiation therapy. JOGNN J Obstet Gynecol Neonatal Nurs 38(3):367–374. doi:10.1111/j.1552-6909.2009.01032.x
67. Kershaw T, Northouse L, Kritpracha C, Schafenacker A, Mood D (2004) Coping strategies and quality of life in women with advanced breast cancer and their family caregivers. Psychol Health 19(2):139–155
68. Barber FD (2013) Effects of social support on physical activity, self-efficacy, and quality of life in adult cancer survivors and their caregivers. Oncol Nurs Forum 40(5):481
69. Humpel N, Magee C, Jones SC (2007) The impact of a cancer diagnosis on the health behaviors of cancer survivors and their family and friends. Support Care Cancer 15(6):621–630
70. Matthews BA (2003) Role and gender differences in cancer-related distress: a comparison of survivor and caregiver self-reports. Oncol Nurs Forum 30(3):493–499. doi:10.1188/03.ONF.493-499
71. Sklenarova H, Krumpelmann A, Haun MW, Friederich HC, Huber J, Thomas M, Winkler EC, Herzog W, Hartmann M (2015) When do we need to care about the caregiver? Supportive care needs, anxiety, and depression among informal caregivers of patients with cancer and cancer survivors. Cancer 121(9):1513–1519. doi:10.1002/cncr.29223
72. Price MA, Butow PN, Costa DS, King MT, Aldridge LJ, Fardell JE, DeFazio A, Webb PM, Australian Ovarian Cancer Study Group Quality of Life Study I (2010) Prevalence and predictors of anxiety and depression in women with invasive ovarian cancer and their caregivers. Med J Aust 193(5 Suppl):S52–57 [Erratum appears in Med J Aust. 2011 Aug 15;195(4):232]
73. Mitchell AJ, Ferguson DW, Gill J, Paul J, Symonds P (2013) Depression and anxiety in long-term cancer survivors compared with spouses and healthy controls: a systematic review and meta-analysis. Lancet Oncol 14(8):721–732. doi:10.1016/S1470-2045(13)70244-4
74. Park B, Kim SY, Shin JY, Sanson-Fisher RW, Shin DW, Cho J, Park JH (2013) Prevalence and predictors of anxiety and depression among family caregivers of cancer patients: a nationwide survey of patient-family caregiver dyads in Korea. Support Care Cancer 21(10):2799–2807. doi:10.1007/s00520-013-1852-1
75. Gorji MA, Bouzar Z, Haghshenas M, Kasaeeyan AA, Sadeghi MR, Ardebil MD (2012) Quality of life and depression in caregivers of patients with breast cancer. BMC research notes 5:310
76. Haun MW, Sklenarova H, Villalobos M, Thomas M, Brechtel A, Lowe B, Herzog W, Hartmann M (2014) Depression, anxiety and disease-related distress in couples affected by advanced lung cancer. Lung Cancer 86(2):274–280. doi:10.1016/j.lungcan.2014.09.009
77. Boyes A, Girgis A, D'Este C, Zucca A (2011) Flourishing or floundering? Prevalence and correlates of anxiety and depression among a population-based sample of adult cancer survivors 6 months after diagnosis. J Affect Disord 135:184–192
78. Kurtz M, Kurtz JC, Given C, Given B (2004) Depression and physical health among family caregivers of geriatric patients with cancer—a longitudinal view. Med Sci Monit 10(8):447–456
79. Tuinstra J, Hagedoorn M, Van Sonderen E, Ranchor AV, Van den Bos GAM, Nijboer C, Sanderman R (2004) Psychological distress in couples dealing with colorectal cancer: Gender and role differences and intracouple correspondence. Brit J Health Psychol 9(4):465–478
80. Baider L, Andritsch E, Goldzweig G, Uziely B, Ever-Hadani P, Hofman G, Krenn G, Samonigg H (2004) Changes in psychological distress of women with breast cancer in long-term remission and their husbands. Psychosomatics 45(1):58–68. doi:10.1176/appi.psy.45.1.58

81. Couper J, Bloch S, Love AW, Duchesne G, Macvean M, Kissane DW (2006) The psychosocial impact of prostate cancer on patients and their partners. Med J Aust 185 (8):428–432
82. Bayman N, Bigatti S (2010) Relationship between coping strategies and distress among breast cancer patients and their partners. Psycho-Oncology 19:S40. doi:10.1002/pon.1689
83. Hagedoorn M, Sanderman R, Bolks HN, Tuinstra J, Coyne JC (2008) Distress in couples coping with cancer: a meta-analysis and critical review of role and gender effects. Psychol Bull 134(1):1–30. doi:10.1037/0033-2909.134.1.1
84. Mystakidou K, Parpa E, Panagiotou I, Tsilika E, Galanos A, Gouliamos A (2013) Caregivers' anxiety and self-efficacy in palliative care. Eur J Cancer Care 22(2):188–195. doi:10.1111/ecc.12012
85. Dunn LB, Aouizerat BE, Langford DJ, Cooper BA, Dhruva A, Cataldo JK, Baggott CR, Merriman JD, Dodd M, West C, Paul SM, Miaskowski C (2013) Cytokine gene variation is associated with depressive symptom trajectories in oncology patients and family caregivers. Eur J Oncol Nurs 17(3):346–353. doi:10.1016/j.ejon.2012.10.004
86. Rhee YS, Yun YH, Park S, Shin DO, Lee KM, Yoo HJ, Kim JH, Kim SO, Lee R, Lee YO, Kim NS (2008) Depression in family caregivers of cancer patients: the feeling of burden as a predictor of depression. J Clin Oncol 26(36):5890–5895
87. Fririksdottir N, Saevarsdottir T, Halfdanardottir SI, Jonsdottir A, Magnusdottir H, Olafsdottir KL, Gumundsdottir G, Gunnarsdottir S (2011) Family members of cancer patients: needs, quality of life and symptoms of anxiety and depression. Acta Oncol 50 (2):252–258. doi:10.3109/0284186X.2010.529821
88. Mystakidou K, Tsilika E, Parpa E, Galanos A, Vlahos L (2007) Caregivers of advanced cancer patients: feelings of hopelessness and depression. Cancer Nurs 30(5):412–418
89. Sahadevan S, George TM, Sudheeran PC, Sreekumar D, Namboodiri V (2015) Determinants of depression in principal caregivers of patients with cancer. Indian J Psychiatry 1:S28
90. Given B, Wyatt G, Given C, Sherwood P, Gift A, DeVoss D, Rahbar M (2004) Burden and depression among caregivers of patients with cancer at the end of life. Oncol Nurs Forum 31 (6):1105–1117. doi:10.1188/04.ONF.1105-1117
91. Dalton WT, Nelson DV, Brobst JB, Lindsay JE, Friedman LC (2007) Psychosocial variables associated with husbands' adjustment three months following wives' diagnosis of breast cancer. J Cancer Educ 22(4):245–249
92. Bigatti SM, Wagner CD, Lydon-Lam JR, Steiner JL, Miller KD (2011) Depression in husbands of breast cancer patients: relationships to coping and social support. Support Care Cancer 19(4):455–466. doi:10.1007/s00520-010-0835-8
93. Ownsworth T, Henderson L, Chambers SK (2010) Social support buffers the impact of functional impairments on caregiver psychological well-being in the context of brain tumor and other cancers. Psycho-Oncology 19(10):1116–1122. doi:10.1002/pon.1663
94. Regan TW, Lambert SD, Kelly B, McElduff P, Girgis A, Kayser K, Turner J (2014) Cross-sectional relationships between dyadic coping and anxiety, depression, and relationship satisfaction for patients with prostate cancer and their spouses. Patient Educ Couns 96(1):120–127. doi:10.1016/j.pec.2014.04.010
95. Regan T, Lambert SD, Kelly B, Falconier M, Kissane D, Levesque JV (2015) Couples coping with cancer: exploration of theoretical frameworks from dyadic studies. Psycho-Oncology 24(12):1605–1617
96. Hodges L, Humphris G, Macfarlane G (2005) A meta-analytic investigation of the relationship between the psychological distress of cancer patients and their carers. Soc Sci Med 60(1):1–12. doi:10.1016/j.socscimed.2004.04.018
97. Lee Y-H, Liao Y-C, Liao W-Y, Shun S-C, Liu Y-C, Chan J-C, Yu C-J, Yang P-C, Lai Y-H (2013) Anxiety, depression and related factors in family caregivers of newly diagnosed lung cancer patients before first treatment. Psycho-Oncology 22(11):2617–2623. doi:10.1002/pon.3328

98. Badr H, Gupta V, Sikora A, Posner M (2014) Psychological distress in patients and caregivers over the course of radiotherapy for head and neck Cancer. Oral Oncol 50 (10):1005–1011. doi:10.1016/j.oraloncology.2014.07.003
99. Oechsle K, Goerth K, Bokemeyer C, Mehnert A (2013) Anxiety and depression in caregivers of terminally ill cancer patients: impact on their perspective of the patients' symptom burden. J Palliat Med 16(9):1095–1101. doi:10.1089/jpm.2013.0038
100. Hagedoorn M (2008) Gender differences in distress in partners of patients with cancer: an overview of empirical studies. Psycho-Oncology 17:S105–S106
101. Litzelman K, Kent EE, Rowland JH (2016) Social factors in informal cancer caregivers: the interrelationships among social stressors, relationship quality, and family functioning in the CanCORS data set. Cancer 122(2):278–286. doi:10.1002/cncr.29741
102. Dorval M, Guay S, Mondor M, Masse B, Falardeau M, Robidoux A, Deschenes L, Maunsell E (2005) Couples who get closer after breast cancer: frequency and predictors in a prospective investigation. J Clin Oncol Official J Am Soc Clin Oncol 23(15):3588–3596
103. Meyerowitz BE, Oh S (2009) Psychosocial response to cancer diagnosis and treatment. In: Miller SM, Bowen DJ, Croyle RT, Rowland JH (eds) Handbook of cancer control and behavioral science: a resource for researchers, practitioners, and policymakers. American Psychological Association, Washington, DC, pp 361–389
104. Galbraith ME (2005) Couples surviving prostate cancer: quality of life and relationship issues. Commun Nurs Res 38:308
105. Fergus KD, Gray RE (2009) Relationship vulnerabilities during breast cancer: patient and partner perspectives. Psycho-Oncology 18(12):1311–1322. doi:10.1002/pon.1555
106. Langer SL, Yi JC, Storer BE, Syrjala KL (2010) Marital adjustment, satisfaction and dissolution among hematopoietic stem cell transplant patients and spouses: a prospective, five-year longitudinal investigation. Psycho-Oncology 19(2):190–200. doi:10.1002/pon.1542
107. Laitala VS, Saarto T, Einio EK, Martikainen P, Silventoinen K (2015) Early-stage breast cancer is not associated with the risk of marital dissolution in a large prospective study of women. Br J Cancer 113(3):543–547. doi:10.1038/bjc.2015.216
108. Bishop MM, Beaumont JL, Hahn EA, Cella D, Andrykowski MA, Brady MJ, Horowitz MM, Sobocinski KA, Rizzo JD, Wingard JR (2007) Late effects of cancer and hematopoietic stem-cell transplantation on spouses or partners compared with survivors and survivor-matched controls. J Clin Oncol 25(11):1403–1411
109. Nijboer C, Tempelaar R, Triemstra M, van den Bos GA, Sanderman R (2001) The role of social and psychologic resources in caregiving of cancer patients. Cancer 91(5):1029–1039
110. Hanly P, Céilleachair AO, Skally M, O'Leary E, Kapur K, Fitzpatrick P, Staines A, Sharp L (2013) How much does it cost to care for survivors of colorectal cancer? Caregiver's time, travel and out-of-pocket costs. Support Care Cancer 21(9):2583–2592. doi:10.1007/s00520-013-1834-3
111. Hanly P, Ceilleachair AO, Skally M, O'Leary E, Staines A, Kapur K, Fitzpatrick P, Sharp L (2013) Time costs associated with informal care for colorectal cancer: an investigation of the impact of alternative valuation methods. Appl Health Econ Health Policy 11(3):193–203. doi:10.1007/s40258-013-0013-5
112. Hanratty B, Holland P, Jacoby A, Whitehead M (2007) Financial stress and strain associated with terminal cancer–a review of the evidence. Palliat Med 21(7):595–607
113. Carey M, Paul C, Cameron E, Lynagh M, Hall A, Tzelepis F (2012) Financial and social impact of supporting a haematological cancer survivor. Eur J Cancer Care 21(2):169–176. doi:10.1111/j.1365-2354.2011.01302.x
114. Van Houtven CH, Ramsey SD, Hornbrook MC, Atienza AA, van Ryn M (2010) Economic burden for informal caregivers of lung and colorectal cancer patients. Oncologist 15(8):883–893. doi:10.1634/theoncologist.2010-0005
115. Longo CJ, Fitch M, Deber RB, Williams AP (2006) Financial and family burden associated with cancer treatment in Ontario, Canada. Support Care Cancer 14(11):1077–1085. doi:10.1007/s00520-006-0088-8

116. Grunfeld E, Coyle D, Whelan T, Clinch J, Reyno L, Earle CC, Willan A, Viola R, Coristine M, Janz T, Glossop R (2004) Family caregiver burden: results of a longitudinal study of breast cancer patients and their principal caregivers. CMAJ Can Med Assoc J 170 (12):1795–1801
117. Cohen CA, Colantonio A, Vernich L (2002) Positive aspects of caregiving: rounding out the caregiver experience. Int J Geriatr Psychiatry 17(2):184–188
118. Levesque J (2012) Benefit finding in parental cancer: types and predictors of benefits and their influence on depression and well-being. Charles Sturt University
119. Weiss T (2002) Posttraumatic growth in women with breast cancer and their husbands: an intersubjective validation study. J Psychosoc Oncol 20(2):65–80
120. Li Q, Loke AY (2013) The positive aspects of caregiving for cancer patients: a critical review of the literature and directions for future research. Psycho-Oncology 22(11):2399–2407. doi:10.1002/pon.3311
121. Kim Y, Schulz R, Carver CS (2007) Benefit fidning in the cancer caregiving experience. Psychosom Med 69:283–291
122. Cassidy T (2013) Benefit finding through caring: the cancer caregiver experience. Psychol Health 28(3):250–266. doi:10.1080/08870446.2012.717623
123. Levesque JV, Maybery D (2014) Predictors of benefit fidning in the adult children of patients with cancer. J Psychosoc Oncol 32:535–554
124. Levesque JV, Maybery D (2012) Parental cancer: catalyst for positive growth and change. Qual Health Res 22(3):397–408. doi:10.1177/1049732311421617
125. Teixeira RJ, Pereira G (2013) Factors contributing to posttraumatic growth and its buffering effect in adult children of cancer patients undergoing treatment. J Psychosoc Oncol 31:235–265
126. Kim Y, Carver CS, Schulz R, Lucette A, Cannady RS (2013) Finding benefit in bereavement among family cancer caregivers. J Palliat Med 16:1040–1047
127. Koop PM, Strang VR (2003) The bereavement experience following home-based family caregiving for persons with advanced cancer. Clin Nurs Res 2:127–144
128. Wong WK, Ussher J (2009) Bereaved informal cancer carers making sense of their palliative care experiences at home. Health Soc Care Community 17(3):274–282. doi:10.1111/j.1365-2524.2008.00828.x
129. Carbonneau H, Caron C, Desrosiers J (2010) Development of a conceptual framework of positive aspects of caregiving in dementia. Dement Geriatr Cogn Disord 9:327–353
130. Kramer B (1997) Gain in the caregiving experience: where are we? What next? Gerontologist 37:218–232
131. Lechner SC, Tennen H, Affleck G (2009) Benefit finding and growth. In: Lopez S, Snyder CR (eds) Oxford handbook of positive psychology. Oxford University Press, New York, pp 633–640
132. Coyne JC, Tennen H (2010) Positive psychology in cancer care: bad science, exaggerated claims, and unproven medicine. Ann Behav Med 39(1):16–26. doi:10.1007/s12160-009-9154-z
133. Sawyer A, Ayers S, Field A (2010) Posttraumatic growth and adjustment among individuals with cancer or HIV/AIDS: a meta-analysis. Clin Psychol Rev 30:436–447
134. Molassiotis A, Wilson B, Blair S, Howe T, Cavet J (2011) Unmet supportive care needs, psychological well-being and quality of life in patients living with multiple myeloma and their partners. Psycho-Oncology 20(1):88–97. doi:10.1002/pon.1710
135. Sanson-Fisher R, Girgis A, Boyes A, Bonevski B, Burton L, Cook P (2000) The unmet supportive care needs of patients with cancer. Cancer 88(1):226–237
136. Lambert SD, Harrison JD, Smith E, Bonevski B, Carey M, Lawsin C, Paul C, Girgis A (2012) The unmet needs of partners and caregivers of adults diagnosed with cancer: a systematic review. BMJ Support Palliat Care 2(3):224–230. doi:10.1136/bmjspcare-2012-000226
137. Park SM, Kim YJ, Kim S, Choi JS, Lim HY, Choi YS, Hong YS, Kim SY, Heo DS, Kang KM, Jeong HS, Lee CG, Moon do H, Choi JY, Kong IS, Yun YH, Park SM, Kim YJ,

Kim S, Choi JS, Lim H-Y, Choi YS, Hong YS, Kim S-Y, Heo DS, Kang KM, Jeong HS, Lee CG, Moon DH, Choi J-Y, Kong IS, Yun YH (2010) Impact of caregivers' unmet needs for supportive care on quality of terminal cancer care delivered and caregiver's workforce performance. Support Care Cancer 18(6):699–706

138. Janda M, Steginga S, Dunn J, Langbecker D, Walker D, Eakin E (2008) Unmet supportive care needs and interest in services among patients with a brain tumour and their carers. Patient Educ Couns 71(2):251–258. doi:10.1016/j.pec.2008.01.020
139. Hodgkinson K, Butow P, Hunt GE, Wyse R, Hobbs KM, Wain G (2007) Life after cancer: couples' and partners' psychological adjustment and supportive care needs. Support Care Cancer 15(4):405–415. doi:10.1007/s00520-006-0148-0
140. Kim Y, Kashy DA, Spillers RL, Evans TV (2010) Needs assessment of family caregivers of cancer survivors: three cohorts comparison. Psycho-Oncology 19(6):573–582. doi:10.1002/pon.1597
141. Harrison J, Young J, Price M, Butow P, Solomon M (2009) What are the unmet supportive care needs of people with cancer? A systematic review. Support Care Cancer 17(8):1117–1128. doi:10.1007/s00520-009-0615-5
142. Buscemi V, Font A, Viladricht C (2010) Focus on relationship between the caregivers unmet needs and other caregiving outcomes in cancer palliative care. Psicooncologia 7(1):109–125
143. Butow P, Price M, Bell M, Webb P, De Fazio A, Friedlander M (2013) Caring for women with ovarian cancer in the last year of their life: impact on the caregiver. Asia Pac J Clin Oncol 9:103. doi:10.1111/ajco.12145
144. Sanson-Fisher R, Carey M, Paul C (2009) Measuring the unmet needs of those with cancer: a critical overview. Cancer Forum 33(3):198–201
145. Eriksson E, Lauri S (2000) Informational and emotional support for cancer patients' relatives. Eur J Cancer Care (Engl) 9(1):8–15
146. Ross S, Mosher CE, Ronis-Tobin V, Hermele S, Ostroff JS, Ross S, Mosher CE, Ronis-Tobin V, Hermele S, Ostroff JS (2010) Psychosocial adjustment of family caregivers of head and neck cancer survivors. Support Care Cancer 18(2):171–178
147. Girgis A, Lambert SD, McElduff P, Bonevski B, Lecathelinais C, Boyes A, Stacey F (2013) Some things change, some things stay the same: a longitudinal analysis of cancer caregivers' unmet supportive care needs. Psycho-Oncology 22(7):1557–1564. doi:10.1002/pon.3166
148. Mason TM (2008) Wives of men with prostate cancer postbrachytherapy: perceived Information Needs and Degree of Being Met. Cancer Nurs 31(1):32–37. doi:10.1097/01.NCC.0000305674.06211.03
149. Mason TM, Mason TM (2005) Information needs of wives of men following prostatectomy. Oncol Nurs Forum 32(3):557–563
150. Fridriksdottir N, Sigurdardottir V, Gunnarsdottir S (2006) Important needs of families in acute and palliative care settings assessed with the family inventory of needs. Palliat Med 20 (4):425–432
151. Eriksson E, Arve S, Lauri S, Eriksson E, Arve S, Lauri S (2006) Informational and emotional support received by relatives before and after the cancer patient's death. Eur J Oncol Nurs 10 (1):48–58
152. Hodgkinson K, Butow P, Hobbs KM, Hunt GE, Lo SK, Wain G (2007) Assessing unmet supportive care needs in partners of cancer survivors: the development and evaluation of the Cancer Survivors' Partners Unmet Needs measure (CaSPUN). Psycho-Oncology 16(9):805–813
153. Stafford L, Judd F, Stafford L, Judd F (2010) Partners of long-term gynaecologic cancer survivors: psychiatric morbidity, psychosexual outcomes and supportive care needs. Gynecol Oncol 118(3):268–273
154. Soothill K, Morris SM, Thomas C, Harman JC, Francis B, McIllmurray MB (2003) The universal, situational, and personal needs of cancer patients and their main carers. Eur J Oncol Nurs 7(1):5–16
155. Turner D, Adams E, Boulton M, Harrison S, Khan N, Rose P, Ward A, Watson EK (2013) Partners and close family members of long-term cancer survivors: health status, psychosocial

well-being and unmet supportive care needs. Psycho-Oncology 22(1):12–19. doi:10.1002/pon.2050
156. Nikoletti S, Kristjanson LJ, Tataryn D, McPhee I, Burt L, Nikoletti S, Kristjanson LJ, Tataryn D, McPhee I, Burt L (2003) Information needs and coping styles of primary family caregivers of women following breast cancer surgery. Oncol Nurs Forum 30(6):987–996
157. Applebaum AJ, Farran CJ, Marziliano AM, Pasternak AR, Breitbart W (2014) Preliminary study of themes of meaning and psychosocial service use among informal cancer caregivers. Palliat Support Care 12:139–148
158. Cherlin EJ, Barry CL, Prigerson HG, Green DS, Johnson-Hurzeler R, Kasl SV, Bradley EH (2007) Bereavement services for family caregivers: how often used, why, and why not. J Palliat Med 10(1):148–158
159. Lichtenthal WG, Nilsson M, Kissane DW, Breitbart W, Kacel E, Jones EC, Prigerson HG (2011) Underutilization of mental health services among bereaved caregivers with prolonged grief disorder. Psychiatric Services 62(10):1225–1229
160. Mosher C, Given B, Ostroff J (2015) Barriers to mental health service use among distressed family caregivers of lung cancer patients. Eur J Cancer Care 24(1):50–59. doi:10.1111/ecc.12203
161. Son KY, Park SM, Lee CH, Choi GJ, Lee D, Jo S, Lee SH, Cho B (2011) Behavioral risk factors and use of preventative screening services among spousal caregivers of cancer patients. Support Care Cancer 19:919–927
162. Reeves KW, Bacon K, Fredman L (2012) Caregiving associated with selected cancer risk behaviors and screening utilization among women: cross-sectional results of the 2009 BRFSS. BMC Public Health 12:685. doi:10.1186/1471-2458-12-685
163. Lee C, Gramotnev H (2007) Transitions into and out of caregiving: health and social characteristics of mid-age Australian women. Psychol Health 22:193–209
164. Mosher CE, Champion VL, Hanna N, Jalal SI, Fakiris AJ, Birdas TJ, Okereke IC, Kesler KA, Einhorn LH, Given BA, Monahan PO, Ostroff JS (2013) Support service use and interest in support services among distressed family caregivers of lung cancer patients. Psycho-Oncology 22(7):1549–1556. doi:10.1002/pon.3168
165. Applebaum A, Marziliano A, Pasternak A, Breitbart W (2013) Psychosocial service use of cancer caregivers: caregiver and patient perspectives. Psycho-Oncology 22:69. doi:10.1002/pon.3245
166. Harding R, List S, Epiphaniou E, Jones H (2012) How can informal caregivers in cancer and palliative care be supported? An updated systematic literature review of interventions and their effectiveness. Palliat Med 26(1):7–22. doi:10.1177/0269216311409613
167. Li Q, Loke AY (2014) A systematic review of spousal couple-based intervention studies for couples coping with cancer. Direction for the development of interventions. Psycho-Oncology 23(7):731–739. doi:10.1002/pon.3535
168. Waldron EA, Janke E, Bechtel CF, Ramirez M, Cohen A (2013) A systematic review of psychosocial interventions to improve cancer caregiver quality of life. Psycho-Oncology 22(6):1200–1207. doi:10.1002/pon.3118
169. Wootten A, Abbott J, Farrell A, Austin D, Klein B (2014) Psychosocial interventions to support partners of men with prostate cancer: a systematic and critical review of the literature. J Cancer Surviv 8(3):472–484. doi:10.1007/s11764-014-0361-7
170. Badr H, Krebs P (2012) A systematic review and meta-analysis of psychosocial interventions for couples coping with cancer. Psycho-Oncology 22(8):1688–16704. doi:10.1002/pon.3200
171. Baik OM, Adams KB (2011) Improving the well-being of couples facing cancer: a review of couples-based psychosocial interventions. J Marital Fam Ther 37(2):250–266. doi:10.1111/j.1752-0606.2010.00217.x
172. Badr H, Acitelli LK, Taylor CL (2008) Does talking about their relationship affect couples' martial and psychological adjustment to lung cancer? J Cancer Surviv 2(1):53–64
173. Regan T, Lambert SD, Girgis A, Kelly B, Turner J, Kayser K (2012) Do couple-based interventions make a difference for couples affected by cancer? BMC Cancer 12:279. doi:10.1186/1471-2407-12-279

174. Brandão T, Schulz MS, Matos PM (2014) Psychological intervention with couples coping with breast cancer: a systematic review. Psychol Health 29(5):491–516. doi:10.1080/08870446.2013.859257
175. Hudson P (2004) A critical review of supportive interventions for family caregivers of patients with palliative-stage cancer. J Psychosoc Oncol 22(4):77–92. doi:10.1300/J077v22n04_05
176. Rehse B, Pukrop R (2003) Effects of psychosocial interventions on quality of life in adult cancer patients: meta analysis of 37 published controled outcome studies. Patient Educ Couns 50:179–186
177. Carter PA (2006) A brief behavioral sleep intervention for family caregivers of persons with cancer. Cancer Nurs 29(2):95–103
178. Kuijer RG, Buunk BP, De Jong GM, Ybema JF, Sanderman R (2004) Effects of a brief intervention program for patients with cancer and their partners on feelings of inequity, relationship quality and psychological distress. Psycho-Oncology 13(5):321–334. doi:10.1002/pon.749
179. Northouse L, Kershaw T, Mood D, Schafenacker A (2005) Effects of a family intervention on the quality of life of women with recurrent breast cancer and their family caregivers. Psycho-Oncology 14(6):478–491. doi:10.1002/pon.871
180. Baucom DH, Porter LS, Kirby JS, Hudepohl J (2012) Couple-based interventions for medical problems. Behav Ther 43(1):61–76. doi:10.1016/j.beth.2011.01.008
181. Ussher JM, Perz J, Hawkins Y, Brack M (2009) Evaluating the efficacy of psycho-social interventions for informal carers of cancer patients: a systematic review of the research literature. Health Psychology Review 3(1):85–107. doi:10.1080/17437190903033401
182. Lipsey MW, Wilson DB (2001) Practical meta-analysis, vol 49. Sage Publication, Inc.
183. Meyer TJ, Mark MM (1995) Effects of psychosocial interventions with adult cancer patients: a meta-analysis of randomized experiments. Health Psychol 14(2):101–108
184. Sheard T, Maguire P (1999) The effect of psychological interventions on anxiety and depression in cancer patients: results of two meta-analyses. Br J Cancer 80(11):1770–1780
185. Lazarus R, Folkman S (1984) Stress, appraisal, and coping. Springer Publishing Company Inc, New York
186. Kayser K (2005) Enhancing dyadic coping during a time of crisis: a theory-based intervention with breast cancer patients and their partners. American Psychological Association, Washington, DC
187. Heinrichs N, Zimmermann T, Huber B, Herschbach P, Russell DW, Baucom DH (2012) Cancer distress reduction with a couple-based skills training: a randomized controlled trial. Ann Behav Med 43(2):239–252. doi:10.1007/s12160-011-9314-9
188. Osborne R, Elsworth G, Whitfield K (2007) The Health Education Impact Questionnaire (heiQ): an outcomes and evaluation measure for patient education and self-management interventions for people with chronic conditions. Patient Educ Couns 66(2):192–201
189. Scott JL, Halford W, Ward BG (2004) United we stand? The effects of a couple-coping intervention on adjustment to early stage breast or gynecological cancer. J Consult Clin Psychol 72(6):1122–1135. doi:10.1037/0022-006X.72.6.1122
190. Nezu AM, Nezu CM, Felgoise SH, McClure KS, Houts PS (2003) Project Genesis: assessing the efficacy of problem-solving therapy for distressed adult cancer patients. J Consult Clin Psychol 71(6):1036–1048
191. Hopkinson JB, Brown JC, Okamoto I, Addington-Hall JM (2012) The effectiveness of patient-family carer (couple) intervention for the management of symptoms and other health-related problems in people affected by cancer: a systematic literature search and narrative review. J Pain Symptom Manage 43(1):111–142. doi:10.1016/j.jpainsymman.2011.03.013
192. Regan T, Lambert SD, Kelly B (2013) Uptake and attrition in couple-based interventions for cancer: perspectives from the literature. Psycho-Oncology 22(12):2639–2647. doi:10.1002/pon.3342

193. Lambert SD, Girgis A, Turner J, Regan T, Candler H, Britton B, Chambers S, Lawsin C, Kayser K (2013) "You need something like this to give you guidelines on what to do": patients' and partners' use and perceptions of a self-directed coping skills training resource. Support Care Cancer 21(12):3451–3460. doi:10.1007/s00520-013-1914-4
194. Cochrane BB, Lewis FM (2005) Partner's adjustment to breast cancer: a critical analysis of intervention studies. Health Psychol 24(3):327–332. doi:10.1037/0278-6133.24.3.327
195. Chan RJ, Webster J, Marquart L (2011) Information interventions for orienting patients and their carers to cancer care facilities. Cochrane database of systematic reviews (Online) 12: CD008273
196. Warburton DER, Nicol CW, Bredin SSD (2006) Health benefits of physical activity: The evidence. CMAJ 174:801–809
197. Fitzpatrick TR, Edgar L, Holcroft C (2012) Assessing the relationship between physical fitness activities, cognitive health and quality of life among older breast cancer survivors. J Psychosoc Oncol 30:556–572
198. Lambert SD, Duncan L, Bruson AM, Kapellas S, Myrand M, Santa Mina D, Culos-Reed N, Lambrou A (2015) The effect of exercise on caregivers' psychosocial and physical activity outcomes: a systemic review. Psycho-Oncology Suppl 2:133
199. Beatty L, Lambert S (2013) A systematic review of internet-based self-help therapeutic interventions to improve distress and disease-control among adults with chronic health conditions. Clin Psychol Rev 33(4):609–622. doi:10.1016/j.cpr.2013.03.004
200. Tang W, Chan C, So W, Leung D (2014) Web-based interventions for caregivers of cancer patients: A review of literatures. Asia Pac J Oncol Nurs 1:9–15
201. Mitchell G, Girgis A, Jiwa M, Sibbritt D, Burridge L (2010) A GP caregiver needs toolkit versus usual care in the management of the needs of caregivers of patients with advanced cancer: a randomized controlled trial. Trials 11:115. doi:10.1186/1745-6215-11-115
202. Mitchell GK, Girgis A, Jiwa M, Sibbritt D, Burridge LH, Senior HE (2013) Providing general practice needs-based care for carers of people with advanced cancer: a randomised controlled trial. Br J Gen Pract 63(615):683–690. doi:10.3399/bjgp13X673694
203. Waller A, Girgis A, Currow D, Lecathelinais C, Team PCRP (2008) Development of the palliative care needs assessment tool (PC-NAT) for use by multi-disciplinary health professionals. Palliat Med 22(8):956–964. doi:10.1177/0269216308098797
204. Stetz KM, Brown M (2004) Physical and psychosocial health in family caregiving: a comparison of AIDS and cancer caregivers. Public Health Nurs 21(6):533–540
205. Burton AM, Sautter JM, Tulsky JA, Lindquist JH, Hays JC, Olsen MK, Zimmerman SI, Steinhauser KE (2012) Burden and well-being among a diverse sample of cancer, congestive heart failure, and chronic obstructive pulmonary disease caregivers. J Pain Symptom Manage 44(3):410–420. doi:10.1016/j.jpainsymman.2011.09.018
206. Garlo K, O'Leary JR, Van Ness PH, Fried TR (2010) Burden in caregivers of older adults with advanced illness. J Am Geriatr Soc 58(12):2315–2322. doi:10.1111/j.1532-5415.2010.03177.x
207. Campbell LC, Keefe FJ, Scipio C, McKee DC, Edwards CL, Herman SH, Johnson LE, Colvin OM, McBride CM, Donatucci C (2007) Facilitating research participation and improving quality of life for African American prostate cancer survivors and their intimate partners. A pilot study of telephone-based coping skills training. Cancer 109(2 Suppl):414–424. doi:10.1002/cncr.22355
208. Mokuau N, Braun KL, Wong LK, Higuchi P, Gotay CC (2008) Development of a family intervention for native Hawaiian women with cancer: a pilot study. Soc Work 53(1):9–19

Further Reading

209. Hagedoorn M, Sanderman R, Bolks HN, Tuinstra J, Coyne JC (2008) Distress in couples coping with cancer: a meta-analysis and critical review of role and gender effects. Psychol Bull 134(1):1–30. doi:10.1037/0033-2909.134.1.1
210. Kim Y, Spillers RL, Hall DL (2012) Quality of life of family caregivers 5 years after a relative's cancer diagnosis: follow-up of the national quality of life survey for caregivers. Psycho-Oncology 21(3):273–281. doi:10.1002/pon.1888
211. Lambert SD, Harrison JD, Smith E, Bonevski B, Carey M, Lawsin C, Paul C, Girgis A (2012) The unmet needs of partners and caregivers of adults diagnosed with cancer: a systematic review. BMJ Support Palliat Care 2(3):224–230. doi:10.1136/bmjspcare-2012-000226
212. Lambert SD, Jones B, Girgis A, Lecathelinais C (2012) Distressed partners and caregivers do not recover easily: adjustment trajectories among partners and caregivers of cancer survivors. Ann Behav Med 44(2):225–235. doi:10.1007/s12160-012-9385-2
213. Northouse LL, Katapodi MC, Song L, Zhang L, Mood DW (2010) Interventions with family caregivers of cancer patients: meta-analysis of randomized trials. CA Cancer J Clin 60 (5):317–339. doi:10.3322/caac.20081
214. Regan T, Lambert SD, Kelly B (2013) Uptake and attrition in couple-based interventions for cancer: perspectives from the literature. Psycho-Oncology 22(12):2639–2647. doi:10.1002/pon.3342

Chapter 7
Prevention of Chronic Conditions and Cancer

Alexandra McCarthy, Tina Skinner, Michael Fenech and Shelley Keating

Abstract A scan of any cancer, diabetes, cardiovascular disease or kidney health guideline underscores the importance of preventive strategies to offset the risk of developing chronic conditions. It also highlights the commonalities amongst preventive strategies for these conditions. In this chapter, we focus on the lifestyle practices that increase or reduce the risk of developing common chronic conditions. We examine how modifying individual-level determinants of health, such as exercise and dietary habits, environmental exposures, and alcohol and medication intake could help prevent them. Throughout this chapter we will discuss how these determinants of health can also work in synergy to influence risk. We will particularly focus on the complementary roles of diet and exercise in reducing body fatness and subsequently in reducing many of the risks associated with chronic disease. This chapter concludes with sections on pharmacoprevention and potential approaches to enhance the uptake of, and adherence to, health-promoting behaviours that can prevent the development of chronic conditions and cancer.

Keywords Risk reduction · Lifestyle practices · Body fatness · Nutrition · Exercise · Pharmacoprevention · Environmental exposures

A. McCarthy (✉)
Division of Cancer Services, Princess Alexandra Hospital, Brisbane, Australia
e-mail: Alexandra.McCarthy@health.qld.gov.au; al.mccarthy@qut.edu.au

T. Skinner · S. Keating
School of Human Movement and Nutrition Sciences, The University of Queensland, Brisbane, Australia
e-mail: t.skinner@uq.edu.au

S. Keating
e-mail: s.keating@uq.edu.au

M. Fenech
Genome Health and Personalised Nutrition Laboratory, Adelaide, Australia
e-mail: Michael.Fenech@csiro.au

B. Koczwara (ed.), *Cancer and Chronic Conditions*,
DOI 10.1007/978-981-10-1844-2_7

Key Points

- Research increasingly indicates that cancer and other chronic conditions tend to share common risk factors.
- While many drugs have the potential to limit the risk of chronic disease and cancer, the most feasible and economic determinants of health to target are often lifestyle-related.
- The risks associated with cancer and chronic conditions are often amenable to lifestyle modifications that reduce body fatness, maximise physical activity, promote good nutrition that emphasises plant-based sources, and minimise alcohol intake.
- Many health-promoting lifestyle practices have numerous benefits, operating in synergy to modify risk. In particular, good nutrition and optimum physical activity tend to work in a complementary way to reduce body fatness, which, along with tobacco smoking and high alcohol consumption, embodies an enormous risk to health.
- Adherence to diet, exercise and pharmacotherapy is complex, and remains problematic in the context of preventing chronic disease.

7.1 Introduction: Why Prevention Matters

The incidence of chronic conditions such as cardiovascular and kidney disease, diabetes and cancer is rising. The World Health Organisation argues that these chronic conditions affect not only individual quality of life; they are also an under-appreciated cause of poverty and a significant impediment to the economic development of many countries [1]. The WHO Global Report on chronic diseases and health promotion estimated that preventive strategies could result in an additional 2 % reduction in chronic disease death rates worldwide each year, with the potential to prevent 36 million premature deaths by 2015 [1]. The substantial personal and societal costs of chronic disease and cancer have prompted governments to recognise that systemic collaborative action is needed to target chronic disease prevention [2, 3]. Fortunately, there are solutions to the problem that are both efficacious and highly cost-effective [1]. These solutions are the focus of this chapter.

7.2 Defining Prevention

Prevention in the context of chronic conditions and cancer is broadly defined as "approaches and activities aimed at reducing the likelihood that a disease or disorder will affect an individual, interrupting or slowing the progress of the disorder or reducing disability" [4]. Given that many chronic conditions can take decades to become fully established and tend to occur for a long time once they appear, strategies to prevent them are classified into three stages [2]:

- Primary prevention, which reduces the likelihood of developing a disease or disorder
- Secondary prevention, which interrupts, prevents or minimises the progress of a disease or disorder at an early stage
- Tertiary prevention, which halts the progression of damage already done [2].

The good news is that most of the strategies discussed in this chapter are beneficial irrespective of the individual's position on this continuum of prevention.

7.3 Modifying Individual-Level Determinants of Health to Prevent Chronic Disease and Cancer

The elements that influence whether and how an individual develops a chronic condition, and which are often the target of preventive strategies, are known as the determinants of health. Determinants comprise a range of factors: the broader features of the society in which the individual is situated, their socioeconomic characteristics, their individual knowledge and practise of health behaviours, and their biomedical characteristics, such as birth weight, immune status and genetic inheritance.

There are many inter-relationships between the determinants of health. That is, many determinants such as diet, physical activity and genetic inheritance tend to co-exist, working synergistically to potentiate or modify the risk of developing a chronic condition. Adding to this complexity, a single adverse determinant of health can be implicated in the development of several different chronic conditions, which increases the likelihood that comorbidities will develop. Tobacco smoking for example is implicated in the development of type 2 diabetes, ischaemic heart disease, stroke, kidney disease, arthritis, osteoporosis, lung and colorectal cancer, chronic obstructive pulmonary disease, asthma, depression and compromised oral health [5]. Existing disease states are also determinants of health, as they can compound the risk of multiple chronic diseases. For example, diabetes is linked to the subsequent development of cardiovascular, eye and kidney disease [1], while women previously treated for breast cancer are more likely to develop cardiovascular disease or osteoporosis.

To account for this complexity, the World Health Organisation classifies strategies to modify determinants of health into twelve broad areas that range from the universal to the individual: laws and regulations, tax and price interventions, improving the built environment, advocacy, community-based interventions, school-based interventions, workplace interventions, screening, clinical prevention, disease management, rehabilitation, and palliative care [1]. Prevention strategies often work best when they simultaneously target universal-, intermediate- and individual-level determinants of health [3]. Successfully reducing lung cancer rates, for example, commonly involves widespread regulations to restrict the sale of tobacco complemented by confronting anti-tobacco marketing, increased tobacco excise, public health education, individual support via Quit programs and systemic screening programs for those at risk [3]. Given the clinical focus of this book, however, in this chapter we concentrate on the preventive strategies that are most amenable to health professional intervention at the individual level.

Tables 7.1, 7.2 and 7.3 highlight that most of the rigorous evidence related to the individual determinants of chronic disease pertain to cancer, although research increasingly indicates that cancer and other chronic conditions tend to share common risk factors. The three "focus" health determinants for individual-level chronic disease and cancer prevention are risky alcohol consumption, tobacco smoking, and unhealthy diet coupled with excessive energy intake [1, 3]. These determinants are often expressed through the intermediate risk factors of hypertension, abnormal blood lipids and body fatness [1].

In the next sections, we tease out how the individual risk factors presented in these tables operate in the primary, secondary and tertiary continuum of chronic disease and cancer prevention. We discuss the modification of exercise, nutrition, environmental exposures and medications in light of compelling recent evidence that explains the pathophysiology of risk, and how lifestyle modifications work to reduce risk. We also discuss the evidence underpinning strategies to modify the risk of developing chronic diseases and cancer.

7.4 Exercise, Chronic Disease and Cancer

7.4.1 Primary Prevention

In the context of chronic disease, physical activity should be considered as potent a medicine as many preventative drugs [6]. Physical activity is defined as movement that increases metabolic rate and can be categorised in relation to the energy cost of the activity (termed metabolic equivalent, MET, which is the ratio of the work metabolic rate to the resting metabolic rate). There is 'convincing grade' evidence for the beneficial role of physical activity in the primary prevention of dementia [7], type 2 diabetes [8, 9], cardiovascular disease [10, 11] and colorectal cancer [12], and 'probable'-grade evidence in postmenopausal breast cancer and endometrial cancer [13] (Table 7.1).

For the primary prevention of breast cancer in postmenopausal women, a 3 % decreased risk is observed per 7 MET-hours (METs used per hour) of recreational activity/week [13]. Every 5 MET-hours/day is associated with a decreased risk of developing colorectal cancer and colon cancer by 3 and 8 %, respectively [14]. Interestingly, the same relationship does not appear to exist in rectal cancer [14]. While it is not yet possible to determine the dose-response relationship of exercise

Table 7.1 Strong evidence associated with *reduction* of risk of chronic conditions and cancer

Variable	Condition	Strength of evidence
Lifestyle outcome		
Reduced body fatness	Premenopausal breast cancer	Probable [13]
Weight loss	Type 2 diabetes	Level 1 [206]
Lifestyle behaviour		
Increased physical activity	Postmenopausal breast cancer	Probable [13]
	Endometrial cancer	Probable [5]
	Colorectal cancer	Convincing [5]
	Type 2 diabetes	Level 1 [206]
	Cardiovascular disease	Level 1 [207]
	Dyslipidemia	Level 1 [50]
	Hypertension	Level 1 [208]
	Obesity	Level 1 [166]
	Non-alcoholic fatty liver disease	Level 2 [209]
	Osteoporosis	Level 1 [210]
	Chronic kidney disease	Level 1 [211]
	Dementia	Level 1 [7]
Diet		
Consumption of alcoholic drinks	Kidney cancer	Probable [212]
Consumption of foods containing dietary fibre (cereals, grains, roots, tubers and plantains)	Colorectal cancer	Convincing [5]
Consumption of non-starchy vegetables	Cancers of the mouth, pharynx, larynx, oesophagus, stomach	Probable [5]
Consumption of allium vegetables	Stomach cancer	Probable [5]
Fruit consumption	Cancers of the mouth, pharynx, larynx, oesophagus, stomach	Probable [5]
Consumption of foods containing folate	Cancers of the pancreas	Probable [5]
Consumption of foods containing carotenoids	Cancers of the mouth, pharynx, larynx, lung	Probable [5]
Consumption of foods containing beta-carotene	Oesophageal cancer	Probable [5]
Consumption of foods containing lycopene	Prostate cancer	Probable [213]
Consumption of foods containing Vitamin C	Oesophageal cancer	Probable [5]
Consumption of foods containing selenium	Prostate cancer	Probable [213]
Milk consumption	Colorectal cancer	Probable [5]
Calcium consumption	Colorectal cancer	Probable [5]
Coffee consumption	Endometrial cancer	Probable [5]
	Liver cancer	Probable [5]
Calcium dietary supplement consumption	Colorectal cancer	Probable [5]
Selenium dietary supplement consumption	Prostate cancer	Probable [213]
Diet adhering to NHMRC or similar guidelines	Type 2 diabetes	Level 1 [206]

(continued)

Table 7.1 (continued)

Variable	Condition	Strength of evidence
Pharmaceuticals		
Prophylactic dexrazoxane	Prevention of heart failure in adult patients receiving anthracycline-containing chemotherapy	Level 1 [181]
Tamoxifen	Prevention of breast cancer in post-menopausal women diagnosed with high-risk and ER positive breast cancer, and in premenopausal women diagnosed with DCIS	Level 2 [172]
Raloxifene	Prevention of post-menopausal breast cancer in at-risk women	Level 2 [172]
Aromatase inhibitors	Prevention of post-menopausal breast cancer in at-risk women	Level 2 [214]
Beta blockers	Prevention of cardiovascular disease in patients with pre-existing cardiovascular disease, given during and after cardiotoxic cancer treatment	Level 1 [180]
Prophylactic beta blockers	Prevention of cardiovascular disease in adults with no known cardiovascular disease who are treated with anthracycline or trastuzamab therapy for cancer	Level 1 [182]
Angiotensin antagonists	Prevention of cardiovascular disease in patients with and without pre-existing cardiovascular disease, given during and after cardiotoxic cancer treatment	Level 1 [180, 182]
	Prevention of chronic kidney disease in the context of pre-existing diabetes	Level A [215]
Statin therapy	Prevention of cardiovascular disease in adults with no known cardiovascular disease who are treated with anthracycline or trastuzamab therapy for cancer	Level 1 [182]
Metformin	Type 2 diabetes	Level 1 [206]
Acarbose	Type 2 diabetes	Level 1 [206]
Rosiglitazone	Type 2 diabetes	Level 1 [206]
Orlistat	Type 2 diabetes	Level 1 [206]
Aspirin	Cardiovascular disease	Level 1 [193]
Physiological life event		
Lactation	Pre- and postmenopausal breast cancer	Convincing [13]
Blood pressure of people with type 2 diabetes maintained within the target range	Chronic kidney disease	Level A [215]

Key 'Level': National Health and Medical Research Council (NHMRC) Level of Evidence, I-IV. Level 1 is evidence derived from meta-analyses and systematic reviews, Level 2 from good quality RCTs
'Level A' is used by NHMRC to indicate that the "body of evidence can be trusted to guide practice"
'Probable' and 'convincing' are used by the World Cancer Research Fund to indicate causative links between exposure and the development of cancer. These terms refer to the strength of evidence derived from meta-analyses and systematic reviews, plus good quality RCTs and large scale epidemiological studies

Table 7.2 Strong evidence associated with *increased* risk of developing chronic conditions and cancer

Variable	Condition	Strength of evidence
Lifestyle outcome		
Adult weight gain	Postmenopausal breast cancer	Probable [13]
Increased body fatness	Postmenopausal breast cancer	Convincing [13]
	Colorectal cancer	Convincing [5]
	Pancreatic cancer	Convincing [5]
	Endometrial cancer	Convincing [5]
	Ovarian cancer	Probable [5]
	Advanced prostate cancer	Probable [5]
	Gallbladder cancer	Probable [5]
	Kidney cancer	Convincing [5]
	Liver cancer	Convincing [216]
	Pancreatic cancer	Convincing [5]
Increased abdominal fatness	Postmenopausal breast cancer	Probable [13]
	Colorectal cancer	Convincing [5]
	Type 2 diabetes	Level 1 [206]
	Non-alcoholic fatty liver disease	Level 2 [162]
	Cardiovascular disease	Level 1 [163]
Lifestyle behaviour		
Tobacco smoking	Cancers of the lung, oral cavity, pharynx, nasal cavity and accessory sinuses, larynx, oesophagus, stomach, pancreas, colorectum, liver, kidney (body and pelvis), ureter, urinary bladder, uterine cervix and ovary (mucinous), myeloid leukaemia	Sufficient [217]
Sedentary behaviour	Colorectal cancer (survival)	Probable [218]
	Type 2 diabetes mellitus	Level 1 [219]
	Cardiovascular disease	Level 2 [220]
Environmental exposures		
Solar and ultraviolet radiation	Melanoma, basal cell and squamous cell carcinomas of the skin	Sufficient [195]
Ultraviolet emitting tanning devices	Melanoma of the skin and eye	Sufficient [195]
Second-hand smoke	Lung cancer	Sufficient [217]
Diet		
Alcoholic drinks	Pre- and postmenopausal breast cancer	Convincing [13]
	Liver cancer	Convincing [216]
	Colorectal cancer (men)	Convincing [5]
	Colorectal cancer (women)	Probable [5]
Red meat, processed meat	Colorectal cancer	Convincing [5]
Cantonese-style salted fish	Nasopharyngeal cancer	Probable [5]
Glycaemic load	Endometrial cancer	Probable [5]
Diet high in calcium and dairy food	Prostate cancer	Probable [213]
Salt, salted and salted foods	Stomach cancer	Probable [5]
Fungal aflatoxin contamination of cereals, grains, roots, tubers, plantains, legumes (especially peanuts)	Liver cancer	Convincing [216]

(continued)

Table 7.2 (continued)

Variable	Condition	Strength of evidence
Arsenic in drinking water	Lung cancer	Convincing [5]
Arsenic in drinking water	Skin cancer	Probable [5]
Maté (caffeine rich infusion of the leaves of a South American shrub)	Oesophageal cancer	Probable [5]
High-dose beta carotene supplements	Lung cancer	Convincing [5]
Pharmaceuticals		
Doxorubicin >500 mg/m^2; liposomal doxorubicin >900 mg/m^2; epirubicin >720 mg/m^2; mitoxantrone >120 mg/m^2; idarubicin >90 mg/m^2	Chemotherapy-associated heart failure	Level 1 [180]
Combination hormone therapy	Breast cancer	Level 2 [172]
Viral infections		
Human papilloma virus	Cancers of the cervix, vulva, vagina, penis, anus, oral cavity, oropharynx, tonsil	Sufficient evidence [198]
Hepatitis B (HBV) and Hepatitis C (HCV)	Hepatocellular (liver) cancer, non-Hodgkin lymphoma (HCV only)	Sufficient [198]
Life events		
Adult attained height	Postmenopausal breast cancer	Convincing [13]
	Premenopausal breast cancer	Probable [13]
	Colorectal cancer	Convincing [5]
	Ovarian cancer	Convincing [5]
	Prostate cancer	Probable [213]
	Kidney cancer	Probable [5]
Greater birth weight	Premenopausal breast cancer	Probable [13]
Greater childhood growth	Pancreatic cancer	Convincing [5]

Key 'Level': NHMRC Level of Evidence, I-IV. Level 1 is evidence derived from meta-analyses and systematic reviews, Level 2 from good quality RCTs

'Probable' and 'convincing' are used by the World Cancer Research Fund to indicate causative links between exposure and the development of cancer. These terms refer to the strength of evidence derived from meta-analyses and systematic reviews, plus good quality RCTs and large scale epidemiological studies

'Sufficient' evidence is the highest level of evidence for the International Agency for Research on Cancer (IARC). In many instances, e.g. solar and ultraviolet radiation, and tobacco smoking, evidence is derived from large epidemiological and case-control studies rather than RCTs, systematic reviews or meta-analyses

in endometrial cancer due to differences in physical activity assessment across studies, individuals engaging in the greatest amount of recreational, occupational and/or incidental physical activity demonstrate a reduced risk of cancer of the endometrium compared to those engaging in the lowest levels of activity [15].

The effects of physical activity on the primary prevention of colorectal, endometrial and postmenopausal breast cancers are likely pleiotropic (i.e. have multiple, seemingly unrelated effects) and involve a combination of host pathways [16]. Research suggests that physical activity could reduce the risk of these cancers through a number of pathways, including the modulation of body composition, metabolic hormones, sex-steroid hormones, alterations in immune function, levels of oxidative stress as well as the balance of markers of inflammation and cytokines [17].

Table 7.3 Diet-related recommendations for cancer and chronic disease prevention[a]

Diet or lifestyle factor	Recommendation
Body fatness	Be as lean as possible within the normal range of body weight
Foods and drinks that promote weight gain	Limit consumption of energy-dense foods. Avoid sugary drinks
Plant foods	Eat mostly foods of plant origin
Animal foods	Limit intake of red meat and avoid processed meat
Alcoholic drinks	Limit intake of alcoholic drinks
Preservation, processing, preparation of food	Limit consumption of salt. Avoid mouldy cereals, grains, pulses or legumes[b]
Dietary supplements	Aim to meet nutritional needs through diet alone (if possible)[c]
Breastfeeding	Mothers to breastfeed; children to be breast fed
Cancer survivors	Follow the recommendations for cancer prevention

[a]Adapted from http://www.wcrf.org/int/research-we-fund/our-cancer-prevention-recommendations 2016
[b]There is considerable evidence that high temperature cooking of protein-rich and fat-rich foods may generate carcinogenic polycyclic aromatic hydrocarbons and heterocyclic amines [128]
[c]Dietary supplementation is only required when there is risk of specific micronutrient deficiency due to dietary restrictions or malabsorption of nutrients [128]

The most widely investigated pathway linking physical activity to cancer risk is the effect of exercise on circulating metabolic factors. Changes in metabolic status mediated through the insulin-like growth factor (IGF) axis represent one of the most plausible host pathways through which physical activity is linked to colorectal cancer [17–19]. For example, Chi and colleagues [20] reported a positive association between the risk of colorectal cancer incidence and circulating levels of IGF-1 (OR = 1.25; $p = 0.003$) and IGF-2 (OR = 1.52; $p = 0.003$). Exercise has a likely hormetic ("U" shaped) effect on the IGF axis, and possibly reduces IGF concentrations in states of systemic overabundance, effectively reducing IGF-1 receptor-mediated signalling; cancer outcomes are subsequently improved with exercise through ablation of this mitotic signalling pathway [21]. Moreover, muscle contraction during exercise induces molecular signalling and involves a variety of signalling molecules, including adenosine monophosphate-activated protein kinase (AMPK; a master regulator of cellular energy homeostasis) [22]. In response to increased energy demands during exercise, AMPK conserves adenosine triphosphate via inhibition of the biosynthetic and anabolic pathways, directly contributing to control of cancer cell growth [23]. Indeed, AMPK is reported to be differentially up-regulated following exercise in tumour-bearing mice [24].

Cytokines, which are proteins vital for immune system regulation, also have anti-tumour properties [25]. Deregulation of cytokine production or activity can lead to detrimental acceleration of inflammation, angiogenesis and cell proliferation; hence cytokines can be cancer-promoting factors [25–27]. In pre-existing cancer cells, an abundance of cytokines can stimulate tumour growth and cell proliferation [25]. As such, chronically elevated serum cytokines could potentiate tumour development and progression.

The effects of acute versus chronic exercise on plasma cytokine responses are seemingly paradoxical. Acute exercise results in a transient increase in circulating levels of cytokines produced by myoblasts [28–31]. The underlying mechanism behind this acute increase is the development of a hypoxic microenvironment within the muscle cells [32, 33]. Hypoxia results in the production of reactive oxygen species [32, 33] that stimulate the AP-1 and NF-κB pathways, the primary sources of cytokine production, such as interleukin-8 (IL-8) [34–36]. It is postulated that IL-8 acts locally to stimulate angiogenesis within the muscle, a known adaptation to exercise [37]. An increase in IL-8 is accompanied by a concomitant increase in CXCR2 (a protein coding gene) expression following exercise in the proximate endothelial cells resulting in angiogenesis in the muscle microvasculature [38]. In contrast to the increase in cytokine response to acute exercise, chronic exposure to exercise can normalise circulating cytokine concentrations [39, 40], reducing the perturbations in homeostasis following acute exercise [41]. Given that hypoxia is the primary trigger of cytokine production during exercise, it is reasonable to assume that following regular exercise training, improved delivery of oxygen to the exercising muscles coupled with greater mitochondrial volume results in less hypoxic stress, plus reduced production of cytokine from the muscles. This is supported by numerous studies showing that athletic populations characterised by greater levels of aerobic fitness have dampened immune responses to exercise than their sedentary counterparts [41–44].

Physical activity also plays a role in the prevention of weight gain, which is associated with independent, 'probable' level evidence for the primary prevention of postmenopausal breast cancer. Indeed, the reduced risk of endometrial and postmenopausal breast cancers associated with physical activity can be explained, at least in part, by the enhanced balance of circulating oestrogens, progesterone and androgens that are either a direct result of exercise, or secondary to improvements in body composition that accompany exercise [45, 46]. The modulation of body composition, in particular the reduction of visceral adipose tissue, with regular exercise can also lead to reductions in circulating cytokine levels. Indeed, obesity is associated with higher levels of circulating IL-8 [47, 48] and the reductions in IL-8 found by Troseid and colleagues [40] were associated with reductions in body mass index and waist circumference.

7.4.2 Secondary and Tertiary Prevention

Exercise (planned and structured physical activity) has been touted as a 'polypill' for chronic disease management [49] due to its ability to concomitantly improve the modifiable risk factors associated with the development of type 2 diabetes, cardiovascular disease and some cancers [16]. This includes improvements in atherogenic dyslipidemia [50], insulin resistance [51], hypertension [52], low-grade systemic inflammation [53], central obesity [54], and intrahepatic lipids [55].

Patients with cancer have an increased risk of developing co-morbid chronic diseases including chronic kidney disease (CKD) [56] and coronary heart disease [57], and can also have more cardiovascular disease risk factors than the general population [58]. Indeed, most exercise oncology research has focussed on secondary prevention of chronic conditions, and the modification of the disease- and treatment-related side effects of cancer. Level 1 evidence for the benefits of exercise for cancer patients and survivors indicates it improves psychological wellbeing and quality of life [59], cancer-related fatigue [60], physical functioning [61], body weight and composition [62], muscle strength and endurance [61, 62], immune function [63], and cardiovascular fitness [64].

Treatments for certain cancers, such as selective estrogen receptor modulators (SERMs) for breast cancer and androgen deprivation therapy for prostate cancer, can promote abnormal body composition by increasing fat mass and reducing lean muscle mass [65]. Observational studies have associated abnormal body composition with a poorer prognosis of cancer [66], including hepatocellular carcinoma [67]. Sarcopenia (age-associated loss of skeletal muscle mass and function) is also an independent predictor of mortality after controlling for body mass index, age and tumour stage (HR: 5.19; 95 % CI: 2.58, 10.43) [67]. Regular aerobic exercise training increases energy expenditure and induces lipolysis, which can reduce fat mass, while progressive resistance training induces muscular hypertrophy and prevents the loss of muscle mass commonly associated with hypo-caloric diets [68, 69].

Evidence for 'exercise as medicine' is emerging for a range of secondary sequelae from cancer and its treatments, such as cardiovascular disease [70]. For example, both cellular (e.g. mitigation of mitochondrial dysfunction [71] and reactive oxygen species emission from cardiac mitochondria [72]) and functional (e.g. attenuation of decrements in left ventricular function [73]) mechanisms are implicated in animal models to explain the protection from anthracycline-induced cardiotoxicity afforded by exercise.

Strong associations are also reported between type 2 diabetes and the incidence and prognosis of cancer, especially of the colon, liver and pancreas [74, 75]. Increases in plasma IGF-1 and IGF-2 as a result of hyperinsulinemia activate their respective receptors and initiate mitogenic behaviour within cancerous cells [76, 77]. Exercise training improves peripheral insulin sensitivity [76] and is the most potent stimulus to increase skeletal muscle glucose transporter 4 (GLUT4) expression and subsequent improvement of insulin action, glucose disposal and muscle glycogen storage [22]. In combination with nutritional and pharmacological interventions, exercise training can prevent the progression of impaired glucose tolerance and impaired fasting glucose (conditions indicative of pre-diabetes) to type 2 diabetes. For patients with type 2 diabetes, exercise training can decrease HbA1c levels [8, 78] and prevent further complications associated with poor glycaemic control such as renal and ophthalmic diseases [79].

The improvements in insulin sensitivity and body composition linked with exercise training further reduce the delivery of free fatty acids and glucose to the liver and are associated with improvement of non-alcoholic fatty liver disease (NAFLD). The benefits of exercise on NAFLD arise through numerous mechanisms involving the liver, muscle and adipose tissue, including the abovementioned activation of AMPK. For example, exercise-induced activation of AMPK reduces intrahepatic lipid content by inhibiting lipid synthesis and increasing fatty acid oxidation within the liver [80]. Insulin resistance is a hallmark feature of non-alcoholic steatohepatitis (NASH), a progressive form of NAFLD, characterised by inflammatory changes, hepatocyte ballooning and a variable degree of fibrosis. While there is no evidence demonstrating the reversal of NASH with exercise alone, exercise could prevent the progression of simple steatosis to NASH [81].

There are several other chronic diseases that can arise secondary to the disease- and treatment-related effects of cancer, such as chronic kidney disease CKD, osteoporosis and cognitive impairment. For example, there is a bidirectional relationship between the incidence of CKD and cancer [82]. Physical inactivity is a major risk factor for the development of CKD [83] and there is 'probable'-grade evidence to suggest that exercise improves estimated glomerular filtration rate (eGFR) indicating an improvement in kidney function [84]. Initiation of androgen deprivation therapy (ADT) in men with prostate cancer is reported to result in a 5- to 10-fold increased loss of bone mineral density in multiple skeletal sites [85, 86]. This bone loss and accompanying decrease in muscle mass increases the risk of osteoporosis, falls, and fractures. Indeed, a fracture risk of up to 20 % is reported after 5 years on ADT, nearly twice the risk of healthy men or men with prostate cancer not receiving ADT [87]. This ADT-related increased risk of osteoporosis and osteoporotic fractures arises from the suppression of testosterone and oestrogen, two hormones that have vital direct and indirect roles in the regulation of bone metabolism [88] and microarchitectural decay [89]. Exercise training, specifically resistance training and impact-loading exercises that involve mechanical loading of the skeleton from ground reaction forces and muscle pull, can positively influence bone health [90]. However, while early results are encouraging [91], further research is needed to confirm the skeletal benefits of exercise during or after cancer treatment. Similarly, there is growing evidence to suggest that aromatase inhibitor therapy may be associated with long-term cognitive impairment in some cancer patients, especially in breast cancer survivors [92–94]. Exercise is well-known to improve cognitive function and prevent age- and disease-related cognitive decline, with recent evidence suggesting this may include oestrogen deficiency-induced cognitive impairment [95, 96].

7.4.3 Physical Activity Recommendations

Given that physical inactivity is the fourth leading cause of death due to non-communicable diseases (contributing to over three million preventable deaths per year [97]), it is an important target for the prevention of chronic diseases. Indeed, yielding a physical activity energy expenditure of 1000 kcal/week (a level considered 'minimal adherence' to physical activity guidelines as outlined below) is associated with a 20–30 % reduction in risk of all-cause mortality, with greater energy expenditures yielding further reductions [98–100]. Poor cardiorespiratory fitness is suggested to be a potent risk factor for all-cause mortality, cardiovascular disease [99] and the incidence of metabolic syndrome [100]. Importantly, improving cardiorespiratory fitness by just one MET is associated with 13 and 15 % reductions in all-cause mortality and risk of cardiovascular events, respectively [101], and these associations are independent of body mass [102].

Cancer survivors are advised to undertake 150 min per week of moderate or 75 min per week of vigorous aerobic exercise or an equivalent combination; and perform resistance exercise of moderate or high intensity on two or more days per week [103, 104]. Exercise prescription guidelines for a range of chronic conditions are available as position statements and reports from a variety of sources, including the American College of Sports Medicine and Exercise and Sports Science Australia. Consistent across all exercise guidelines for health and fitness is the recommendation for adults to undertake both aerobic exercise and progressive resistance training. Emerging evidence suggests that higher intensity exercise may achieve comparable or even superior benefits for a range of cardio-metabolic risk variables including cardiorespiratory fitness and glycaemic control [105] with less time commitment. Progressive resistance training is important for improvements in lean muscle mass, muscle strength and function [79] and may optimise insulin sensitivity; thus the current Australian guidelines for the prevention or management of type 2 diabetes advocate that at least 60 min of the recommended 210 min of moderate, or 125 min of vigorous intensity exercise be performed as progressive resistance training each week [79]. For more specific exercise prescriptions and for complex conditions where there are competing demands, referral to an exercise specialist is recommended to ensure the prioritisation of key components pertinent to the individual's specific needs [e.g. Accredited Exercise Physiologists (Australia), Certified Exercise Physiologists (Canada) or Clinical Exercise Physiologists (United States of America)].

Despite the evidence for the effectiveness of physical activity in enhancing wellness irrespective of health status, people with chronic disease appear to be even less likely than the general population to meet physical activity guidelines e.g. only 12 % of prostate cancer survivors [106] meet contemporary exercise recommendations. Multi-faceted cognitive behavioural strategies to promote the uptake of lifestyle, environmental exposure, diet, exercise and medication recommendations are essential to successful behaviour change. These strategies enable people to modify their lifestyle by changing the way that they think about themselves, their behaviours and their circumstances [107]. While a detailed discussion of these is beyond scope, interventions that use the cognitive behavioural approach generally incorporate two or more of the following processes: mutual goal setting; increasing self-awareness through self-monitoring of enablers and barriers to change; frequent and prolonged contact through scheduled follow-up; feedback and reinforcement by health professionals to guide behaviour; enhancement of self-efficacy; exposure to credible role-modelling; mutual problem solving; and motivational interviewing comprising goal-oriented and individualised counselling [107]. Research demonstrates that when two or more of these strategies are used, particularly favourable results are attained [107].

The following recommendations are provided to encourage increased physical activity of individuals, including those with chronic disease:

1. Referral to exercise professionals specialising in disease-related exercise e.g. clinical exercise physiologists, is recommended to ensure safe, individualised, supervised exercise programs are prescribed to cancer patients and survivors.
2. If individuals are currently sedentary or have low levels of physical activity, build gradually towards the physical activity guidelines.
3. Encourage the incorporation of active transport into the daily routine, such as walking or cycling rather than driving a car.
4. The use of activity trackers can be recommended as an objective tool to enable self-monitoring and gradual improvements in physical activity e.g. 10 % in average steps per week.
5. Encourage individuals to break up long periods of sitting as often as possible and be aware of time spent in front of the computer screen.

At the community level, the following environmental changes and policy-related activities are suggested to increase physical activity, prevent disease or promote health in groups of people [108]:

1. Using the media to deliver community-wide, large-scale, multicomponent physical activity campaigns.
2. Implementing point-of-decision prompts (e.g. signs posted by elevators and escalators) to encourage use of stairs.
3. Focus on building, strengthening, and maintaining social networks to enhance social support interventions in community settings.
4. Creation of or enhanced access to places for physical activity combined with informational outreach activities.
5. Street- or community-scale urban design (e.g. ensuring sidewalk continuity) and land-use policies (e.g. mixed land-use zoning) and practices to support physical activity participation.
6. Transportation and travel policies and practices to encourage active transport by facilitating walking, bicycling, and public transportation use.

7.5 Nutrition, Cancer and Chronic Disease

Nutrition can have a profound impact on both cancer and chronic diseases because the same nutritional deficiencies or excesses that increase the risk of cancer can also initiate or enhance susceptibility to the chronic degenerative diseases of ageing such as diabetes, cardiovascular disease and dementia [109]. An example at the micronutrient level is folate deficiency, which increases the risk of colorectal, breast, ovary, pancreas, brain, lung and cervical cancers [110] as well as neural tube defects and anaemia [111]. The reason folate deficiency is associated with cancer is because it causes a high level of DNA damage (e.g. DNA strand breaks, chromosome aberrations, micronuclei), chromosomal instability and DNA hypomethylation, which accelerates the number of cells with abnormal genomes and/or epigenomes from which cancers can evolve [110, 112]. In addition, folate deficiency causes an elevation in homocysteine concentration, which is a risk factor for diabetic retinopathy and nephropathy in type 1 diabetes, cardiovascular disease and dementia [111, 113–115]. At the macronutrient level, the available evidence suggests that excess caloric intake leading to obesity could increase the risk for several cancers (e.g. oesophagus, breast, prostate, pancreas and colorectum), as well as the propensity to develop diabetes, cardiovascular disease and cognitive impairment [12, 116–118]. The mechanism by which obesity increases the risk of cancer, diabetes cardiovascular disease and cognitive decline is not clear but obesity and all of the above chronic conditions are associated with increased DNA damage at the chromosomal, telomere, and mitochondrial DNA level. This suggests a common DNA damage mechanism, which is most likely to be a combination of increased oxidative stress due to inflammation, excessive intake of dietary genotoxins and perhaps deficiency in the micronutrients needed for DNA replication and/or repair [98, 112, 119–121]. Furthermore, as indicated above, obesity increases IGF-1 and IGF-2, which may promote the growth of initiated cancer cells.

A significant cause of cancer is damage to the genome leading to abnormal gene expression [122–127]. DNA damage can occur at the chromosomal, gene sequence, telomere and mitochondrial DNA level and could also involve alterations in DNA methylation, which accelerate the evolution of the genomically unstable cells that can more easily transform into cancers and divide abnormally. In this regard, from a cancer prevention perspective, nutrition is important in ensuring healthy cell function and reproduction with respect to the supply of:

1. Co-factors required for DNA synthesis (e.g. folate, vitamin B12, vitamin B6)
2. Co-factors required for DNA repair (e.g. niacin, zinc, magnesium)
3. Antioxidants to prevent oxidation of DNA (e.g. vitamin C, lycopene, polyphenols)
4. Methyl donors to maintain epigenetic control of gene expression (e.g. folate, choline)
5. Natural or man-made genotoxins that damage DNA (e.g. hetrocyclic amines, alcohol)
6. Excess calories that promote obesity and oxidative stress
7. Phytonutrients that promote apoptosis of cells with damaged DNA (e.g. retinoids, polyphenols)
8. Nutrients that may promote the growth of initiated cancers (e.g. methionine, folic acid).

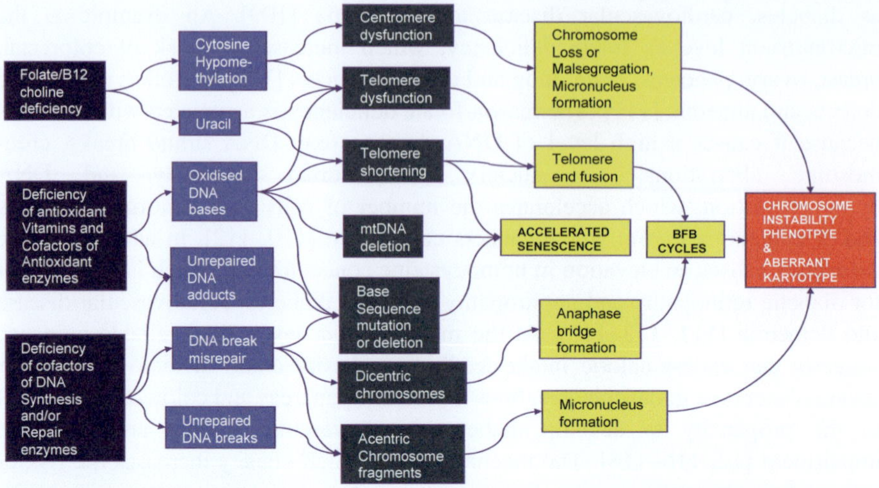

Fig. 7.1 Mechanisms by which micronutrient deficiencies could cause damage to the genome. *BFB* Breakage-fusion-bridge cycles

Figure 7.1 summarises the impact of key nutrient deficiencies that can affect genome integrity via multiple mechanisms. These include the defective maintenance of methylated DNA, causation of damage to DNA bases, and impairment of DNA repair leading to chromosomal instability and aberrant karyotypes which fuel the evolution of malignant cancers [112, 127].

The 2014 World Cancer Research Fund report provides the most comprehensive assessment of the level of evidence for the impact of nutrition on reducing or increasing cancer risk [13]. Tables 7.1 and 7.2 provide a summary of the key outcomes of the meta-analyses that were performed with regards to food and beverage groups and some of the minor dietary components that also affect the risk of other degenerative diseases (e.g. salt, which also affects cardiovascular disease risk and mortality). Based on current evidence, there is (i) convincing evidence that increased intake of foods contaminated with aflatoxins, red meat and processed meat, water contaminated with arsenic, alcoholic drinks, and high dose beta-carotene supplements increase the risk of cancer and (ii) evidence of a probable decreased risk for cancer with increased intake of plant foods including those rich in fibre (cereals, grains, roots, tubers, plantains) and non-starchy vegetables, fruits, pulses, legumes, nuts, seeds, herbs, spices. In addition, breastfeeding (lactation) is convincingly associated with reduced breast cancer risk of the mother and more recently evidence has emerged that childhood leukaemia incidence could be reduced by breastfeeding for 6 months or more [128, 129].

Although there is some evidence that certain dietary patterns (e.g. Mediterranean diet [130]) protect against cardiovascular disease, dementia and cancer there are too few robustly-designed epidemiological prospective studies to provide convincing evidence that a specific dietary pattern aggravates cancer risk to a significantly different extent, relative to another dietary pattern. The main difficulty is that even within a single dietary pattern there can be large differences in micronutrient composition and caloric intake, depending on the food items within the same food group that are included in the pattern. For example, in the case of vegetables one would have to consume 2.5 kg per day if choosing roots, tubers and 'fruit' vegetables but only 0.4 kg per day if one consumed pulses, legumes, leafy and cruciferous vegetables to achieve the recommend intake of folate [131]. Therefore it is plausible that the choice of vegetables influences micronutrient intake and possibly cancer risk. With regards to flesh foods, in October 2015, based on robust epidemiological evidence and strong mechanistic plausibility, the WHO International Agency for Research on Cancer (IARC) classified consumption of processed meat as "carcinogenic to humans" (Group 1 carcinogen) and consumption of red meat as "probably carcinogenic to humans" (Group 2A carcinogen) [132]. This provides an important indication for choosing dietary patterns that are mainly plant-based and low in processed meat and/or red meat. The consumption of alcoholic drinks varies between cultures and has one of the most profound impacts on cancer risk, particularly amongst those with genetic defects in detoxifying acetaldehyde [133, 134], a genotoxic metabolite generated directly from alcohol in the body, which has been classified as a Group 1 carcinogen by IARC [135, 136].

Intake of alcoholic drinks is convincingly associated with cancers of the mouth, pharynx, larynx, oesophagus, colorectum (in men), breast (pre- and post-menopausal) and probably with liver and colorectum (women) [132]. The consumption of alcoholic drinks varies between cultures and has one of the most profound impacts on cancer risk, particularly amongst those with genetic defects in the ALDH2 enzyme required to detoxify acetaldehyde, a genotoxic metabolite generated directly from alcohol in the body. Acetaldehyde has been classified as a Group 1 carcinogen by IARC [133, 135, 136]. Acetaldehyde exerts its carcinogenic effects via a genotoxicity mechanism which causes DNA adducts, DNA-protein cross-links, chromosome aberrations and micronuclei and these effects are stronger in those with defective capacity in detoxifying acetaldehyde to acetate or if cells are deficient in folate [133, 134, 137–139].

To date, there is no conclusive direct evidence to support the association of caloric intake with human cancer risk, even though it is evident from several studies that caloric restriction appears to increase life-span and postpone the onset of degenerative diseases across mammalian species [140, 141]. Therefore, current guidelines suggest that irrespective of whether an individual is at the primary, secondary or tertiary stage of chronic disease prevention, all individuals should eat a diet consistent with the relevant national guidelines and avoid physical inactivity. Table 7.3, which is adapted from the World Cancer Research Fund guidelines, outlines lifestyle recommendations germane to most chronic conditions.

7.6 Reducing Body Fatness: The Synergy of Diet and Exercise in Preventing Chronic Disease Risk

Obesity, the excessive accumulation of body fat, is associated with the development of many chronic diseases. The central distribution of excess body fat (i.e., increased levels of visceral adipose tissue) and the ectopic storage of excess fat (e.g., within the liver, pancreas and muscle) are particularly linked to an increased risk of cardiometabolic disease [142–144]. As pharmacological agents do not specifically reduce fat from these regions, or are unsuitable for the long-term treatment of obesity, the synergy of diet and exercise is the cornerstone of obesity management.

7.6.1 Dietary Interventions to Prevention of Body Fat Gain and Promote Body Fat Loss

The most successful dietary interventions to prevent weight gain or promote weight loss are generally based on dietary patterns that meet nutritional requirements for health without excess calories, or marginally fewer calories (in the case of weight loss) than what is needed to meet energy requirements or achieve energy balance [145–147]. Good examples are the Mediterranean diet and the Dietary Approaches to Stop Hypertension [DASH] program. Weight loss in those who are overweight or obese can be achieved by reducing the portion sizes of habitual foods or by replacing high caloric density foods that are poor in micronutrients with foods containing less calories, but which are richer in vitamins and other essential micronutrients [148, 149].

A higher intake of plant foods is usually associated with leaner body mass [150, 151]. Evidence is also accumulating in support of novel higher-protein (>20 % of energy) diets for successful weight loss maintenance and the prevention of type 2 diabetes [152, 153]. Higher protein and plant-based diets have the advantage of having relatively low energy density and aiding longer-term appetite suppression [150, 151, 153]. Success in caloric restriction is improved by selecting foods that are most effective with respect to satiety. A recent systematic review found 'probable' evidence for high intake of dietary fibre and nuts predicting less weight gain, and for high intakes of meat in predicting more weight gain [154].

Low calorie meal replacements provide a practical approach to achieving and maintaining successful control of body weight and preventing weight regain in the longer term [155, 156]. Although there are concerns about weight cycling due to difficulty in maintaining a lower or healthier body weight, Level 1 evidence indicates that the risks related to weight cycling, cancer or cardiometabolic disease and mortality is small, if not non-existent [157, 158].

The WHO recommendations to prevent weight gain are as follows [159]:

- Energy intake (calories) should be in balance with energy expenditure. Total fat should not exceed 30 % of total energy intake to avoid unhealthy weight gain, with a shift in fat consumption away from saturated fats to unsaturated fats, and towards the elimination of industrial transfats.
- Limiting intake of free sugars to less than 10 % of total energy intake is part of a healthy diet. A further reduction to less than 5 % of total energy intake is suggested for additional health benefits.

7.6.2 Physical Activity Recommendations for Reducing and Preventing Increases in Body Fatness

Physical activity can also prevent an increase in body fatness, in particular visceral adipose tissue, which is linked with numerous chronic health conditions including type 2 diabetes [160, 161], non-alcoholic fatty liver disease [162], and cardiovascular disease [163], as well as several cancers (Table 7.2). Increased levels of physical activity independently predict lower waist circumference (a clinical indicator of central fat distribution, which includes both subcutaneous and visceral adipose tissue) [164]. Moreover, epidemiological data indicate that for individuals with the same body mass index, those with moderate levels of cardiorespiratory fitness have lower levels of total and visceral adipose tissue than their less fit counterparts [165].

Evidence indicates that 150–250 min/week of moderate intensity physical activity effectively prevents weight gain in adults [69]; however, while physical activity alone can lead to small reductions in weight [166], the volume required to lose weight with exercise alone is much larger in the absence of concomitant caloric restriction. The current recommendation for weight loss and the maintenance of weight reduction recommend 60 min per day of low-moderate intensity exercise, totalling ~470 min per week [69].

While caloric restriction is the most effective method for achieving weight reduction [167], epidemiological evidence indicates that physical activity plays an important role in the prevention of weight regain, with 90 % of individuals who have successfully maintained weight loss for over 5 years reporting an average of 60 min of exercise per day (mostly walking) [168]. Furthermore, Level 1 evidence indicates that the benefits of aerobic exercise aerobic on visceral adipose tissue reduction [54, 169] can occur at levels below those currently recommended for weight reduction [54]. While the evidence for resistance training for the reduction of visceral adipose tissue is less clear [54, 62], resistance training is the only antidote for muscle loss associated with caloric restriction [170]. Therefore, the combination of caloric restriction and increased physical activity is undoubtedly the most effective method for weight loss and body fat reduction.

7.7 Pharmacoprevention

Pharmacoprevention is the use of drugs to reduce the risk of chronic diseases and cancer [171]. In this section, we begin with a discussion of drugs known to prevent cancer or its recurrence. This is followed by an exploration of the drugs used to prevent or manage the chronic diseases that can develop in cancer patients as a result of their cancer treatment, and drugs that offset the impact of cancer treatments on comorbid chronic conditions.

7.7.1 Prevention of Primary Cancer and Cancer Recurrence

In terms of cancer prevention, the most rigorous evidence for prevention applies only to the primary prevention of breast cancer, where risk is high in the following circumstances [171]:

- Multiple relatives affected by breast cancer or ovarian cancer on the same side of the family
- Younger age (i.e. under 40 years) at cancer diagnosis
- Relative with an identified mutation in a high-risk breast cancer gene, e.g. BRAC1 or BRAC2
- Relatives affected by bilateral breast cancer
- Breast and ovarian cancer in the same relative
- Ashkenazi Jewish ancestry.

The *selective oestrogen receptor modulators* (SERMS) tamoxifen and raloxifene are the most common pharmacopreventatives. Both drugs interfere with the carcinogenic actions of oestrogen on breast tissue. Tamoxifen reduces the risk of pre- and post-menopausal women developing oestrogen receptor-positive breast cancer where there is a family history of the disease [171]. Raloxifene is used only in post-menopausal women [172], and has the incidental benefit of reducing the risk of osteoporotic fractures. While they do reduce risk by up to 40 % [171] in the target population, SERMS ultimately have no effect on mortality [172] and are not useful in the case of oestrogen receptor-negative breast cancers.

Aromatase inhibitors: Drugs could also have a role in reducing the risk of cancer recurrence in women previously treated for breast cancer. Aromatase inhibitors such as exemestane, letrozole and anastrozole are currently used to treat hormone receptor–positive breast cancers in postmenopausal women. These drugs decrease oestrogen levels by interfering with the ability of the aromatase enzyme produced by body fat to change naturally circulating androgen into oestrogen. Hence aromatase inhibitors are only useful in post-menopausal women, whose ovaries no longer produce oestrogen. The National Cancer Institute guidelines recommend [172] the use of aromatase inhibitors to reduce the incidence of breast cancer in postmenopausal women with an increased risk (i.e., aged over 60 years, previous ductal carcinoma in situ with mastectomy, or a Gail 5-year risk score >1.66) [172]. The Australian guidelines, on the basis of Level 2 evidence, also recommend their use [173].

Metformin: The literature often states, based on the results of some epidemiological studies, that individuals with type 2 diabetes or insulin resistance are not only at risk of type 1 diabetes and its attendant comorbidities, they are also at risk of developing a range of cancers (primarily cancer of the pancreas, colon and liver) [174]. At this stage, however, the evidence of a causal association between diabetes and cancer is poor [175], as the findings of these studies are predominantly retrospective and non-randomised [176]. If there is a definite association, it could be the result of a common risk factor: body fatness. High levels of body fat, cancer and type 2 diabetes are all associated with increased production of insulin-like growth factor, a hormone critical to cell growth, proliferation and death. This has led to further suggestion that metformin, most commonly used as an anti-hyperglycaemic and insulin sensitiser in type 2 diabetes, could also inhibit the growth and metabolic processes of cancer cells [174]. It therefore is considered a potentially viable agent to prevent cancer, with many clinical trials currently underway [176].

As with all medications, cancer preventives do not come without chronic disease risks of their own. Tamoxifen is associated with the development of endometrial cancer and both drugs are implicated in thromboembolic events [171, 172]. Fortunately both side effects are relatively rare. Aromatase inhibitors accelerate osteoporosis and affect lipid metabolism [173]. More importantly, hormone modulation induces symptoms of menopause, which are often more sudden and more severe than in natural menopause [177]. These side effects influence adherence to the therapy [173], which in turn influences risk reduction, because to achieve their effect these drugs must be taken for 5 years. 46 % of women prescribed tamoxifen do not complete their 5-year course [173].

7.7.2 Drugs to Prevent Development of Other Chronic Diseases After Cancer Treatment

Table 7.2 outlines the chemotherapy drugs most strongly associated with the subsequent development of cardiotoxicity, especially heart failure, after cancer treatment. Anthracyclines and trastuzamab are the agents most commonly associated with cardiotoxicity. Anthracycline chemotherapy is thought to disrupt the normal catalytic cycle of topoisomerase 2β, resulting in mitochondrial dysfunction, the generation of free radicals and DNA disruption. Because it results in cardiomyocyte death, it is largely irreversible [178, 179]. Trastuzamab cardiotoxicity is thought to result from the disruption of the cellular repair pathways the enable cardiomyocyte contractility, causing reversible cell dysfunction rather than cell death [180]. Radiotherapy, if incidentally delivered in the cardiac field, is associated with coronary arteritis and atherosclerosis up to 15 years from treatment completion

[180]. Underlining the synergistic nature of cancer, cancer treatments and other chronic diseases, many of the known risk factors for developing chemotherapy-induced cardiotoxicity are remarkably similar to those for developing cardiovascular disease; namely pre-existing cardiovascular symptoms, family history, diabetes, dyslipidaemia and obesity [178].

Dexrazoxane, an iron-chelating agent, is thought to be cardioprotective during chemotherapy in two ways. The first is by interfering with the iron-mediated generation of free radicals associated with the administration of anthracycline chemotherapy [178, 180]; the second involves interference with anthracycline's ability to inhibit topoisomerase 2β, which results in cell death. A meta-analysis of cardioprotective agents for anthracycline chemotherapy published in 2011 [181] reported ambiguous results for dexrazoxane. While the analysis demonstrated a statistically significant benefit in favour of dexrazoxane for the occurrence of subsequent heart failure, it could not determine differences in survival between the intervention and control groups [181]. A subsequent meta-analysis by Kalem and Marwick [182], however, demonstrated that dexrazoxane given prophylactically to asymptomatic patients receiving chemotherapy could usefully lessen the burden of subsequent cardiotoxicity.

Beta blockers and ACE inhibitors: Based on good evidence, for many years diabetes [183], cardiovascular disease [184, 185] and kidney [186] guidelines have recommended the use of anti-hypertensives to mitigate the risk of renal or cardiovascular comorbidities. More recently, these drugs have played a role in some cancer treatments. The European Guidelines for Medical Oncology (ESMO) note that patients receiving potentially cardiotoxic chemotherapy have a high risk of developing heart failure and could be considered 'Stage A' or asymptomatic heart failure patients [180]. There is therefore a potential role for heart failure drugs during and after cancer treatment, especially angiotensin agonists (ACE-I) and beta blockers. This role was confirmed by a meta-analysis reporting the efficacy of ACE-Is and beta blockers in reducing the incidence of anthracycline-induced cardiotoxicity in patients who were asymptomatic during chemotherapy [182].

Statins have had a long-standing role in reducing the risk of hypertension in individuals pre-disposed to high cholesterol levels, but they are also increasingly used in the primary prevention of cardiovascular disease after cancer treatment. A recent meta-analysis confirmed the potential for statins to prevent cardiotoxicity in asymptomatic patients receiving cardiotoxic cancer treatments [182]. The cardioprotective action of statins in this context is attributed to their capacity to reduce the oxidative stress and cellular inflammation that result from chemo- and radiotherapy, and to delay myocyte apoptosis [182]. It is sometimes argued that cholesterol-lowering drugs, which coincidentally antagonise the cellular processes that control the initiation, growth and metastasis of tumours, could also help prevent melanoma [187], and colorectal [187] and prostate [188] cancers. However this argument is not supported by rigorous evidence, with some experts arguing that the results of animal studies imply that statins are in fact "carcinogenic" [189], and that case-control [189] and placebo-controlled studies [190] in humans indicate that statin therapy is actually associated with a higher incidence of cancer.

7.7.3 Drugs that Offset the Impact of Cancer Drugs on Co-existing Chronic Conditions

Beta blockers and ACE inhibitors: There is strong evidence that beta blockade and ACE-I therapy initiated within 2 months of chemotherapy completion in patients with confirmed anthracycline-induced cardiomyopathy can reverse left ventricular dysfunction [180]. The same recommendations apply to trastuzamab- and radiotherapy-induced cardiac dysfunction [180]. The precise mechanism of action is unknown, but could be because both drugs reduce cardiac afterload [182]. Angiotensin inhibitors also have complex beneficial interactions with cardiomyocyte angiotensin 2 receptors and epidermal growth factors; whilst beta blockers have potential antioxidant effects [182].

Aspirin: Antiplatelet therapy, in conjunction with a healthy lifestyle, can diminish the risk of cardiovascular disease [191, 192]. Mostly recommended in the form of low-dose aspirin, like all drugs it is not without side effects and these must be weighed against its benefits. Low-dose aspirin is recommended for individuals with established cardiovascular disease, or those who have known cardiovascular risk factors (such as previous anthracycline therapy for cancer), to reduce the risk of non-fatal myocardial infarction and non-fatal stroke [193]. This recommendation is made only where an overall benefit exists and clearly outweighs the harm of gastrointestinal bleeding and haemorrhagic stroke. There is no evidence to support the prophylactic use of aspirin in individuals who do not have cardiovascular risk factors [193]. Some studies raise the possibility of aspirin providing protection against colon cancer after five years of use; however the many methodological limitations of these studies mean that the evidence for this use of aspirin is poor.

7.8 Environmental Risk Reduction

7.8.1 Radiation Exposure

Radiation risks fall into two categories: those associated with ionising radiation and those associated with solar and ultraviolet radiation (sun) exposure. Ionising radiation is particularly associated with the development of many malignancies of the blood and solid tissue, and with the DNA damage that leads to a variety of other genetically-based chronic conditions. Exposure to ionising radiation apart from radiotherapy is beyond the lifestyle focus of this chapter. More amenable to lifestyle modification is sun exposure, which is limited to cancer risk.

Solar radiation and ultraviolet (UV) radiation from UV-emitting tanning devices are considered Class 1 carcinogens [194], which are particularly implicated in the development of primary cutaneous malignant melanomas and non-melanocytic skin cancers [195]. Radiotherapy is also innately carcinogenic and is routinely associated with the development of second primary cancers such as melanoma [196]. Although a recent systematic review determined that only a relatively small proportion of second cancer is associated with radiotherapy [197], nonetheless, radiotherapy and some common chemotherapy treatments such as 5-fluorouracil, methotrexate and doxorubicin tend to increase sun sensitivity in the treatment period, and for some time after treatment. Hence the standard preventive approaches of limiting exposure to intense sunlight, regular use of broad spectrum sunscreen, wearing wide-brimmed hats, sunglasses and loose clothing, and avoidance of solarium beds are as critical during treatment as they are before and after cancer treatment [195].

7.8.2 Viral Infections

Many infectious agents induce chronic diseases such as tuberculosis, malaria, some cancers and HIV-AIDS. For example, between 3.3 and 16 % of all cancers are attributed to viral infections [198]. Infectious agents induce long-term conditions in three ways [199]. The first is through progressive tissue pathology or organ decompensation, e.g. when the hepatitis B virus induces chronic liver disease. The second is a result of the initial infection causing permanent lifestyle deficits or disabilities, e.g. poliomyelitis-induced paralysis. The third is by predisposing individuals to chronic outcomes. This is a complex pathway exemplified by maternal infection during pregnancy, which in turn leads to pre-term delivery, that, even when the infant is not infected, increases the child's subsequent risk of respiratory and neurological disabilities [199].

As O'Connor et al. [199] argue, understanding these viral pathways and their synergies affords many opportunities to reduce the impact of chronic disease before its outcomes are irreversible. For example, some forms of the sexually-transmitted human papillomavirus (HPV) are classified as Class I carcinogens, implicated in the development of cancers of the genital organs and the oropharyngeal and anal regions [198]. Infection with the hepatitis B (HBV) and hepatitis C (HCV) viruses, which involve sexual and/or blood-to-blood contact, not only induces chronic liver disease but substantially increases the risk of developing liver cancer, with 80 % of all primary liver cancers associated with hepatitis infection [200]. Gastric cancers are strongly associated with *helicobacter* pylori infection [201].

Inevitably, lifestyle factors working in synergy with these biological agents potentiate risk; hence lifestyle modification again has the potential to positively affect global health outcomes, especially where these cancers are concerned. Safe sexual and drug injection practices substantially modify the risks of HBC and HPV infection [198]; vaccination helps protect against HBV and HPV [198]; while studies indicate that a high salt intake could work in synergy with *helicobacter* to potentiate the risk of gastric cancer [201].

7.9 Encouraging Uptake of Preventive Strategies

Much of the information presented in this chapter is not novel. We know intuitively and from rigorous evidence that lifestyle behaviours affect health. We understand that people have the highest risk of chronic disease when they have several adverse determinants of health. It is equally clear that lifestyle modification and medications can help prevent and modify the risk of chronic disease. But we also know that these factors interact in complex ways. The problem is that there are many desirable behaviour targets: exercise, diet, smoking behaviours, sun avoidance, medication adherence, and sexual practices. Targeting a single behaviour in a time- and resource-poor clinical environment could exclude other, equally important lifestyle variables. The World Health Organisation emphasise that a combination of interventions is often needed to realise the full potential of risk reduction strategies in the context of chronic disease [1]. Moreover, strategies that account for several risk factors at once tend to be more cost-effective than those that only address a single risk factor [1, 3].

The other problem is that making the necessary lifestyle changes is not easy, nor even particularly attractive in a societal context that values novel, highly technical interventions; where 60 % of the population have low levels of health literacy [202]; and when the most socially-disadvantaged are at highest risk because they have less access to health education and services, less opportunity to exercise, and fewer healthy food options [203]. The difficulties in instilling behaviour changes are underscored by the latest Australian census data, which are typical of developed countries. For example, 63 % of men and 73 % of Australian women are either sedentary or engage in the lowest levels of exercise [204]. These levels are incompatible with health. There is also a clear trend in the Australian population to the heavier end of the body mass index, with 70 % of men and 56 % of women now classed as overweight or obese [204]. The Australian Bureau of Statistics (2015) attributes this to "an imbalance between energy consumed and energy expended", a situation not helped by the high Australian rates of alcohol consumption. The census data for 2011–2012 reveal that 29 % of Australian men and 10 % of Australian women have self-reported 'risky' alcohol intakes, which indicates a small but significant increase from previous years [204]. Fortunately, the incidence of tobacco smoking has decreased, but given it is considered the largest single preventable cause of cancer and chronic disease [204], the current rates of 20 % for men and 16 % for women remain problematic [204]. In addition, while medications are therapeutic, they often come with a range of unpleasant or undesirable side effects that individuals might consider outweigh any benefits they confer. How to select which of the many determinants and behaviours to target, how to promote the uptake of those behaviours, and how to ensure adherence, are discussed in the remainder of this chapter.

7.9.1 Adherence

The factors that affect sustained uptake of preventive interventions are remarkably similar to those that determine health status. These are socio-economic, health system, therapy-related, patient-related and condition-related factors [205]. Hence strategies to enhance adherence to medication, lifestyle and other changes need to be equally multifaceted. Despite this complexity, the American College of Preventive Medicine [205] argues that interventions to promote adherence can and should be simple, and that simple interventions are often the most cost-effective. The College recommends the "SIMPLE" approach to improve adherence to medication, but this approach is equally useful in sustaining all of the behaviour changes discussed in Table 7.4.

Table 7.4 The SIMPLE approach to enhancing adherence (adapted from [205])

S	Simplify the regimen	The complexity of the required behaviour change can affect adherence, so simplify the regimen whenever possible. E.g. adjust timing, frequency, amount; match to person's activities of daily living
I	Impart knowledge	Adherence is enhanced when a person understands their risk and the benefits of behaviour change to offset this risk. Education alone does not promote adherence, but change can occur when education is combined with regimen simplification and effective clinician communication, e.g. shared decision-making, simpler person-centred language
M	Modify patient beliefs and human behaviour	Understanding the person's perceptions of susceptibility, severity, benefit and barriers is essential, since knowledge alone is not sufficient to enhance adherence (especially where complex behavioural change is necessary). E.g., empower people to self-manage their condition, ensure they understand the benefits of adherence and the risks of non-adherence, understand the person's needs
P	Provide communication and trust	Modifying a person's beliefs is only possible where a high level of trust, reinforced by a positive communication style, exists. Clinicians should, for example, practise active listening, elicit the person's input during decision-making, provide timely feedback, accurately paraphrase conversation and allow time for questions
L	Leave the bias	Ethnic, minority and socioeconomic disparities operate across all chronic conditions. People from non-dominant or disadvantaged groups experience less person-centred communication from clinicians and more verbal passivity. E.g. tailor education to person's level of health literacy, specifically query about cultural norms to understand them, review communication style to ensure person-centredness
E	Evaluate adherence	The issue of non-adherence is uniformly underestimated by clinicians. If it isn't suspected, it can't be corrected. Measuring adherence can lead to better adherence, e.g. ask person simply and directly if they follow their regimen, ask about adherence behaviour at every encounter

7.10 Conclusion

Human behaviours are powerful factors that increase or reduce the risk of developing common chronic conditions and cancer at the primary, secondary and tertiary levels. While many drugs have the potential to limit the risk of chronic disease and cancer, the most feasible and economic determinants of health to target are often lifestyle-related. Although it can be difficult to persuade people to change their lifestyles and to sustain that change, it is worth the effort. Many health-promoting lifestyle practices have numerous benefits, operating in synergy to modify risk. In particular, good nutrition and optimum physical activity tend to work in a complementary way to reduce body fatness, which along with tobacco smoking and high alcohol intakes, embodies an enormous risk to health.

References

1. World Health Organisation (WHO) (2005) Preventing chronic diseases: a vital investment. WHO, Geneva
2. Australian Institute of Health and Welfare (AIHW) (2014) Preventing and treating ill health. AIHW, Canberra
3. Australian Institute of Health and Welfare (AIHW) (2015) Health behaviours and their role in the prevention of chronic disease. http://www.aihw.gov.au/chronic-disease/risk-factors/ch1/. Accessed 20 Jan 2016
4. World Health Organisation (WHO) (2004) Global Forum on chronic disease prevention and control. WHO, Geneva
5. World Cancer Research Fund International (2016) Continuous update project. http://www.wcrf.org/int/research-we-fund/continuous-update-project-cup. Accessed 20 Feb 2016
6. Naci H, Ioannidis JPA (2013) Comparative effectiveness of exercise and drug interventions on mortality outcomes: metaepidemiological study. BMJ Brit Med J. 347:f5577 (10/0108/22/accepted 2013)
7. Aarsland D, Sardahaee FS, Anderssen S, Ballard C (2010) Is physical activity a potential preventive factor for vascular dementia? A systematic review. Aging Ment Health 14(4): 386–395
8. Boule NG, Haddad E, Kenny GP, Wells GA, Sigal RJ (2001) Effects of exercise on glycemic control and body mass in type 2 diabetes mellitus: a meta-analysis of controlled clinical trials. JAMA 286(10):1218–1227
9. Thomas DE, Elliott EJ, Naughton GA (2006) Exercise for type 2 diabetes mellitus. Cochrane Database Syst Rev 3:Cd002968
10. Pearson TA, Blair SN, Daniels SR et al (2002) AHA guidelines for primary prevention of cardiovascular disease and stroke: 2002 update: consensus panel guide to comprehensive risk reduction for adult patients without coronary or other atherosclerotic vascular diseases. American Heart Association Science Advisory and Coordinating Committee. Circulation 106 (3):388–391
11. Fletcher GF, Balady G, Blair SN et al (1996) Statement on exercise: benefits and recommendations for physical activity programs for all Americans. A statement for health professionals by the Committee on Exercise and Cardiac Rehabilitation of the Council on Clinical Cardiology, American Heart Association. Circulation 94(4):857–862

12. Eheman C, Henley SJ, Ballard-Barbash R et al (2012) Annual Report to the Nation on the status of cancer, 1975–2008, featuring cancers associated with excess weight and lack of sufficient physical activity. Cancer 118(9):2338–2366
13. World Cancer Research Fund and American Institute for Cancer Research (WCRF/AICR) (2010) Continuous update project report summary: food, nutrition and physical activity and the prevention of breast cancer. 2014
14. World Cancer Research Fund/American Institute for Cancer Research (2011) Continuous update project report. Food, nutrition, physical activity, and the prevention of colorectal cancer. http://www.wcrf.org/int/research-we-fund/continuous-update-project-findings-reports/colorectal-bowel-cancer. Accessed 22 Feb 2016
15. World Cancer Research Fund International (2013) Continuous update project report. Food, nutrition, physical activity, and the prevention of endometrial cancer. http://www.dietandcancerreport.org
16. Pedersen L, Christensen JF, Hojman P (2015) Effects of exercise on tumor physiology and metabolism. Cancer J 21(2):111–116
17. Betof AS, Dewhirst MW, Jones LW (2013) Effects and potential mechanisms of exercise training on cancer progression: a translational perspective. Brain Behav Immun 30(Suppl): S75–S87
18. Ballard-Barbash R, Friedenreich CM, Courneya KS, Siddiqi SM, McTiernan A, Alfano CM (2012) Physical activity, biomarkers, and disease outcomes in cancer survivors: a systematic review. J Natl Cancer Inst 104(11):815–840
19. Buffart LM, Galvao DA, Brug J, Chinapaw MJ, Newton RU (2014) Evidence-based physical activity guidelines for cancer survivors: current guidelines, knowledge gaps and future research directions. Cancer Treat Rev 40(2):327–340
20. Chi F, Wu R, Zeng YC, Xing R, Liu Y (2013) Circulation insulin-like growth factor peptides and colorectal cancer risk: an updated systematic review and meta-analysis. Mol Biol Rep 40(5):3583–3590
21. Devin JL, Bolam KA, Jenkins DG, Skinner TL (2015) The influence of exercise on the insulin-like growth factor axis in oncology: physiological basis, current, and future perspectives. Cancer Epidemiol Biomarkers Prev
22. Richter EA, Hargreaves M (2013) Exercise, GLUT4, and skeletal muscle glucose uptake. Physiol Rev 93(3):993–1017
23. Hardie DG, Ross FA, Hawley SA (2012) AMPK: a nutrient and energy sensor that maintains energy homeostasis. Nat Rev Mol Cell Biol 13(4):251–262
24. Jiang W, Zhu Z, Thompson HJ (2009) Effects of physical activity and restricted energy intake on chemically induced mammary carcinogenesis. Cancer Prev Res (Phila) 2(4): 338–344
25. Dranoff G (2004) Cytokines in cancer pathogenesis and cancer therapy. Nat Rev Cancer 4(1):11–22
26. Hiscott J, Ware C (2011) Cytokines. Curr Opin Immunol 23(5):561–563 (10)
27. Lippitz BE (2013) Cytokine patterns in patients with cancer: a systematic review. Lancet Oncol 14(6):e218–e228
28. Chan MH, Carey AL, Watt MJ, Febbraio MA (2004) Cytokine gene expression in human skeletal muscle during concentric contraction: evidence that IL-8, like IL-6, is influenced by glycogen availability. Am J Physiol Regul Integr Comp Physiol 287(2):R322–R327
29. Louis E, Raue U, Yang Y, Jemiolo B, Trappe S (2007) Time course of proteolytic, cytokine, and myostatin gene expression after acute exercise in human skeletal muscle. J Appl Physiol (1985) 103(5):1744–1751
30. Akerstrom T, Steensberg A, Keller P, Keller C, Penkowa M, Pedersen BK (2005) Exercise induces interleukin-8 expression in human skeletal muscle. J Physiol 563(Pt 2):507–516
31. Nieman DC, Davis JM, Henson DA et al (2003) Carbohydrate ingestion influences skeletal muscle cytokine mRNA and plasma cytokine levels after a 3-h run. J Appl Physiol (1985) 94 (5):1917–1925

32. Ali MH, Schlidt SA, Chandel NS, Hynes KL, Schumacker PT, Gewertz BL (1999) Endothelial permeability and IL-6 production during hypoxia: role of ROS in signal transduction. Am J Physiol 277(5 Pt 1):L1057–L1065
33. Ito K, Hanazawa T, Tomita K, Barnes PJ, Adcock IM (2004) Oxidative stress reduces histone deacetylase 2 activity and enhances IL-8 gene expression: role of tyrosine nitration. Biochem Biophys Res Commun 315(1):240–245
34. Droge W (2002) Free radicals in the physiological control of cell function. Physiol Rev 82(1):47–95
35. Kim YM, Reed W, Wu W, Bromberg PA, Graves LM, Samet JM (2006) Zn2+-induced IL-8 expression involves AP-1, JNK, and ERK activities in human airway epithelial cells. Am J Physiol Lung Cell Mol Physiol 290(5):L1028–L1035
36. Yamamoto S, Shimizu S, Kiyonaka S et al (2008) TRPM2-mediated Ca2+ influx induces chemokine production in monocytes that aggravates inflammatory neutrophil infiltration. Nat Med 14(7):738–747
37. Pedersen BK, Akerstrom TC, Nielsen AR, Fischer CP (2007) Role of myokines in exercise and metabolism. J Appl Physiol (1985) 103(3):1093–1098
38. Frydelund-Larsen L, Penkowa M, Akerstrom T, Zankari A, Nielsen S, Pedersen BK (2007) Exercise induces interleukin-8 receptor (CXCR2) expression in human skeletal muscle. Exp Physiol 92(1):233–240
39. Della Gatta PA, Garnham AP, Peake JM, Cameron-Smith D (2014) Effect of exercise training on skeletal muscle cytokine expression in the elderly. Brain Behav Immun 39: 80–86 (7)
40. Troseid M, Lappegard KT, Claudi T et al (2004) Exercise reduces plasma levels of the chemokines MCP-1 and IL-8 in subjects with the metabolic syndrome. Eur Heart J 25(4):349–355
41. Croft L, Bartlett JD, MacLaren DP et al (2009) High-intensity interval training attenuates the exercise-induced increase in plasma IL-6 in response to acute exercise. Appl Physiol Nutr Metab 34(6):1098–1107
42. Ambarish V, Chandrashekara S, Suresh KP (2012) Moderate regular exercises reduce inflammatory response for physical stress. Indian J Physiol Pharmacol 56(1):7–14
43. Fischer CP, Plomgaard P, Hansen AK, Pilegaard H, Saltin B, Pedersen BK (2004) Endurance training reduces the contraction-induced interleukin-6 mRNA expression in human skeletal muscle. Am J Physiol Endocrinol Metab 287(6):E1189–E1194
44. Gokhale R, Chandrashekara S, Vasanthakumar KC (2007) Cytokine response to strenuous exercise in athletes and non-athletes–an adaptive response. Cytokine 40(2):123–127
45. McTiernan A, Tworoger SS, Ulrich CM et al (2004) Effect of exercise on serum estrogens in postmenopausal women: a 12-month randomized clinical trial. Cancer Res 64(8):2923–2928
46. McTiernan A (2008) Mechanisms linking physical activity with cancer. Nat Rev Cancer 8 (3):205–211
47. Bruun JM, Verdich C, Toubro S, Astrup A, Richelsen B (2003) Association between measures of insulin sensitivity and circulating levels of interleukin-8, interleukin-6 and tumor necrosis factor-alpha. Effect of weight loss in obese men. Eur J Endocrinol 148(5):535–542
48. Straczkowski M, Dzienis-Straczkowska S, Stepien A, Kowalska I, Szelachowska M, Kinalska I (2002) Plasma interleukin-8 concentrations are increased in obese subjects and related to fat mass and tumor necrosis factor-alpha system. J Clin Endocrinol Metab 87(10):4602–4606
49. Fiuza-Luces C, Garatachea N, Berger NA, Lucia A (2013) Exercise is the real polypill. Physiology (Bethesda) 28(5):330–358
50. Mann S, Beedie C, Jiminez A (2014) Differential effects of aerobic exercise, resistance training and combined exercise modalities on cholesterol and the lipid profile: review, synthesis and recommendations. Sports Medicine 44(2):211–221
51. Hawley JA (2004) Exercise as a therapeutic intervention for the prevention and treatment of insulin resistance. Diabetes Metab Res Rev 20(5):383–393

52. Sharman JE, Stowasser M (2009) Australian association for exercise and sports science position statement on exercise and hypertension. J Sci Med Sport. 12(2):252–257
53. Gleeson M, Bishop NC, Stensel DJ, Lindley MR, Mastana SS, Nimmo MA (2011) The anti-inflammatory effects of exercise: mechanisms and implications for the prevention and treatment of disease. Nat Rev Immunol 11(9):607–615
54. Ismail I, Keating SE, Baker MK, Johnson NA (2012) A systematic review and meta-analysis of the effect of aerobic vs. resistance exercise training on visceral fat. Obes Rev 13(1):68–91
55. Keating SE, Hackett DA, George J, Johnson NA (2012) Exercise and non-alcoholic fatty liver disease: a systematic review and meta-analysis. J Hepatol 57(1):157–166
56. Shin HY, Linton JA, Shim JY, Kang HT (2015) Cancer survivors aged 40 years or elder are associated with high risk of chronic kidney disease: the 2010–2012 Korean National Health and Nutrition Examination Survey. Asian Pac J Cancer Prev 16(4):1355–1360
57. Fairley TL, Hawk H, Pierre S (2010) Health behaviors and quality of life of cancer survivors in Massachusetts, 2006: data use for comprehensive cancer control. Prev Chronic Dis 7(1):A09
58. Weaver KE, Foraker RE, Alfano CM et al (2013) Cardiovascular risk factors among long-term survivors of breast, prostate, colorectal, and gynecologic cancers: a gap in survivorship care? J Cancer Surviv 7(2):253–261
59. Mishra SI, Scherer RW, Snyder C, Geigle P, Gotay C (2014) Are exercise programs effective for improving health-related quality of life among cancer survivors? A systematic review and meta-analysis. Oncol Nurs Forum 41(6):E326–E342
60. Meneses-Echavez JF, Gonzalez-Jimenez E, Correa-Bautista JE, Valle JS, Ramirez-Velez R (2015) Effectiveness of physical exercise on fatigue in cancer patients during active treatment: a systematic review and meta-analysis. Cad Saude Publica 31(4):667–681
61. Cheema BS, Kilbreath SL, Fahey PP, Delaney GP, Atlantis E (2014) Safety and efficacy of progressive resistance training in breast cancer: a systematic review and meta-analysis. Breast Cancer Res Treat 148(2):249–268
62. Strasser B, Steindorf K, Wiskemann J, Ulrich CM (2013) Impact of resistance training in cancer survivors: a meta-analysis. Med Sci Sports Exerc 45(11):2080–2090
63. Kruijsen-Jaarsma M, Revesz D, Bierings MB, Buffart LM, Takken T (2013) Effects of exercise on immune function in patients with cancer: a systematic review. Exerc Immunol Rev 19:120–143
64. Schmitz KH, Holtzman J, Courneya KS, Masse LC, Duval S, Kane R (2005) Controlled physical activity trials in cancer survivors: a systematic review and meta-analysis. Cancer Epidemiol Biomarkers Prev 14(7):1588–1595
65. Haseen F, Murray LJ, Cardwell CR, O'Sullivan JM, Cantwell MM (2010) The effect of androgen deprivation therapy on body composition in men with prostate cancer: systematic review and meta-analysis. J Cancer Surviv 4(2):128–139
66. Gonzalez MC, Pastore CA, Orlandi SP, Heymsfield SB (2014) Obesity paradox in cancer: new insights provided by body composition. Am J Clin Nutr 99(5):999–1005
67. Fujiwara N, Nakagawa H, Kudo Y et al (2015) Sarcopenia, intramuscular fat deposition, and visceral adiposity independently predict the outcomes of hepatocellular carcinoma. J Hepatol 63(1):131–140
68. Pines A (2012) Weight loss, weight regain and bone health. Climacteric 15(4):317–319
69. Donnelly JE, Blair SN, Jakicic JM, Manore MM, Rankin JW, Smith BK (2009) American College of Sports Medicine Position Stand. Appropriate physical activity intervention strategies for weight loss and prevention of weight regain for adults. Med Sci Sports Exerc 41(2):459–471
70. Sturgeon KM, Ky B, Libonati JR, Schmitz KH (2014) The effects of exercise on cardiovascular outcomes before, during, and after treatment for breast cancer. Breast Cancer Res Treat 143(2):219–226
71. Ascensao A, Lumini-Oliveira J, Machado NG et al (2011) Acute exercise protects against calcium-induced cardiac mitochondrial permeability transition pore opening in doxorubicin-treated rats. Clin Sci (Lond) 120(1):37–49

72. Kavazis AN, Smuder AJ, Min K, Tumer N, Powers SK (2010) Short-term exercise training protects against doxorubicin-induced cardiac mitochondrial damage independent of HSP72. Am J Physiol Heart Circ Physiol 299(5):H1515–H1524
73. Chicco AJ, Schneider CM, Hayward R (2005) Voluntary exercise protects against acute doxorubicin cardiotoxicity in the isolated perfused rat heart. Am J Physiol Regul Integr Comp Physiol 289(2):R424–R431
74. Giovannucci E, Harlan DM, Archer MC et al (2010) Diabetes and cancer: a consensus report. CA Cancer J Clin 60(4):207–221
75. Vigneri P, Frasca F, Sciacca L, Pandini G, Vigneri R (2009) Diabetes and cancer. Endocr Relat Cancer 16(4):1103–1123
76. Sandhu MS, Dunger DB, Giovannucci EL (2002) Insulin, insulin-like growth factor-I (IGF-I), IGF binding proteins, their biologic interactions, and colorectal cancer. J Natl Cancer Inst 94(13):972–980
77. Ahmed RL, Thomas W, Schmitz KH (2007) Interactions between insulin, body fat, and insulin-like growth factor axis proteins. Cancer Epidemiol Biomarkers Prev 16(3):593–597
78. Sigal RJ, Kenny GP, Wasserman DH, Castaneda-Sceppa C (2004) Physical activity/exercise and type 2 diabetes. Diabetes Care 27(10):2518–2539
79. Hordern MD, Dunstan DW, Prins JB, Baker MK, Singh MA, Coombes JS (2012) Exercise prescription for patients with type 2 diabetes and pre-diabetes: a position statement from Exercise and Sport Science Australia. J Sci Med Sport 15(1):25–31
80. Rector RS, Uptergrove GM, Morris EM et al (2011) Daily exercise vs. caloric restriction for prevention of nonalcoholic fatty liver disease in the OLETF rat model. Am J Physiol Gastrointest Liver Physiol 300(5):G874–G883
81. Berzigotti A, Saran U, Dufour JF (2015) Physical activity and liver diseases. Hepatology
82. Stengel B (2010) Chronic kidney disease and cancer: a troubling connection. J Nephrol 23(3):253–262
83. White SL, Dunstan DW, Polkinghorne KR, Atkins RC, Cass A, Chadban SJ (2011) Physical inactivity and chronic kidney disease in Australian adults: the AusDiab study. Nutr Metab Cardiovasc Dis 21(2):104–112
84. Heiwe S, Jacobson SH (2011) Exercise training for adults with chronic kidney disease. Cochrane Database Syst Rev 10:Cd003236
85. Israeli RS, Ryan CW, Jung LL (2008) Managing bone loss in men with locally advanced prostate cancer receiving androgen deprivation therapy. J Urol 179(2):414–423
86. Greenspan SL, Coates P, Sereika SM, Nelson JB, Trump DL, Resnick NM (2005) Bone loss after initiation of androgen deprivation therapy in patients with prostate cancer. J Clin Endocrinol Metab 90(12):6410–6417
87. Lattouf JB, Saad F (2010) Bone complications of androgen deprivation therapy: screening, prevention, and treatment. Curr Opin Urol 20(3):247–252
88. Clarke BL, Khosla S (2009) Androgens and Bone. Steroids 74(3):296–305 (10/17)
89. Hamilton EJ, Ghasem-Zadeh A, Gianatti E et al (2010) Structural decay of bone microarchitecture in men with prostate cancer treated with androgen deprivation therapy. J Clin Endocrinol Metab 95(12):E456–E463
90. Guadalupe-Grau A, Fuentes T, Guerra B, Calbet JA (2009) Exercise and bone mass in adults. Sports Med 39(6):439–468
91. Winters-Stone KM, Schwartz A, Nail LM (2010) A review of exercise interventions to improve bone health in adult cancer survivors. J Cancer Surviv 4(3):187–201
92. Schilder CM, Eggens PC, Seynaeve C et al (2009) Neuropsychological functioning in postmenopausal breast cancer patients treated with tamoxifen or exemestane after AC-chemotherapy: cross-sectional findings from the neuropsychological TEAM-side study. Acta Oncol 48(1):76–85
93. Jenkins V, Shilling V, Fallowfield L, Howell A, Hutton S (2004) Does hormone therapy for the treatment of breast cancer have a detrimental effect on memory and cognition? A pilot study. Psychooncology 13(1):61–66

94. Collins B, Mackenzie J, Stewart A, Bielajew C, Verma S (2009) Cognitive effects of hormonal therapy in early stage breast cancer patients: a prospective study. Psychooncology 18(8):811–821
95. Gomez-Pinilla F, Hillman C (2013) The influence of exercise on cognitive abilities. Compr Physiol 3(1):403–428
96. Li C, Zhou C, Li R (2015) Can exercise ameliorate aromatase inhibitor-induced cognitive decline in breast cancer patients? Mol Neurobiol
97. World Health Organisation (WHO) (2009) Mortality and burden of disease attributable to selected major risks. Global health risks. WHO, Geneva
98. Lee IM, Skerrett PJ (2001) Physical activity and all-cause mortality: what is the dose-response relation? Med Sci Sports Exerc 33(6 Suppl):S459–S471 (discussion S493–454)
99. Haapanen-Niemi N, Miilunpalo S, Pasanen M, Vuori I, Oja P, Malmberg J (2000) Body mass index, physical inactivity and low level of physical fitness as determinants of all-cause and cardiovascular disease mortality–16 y follow-up of middle-aged and elderly men and women. Int J Obes Relat Metab Disord 24(11):1465–1474
100. LaMonte MJ, Barlow CE, Jurca R, Kampert JB, Church TS, Blair SN (2005) Cardiorespiratory fitness is inversely associated with the incidence of metabolic syndrome: a prospective study of men and women. Circulation 112(4):505–512
101. Kodama S, Saito K, Tanaka S et al (2009) Cardiorespiratory fitness as a quantitative predictor of all-cause mortality and cardiovascular events in healthy men and women: a meta-analysis. JAMA 301(19):2024–2035
102. Barry VW, Baruth M, Beets MW, Durstine JL, Liu J, Blair SN (2014) Fitness vs. fatness on all-cause mortality: a meta-analysis. Prog Cardiovasc Dis 56(4):382–390 (1)
103. Rock CL, Doyle C, Demark-Wahnefried W et al (2012) Nutrition and physical activity guidelines for cancer survivors. CA Cancer J Clin 62(4):242–274
104. Schmitz KH, Courneya KS, Matthews C et al (2010) American College of Sports Medicine roundtable on exercise guidelines for cancer survivors. Med Sci Sports Exerc 42(7): 1409–1426
105. Ross R, Hudson R, Stotz PJ, Lam M (2015) Effects of exercise amount and intensity on abdominal obesity and glucose tolerance in obese adults: a randomized trial. Ann Intern Med 162(5):325–334
106. Galvao DA, Newton RU, Gardiner RA et al (2015) Compliance to exercise-oncology guidelines in prostate cancer survivors and associations with psychological distress, unmet supportive care needs, and quality of life. Psychooncology
107. Artinian NT, Fletcher GF, Mozaffarian D et al (2010) Interventions to promote physical activity and dietary lifestyle changes for cardiovascular risk factor reduction in adults: a scientific statement from the American Heart Association. Circulation 122(4):406–441
108. Centers for Disease Control and Prevention (2011) The CDC Guide to Strategies to Increase Physical Activity in the Community. In: Services DoHaH (ed) Atlanta, US
109. Kiefte-de Jong JC, Mathers JC, Franco OH (2014) Nutrition and healthy ageing: the key ingredients. Proc Nutr Soc 73(2):249–259
110. Duthie SJ (2011) Folate and cancer: how DNA damage, repair and methylation impact on colon carcinogenesis. J Inherit Metab Dis 34(1):101–109
111. McKay JA, Mathers JC (2016) Maternal folate deficiency and metabolic dysfunction in offspring. Proc Nutr Soc 75(1):90–95
112. Fenech MF (2010) Dietary reference values of individual micronutrients and nutriomes for genome damage prevention: current status and a road map to the future. Am J Clin Nutr 91 (5):1438s–1454s
113. Xu C, Wu Y, Liu G, Liu X, Wang F, Yu J (2014) Relationship between homocysteine level and diabetic retinopathy: a systematic review and meta-analysis. Diagnostic Pathology. 9:167 (09/26 06/26/received 08/16/accepted 2014)
114. Douaud G, Refsum H, de Jager CA et al (2013) Preventing Alzheimer's disease-related gray matter atrophy by B-vitamin treatment. Proceedings of the National Academy of Sciences. 110(23):9523–9528

115. Oulhaj A, Refsum H, Beaumont H et al (2010) Homocysteine as a predictor of cognitive decline in Alzheimer's disease. Int J Geriatr Psychiatry 25(1):82–90
116. Nguyen JCD, Killcross AS, Jenkins TA (2015) Obesity and cognitive decline: role of inflammation and vascular changes. Frontiers in Neuroscience 8:375 (11/1910/06/received 10/31/accepted 2014)
117. Dufouil C, Seshadri S, Chene G (2014) Cardiovascular risk profile in women and dementia. J Alzheimers Dis 42(Suppl 4):S353–S363
118. Anderson AS, Key TJ, Norat T et al (2015) European Code against Cancer 4th Edition: Obesity, body fatness and cancer. Cancer Epidemiol 39(Suppl 1):S34–S45
119. Matyszewski A, Czarnecka AM, Solarek W et al (2015) Molecular basis of carcinogenesis in diabetic patients (review). Int J Oncol 46(4):1435–1443
120. Cerda C, Sanchez C, Climent B et al (2014) Oxidative stress and DNA damage in obesity-related tumorigenesis. Adv Exp Med Biol 824:5–17
121. Armani C, Botto N, Andreassi MG, Centaro E (2013) Molecular markers of cardiovascular damage in hypertension. Curr Pharm Des 19(13):2341–2350
122. Benayoun BA, Pollina EA, Brunet A (2015) Epigenetic regulation of ageing: linking environmental inputs to genomic stability. Nat Rev Mol Cell Biol 16(10):593–610
123. Macheret M, Halazonetis TD (2015) DNA replication stress as a hallmark of cancer. Annu Rev Pathol 10:425–448
124. López-Otín C, Blasco MA, Partridge L, Serrano M, Kroemer G (2013) The Hallmarks of Aging. Cell.153(6):1194–1217
125. Hanahan D, Weinberg Robert A (2011) Hallmarks of cancer: the next generation. Cell 144(5):646–674
126. Maslov AY, Vijg J (2009) Genome instability, cancer and aging. Biochim Biophys Acta 1790(10):963–969
127. Fenech M (2002) Chromosomal biomarkers of genomic instability relevant to cancer. Drug Discov Today 7(22):1128–1137
128. World Cancer Research Fund/American Institute for Cancer Research (2007) Food, nutrition, physical activity, and the prevention of cancer: a global perspective. AICR, Washington DC
129. Amitay EL, Keinan-Boker L (2015) Breastfeeding and childhood leukemia incidence: A meta-analysis and systematic review. JAMA Pediatrics 169(6):e151025
130. Sofi F, Cesari F, Abbate R, Gensini GF, Casini A (2008) Adherence to Mediterranean diet and health status: meta-analysis. BMJ 337 (2008-09-11 23:05:19 2008)
131. Fenech MF (2014) Nutriomes and personalised nutrition for DNA damage prevention, telomere integrity maintenance and cancer growth control. Cancer Treat Res 159:427–441
132. World Health Organisation/International Agency for Research on Cancer (2015) Continuous Update. http://www.iarc.fr/en/media-centre/iarcnews/pdf/Monographs-Q&A_Vol114.pdf. Accessed 18 Feb 2016
133. Brooks PJ, Zakhari S (2014) Acetaldehyde and the genome: beyond nuclear DNA adducts and carcinogenesis. Environ Mol Mutagen 55(2):77–91
134. Brooks PJ, Theruvathu JA (2005) DNA adducts from acetaldehyde: implications for alcohol-related carcinogenesis. Alcohol 35(3):187–193
135. International Agency for Research on Cancer (IARC) (2010) Alcohol consumption and ethyl carbamate. IARC, Lyon
136. International Agency for Research on Cancer (IARC) (2012) IARC Monographs on the Evaluation of Carcinogenic Risk to Humans. IARC, Lyon
137. Yu HS, Oyama T, Isse T et al (2010) Formation of acetaldehyde-derived DNA adducts due to alcohol exposure. Chem Biol Interact 188(3):367–375
138. Iarmarcovai G, Bonassi S, Botta A, Baan RA, Orsiere T (2008) Genetic polymorphisms and micronucleus formation: a review of the literature. Mutat Res 658(3):215–233
139. Teo T, Fenech M (2008) The interactive effect of alcohol and folic acid on genome stability in human WIL2-NS cells measured using the cytokinesis-block micronucleus cytome assay. Mutat Res 657(1):32–38

140. Fontana L, Partridge L (2015) Promoting health and longevity through diet: from model organisms to humans. Cell 161(1):106–118
141. Rizza W, Veronese N, Fontana L (2014) What are the roles of calorie restriction and diet quality in promoting healthy longevity? Ageing Res Rev 13:38–45
142. Tchernof A, Despres JP (2013) Pathophysiology of human visceral obesity: an update. Physiol Rev 93(1):359–404
143. Snel M, Jonker JT, Schoones J et al (2012) Ectopic Fat and Insulin Resistance: Pathophysiology and Effect of Diet and Lifestyle Interventions. Int J Endocrinol 2012:18
144. Hocking S, Samocha-Bonet D, Milner KL, Greenfield JR, Chisholm DJ (2013) Adiposity and insulin resistance in humans: the role of the different tissue and cellular lipid depots. Endocr Rev 34(4):463–500
145. Mancini JG, Filion KB, Atallah R, Eisenberg MU (2015) Systematic review of the Mediterranean diet for long-term weight loss. Am J Med S0002-9343(15):3027–3029
146. Hill AM, Harris Jackson KA, Roussell MA, West SG, Kris-Etherton PM (2015) Type and amount of dietary protein in the treatment of metabolic syndrome: a randomized controlled trial. Am J Clin Nutr 102(4):757–770
147. Razavi ZM, Telkabadi MH, Bahmani F, Salehi B, Farshbaf S, Asemi Z (2015) The effects of DASH diet on weight loss and metabolic status in adults with non-alcoholic fatty liver disease: a randomized clinical trial. Liver Int. doi:10.1111/liv.12990 [Epub ahead of print]
148. Ello-Martin JA, Ledikwe JH, Rolls BJ (2005) The influence of food portion size and energy density on energy intake: implications for weight management. Am J Clin Nutr 82(Suppl. 1): S236–S241
149. Rolls BJ (2014) What is the role of portion control in weight management? Int J Obes 38(Suppl. 1):S1–S8
150. Barnard ND, Levin SM, Yokoyama Y (2015) A systematic review and meta-analysis of changes in body weight in clinical trials of vegetarian diets. J Acad Nutr Diet 115(6): 954–969
151. Sabate J, Wien M (2010) Vegetarian diets and childhood obesity prevention. Am J Clin Nutr 91(5):S1525–S1529
152. Tay J, Luscombe-Marsh ND, Thompson CH et al (2015) Comparison of low- and high-carbohydrate diets for type 2 diabetes management: a randomized trial. Am J Clin Nutr 102(4):780–790
153. Neacsu M, Fyfe C, Horgan G, Johnstone AM (2014) Appetite control and biomarkers of satiety with vegetarian (soy) and meat-based high-protein diets for weight loss in obese men: a randomized crossover trial. Am J Clin Nutr 100(2):548–558
154. Fogelholm M, Anderssen S, Gunnarsdottir I, Lahti-Koski M (2012) Dietary macronutrients and food consumption as determinants of long-term weight change in adult populations: a systematic literature review. Food Nutr Res 56. doi:10.3402/fnr.v56i0.19103 (Epub 2012 Aug 13)
155. Keogh JB, Clifton PM (2012) Meal replacements for weight loss in type 2 diabetes in a community setting. J Nutr Metab. doi:10.1155/2012/918571
156. Carney D, Schultz S, Lim J, Walters W (2015) Successful medical weight loss in a community setting. J Obes Weightloss Ther 5(1):pii:248
157. Mehta T, Smith DL, Muhammad J, Casazza K (2014) Impact of weight cycling on risk of morbidity and mortality. Obes Rev 15(11):870–881
158. Stevens VL, Jacobs EJ, Patel AV et al (2015) Weight cycling and cancer incidence in a large prospective US cohort. Am J Epidemiol 182(5):394–404
159. World Health Organisation (WHO) (2003) Population nutrient intake goals for preventing diet-related chronic diseases. Accessed 29 Feb 2016
160. Despres JP (1993) Abdominal obesity as important component of insulin-resistance syndrome. Nutrition 9(5):452–459
161. Goodpaster BH, Krishnaswami S, Resnick H et al (2003) Association between regional adipose tissue distribution and both type 2 diabetes and impaired glucose tolerance in elderly men and women. Diabetes Care 26(2):372–379

162. Park BJ, Kim YJ, Kim DH et al (2008) Visceral adipose tissue area is an independent risk factor for hepatic steatosis. J Gastroenterol Hepatol 23(6):900–907
163. Yusuf S, Hawken S, Ounpuu S et al (2005) Obesity and the risk of myocardial infarction in 27,000 participants from 52 countries: a case-control study. Lancet 366(9497):1640–1649
164. Ekelund U, Besson H, Luan J et al (2011) Physical activity and gain in abdominal adiposity and body weight: prospective cohort study in 288,498 men and women. Am J Clin Nutr 93(4):826–835
165. Janssen I, Katzmarzyk PT, Ross R et al (2004) Fitness alters the associations of BMI and waist circumference with total and abdominal fat. Obes Res 12(3):525–537
166. Shaw K, Gennat H, O'Rourke P, Del Mar C (2006) Exercise for overweight or obesity. Cochrane Database Syst Rev 4:Cd003817
167. Franz MJ, VanWormer JJ, Crain AL et al (2007) Weight-loss outcomes: a systematic review and meta-analysis of weight-loss clinical trials with a minimum 1-year follow-up. J Am Diet Assoc 107(10):1755–1767
168. Brown Medical School/The Miriam Hospital Weight Control, Diabetes Research Center (2016) The National Weight Control Registry. http://www.nwcr.ws/Research/default.htm. Accessed 22 Feb 2016
169. Vissers D, Hens W, Taeymans J, Baeyens J-P, Poortmans J, Van Gaal L (2013) The effect of exercise on visceral adipose tissue in overweight adults: a systematic review and meta-analysis. PLoS ONE 8(2):e56415
170. Bryner RW, Ullrich IH, Sauers J et al (1999) Effects of resistance vs. aerobic training combined with an 800 calorie liquid diet on lean body mass and resting metabolic rate. J Am Coll Nutr 18(2):115–121
171. Cancer Australia (2011) Risk-reducing Medication for Women at Increased Risk of Breast Cancer Due to Family History. In: Australia C (ed) Australian Government
172. National Cancer Institute (2015) Breast cancer prevention for health professionals. http://www.cancer.gov/types/breast/hp/breast-prevention-pdq#section/_1. Accessed 19 Oct 2015
173. Australia Cancer (2011) Recommendations for aromatase inhibitors as adjuvant endocrine therapy for post-menopausal women with hormone receptor-positive early breast cancer. National Breast Cancer Centre, Camperdown
174. Morales D, Morris AD (2015) Metformin in cancer treatment and prevention. Annu Rev Med 66(1):17–29
175. Vestergaard P, Starup-Linde J (2013) Diabetes, cancer and treatment—A mini-review. Curr Drug Saf 8(5):292–295
176. Pollak MN (2012) Investigating metformin for cancer prevention and treatment: the end of the beginning. Cancer Discov 2(9):778–790
177. McCarthy AL, Tramm R, Shaban RZ, Yates P (2013) Factors influencing health behaviors of younger women after menopause-inducing cancer treatment. Public Health Nurs 30(2): 106–116
178. Vejpongsa P, Yeh ETH (2014) Prevention of Anthracycline-Induced Cardiotoxicity: Challenges and Opportunities. J Am Coll Cardiol 64(9):938–945
179. Todaro MC, Oreto L, Qamar R, Paterick TE, Carerj S, Khandheria BK (2013) Cardioncology: state of the heart. Int J Cardiol 168(2):680–687
180. Curigliano G, Cardinale D, Suter T et al (2012) Cardiovascular toxicity induced by chemotherapy, targeted agents and radiotherapy: ESMO Clinical Practice Guidelines. Ann Oncol 23(Suppl 7):vii155–vii166
181. van Dalen EC, Caron HN, Dickinson HO, Kremer LC (2008) Cardioprotective interventions for cancer patients receiving anthracyclines. Cochrane Database Syst Rev 2:Cd003917
182. Kalam K, Marwick T (2013) Role of cardioprotective therapy for prevention of cardiotoxicity with chemotherapy: a systematic review and meta-analysis. Eur J Cancer 49:2900–2909
183. Colagiuri B, Roscoe JA, Morrow GR, Atkins JN, Giguere JK, Colman LK (2008) How do patient expectancies, quality of life, and postchemotherapy nausea interrelate? Cancer 113(3):654–661

184. National Heart Foundation of Australia and the Cardiac Society of Australia and New Zealand (2012) An expert guide to clinical practice for secondary prevention of coronary heart disease. Reducing risk in heart disease. National Heart Foundation of Australia, Melbourne
185. National Heart Foundation of Australia and the Cardiac Society of Australia and New Zealand (Chronic Heart Failure Guidelines Expert Writing Panel) (2011) Guidelines for the prevention, detection and management of chronic heart failure in Australia. National Heart Foundation of Australia
186. Kidney Health Australia (2015) Prevention. http://www.kidney.org.au/KidneyDisease/Prevention/tabid/820/Default.aspx. Accessed 21 Oct 2015
187. Demierre MF, Higgins PD, Gruber SB, Hawk E, Lippman SM (2005) Statins and cancer prevention. Nat Rev Cancer 5(12):930–942
188. Lustman A, Nakar S, Cohen AD, Vinker S (2014) Statin use and incident prostate cancer risk: does the statin brand matter? A population-based cohort study. Prostate Cancer Prostatic Dis 17(1):6–9
189. Ravnskov U, Rosch PJ, McCully KS (2015) Statins do not protect against cancer: quite the opposite. J Clin Oncol
190. Goldstein MR, Mascitelli L, Pezzetta F (2008) Do statins prevent or promote cancer? Curr Oncol 15(2):76–77
191. Heart Foundation (2009) Aspirin. http://www.heartfoundation.org.au/SiteCollection Documents/Aspirin.pdf. Accessed 20 Oct 2015
192. American Heart Foundation (2015) Aspirin and heart disease. American Heart Foundation, Dallas
193. Hung J (2003) Aspirin for cardiovascular disease prevention. Med J Aust 179(3):147–152
194. International Agency for Research on Cancer (1992) (IARC). IARC monographs on the evaluation of carcinogenic risks to humans. Solar and ultraviolet radiation. IARC Monogr Eval Carcinog Risks Hum 55:1–316
195. CancerAustralia (2015) UV radiation. Cancer Australia, Sydney
196. Morton LM, Onel K, Curtis RE, Hungate EA, Armstrong GT (2014) The rising incidence of second cancers: patterns of occurrence and identification of risk factors for children and adults. Am Soc Clin Oncol Educ Book e57–e67
197. Berrington DGA, Curtis RE, Kry SF et al (2011) Proportion of second cancers attributable to radiotherapy in adults: a cohort study in the US SEER cancer registries. Lancet Oncol 12(4):353–360
198. Cancer Australia (2015) Infections. Cancer Australia, Sydney
199. O'Connor SM, Taylor CE, Hughes JM (2006) Emerging infectious determinants of chronic diseases. Emerg Infect Dis 12(7):1051–1057
200. Hepatitis B Foundation (2014) Hepatitis B and Primary Liver Cancer. http://www.hepb.org/professionals/hepb_and_liver_cancer.htm. Accessed 20 Oct 2015
201. Wroblewski LE, Peek RM Jr, Wilson KT (2010) Helicobacter pylori and gastric cancer: factors that modulate disease risk. Clin Microbiol Rev 23(4):713–739
202. Australian Commission on Saftey and Quality in Health Care (ACSQHC) (2015) Health literacy: a summary for clinicians. ACSQHC, Sydney
203. Australian Bureau of Statistics (2010) Health and socioeconomic disadvantage. Australian Social Trends, cat. no. 4102.0. http://www.abs.gov.au/AUSSTATS/abs@.nsf/Lookup/4102.0Main+Features30Mar+2010. Accessed 21 Oct 2015
204. Australian Bureau of Statistics (ABS) (2015) Health risk factors. http://www.abs.gov.au/ausstats/abs@.nsf/Lookup/4364.0.55.001Chapter4002011-12. Accessed 18 Feb 2016
205. American College of Preventative Medicine (2011) Medication adherence time tool: medication adhereance—Improving health outcomes. http://www.acpm.org/?MedAdhereTT Providers. Accessed 8 Feb 2016
206. Colagiuri R, Girgis S, Gomez M, Walker K, Colagiuri S, O'Dea K (2009) National evidence based guideline for the primary prevention of type 2 diabetes. Diabetes Australia and the NHMRC, Canberra

207. Kohl HW, 3rd (2001) Physical activity and cardiovascular disease: evidence for a dose response. Med Sci Sports Exerc 33(6 Suppl):S472–S483 (discussion S493–474)
208. Whelton SP, Chin A, Xin X, He J (2002) Effect of aerobic exercise on blood pressure: a meta-analysis of randomized, controlled trials. Ann Intern Med 136(7):493–503
209. Zelber-Sagi S, Nitzan-Kaluski D, Goldsmith R et al (2008) Role of leisure-time physical activity in nonalcoholic fatty liver disease: a population-based study. Hepatology 48(6): 1791–1798
210. Marques EA, Mota J, Carvalho J (2012) Exercise effects on bone mineral density in older adults: a meta-analysis of randomized controlled trials. Age (Dordr) 34(6):1493–1515
211. Barcellos FC, Santos IS, Umpierre D, Bohlke M, Hallal PC (2015) Effects of exercise in the whole spectrum of chronic kidney disease: a systematic review. Clin Kidney J 8(6):753–765
212. World Cancer Research Fund International (2015) Kidney cancer 2015 report. http://www.wcrf.org/int/researche-we-find/continuous-update-project-findings-reports/kidney-cancer. Accessed 21 Sep 2015
213. World Cancer Research Fund International (2015) Prostate cancer report 2014 report. http://www.wcrf.org/int/researche-we-find/continuous-update-project-findings-reports/prostate-cancer. Accessed 29 Sep 2015
214. Goss PE, Ingle JN, Alés-Martínez JE et al (2011) Exemestane for breast-cancer prevention in postmenopausal women. N Engl J Med 364(25):2381–2391
215. Chadban S, Howell M, Twigg S et al (2010) The CARI guidelines. Prevention and management of chronic kidney disease in type 2 diabetes. Nephrology (Carlton) 15(Suppl 1): S162–S194
216. World Cancer Research Fund International (2015) Liver cancer 2015 report. http://www.wcrf.org/int/researche-we-find/continuous-update-project-findings-reports/liver-cancer. Accessed 29 Sep 2015
217. Australia Cancer (2015) Tobacco. Cancer Australia, Sydney
218. Campbell PT, Patel AV, Newton CC, Jacobs EJ, Gapstur SM (2013) Associations of recreational physical activity and leisure time spent sitting with colorectal cancer survival. J Clin Oncol 31(7):876–885
219. Biswas A, Oh PI, Faulkner GE et al (2015) Sedentary time and its association with risk for disease incidence, mortality, and hospitalization in adults: a systematic review and meta-analysis. Ann Intern Med 162(2):123–132
220. Bauman AE, Chau JY, Ding D, Bennie J (2013) Too much sitting and cardio-metabolic risk: an update of epidemiological evidence. Curr Cardiovasc Risk Rep 7(4):293–298

Further Reading

221. American college of sports medicine. http://www.acsm.org/public-information/position-stands
222. Exercise and sports science Australia. https://www.essa.org.au/for-media/position-statements/
223. World cancer research fund international. http://www.wcrf.org/int/research-we-fund/our-cancer-prevention-recommendations
224. World cancer research fund international. http://www.wcrf.org/int/research-we-fund/continuous-update-project-cup

Chapter 8
Chronic Condition Management Models for Cancer Care and Survivorship

Sharon Lawn and Malcolm Battersby

Abstract Improvements in the treatment of cancer have meant that the number of cancer survivors is growing. This group is now more likely to be living with the longer-term adverse effects of cancer on their overall health and wellbeing, and to develop comorbid chronic conditions that require ongoing care in the community, beyond the cancer clinic. People with chronic conditions are also generally living longer due to improvements in treatment, care and support options and therefore are at risk of developing cancer as they age. This chapter outlines a range of chronic condition management models likely to be necessary for effective self-management support to cancer patients and survivors who suffer from and develop chronic conditions, or have risk factors for their development, and people with chronic conditions who also go on to develop cancer. Integrated care and communication issues across healthcare transitions are briefly discussed.

Keywords Cancer patients and survivors · Chronic condition management · Self-management · Models of care · Care coordination

Key Points

- Chronic condition management models available to support chronic condition self-management are also relevant to cancer patients and survivors.
- Integration of care across transitions from acute cancer treatment to longer term care in the community continues to be an issue for cancer patients, despite their high rates of comorbid chronic health conditions.

S. Lawn (✉) · M. Battersby
Department of Psychiatry, Flinders Human Behaviour and Health Research Unit, Margaret Tobin Centre, Flinders University, Adelaide, Australia
e-mail: Sharon.lawn@flinders.edu.au

B. Koczwara (ed.), *Cancer and Chronic Conditions*,
DOI 10.1007/978-981-10-1844-2_8

- Peer support, nurse-led clinics in primary care, coordinated care across transitions, and chronic condition self-management care planning are some of the range of approaches that show promise for people living with chronic conditions and cancer.

8.1 Introduction

Many people with cancer have coexisting chronic conditions and many cancer survivors subsequently develop them because they share many risk factors and several chronic conditions are causally linked with increased risk of cancer [1]. Therefore, how chronic conditions are managed is very relevant to cancer and together, they pose many challenges to traditional siloed models of care. Cancer in its treatment phase, in the management of co-existing chronic diseases and the increased risk of acquiring chronic diseases as a consequence of treatment, suggests that the concepts and models of care developed for chronic condition management internationally should be applied to cancer management. During the diagnosis and treatment phase of cancer, coping with the stress of the diagnosis, understanding the medical aspects of the condition and the treatment options, and managing the daily impacts of the disease and its treatment are similar to dealing with any chronic disease. The most internationally recognised approach to chronic disease management is the Chronic Care Model [2, 3], an evidenced based framework describing six elements at the health system and the practice level which aim to assist a patient to be activated through the support of a collaborative multidisciplinary team (see below). Like patients with chronic conditions more broadly, the current care provided to cancer patients is often delivered within the specialist silo of the oncology clinic. Their other chronic care needs may become a lesser priority and coordination of treatments and needs across the specialist chronic disease areas can be challenging for all concerned.

With improvements in screening, early detection and treatment of many cancers, survival rates have likewise improved significantly; and the cancer survivorship trajectory has changed significantly [4]. Cancer survivors are simply living longer and are a growing population within the community [5, 6]. This has meant that many cancer survivors must accommodate the management of a number of complicating late effects of cancer and its treatments that can contribute to the development of chronic health conditions. Like other groups in the population, cancer survivors might also have existing chronic conditions that pre-date their cancer diagnosis that also must be managed. Alternatively, and in line with others in the population, cancer survivors might also develop chronic conditions due to hereditary markers for certain conditions, the influence of a range of lifestyle risk factors (such as smoking and low levels of physical activity), and the natural course of aging. Conversely, as more people are living longer due to improvements in medical treatment and care, they are likely to develop a range of comorbid chronic health conditions in older age, including various types of cancers. Together, these circumstances can create a complex and unique picture of comorbidity and risk factors that requires longer-term management across the person's lifespan. The cancer journey for many people who experience it is recognised as involving a continuum from prevention, early detection, diagnosis, treatment, survivorship, to end of life care [7]. This change in the cancer survivorship trajectory requires a commensurate change in how both cancer care and chronic condition care in the community are structured and delivered.

Effective management of cancer by health services requires effective integration of care at all stages of disease trajectory and begins with how cancer care providers view their roles and responsibilities in communicating with other stakeholders in care, and how they view the role of cancer patients in care, as either active or passive participants. In the early stages of diagnosis and treatment, doctors are the experts and patients are very dependent on the knowledge and skill of the clinician; however, patients should be engaged as early as possible in their own care through shared decision-making. As the course of treatment evolves, patients should be encouraged to share their knowledge of the condition and its impacts on them, and how they manage the condition and its treatment on a daily basis. Principles of patient centred care should be central to the clinician-patient relationship at all stages of the treatment and management of the condition. Integration of care refers to how health providers take into account other medical and psychiatric co-morbidities, the psychosocial aspects of the patient's circumstances and how other health providers and community services are integrated into the patient's care.

Integration of care is also important after treatment is completed, to mitigate the impact of chronic conditions that might develop as a result of the cancer treatment. However, cancer care is usually focused on management of cancer specific issues with less emphasis on management of other health problems [8]. Strategies such as self-management support, which are recognised as effective for the management of other chronic conditions, such as diabetes and arthritis [9, 10], are rarely utilised with cancer patients and cancer survivors. This is despite research confirming the importance of encouraging self-management and patient autonomy for improved outcomes for cancer survivors, and improved quality of life regardless of where the person sits on the cancer trajectory from prevention to palliation [11, 12]. There is also less emphasis on prevention strategies and lifestyle modification for cancer survivors. Chronic condition management is often not considered a priority by cancer care providers or cancer patients as the fear of cancer is considered the immediate priority for treatment and care. Additionally, cancer care providers have limited skills in chronic condition management and self-management support to patients, and health care systems are not always designed to support integrated care of cancer and other chronic conditions [13, 14]. Likewise, general practitioners (GPs) and other health care professionals within primary care may be well-versed at coordinating care for a their patients with a broad range of chronic health conditions though they may be more tentative in providing care to cancer patients during their more acute treatment phase, instead deferring to specialist oncology services [14–16].

This is also so for cancer survivors, once their care moves from the cancer care services to broader community and primary care services where care often occurs within health systems designed to provide episodic, acute health care and fails to address self-management, prevention and health promotion, and to provide sufficiently coordinated systems for follow-up [17]. Current approaches to cancer care do not adequately engage cancer patients in self-management; their focus is on the immediate need to treat the cancer. This is despite emerging evidence that cancer patients can be engaged earlier in their cancer trajectory [18] and longstanding advocacy from consumer support organisations that many cancer patients desire and indeed do undertake a range of activities to build their knowledge and alter their lifestyle in order to help maximize their health outcomes following a cancer diagnosis [14].

Likewise, current approaches do not adequately engage cancer survivors to self-manage their long-term needs, non-cancer issues such as health lifestyle management or management of comorbidity [13, 15, 16]. We know that many cancer survivors continue to have unmet physical and emotional needs within existing models of care [19–21]. Chronic conditions require delivery of a different kind of health care; one that is more holistic and more fully includes the person and their informal supports, and which improves the coordination and communication of care across a range of healthcare providers and, where relevant, psychosocial support providers.

Recognising cancer as a chronic condition requires a shift in how care is provided to these patients. Cure or amelioration of the immediate threat to the person's life is no longer the only priority. Models of care must now consider and place greater emphasis on the cancer survivor's active involvement in decisions made about their care, acknowledging their 'lived experience' expertise. This is also relevant for patients still in active treatment for their cancer and those people who are receiving palliative care for their cancer and/or other chronic conditions. Because cancer survivors' care will be delivered largely in the communities in which they live, health professionals and services in the community and primary health services and non-government consumer-engaged organisations now play an even more important role in providing that support and care than previously, when care was predominantly centred around acute care within tertiary hospital oncology departments. This shift has required a commensurate focus on models that emphasise greater patient empowerment, health literacy and self-management; as well as greater coordination of care between health professionals and between services, involving multidisciplinary and interprofessional care, and continuity of care. The acute model of care in which the oncology, respiratory, cardiac or other chronic disease specialist is the primary care provider is no longer the only approach to care that is required. Hence, there has been a growing focus on models of care that involve chronic condition management and self-management support care planning for cancer survivors [14]. These have relevance to cancer patients more broadly, regardless of their stage of treatment, especially if they have other comorbid chronic physical and/or mental health conditions. Cancer patients have different needs at different points in their cancer journey, as the following diagram shows; they move between these care points, according to the stage, severity and complexity of those needs (see Fig. 8.1).

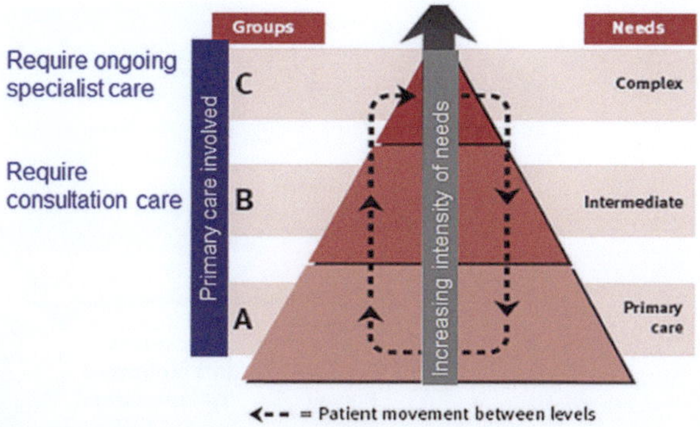

Fig. 8.1 The cancer patient's journey within healthcare systems (reproduced with permission from: Palliative Care Australia (2005) A guide to palliative care service development: a population based approach. Canberra: Palliative Care Australia)

8.2 Chronic Condition Management Models for Cancer Patients and Cancer Survivors

Chronic condition management models of care emphasise the sharing of information between the person with the chronic condition, their informal supports, such as family members (where applicable), and service providers. They place emphasis on linkage and transparent communication of consistent and timely information. The various models differ in how that communication is organised, who leads the communication and how it is shared. Several of the following models are not mutually exclusive; they are likely to form necessary parts of a comprehensive system response to the chronic care needs of cancer patients regardless of where they sit in the cancer survivor journey. The Chronic Care Model [2, 3] provides an overarching framework for the management of chronic diseases and conditions within systems of care, internationally.

8.2.1 The Chronic Care Model

The Chronic Care Model, developed by the McColl Institute for Healthcare Innovation in the United States [2, 3], is an internationally recognised, evidence-based guide to the comprehensive, integrated re-organisation of care delivery needed to support chronic condition self-management. It has been expanded to include a greater focus on community resources, population health and health promotion; all issues of relevance to the service providers and systems that support people with chronic conditions who develop cancer and to cancer survivors at risk of developing comorbid chronic conditions (see Fig. 8.2). It acknowledges three important domains of influence which interact and influence each other, and which influence the quality of chronic condition management and self-management support:

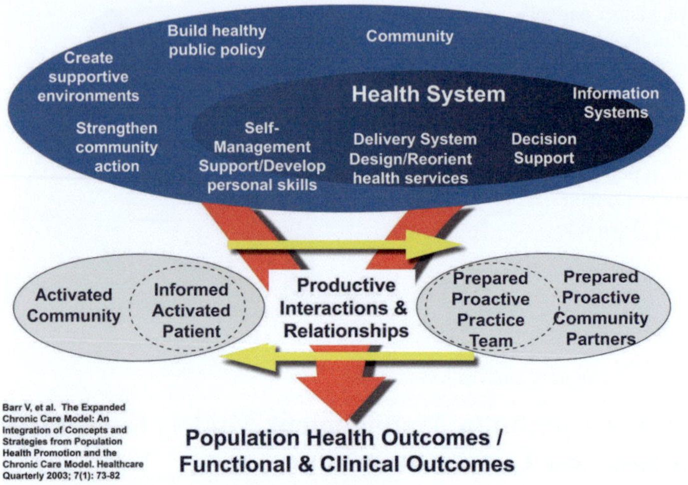

Fig. 8.2 The expanded chronic care model: integrating population health promotion

1. The Macro level of healthcare aims to coordinate and maintain the overall values, principles and strategies for the development of the national healthcare system. It is also the role of this level to allocate funding and resources to the appropriate sectors, to set national standards for care provision and professional practice, strengthen community action, and establish broad population health and public health frameworks.
2. The Meso level of healthcare involves the necessary service delivery structures that connect policy and principles at the macro level to the actions of individual providers at the micro level. It includes the following:

   - Self-management support training and education to health professionals
   - Delivery system design to enhance service team and inter-agency communications
   - Decision support tools established to monitor and guide practice (including evidence-based guidelines)
   - Clinical information systems to enhance the recording, storage, retrieval and communication of patient data.

3. The Micro level of healthcare involves the interactions between the health professional and the patient. The World Health Organisation (WHO) asserts that the two most common issues that occur at the micro-level are the failure of healthcare providers to adequately empower patients and a lack of emphasis on quality interactions between the patient and healthcare providers [17].

Research has shown that many processes within the Chronic Care Model are inadequate for cancer patients. A Norwegian survey, for example, with cancer patients and health professionals found that few services or training programmes had been offered to these patients after their treatment was completed. Patient participants also reported poor communication to them by service providers and their follow-up care, and also between service providers. This left cancer patients confused about which service they should contact for follow-up. Many patients reported wanting, "a more systematic post-treatment programme, as well as clear guidelines delineating the specific areas of responsibility assigned to hospitals and the local public health services" (p. 56) [22].

We describe below, programs and models of care that have been shown to improve outcomes in chronic condition management and are applicable to cancer management.

8.2.1.1 Self-help Group Programs

Patients receiving active treatment for their cancer and cancer survivors have valid forms of knowledge and expertise that are inherent in their experience as cancer patients. This expertise can inform the delivery of care and priorities for research [23, 24]. Finding cures and effective treatments for cancer, while essential, are only one aspect of the evolving picture of cancer survivorship and have given rise to a broad range of peer support networks specific to cancer survivors and cancer patients in the active stages of cancer treatment. These are both formal and informal and have reciprocity of support by others with lived experience at their core [25], similar to support groups for people with lived experience of chronic health conditions, more broadly. Arthritis, Parkinson's disease and mental health support networks are notable examples. Peer support is well known to contribute to reduced feelings of isolation and greater feelings of empowerment through exchange of information and emotional support between peers [26–28]. The evidence for the value of patient empowerment [29] and peer support between patients with chronic health conditions is now well established [28, 30], though the evidence for psychosocial benefit for cancer patients is mixed and requires further research [31, 32].

As the cancer survivor population grows, the general community's literacy regarding cancer survivorship needs to also grow and shift from attitudes largely driven by fear and despondency about cancer diagnoses and future survival [14], to one in which they embrace support and inclusion of cancer survivors in the community. This required shift in attitude also applies to cancer survivors given that research has shown that those who self-identify as survivors have better psychological well-being, sense of control and hope than those who relinquish responsibility for their health to health care providers [33]. This shift in perception within the community might also help to address the exclusion, isolation and stigma that some cancer patients and cancer survivors experience in the community [34, 35]. Many countries have responded to this shifting need by establishing a range of cancer advocacy, research and community information services. In Australia, Cancer Foundations exist in each jurisdiction, as do a comprehensive network of cancer support groups such as Cancer Voices Australia, CanTeen, and Foundations for specific types of cancers [36]. In the UK, Macmillan Cancer Support is an example of an organisation undertaken a range of these roles.

The Stanford Chronic Disease Self-Management Course, developed by Kate Lorig and colleagues at Stanford University in the United State, is a prominent example of a peer-led group based program for people with chronic conditions [37, 38]. In the UK, it is known as the Expert Patient Program [39]. This group-based program has been used with cancer survivors in a range of contexts with positive outcomes [26, 40, 41] and have included web-based program delivery [42]. In the UK, Risendal et al. [43] delivered 27 workshops to 22 Cancer Thriving and Surviving (CTS) leaders and 244 cancer survivors to test their feasibility and acceptability for this population. They found 95% satisfaction with this approach and concluded that it represents, “a powerful tool toward improving health-related outcomes in this at-risk population” (p. 771) [see also 44]. Salvatore et al. [41] undertook a comparative study with 116 cancer survivors and 1054 non-cancer patients with other chronic conditions investigating the applicability of this program with cancer survivors and program outcomes. They found general health, depression, sleep, communication with health professionals, medication compliance and physical activity improved significantly, and were sustained at 12 months.

8.2.1.2 Cancer Patients and Cancer Survivors as Navigators of Existing Healthcare Systems

Central to chronic condition management is the active role of the person with the health conditions in the communication loop, given that they or their informal supports are the primary navigator across services in order to get their healthcare needs met. However, in order to do this, cancer patients need access to their health information. Hence, Cancer Council Australia [45] recommend that every cancer survivor request a comprehensive care summary and follow-up plan from their specialist once they complete their cancer treatment. For cancer patients with existing chronic health conditions, this would also include the need for care summaries and routine communication about progress between oncology specialists and primary care providers with continuing responsibility for the coordination of care for the person’s other health conditions and non-cancer related acute health needs. Currently, this system navigation and communication of information between providers is done, largely, by the cancer patient; though many cancer patients may not have adequate capacity, access to their own health information or sufficient health literacy or confidence to perform these roles. The Cancer Council Australia, for example, provides a range of resources to assist cancer patients in this role (see Box 1).

Box 1: Suggested Questions for Cancer Survivors to Ask to their Specialists (Source: Cancer Council Australia [45])

1. What treatments and drugs have I been given?
2. How often should I have a routine visit?
3. Which doctor(s) should I see for my follow-up cancer care?
4. What are the chances that my cancer will come back or that I will get another type of cancer?
5. What follow-up tests, if any, should I have?
6. How often will I need these tests?
7. What symptoms should I watch for?
8. If I develop any of these symptoms, whom should I call?
9. What are the common long-term and late effects of the treatment I received?
10. What should I do to maintain my health and wellbeing?
11. Will I have trouble getting health insurance or keeping a job because of my cancer?
12. Are there support groups I can turn to?

However, this approach assumes that each patient has the capacity to be the navigator of their own care needs. It takes little account of social determinants such as access to and availability of other community resources and services, language and cultural barriers, potential levels of comorbid disability, and other factors.

8.2.1.3 Referral and Coordination of Care Between Service Providers

Research has highlighted that many cancer patients have felt abandoned by the health care system once their specialised cancer treatment is completed [19, 20]. This represents a failure in care coordination across health and support service boundaries, given that research has also confirmed that the transition period immediately following the conclusion of active cancer treatment is likely to be one of a number of highly distressing points for cancer patients, and that those patients who report higher levels of distress at such times tend to also have longer-term problems with adjustment to life after cancer [19]. Reasons for this transition stress in cancer patients relate to the loss of a safety net that was previously present through intense contact with cancer treatment providers and potentially also other cancer patients [11, 46].

In an effort to address some of these healthcare system-based communication and coordination concerns, some governments have attempted to introduce more system integration measures. Across England, for example, Cancer Networks funded centrally and through local bodies were established in 2000. The various National Health Service (NHS) organisations within each of the networks, prior to funding cuts in 2012 that reduced their number from 28 to 12 Networks, aim to work together to deliver high quality, integrated cancer services for their local populations. They bring local area clinicians, patients and managers together, "to deliver the national cancer strategy, to improve performance of cancer services and to facilitate communication and engagement around cancer issues" (p. 5) [47]. Similar networks have been established elsewhere for healthcare delivery more broadly [48]. Most recently, across Australia has been the establishment of Primary Health Networks (PHNs). These are tasked with increasing the efficiency and effectiveness of health services for patients and supporting services to improve the coordination of care for patients within and across health service sectors [49].

Specific to cancer survivorship care, six pilot projects were undertaken in Victoria, Australia to test various models of coordination of care [50]. These included shared care between cancer care services and GPs or discharge for GP follow-up and engagement within primary care. Researchers piloting these approaches reported high levels of acceptability and satisfaction with shared care/discharge to GP follow-up; however, a range of barriers were also reported which included time constraints and GP engagement. Nurse-led clinics were also piloted and included screening, information provision, linkage with other services and transition to GP follow-up; though, no comparison with other models of care was undertaken.

8.2.1.4 Cancer Survivor Care Plans

Various approaches to provision of treatment summaries and survivorship care plans (SCPs) have been explored among cancer survivors [51, 52]. Notably, the focus of these SCPs has been on cancer specific management, rather than patient-led identification of self-management needs, strengths and barriers that may influence their lifestyle behaviour and engagement in care plans [53]. We know that cancer patients' involvement in cancer care can benefit their capacity to live well with cancer, refocusing their lives, "in a positive, purposeful and productive way" [54]. However, initial uncertainty and vulnerability about the longer-term future might hamper the process of cancer patients' active involvement in care planning for the longer-term, at least in the early transition phase for some patients [46].

In a pilot project report by Howell et al. [50], SCPs were positively received by cancer survivors and also perceived as a valuable communication tool by service providers across secondary and primary care. They also found that GPs were more likely to discuss SCPs with cancer survivors where shared care arrangements were in place with secondary care cancer care providers. GPs were also more likely to find SCPs helpful and relevant when information was presented in chronic condition management terms; though, time constraints were reported as a barrier to full integration of this approach.

The Australian Cancer Survivorship Centre [55] undertook an evaluation of SCPs with a large sample of cancer survivors, nurse coordinators and general practitioners (GPs) and concluded that most participants found their SCPs useful. However, over half of cancer survivor participants had not discussed their SCP with their GP. All nurse coordinators felt that SCPs were useful because they improved their communications with the cancer survivor's GP. Most GPs reported receiving a copy of the SCP, most had read it, but few had discussed it with their patient. Few SCPs led to the development of chronic condition self-management care plans. Limited time and resources, competing demands, and inadequate leadership and commitment within the organisation were reported as reasons for limited GP involvement. A range of recommendations were proposed:

- Improved organisational commitment, leaders and multidisciplinary engagement
- Education across all sectors to improve understanding, awareness and practice tools
- Better IT systems to improve communication
- Dedicated resources to enable the implementation of SCPs across clinical services
- More evaluation to provide more rigorous evidence.

8.2.1.5 Nurse-led Clinics

The growth in the scope of role for primary health care nurses offers one (PHCNs) way forward to addressing the barriers to effective chronic condition management [56], more broadly, with primary care, and there has been increasing focus on their role [49]. Within primary care settings where cancer patients will usually begin their contact with the health system for any chronic conditions, and for the screening of risks for cancer [7], the PHCN is an important frontline health worker who could play an important role in the development and delivery of a coordinated holistic model of cancer survivorship care and chronic condition prevention, management and self-management support [57]. McCorkle et al.'s [7] review of self-management approaches for cancer survivorship care stress the complexity of the care continuum for cancer survivors and the need for a champion to provide links between primary care and oncology providers (with relevance also to all cancer patients). This would occur within what they refer to as the 'practice home' in order to make chronic condition care planning possible for this group. In Australia, there are over 10,000 PHCNs within general practice, with more than 60 % of clinics employing a PHCN in Australia today. Their growth has been supported by a range of funding initiative and structural changes to the way general practices are funded, to support them to address the needs of patients with chronic conditions [58, 59].

8.2.1.6 Collaborative Care: Chronic Condition Self-Management Support (The Flinders Program)

Collaborative care has emerged as a significant model in the management of chronic disease. It has both economic drivers but also a social justice focus underpinned by empowerment [60, 61]. This is demonstrated by Lawn et al. [18] who state:

> Self-management support provided through a partnership between the patient and support providers reverses the focus on telling patients what they 'should do' to one where the patient is supported in addressing their own agenda. It is integral in delivering more person-centred care which promotes greater patient autonomy and control, and patient/health professional collaboration, and re-establishing patients' personal ownership of health… This may be especially important for people who have experienced cancer and survived, particularly because many cancer patients report heightened feelings of fear and powerlessness in the face of a cancer diagnosis and the threat of its recurrence (p. 3358) [see also 62, 63].

Reflective of this empowerment framework, the nationally agreed principles underpinning effective chronic condition management and self-management support established for the Australian Government Department of Health and Ageing [64] provide a useful framework in which to position the role of chronic condition management and self-management for cancer survivors.

Box 2: Capabilities and Underlying Principles for Effective Self-Management (KICMRILS)

- **K**now your condition
- Be actively **I**nvolved with the health practitioners to make decisions and navigate the system
- Follow the **C**are plan that is agreed upon with the GP and other health practitioners
- **M**onitor symptoms associated with the condition(s) and **R**espond to, manage and cope with the symptoms
- Manage the physical, emotional and social **I**mpact of the condition(s) on your life
- Live a healthy **L**ifestyle
- Readily access **S**upport services.

Box 3: Underlying Principles and Processes for Effective Self-Management Support

- Assessment of self-management (learn what the patient knows, their actions, strengths and barriers)
- Collaborative problem definition (between patient and their health practitioners)

- Targeting, goal setting and planning (target issues of greatest importance to patient, set realistic goals and develop personalised care plan)
- Self-management training and support services (instruction on disease management, behavioural support, and address physical and emotional demands of chronic condition)
- Active and sustained follow-up (reliable follow-up leads to better outcomes).

One example of how chronic condition self-management support has been operationalized into practice is the Flinders Program of Chronic Condition Care Planning [65] (see Fig. 8.3). This program incorporates the above principles of self-management by the patient and the self-management support by health care providers, families and other support providers in the community. It is an evidence-based, structured interview process, using cognitive behavioral and motivational processes that allow for assessment of self-management behaviors, enablers and barriers to change, and collaborative identification of problems and goals, leading to the development of an individualized person-centered self-management care plan [65, 66]. It includes the following steps:

1. The Partners in Health Scale (PIH): A patient Likert-rated validated questionnaire informed by the WHO and Australian National Chronic Disease Strategy principles of self-management [67, 68]. It enables measurement of perceived change over time where 0 = less favorable and 8 = more favorable self-management capacity. Self-management rated capacities include: knowledge of condition and treatments; quality of relationships with healthcare providers; actions taken to monitor and respond to signs and symptoms; access to services and supports; physical, social and emotional impacts, and lifestyle factors.

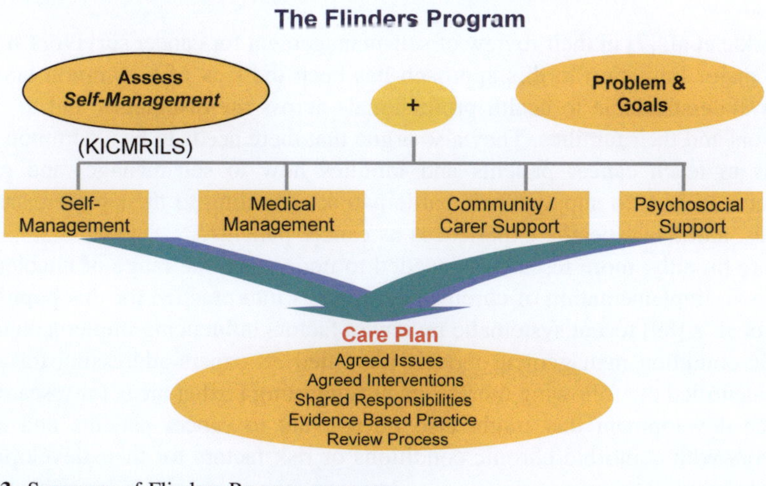

Fig. 8.3 Summary of Flinders Program processes

2. The Cue and Response Interview (C&R): An adjunct to the PIH using open-ended questions or cues to explore the patient's responses to the PIH in more depth, with the patient and worker comparing their Likert-ratings to identify agreed good self-management, agreed issues that need to be addressed, and any discrepancies in views that can then be discussed as part of formulation of a self-management care plan. It enables the strengths and barriers to self-management to be explored, and checks assumptions that either the worker or patient may have, as part of a motivational process.
3. The Problems and Goals (P&G) Assessment: Defines a problem statement from the patient's perspective (the problem, its impact and how it makes them feel) and identifies specific, measurable, achievable, realistic and timely (SMART) goals that they can work towards. It is Likert-rated, allowing measurement of progress over time where 0 = not a problem and 8 = a significant problem; and goal statements: 0 = no progress towards achievement and 8 = achieved.
4. Self-Management Care Plan: Includes self-management issues, aims, steps to achieve them, who is responsible and date for review.

The Flinders Program (adapted for prevention) has been trialled with a small sample of 25 cancer patients being treated with curative intent to investigate the feasibility and acceptability of these care planning tools with this population [18]. Of note, both cancer patients in the active phase of treatment and later in their cancer treatment trajectory found this approach acceptable as a means of helping them to develop and achieve their nutrition and physical activity goals. Building self-management capacity during the active phase of cancer treatment, rather than waiting for treatment to be completed, has appeared to provide health and psychosocial benefits.

8.3 Future Direction for Research and Practice

McCorkle et al. [7] in their review of self-management for cancer survivors stressed that a major limitation to this approach has been the lack of a common language that is understandable to health professionals across the disciplines and to cancer survivors and their families. They also argue that there needs to be a common set of actions to teach cancer patients and families how to self-manage, and greater guidance on how to support their participation according to their preferences and abilities, and their specific experiences as cancer patients.

More broadly, more research is needed to understand the range of enablers and barriers to implementation of chronic care models into practice for this population. Davy et al.'s [69] recent systematic review of factors influencing implementation of chronic condition management models identified 38 papers addressing this issue. They identified the following themes, each suggesting further areas for research and practice development that might also be relevant to cancer patients and cancer survivors with comorbid chronic conditions or risk factors for their development:

- Acceptability of the interventions for healthcare providers and patients
- Preparation of healthcare providers for a CCM approach, including communication needs, necessary incentives for change, skills development and the potential role of leaders and champions
- Supporting patients for a CCM approach, given their diverse needs and preferences in engaging with care
- The resources needed for implementation and sustainability of a CCM approach, including information and communication requirements, funding, collaborations, monitoring and evaluation.

Similar themes were identified by Mitchell et al. [70] in their systematic review of integrated models of care at the primary-secondary interface. Effective models contained the following elements: interdisciplinary teamwork, communication information exchange, shared care guidelines or pathways, training and education, access and acceptability for patients, and a viable funding model.

Other considerations that represent clear gaps in current knowledge and practice, for cancer patients, cancer survivors and patients with chronic conditions more broadly, are also worthy of mention:

- What is the role of palliative care in the chronic disease continuum for cancer patients and patients with chronic conditions more broadly?
- What role should chronic condition management models play for people with chronic conditions who are then diagnosed with cancer or going through acute cancer treatment, or dying of cancer?
- How could Advance Care Directives be incorporated into chronic condition management models involving cancer patients and cancer survivors and more broadly [71]?
- What is the role of information technology systems solutions to address fragmented care and enhance coordination and communication across the cancer care/chronic care continuum?
- What would sustainable models of shared care that include the role of PHCNs look like?

Overall, further translational research is also needed to determine the acceptability and feasibility of these approaches with cancer patients during active treatment for their cancer and for cancer survivors, and to better understand enablers and barriers for clinicians embedding these approaches into routine chronic condition care and cancer survivorship care.

References

1. Sarfati D, Koczwara B, Jackson C (2016) The impact of comorbidity on cancer and its treatment. CA Cancer J Clin Early Online. doi:10.3322/caac.21342
2. Wagner E, Austin B, von Korff M (1996) Organizing care for patients with chronic illness. Milbank Q 74:511–514

3. Wagner EH, Austin BT, Davis C, Hindmarsh M, Schaefer J, Bonomi A (2001) Improving chronic illness care: translating evidence into action. Health Aff 20(6):64–78
4. Ferlay J, Shin HR, Bray F, Forman D, Mathers C, Parking D (2010) Cancer incidence and mortality worldwide. International Agency for Research on Cancer, Lyon
5. Australian Institute for Health and Welfare (AIHW) (2012) Cancer survival and prevalence in Australia: period estimates from 1982–2010. AIHW, Canberra. http://www.aihw.gov.au/WorkArea/DownloadAsset.aspx?id=10737422721. Cited 5 Feb 2016
6. de Moor JS, Mariotto AB, Parry C, Alfano CM, Padgett L, Kent EE, Forsythe L, Scoppa S, Hachey M, Rowland JH (2013) Cancer survivors in the United States: prevalence across the survivorship trajectory and implications for care. Cancer Epidemiol Biomar 22(4):561–570
7. McCorkle R, Ercolano E, Lazenby M, Schulman-Green D, Schilling LS, Lorig K, Wagner EH (2011) Self-management: enabling and empowering patients living with cancer as a chronic illness. CA Cancer J Clin 61(1):50–62
8. Institute of Medicine (2013) Delivering high-quality cancer care: charting a new course for a system in crisis. The National Academics Press, Washington, DC
9. Boger E, Ellis J, Latter S, Foster C, Kennedy A, Jones F, Feneerty V, Kellar I, Demain S (2015) Self-management and self-management support outcomes: a systematic review and mixed research synthesis of stakeholder views. PLoS ONE 10(7):e0120990. doi:10.1371/journal.pone.0130990
10. Taylor S, Pinnock H, Epiphanou E, Pearce G, Parke H, Schwappach A et al (2014) A rapid synthesis of the evidence on interventions supporting self-management for people with long-term conditions: PRISMS—Practical systematic Review of Self-Management Support for long-term conditions. Health Serv Delivery Res 2(53). http://www.journalslibrary.nihr.ac.uk/hsdr/volume-2/issue-53#scientific-summary. Cited 11 Mar 2016
11. Jefford M, Lofti-Jam K, Baravelli C, Grogan S, Rogers M, Krishnasamy M et al (2011) Development and pilot testing of a nurse-led posttreatment support package for bowel cancer survivors. Cancer Nurs 34(3):E1–E10
12. Karahalios A, Baravelli C, Carey M, Schofield P, Pollard A, Aranda S et al (2007) An audiovisual information resource to assist in the transition from completion of potentially curative treatment for cancer through to survivorship: a systematic development process. J Cancer Survivorship 1:226–236
13. Earle CC, Ganz PA (2012) Cancer survivorship care: don't let the perfect be the enemy of the good. J Clin Oncol 30:3764–3768
14. Macmillan Cancer Support (2013) Routes from diagnosis. http://www.macmillan.org.uk/Documents/AboutUs/Research/Researchandevaluationreports/Routes-from-diagnosis-report.pdf. Cited 5 Feb 2016
15. Del Guidice ME, Grunfeld E, Harvey BJ, Piliotis E, Verma S (2009) Primary care physicians' views of routine follow-up care of cancer patients. J Clin Oncol 27:3338–3345
16. Hewitt M, Greenfield S, Stovall E (2005) From cancer patient to cancer survivor: lost in transition. National Academies Press, Washington DC
17. World Health Organization (WHO) (2002) Innovative care for chronic conditions. WHO, Geneva. http://whqlibdoc.who.int/hq/2002/WHO_NMC_CCH_02.01.pdf. Cited 5 Feb 2016
18. Lawn S, Zrim S, Leggett S, Miller M, Woodman R, Jones L, Kichenadasse G, Sukumaran S, Karapetis C, Koczwara B (2015) Is self-management feasible and acceptable for addressing nutrition and physical activity needs of cancer survivors? Health Expect 18(6):3358–3373
19. Allen J, Savadatti S, Levy A (2009) The transition from breast cancer 'patient' to 'survivor'. Psycho-Oncology 18:71–78
20. Jefford M, Karahalios E, Pollard A, Baravelli C, Carey M, Franklin J et al (2008) Survivorship issues following treatment completion—Results from focus groups with Australian cancer survivors and health professionals. J Cancer Survivorship 2:20–32
21. Lance Armstrong Foundation (2010) "I learned to live with it" is not good enough: challenges reported by post-treatment cancer survivors in the Livestrong surveys. A Livestrong Report. Lance Armstrong Foundation, Austin, Texas. https://assets-livestrong-org.s3.amazonaws.com/media/site_proxy/data/a54320d560396f8742fa490257c442829f5be4b2.pdf. Cited 5 Feb 2016

22. Saegrov S, Lorensen M (2006) Cancer patients' opinions concerning post-treatment follow up. Eur J Cancer Care 15:56–64
23. Brett J, Staniszewska S, Mockford C, Herron-Marx S, Hughes J, Tysall C, Suleman R (2014) A systematic review of impact of patient and public involvement on service users, researchers and communities. Patient 7:387–395
24. Ward PR, Thompson J, Barber R, Armitabe CJ, Boote JD, Cooper CL, Jones GL (2010) Critical perspectives on 'consumer involvement' in health research: epistemological dissonance and the know-do gap. J Sociol 46:63–82
25. Solomon P (2004) Peer support/peer provided services underlying processes, benefits, and critical ingredients. Psychiat Rehab J 27:392–401
26. Beckmann K, Strassnick K, Abell L, Hermann J, Oakley B (2007) Is a chronic disease self-management program beneficial to people affected by cancer? Aust J Prim Health 13:36–44
27. Dennis C (2003) Peer support within a health care context: a concept analysis. Int J Nurs Stud 40:321–332
28. Embuldeniya G, Veinot P, Bell E, Bell M, Nyhof-Young J, Sale JEM, Britton N (2013) The experience and impact of chronic disease peer support interventions: a qualitative synthesis. Patient Educ Couns 92(1):3–12
29. Anderson R, Funnell M (2010) Patient empowerment: myths and misconceptions. Pat Educ Couns 79:277–282
30. Funnell MM (2010) Peer-based behavioural strategies to improve chronic disease self-management and clinical outcomes: evidence, logistics, evaluation considerations and needs for future research. Fam Pract Suppl 1:i17–i22
31. Hoeya LM, Ieropolia SC, Whitea VM, Jefford M (2008) Systematic review of peer-support programs for people with cancer. Patient Educ Couns 70(3):315–337
32. Carlsson C, Nilbert M, Nilsson K (2005) Supporter or obstructer; experiences from contact person activities among Swedish women with breast cancer. BMC Health Serv Res 5:9–17
33. Park C, Zlateva I, Blank T (2009) Self-identity after cancer: "survivor", "victim", "patient", and "person with cancer". J Gen Internal Med 2(2):430–435
34. Carlisle D (2011) Vocational rehabilitation: A job that is worth doing well. Health Serv J 121 (6252):10–11
35. Lebel S, Devins GM (2008) Stigma in cancer patients whose behavior may have contributed to their disease. Future Oncol 4(5):717–733
36. Australian Government/Cancer Australia (2015) Cancer support organisations. Australian Government/Cancer Australia, Canberra. https://canceraustralia.gov.au/affected-cancer/cancer-support-organisations. Cited 5 Feb 2016
37. Lorig KR, Ritter P, Stewart AL, Sobel DS, Brown BW, Bandura A, González VM, Laurent DD, Holman HR (2001) Chronic disease self-management program: 2-year health status and health care utilization outcomes. Med Care 39(11):1217–1223
38. Stanford Patient Education Research Centre (2015) Chronic disease self-management program. http://patienteducation.stanford.edu/programs/cdsmp.html. Cited 5 Feb 2016
39. Wilson PM, Kendall S, Brooks F (2007) The Expert Patients Programme: a paradox of patient empowerment and medical dominance. Health Soc Care Comm 15(5):426–438
40. Kravitz RL, Tancredi DJ, Grennan T, Kalauokalani D, Street RL, Slee CK, Wun T, Wright Oliver J, Lorig K, Franks P (2011) Cancer health empowerment for living without pain (Ca-Help): effects of a tailored education and coaching intervention on pain and impairment. Pain 152(7):1572–1582
41. Salvatore AL, Ahn S, Jiang L, Lorig K, Ory MG (2014) National study of chronic disease self-management: six- and twelve-month findings among cancer survivors and non-cancer survivors. Fron Public Health 2:214 (eCollection)
42. Bantum EO, Albright CL, White KK, Berenberg JL, Layi G, Ritter PL, Laurent D, Plant K, Lorig K (2014) Surviving and thriving with cancer using a web-based health behavior change intervention: Randomized controlled trial. J Med Internet Res 16(2):e54
43. Risendal BC, Dwyer A, Lorig K, Coombs L, Kellar-Guenther Y, Warren L, Franco A, Ory MG (2014) Adaptation of the chronic disease self-management program for cancer

survivors: feasibility, acceptability, and lessons for implementation. J Cancer Educ 29(4): 762–771
44. Risendal BC, Dwyer A, Seidel RW, Lorig K, Coombs L, Ory MG (2015) Meeting the challenge of cancer survivorship in public health: results from the evaluation of the chronic disease self-management program for cancer survivors. Psycho-Oncol (ePub). doi: 10.1002/pon.3783
45. Cancer Council Australia (2015) Cancer in general practice—a practical guide for primary health care nurses. http://gp.cancer.org.au/video/cancer-in-general-practice-a-practical-guide-for-primary-health-care-nurses-3-of-3/. Cited 5 Feb 2016
46. Shaha M, Cox CL, Belcher A, Cohen MZ (2011) Transitoriness: patients' perception of life after a diagnosis of cancer. Cancer Nurs Pract 10(4):24–27
47. Macmillan Cancer Support (2012) The role of cancer networks in the new NHS. Report. http://www.macmillan.org.uk/Documents/GetInvolved/Campaigns/TheroleofcancernetworksinthenewNHS.pdf. Cited 5 Feb 2016
48. Hutchison B, Levsque J, Strumpf E, Coyle N (2011) Primary health care in Canada: systems in motion. Milbank Q 89(2):256–288
49. Department of Health (2015) Primary health networks (PHNs). Department of Health, Canberra. http://www.health.gov.au/internet/main/publishing.nsf/content/primary_health_networks. Cited 5 Feb 2016
50. Howell P, Kinnane N, Whitfield K (2014) Supporting cancer survivors in Victoria: summary report. Learning from the Victorian Cancer Survivorship Program pilot projects 2011–2014. Department of Health, State Government of Victoria, Melbourne http://www.petermac.org/sites/default/files/Education/Supporting%20cancer%20survivors%20in%20Victoria%20-%20summary%20report.pdf. Cited 5 Feb 2016
51. Ganz PA, Kwan L, Stanton AL, Bower JE, Belin TR (2011) Physical and psychosocial recovery in the year after primary treatment of breast cancer. J Clin Oncol 29:1101–1109
52. Grunfeld E, Julian JA, Pond G et al (2011) Evaluating survivorship care plans: results of a randomized, clinical trial of patients with breast cancer. J Clin Oncol 29:4755–4762
53. Smith TJ, Snyder C (2011) Is it time for (survivorship care) plan B? J Clin Oncol 29:4740–4742
54. Cotterell P, Harlow G, Morris C et al (2011) Service user involvement in cancer care: the impact on service users. Health Expect 14:159–169
55. Australian Cancer Survivorship Centre (2014) Evaluation of the implementation of survivorship care plans at Peter MacCallum Cancer Centre. Australian Cancer Survivorship Centre, Melbourne. http://www.petermac.org/sites/default/files/Education/Evaluation%20fo%20the%20implementation%20of%20survivorship%20care%20plans%20at%20Peter%20Mac_2014.pdf. Cited 5 Feb 2016
56. Australian Practice Nurses Association (APNA) (2016) Definition of the primary health care nurse. http://www.apna.asn.au/scripts/cgiip.exe/WService=APNA/ccms.r?PageId=11012. Cited 5 Feb 2016
57. Anderson DR, St Halaire D, Flinter M (2012) Primary care nursing role and care coordination: an observational study of nursing work in a community health center. Online J Issues Nurs 17 (2) (Manuscript 3)
58. Haji Ali Afzali H, Karnon J, Beilby J, Gray J, Holton C, Banham D (2014) Practice nurse involvement in general practice clinical care: policy and funding issues need resolution. Aust Health Rev 38(3):301–305
59. Kelehera H, Parker R (2013) Health promotion by primary care nurses in Australian general practice. Collegian 20(4):215–221
60. Thille PH, Russell GM (2010) Giving patients responsibility or fostering mutual response-ability: family physicians' constructions of effective chronic illness management. Qual Health Res 20:1343–1352
61. Pulvirenti M, McMillan J, Lawn S (2012) Empowerment, patient centred care and self-management. Health Expect (Early online:1–8)

62. Aujoulat I, Luminet O, Deccache A (2007) The perspective of patients on their experience of powerlessness. Qual Health Res 17:772–785
63. Foster C, Fenlon D (2011) Recovery and self-management support following primary cancer treatment. Brit J Cancer 105:S21–S28
64. Lawn S, Battersby MW (2009) Capabilities for supporting prevention and chronic condition self-management: a resource for educators of primary health care professionals. Flinders University/Australian Government Department of Health and Ageing, Adelaide
65. Flinders Human Behaviour, Health Research Unit (FHBHRU) (2015) 'The Flinders Program™'. FHBHRU, Adelaide. http://www.flinders.edu.au/medicine/sites/fhbhru/self-management.cfm. Cited 5 Feb 2016
66. Battersby MW, Harvey P, Mills PD et al (2007) SA HealthPlus: a controlled trial of a state-wide application of a generic model of chronic illness care. Milbank Q 85:37–67
67. Battersby M, Ask A, Reece M, Markwick M, Collins J (2003) The partners in health scale: the development and psychometric properties of a generic assessment scale for chronic condition self-management. Aust J Prim Health 9:41–52
68. Petkov J, Harvey PW, Battersby MW (2010) The internal consistency and construct validity of the Partners in Health scale: validation of a patient rated chronic condition self-management measure. Qual Life Res 19(7):1079–1085
69. Davy C, Bleasel J, Liu H, Tchan M, Ponniah S, Brown A (2015) Factors influencing the implementation of chronic care models: a systematic literature review. BMC Fam Pract 16:102–113
70. Mitchell GK, Burridge L, Zhang J, Donald M, Scott IA, Dart J, Jackson CL (2015) Systematic review of integrated models of health care delivered at the primary-secondary interface: how effective is it and what determines effectiveness? Aust J Prim Health 21:391–408
71. Lyon ME, Jacobs S, Briggs L, Cheng YI, Wang J (2014) A longitudinal, randomized, controlled trial of advanced care planning for teens with cancer: anxiety, depression, quality of life, advance directives, spirituality. J Adolesc Health 54:710–717

Further Reading

72. Australian Government/Cancer Australia (2016) Promoting self-management. http://cancersurvivorship.net.au/self-management. Cited 5 Feb 2016
73. Cancer Council Australia (2016) Cancer in General Practice: a guide for primary health care nurses. http://gp.cancer.org.au/video/cancer-in-general-practice-a-practical-guide-for-primary-health-care-nurses-3-of-3/. Cited 5 Feb 2016
74. Davies NJ, Batehup L (2010) Self-management support for cancer survivors: guidance for developing interventions—An update of the evidence. Macmillan Cancer Support, London. http://www.ncsi.org.uk/wp-content/uploads/Guidance-for-Developing-Cancer-Specific-Self-Management-Programmes.pdf. Cited 5 Feb 2016
75. Heisler M (2006) Building peer support models to manage chronic disease: seven models for success. http://www.chcf.org/~/media/MEDIA%20LIBRARY%20Files/PDF/PDF%20B/PDF%20BuildingPeerSupportPrograms.pdf. Cited 5 Feb 2016
76. Macmillan Cancer Support (2011) Supported self-management. https://www.macmillan.org.uk/Aboutus/Healthandsocialcareprofessionals/Newsandupdates/MacVoice/Supportedself-management.aspx. Cited 5 Feb 2016
77. National Comprehensive Cancer Network (2016) Managing Cancer as a Chronic Condition. http://www.nccn.org/patients/resources/life_after_cancer/managing.aspx. Cited 5 Feb 2016

Chapter 9
The Management of Polypharmacy in People with Cancer and Chronic Conditions

Justin P. Turner, Ross A. McKinnon and J. Simon Bell

Abstract Polypharmacy has a broad definition, encompassing the use of multiple medications, the use of more medications than necessary, or the use of inappropriate medications. Polypharmacy itself is not necessarily inappropriate, however, it has been associated with negative outcomes in patients with multiple chronic conditions. For people diagnosed with cancer, medications may be prescribed to treat cancer, ameliorate symptoms, improve quality of life and to manage or prevent future complications of chronic diseases. However, the potential benefits of each medication need to be balanced against the potential harms. For example, in studies of older people with cancer, polypharmacy has been associated with greater risk of chemotherapy discontinuation, mortality, grade III-IV toxicity, drug-drug interactions, drug-disease interactions, increased treatment cost and increased use of potentially inappropriate medications (PIMs). Although the possibility confounding by indication cannot be excluded, the results of these studies suggest it is prudent to conduct a comprehensive medication review in patients at risk of adverse drug events. The goal of medication review is not necessarily to reduce a patient's number of medications, but rather to ensure that each medication is appropriate for the patient's goal of care, with an acceptable benefit to risk ratio.

Keywords Polypharmacy · Potentially inappropriate medication · Deprescribing · Drug-drug interactions · Adverse drug events

J.P. Turner (✉) · J.S. Bell
Centre for Medicine Use and Safety, Faculty of Pharmacy and Pharmaceutical Sciences, Monash University, Parkville, VIC, Australia
e-mail: Justin.Turner@monash.edu

J.P. Turner
Centre de Recherche Institut Universitaire de Gériatrie de Montréal, Université de Montreal, Montréal, QC, Canada

R.A. McKinnon
Flinders Centre for Innovation in Cancer, Flinders University, Bedford Park, SA, Australia

B. Koczwara (ed.), *Cancer and Chronic Conditions*,
DOI 10.1007/978-981-10-1844-2_9

Key Points

- Compared to the broader population little is known about polypharmacy in people with chronic conditions and cancer
- The prevalence of polypharmacy in people with cancer ranges from 35 to 50 %. This is higher than the general population. This is potentially due to the additive effect of using medications to treat both cancer and comorbid conditions
- Recent evidence supports defining polypharmacy in older people with cancer as "the use of five or more medications."
- Some chronic conditions (e.g. cardiovascular disease and cerebrovascular disease) are more likely to be associated with polypharmacy than other chronic conditions.
- Drug-drug interactions can occur between medication used to treat cancer and medications used to treat chronic conditions. The higher the number of medications a person uses the higher the likelihood that they will experience a drug-drug interaction. Care should be exercised when prescribing, dispensing or administering any new medication to a person's medication regimen.
- Cancer treatments may lead to the development of chronic conditions (e.g. anthracyclines and cardiovascular disease) or adverse drug events that may be confused with chronic diseases (e.g. coronary spasm with tyrosine kinase inhibitors). Because long term post-marketing safety data are lacking for many newer therapies clinicians and patients should consider new symptoms as potential adverse drug events and investigate accordingly.
- Deprescribing refers to the reduction of medications after consideration of therapeutic goals, benefits, risks and medical ethics.
- Deprescribing should be a patient centered process focusing on the goals of therapy and the risk and benefit for each medication.

9.1 Introduction

As patients accumulate chronic conditions, it stands to reason they will be prescribed medications for symptomatic treatment of their chronic conditions and/or medications used to prevent future complications. These medications are often prescribed in accordance with disease-specific clinical practice guidelines [1], often resulting in positive health outcomes. However, application of disease-specific clinical practice guidelines can result in patients being prescribed a large number of medications [2–4]. For example, application of individual clinical practice guidelines to a hypothetical 79 year old woman with hypertension, diabetes mellitus, osteoporosis, osteoarthritis and COPD would result in 12 separate medications being recommended, to be administered over five dosing intervals throughout the day [2]. Figures 9.1 and 9.2 (adapted from Barnett et al. [5] and Hovstadius et al. [6]) demonstrate how the number of comorbidities and number of medications used increase with age in a comparable manner.

Polypharmacy is highly prevalent in the general population and increases with age to a point, with recent research demonstrating prevalence of polypharmacy reduces in people aged over 95 years [7, 8]. Over one third of older people in Europe, the United States of America (USA), Australia and New Zealand use ≥ 5 medications each day [3, 9–13]. Polypharmacy has been less extensively investigated for people with cancer, with the reported prevalence ranging from 9 to 86 % [14, 15].

The wide variation in the prevalence of polypharmacy in people with cancer is likely due to a culmination of factors, including younger people having a lower number of comorbidities and the various definitions of polypharmacy that have been used [14]. The difficulties in defining polypharmacy are explored in the following section of this chapter. Despite the wide range of reported prevalence, the majority of studies suggest the prevalence of polypharmacy in people diagnosed with cancer ranges between 35 and 50 % [16–26]. This may be a result of patients being prescribed medications to treat cancer and ameliorate symptoms in addition to medications to manage chronic conditions. A population-based study reported medication use increased in the six months prior to cancer diagnosis [23]. This suggests patients may use medications to treat symptoms relating to their cancer before it is diagnosed.

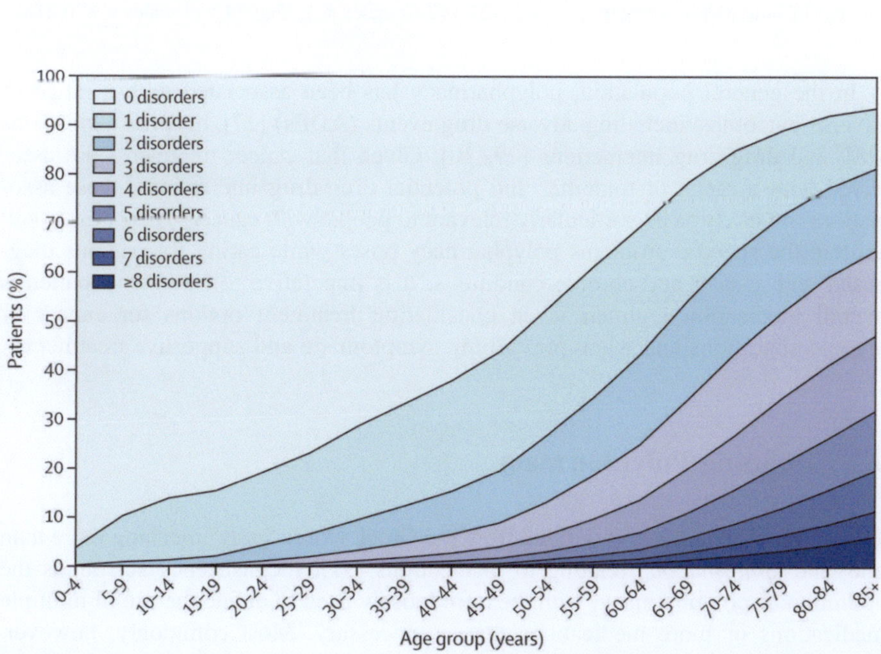

Fig. 9.1 Number of comorbidities with increasing age. Adapted from Barnett et al. [5]

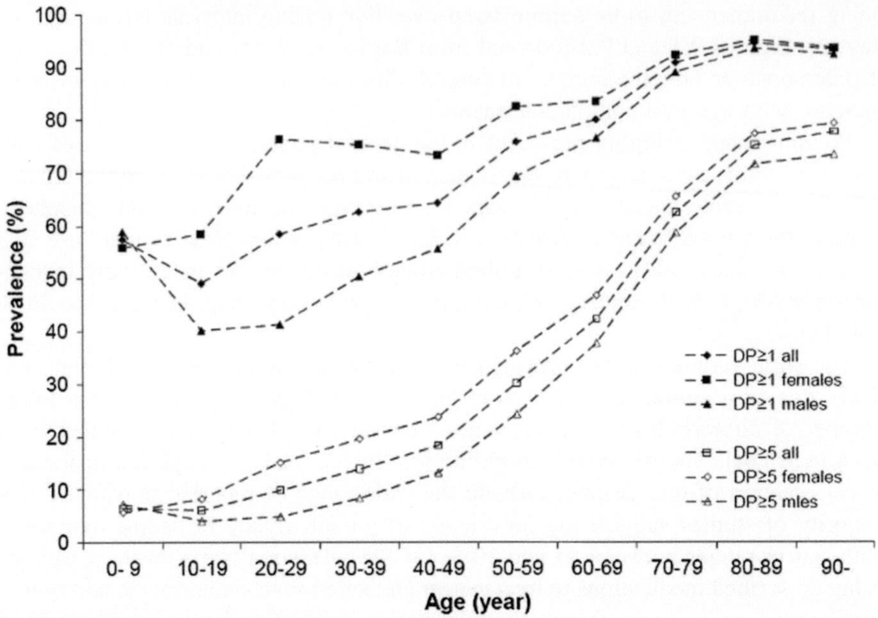

Fig. 9.2 Prevalence of polypharmacy with increasing age. Adapted from Hovstadius et al. [6]. The prevalence of one or more (DPs $\geq$ 1) and five or more (DP $\geq$ 5) dispensed drugs. The prevalence (%) of DP $\geq$ 1 and DP $\geq$ 5 related to sex and age groups in Sweden in 2006. Number of individuals with DP $\geq$ 1 = 6,146,679 (females = 3,466,243 and males = 2,680,436). Number of individuals with DP $\geq$ 5 = 2,227,152 (females = 1,356,934 and males = 870,218)

In the general population, polypharmacy has been associated with a range of adverse outcomes, including adverse drug events (ADEs) [27], hospital admissions [28], and drug-drug interactions [29, 30]. Given that cancer treatments are associated with a range of toxicities and potential drug-drug interactions, these associations are likely to be particularly relevant to people with cancer. This chapter will explore the specific problems polypharmacy poses while caring for patients diagnosed with cancer and chronic conditions. It is imperative to consider a patient's overall medication regimen when considering treatment options for cancer or chronic conditions and when prescribing symptomatic and supportive treatments.

9.2 Defining Polypharmacy

The word polypharmacy is derived from the Greek words "*poly*" meaning more than one, and "*pharmacon*" relating to medications [31]. Inconsistency surrounds the definition of polypharmacy, with the term loosely used to define the use of multiple medications or more medications than is necessary. Most commonly, however, polypharmacy is more specifically defined using a cut-point number [1]. A range of cut points appear in the general literature, including greater than or equal to two [32], four [33], five [34], six [35], seven [36], eight [37], or nine medications [38]. Recently in response to the high prevalence of ten or more medications, two new terms, excessive polypharmacy and hyperpolypharmacy, have been used [39, 40].

Research investigating polypharmacy within groups of people with cancer has used a narrower range of cut-points. The most common definition has been the use of ≥ 5 or more medications. Other studies have used greater than or equal to three [22], four [21], six [41], eight [42], or nine [19] while others have used ranges of medications, for example 0–3, 4–9 and ≥ 10 [24].

The definition of polypharmacy that is most predictive of various adverse events is likely to depend on the clinical characteristics of the patient sample. Recent research used a novel approach to address the question of how to define the polypharmacy cut point number. An Australian study involving community dwelling older people newly diagnosed with cancer, used receiver operating characteristic (ROC) curves to identify which number of medicines had the best balance between sensitivity and specificity for predicting adverse outcomes due to polypharmacy [43]. ROC curves are a graphical plot displaying the balance between sensitivity and specificity for a given test with a binary (yes/no) outcome (Fig. 9.3). ROC curves were originally designed by radar engineers in World War II to improve the detection of enemy objects. They are now widely used to assess the sensitivity and specificity of tests in many fields from medicine to mining. The Australian study concluded that within the patient cohort studied, the definition of five-or-more medications was reasonable for identifying patients who may be at risk of adverse outcomes including frailty, reduced physical function,

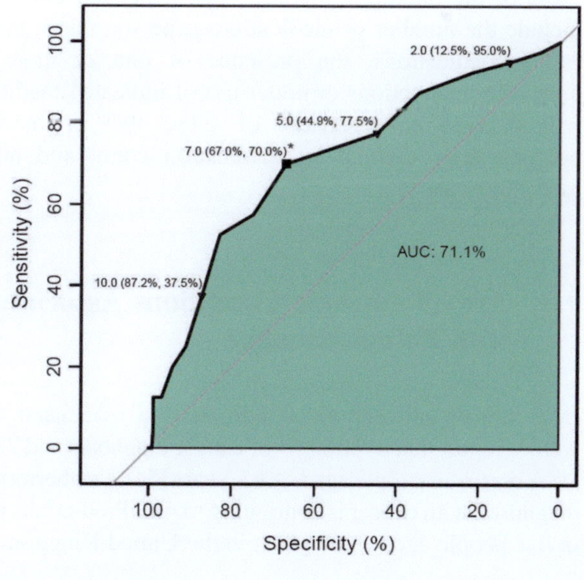

Fig. 9.3 Receiver Operating Characteristic (ROC) curve showing specificity and sensitivity for the association between number of medications and frailty in community dwelling older people with cancer. Adapted from Turner et al. [43] Number of medications (specificity, sensitivity)

falls, exhaustion and reduced performance status (using Karnofsky Performance Scale [KPS] [44]) [43]. The cut-point of five-or-more medications is also supported by research in Japanese and Australian community dwelling older people looking at falls and frailty [45, 46]. To reflect the clinical characteristics of various patient populations, other cut-points may be required. For example, residents of long-term care facilities frequently use nine-or-more medications, thereby in this setting, a higher cut-point may be more useful [47].

A challenge for determining whether or not a patient with cancer has polypharmacy is to know which medications should be included in the medication count. Very few studies on polypharmacy in people with cancer have described the inclusion or exclusion of as-needed (PRN) medications [24, 26, 34, 43], complementary and alternative medications [34, 43, 48], non-prescription medications [24, 34, 43] or chemotherapy [49]. To determine polypharmacy, research in oncology settings has utilized medication chart review, medical records review, or comprehensive geriatric assessment, during which a patient's medication use was verified by a health professional. Additionally, most studies report point prevalent medication use. This is where all medications a person is taking on a specific day are counted. When considering patients with cancer and chronic conditions, an appropriate exposure window should be used to take into account medications that may have been administered recently or medications that are given in a cyclical manner during a course of chemotherapy treatment. This will ensure all potential ADEs or drug-drug interactions are considered (see example of trimethoprim/sulfamethoxazole below) [50].

Polypharmacy has been associated with the use of inappropriate medications. Medications can be considered inappropriate when the likely risks outweigh the benefits, especially when safer alternatives exist. As a result of this association, some of the oncology literature has expanded the definition of polypharmacy to include the number of medications a person takes, the use of one or more unnecessary medications, the presence of one or more inappropriate medications, drug-drug interactions or under use of indicated medications [51–55]. This chapter will provide an overview of these two approaches separately, looking at polypharmacy defined by medication count and also looking at inappropriate medication use.

9.3 Are all Chronic Conditions Associated with Polypharmacy?

Both cancer and chronic conditions are associated with aging. Epidemiological studies report that over 60 % of cancer diagnosis and 70 % of cancer mortality in the USA occurs in people aged ≥ 65 years [54]. Furthermore, the number of older people diagnosed with cancer is continuing to rise. Predictions indicate that by 2030 up to one in five people aged ≥ 65 years in the United Kingdom (UK) will be diagnosed with cancer during their lifetime [56]. This same age group has the highest prevalence of comorbidities and is the highest consumers of medication [57]. Therefore oncologists are likely to encounter patients with multimorbidity and polypharmacy.

The incidence of polypharmacy continues to rise over time [3]. A Swedish population-based study found the prevalence of polypharmacy (defined as ≥ 5 medications) increased by 8 % between 2005 and 2008, with the prevalence of excessive polypharmacy (≥ 10 medications) increasing by 16 % over the same period [7]. Similar observations were made in New Zealand between 2005 and 2013 [3]. This increase in polypharmacy is likely to reflect application of disease-specific clnical practice guidelines to patients with multimorbidity [58]. In 2007, a Scottish population-based study revealed multimorbidity was common in community dwelling people aged ≥ 65 years. Nearly two out of three people (65 %) were diagnosed with multimorbidity, increasing to over four in five (82 %) of those aged ≥ 85 years [5]. One author has described multimorbidity as the most common chronic condition with almost three out of four people in the USA aged ≥ 65 years being diagnosed with three or more chronic conditions [58]. Therefore the number of patients diagnosed with cancer with polypharmacy will continue to rise, making it imperative to balance the goals of treatment for each condition.

However, not all chronic conditions are equally associated with polypharmacy. An Italian hospital based study identified that older people diagnosed with coronary heart disease, cerebrovascular disease and diabetes had greater odds of polypharmacy compared to older people without diabetes and cerebrovascular disease (Odds Ratio [OR] 9.8, 95 % Confidence Interval [95 %CI] 1.3–72.2). This suggested that patients with a diagnosis of coronary heart disease have a higher likelihood of being prescribed polypharmacy [59]. Similar observations have been made in a cross-sectional study investigating community dwelling adults across the USA [60]. The odds of receiving polypharmacy were 68 % greater for people with cardiometabolic and respiratory conditions compared to people with musculoskeletal and respiratory conditions. Therefore when developing treatment plans for patients with cancer and chronic conditions, clinicians should be mindful of which chronic conditions are associated with a greater risk of experiencing polypharmacy.

9.4 Prevalence of Polypharmacy in People with Cancer and Chronic Conditions

A similar range of factors that influence polypharmacy in the general population also impact on the prevalence of polypharmacy in people with cancer. Age had a considerable impact on the prevalence of polypharmacy in a retrospective study of people diagnosed with non-small cell lung cancer. For patients <70 years, only 9 % used ≥ 5 medications, compared to 24 % of patients aged ≥ 70 ($p < 0.001$) [14]. Additionally rates of polypharmacy have been observed to increase at the time of hospital discharge. Research in an acute care hospital ward demonstrated an increase in polypharmacy prevalence (≥ 9 medications) between admission (32 %)

and discharge (38 %). This increase was primarily due to the addition of PRN medications for symptom management [19].

The diagnosis of cancer may also increase the prevalence of polypharmacy compared to patients without cancer. Using the Danish National Health Odense Pharmacoepidemiologic database, Jorgensen et al. [23] compared people with a diagnosis of cancer and matched cases without cancer. People with cancer had a higher prevalence of minor and major polypharmacy (defined as 2–4 and ≥ 5 medications respectively). This suggests that when patients first present to an oncology clinic, a review of the appropriateness of patients medications should be undertaken [34].

9.5 Implications of Polypharmacy in People with Cancer and Chronic Conditions

Most of the time prescribing of medications leads to improved health outcomes [2, 61]. However, despite the benefit that each medication can impart, increased numbers of medications are associated with harms. In community based older people, polypharmacy has been associated with a range of harms including drug-drug interactions, ADEs and hospitalizations. In a cross-sectional study of Canadians aged ≥ 65 years presenting to an emergency department, 31 % of patients using multiple medications had drug-drug interactions [29]. As the number of medications a patient takes increases, the odds of experiencing drug-drug interactions are greater [30, 62]. A different Canadian study investigating polypharmacy in older hospitalized people demonstrated the probability of having ≥ 1 cytochrome-P450 (CYP) mediated drug interaction was 50 % for people using 5–9 medications, 81 % for 10–14 medications, 92 % for 15–19 medications and 100 % for ≥ 20 medications [63]. Across the USA, between 1995 and 2005, patients presenting to hospital using ≥ 5 medications had an 88 % higher risk of experiencing ADEs [27]. Likewise, veterans in the USA using ≥ 5 medications had an almost four-fold increase in unplanned ADE related hospitalisations [28].

Polypharmacy may reflect an extensive medical history, and may be indicative of difficulties choosing the optimal treatment strategy [64]. Therefore it is worth considering that the number or severity of comorbidities may be potential confounders when investigating outcomes associated with polypharmacy [65]. It has been postulated that the outcomes associated with polypharmacy are a reflection of underlying multimorbidity, rather than the number of medications patients use [61, 65, 66]. In a study involving analysis of Scottish primary care data for patients aged ≥ 20 years, the relationships between unplanned hospital admissions and both polypharmacy and multimorbidity were considered [65]. Unplanned hospital admissions were strongly associated with number of medications used, although the association decreased as comorbidity count increased. This highlights the need to consider polypharmacy in the context of the patients' chronic comorbidities and treatment goals.

There have been relatively few studies investigating the harms of polypharmacy in people with cancer compared to people in other settings. Polypharmacy has been investigated in relation to recovery from cancer surgery [16, 67], chemotherapy related toxicity [20], drug-drug interactions [48], and survival [18, 41]. Two studies have investigated the association between polypharmacy and cancer related surgical outcomes [16, 67]. Badgwell et al. [16] studied patients undergoing abdominal cancer surgery and found patients using ≥ 5 medications had two times higher odds of having a prolonged hospital admission following surgery. In breast cancer patients aged ≥ 65 years, Rocco et al. found a 16-fold higher rate of post-operative complications for patients using of ≥ 5 medications [67].

The relationship between polypharmacy and chemotherapy toxicity requires further investigation. In a small prospective longitudinal Italian study (n = 16), Iurlo et al. [22] investigated patients aged ≥ 65 years diagnosed with chronic myeloid leukemia. There was an association between polypharmacy (≥ 3 medications) and tyrosine kinase inhibitor dose reduction due to toxicity. It was postulated that CYP-mediated drug interactions may have been responsible for the toxicity and subsequent dose reduction. In a larger prospective cohort study in the Netherlands, Hamaker et al. [20] investigated polypharmacy in a cohort of older people with breast cancer (n = 78). They identified polypharmacy (≥ 5 medications) was the only factor associated with higher treatment related toxicity, with 57 % of patients with polypharmacy experiencing grade III-IV toxicity. Patients using ≥ 5 medications had six times higher odds of experiencing grade III-IV toxicity compared to patients using <5 medications. The largest study (n = 500) to investigate the association between polypharmacy (4–9 medications) and excessive polypharmacy (≥ 10 medications) and toxicity was conducted by Maggiore et al. in outpatient oncology clinics in the USA. In a retrospective cross-sectional study, they concluded that compared to no polypharmacy (0–3 medications) there was no significant association between polypharmacy or excessive polypharmacy and grade III–V chemotherapy related toxicity or unplanned hospitalisations [24]. Reasons for the difference observed may include the range of cancer types and stages, which may influence the treatment regimens included by each study. Iurlo et al. [22] investigated patients with chronic myeloid leukemia, Hamaker et al. [20] studied patients diagnosed with metastatic breast cancer, while Maggiore et al. [24] investigated patients with any type of solid tumor receiving outpatient chemotherapy (excluding nonmelanoma skin cancer). Furthermore, the retrospective analysis conducted my Maggiore et al. was limited to the data that had been previously collected and, therefore, did not allow for assessment of other clinically important outcomes of toxicity including treatment dose reduction, falls or functional decline. These studies highlight the need for further research that is powered to detect any significant associations between polypharmacy and toxicity, considering a range of clinically important adverse outcomes. The association between polypharmacy and chemotherapy discontinuation has been investigated by both Alexa et al. [14] and Huiart et al. [21]. In patients aged ≥ 70 years with non-small cell lung cancer, Alexa et al. [14] found that compared to patients aged <70 years, polypharmacy (≥ 5 medications) was correlated with early cessation of chemotherapy despite no difference in grade III–IV toxicities. In contrast Huiart et al. [21] found older women with breast cancer who used ≥ 4 medications were 60 % less likely to discontinue their aromatase inhibitor treatment. The difference between these studies lies in the chemotherapy being administered. Alexa et al. investigated the use of platinum based chemotherapy for non-small cell lung cancer, which involves a significant interruption to daily routine, with a high possibility of toxicity, both of which may be seen as harms that outweigh the benefit for older people with polypharmacy due to multimorbidity. Conversely, Huiart et al. investigated daily use of aromatase inhibitors for breast cancer. It is likely that polypharmacy predicted less discontinuation because patients who already have a daily routine for taking multiple medications are unlikely to have a problem adding an aromatase inhibitor to their routine. Conversely, patients not used to taking medications daily may have found adherence difficult.

The association between polypharmacy and mortality in people with cancer is unclear. In a cohort of people undergoing induction therapy for acute myelogenous leukemia, the odds of 30 day mortality increased with each additional medication [18]. For patients receiving ≥ 4 medications compared to ≤ 1, the odds of 30 day mortality were 10 fold higher, with increased overall mortality observed [18]. Freyer et al. [41] also reported reduced overall survival for patients with stage III or IV ovarian cancer using ≥ 6 medications. In contrast to these results Hamaker et al. [20] found no significant association between polypharmacy and mortality in older women with metastatic breast cancer. These studies used similar methodology, adjusting the regression models for variables that were significant in univariate analysis. The difference observed may have been due to small sample sizes or the different cancer types. Alternatively, discontinuation of medications at the end of life setting, would cause an inverse association between polypharmacy and increased mortality. Nevertheless, the variability of results in people with cancer reflects the variability in the broader community [68, 69].

An association between polypharmacy and frailty in older people with cancer has recently been demonstrated. In a recent cross-sectional retrospective analysis of older people newly referred to a senior adult oncology ambulatory center, Nightingale et al. [25] defined frailty as dependence in instrumental activities of daily living (IADLs), significant comorbidities and evidence of geriatric comorbidities. Both polypharmacy (5–9 medications) and excessive polypharmacy (≥ 10) were significantly associated with frailty, more comorbidities and higher Eastern Cooperative Oncology Group Performance Status (ECOG-PS) scores. Similar results were found by Turner et al. [34] who identified polypharmacy was associated with frailty in older community dwelling patients, even after adjusting for age, gender, and Charlson's comorbidity index. In other studies, polypharmacy has been associated with factors that contribute towards frailty. While investigating people newly diagnosed with cancer, Prithviraj et al. [70] collected multiple outcomes assessing functional status, however frailty status was not specifically determined. Despite numerous assessments of functional analysis being performed and investigated, the only significant associations were between polypharmacy and higher ECOG-PS score, higher comorbidity count and greater use of Beers Criteria 2003 medications. While studying the effects of androgen deprivation therapy in older men with prostate cancer, Bylow et al. [17] conducted multiple assessments of functional assessment. The odds of having an abnormal Short Physical Performance Battery score (≤ 9) doubled in patients receiving ≥ 5 medications compared to those receiving <5 medications.

Frailty is an important consideration for patients with cancer and comorbidities because functional impairment can have significant impact on the treatment they receive. A cross-sectional study observed that frailty can alter chemotherapy choice, with frail patients receiving either reduced dose regimens, alternate less toxic regimens or no chemotherapy at all [71]. Similar results were demonstrated in an Australian cohort of older people with metastatic colorectal cancer. Compared to robust patients, vulnerable and frail patients were less likely to receive doublet therapy and had significantly lower rates of survival at 12 months [72]. These studies highlight the potential for polypharmacy to impact on a range of measures used to determine patient's functional capacity and frailty status. This suggests that each medication prescribed for patients with multiple chronic conditions and cancer should be reviewed regularly to ensure its appropriateness.

9.6 Potentially Inappropriate Medications

In the oncology literature, polypharmacy has also been defined as the presence of potentially inappropriate medications (PIMs). This definition of polypharmacy is somewhat unique to the oncology literature. In the pharmacy and clinical pharmacology literature polypharmacy and PIM use are typically distinct concepts.

PIMs may be prescribed in the treatment of chronic conditions, (e.g. amiodarone for arrhythmia) or prescribed to treat cancer symptoms (e.g. amitriptyline used for neuropathic pain), thereby putting patients with both cancer and chronic conditions at risk of being prescribed PIMs. Many definitions for PIMs exist including the use of one or more medications that do not have an indication, or the use of one or more medications where the risk of harm outweighs the potential for benefit [73–75]. For these definitions to be appropriately used in clinical practice, an understanding of the patient's clinical characteristics and chronic conditions is required. Alternatively, both explicit and implicit tools have been defined to identify potentially inappropriate medications where the benefit may be outweighed by the harms.

Implicit criteria have been developed to take into account an individual patient's clinical situation, including the burden of comorbid disease, and a patient's beliefs, values and treatment goals [76]. However, implicit criteria are time consuming to apply and require good knowledge of the patient and their goals of treatment [76]. Although a range of implicit criteria exist, to date, only the medication appropriateness index (MAI) has been researched for use among patients with cancer [15].

In contrast to implicit criteria, explicit criteria are often dichotomous lists of medications to be avoided [76]. Defining PIMs with explicit criteria allows for quality of prescribing to be measured easily and broadly, however, the individual patient's circumstances are not considered [77]. Explicit criteria do not consider that preferred treatment alternatives may have been trialed previously without success, with some medications in the Beers Criteria being considered appropriate by some clinicians as second or third line treatment options [76, 78]. While explicit tools do not consider the clinical situation of individual patients, these tools can be useful to prompt clinicians to be alert for possible ADEs or refer for a comprehensive medication review [79].

Explicit criteria measure inappropriateness via multiple approaches. Medications with an unfavorable benefit to harm profile [80], medications that are associated with specific measurable harmful outcomes [81], or medications that once may have been useful, but due to changes in the patients clinical condition, are now classified as unnecessary or 'futile' [82].

In older people with cancer and multimorbidity, the more medications a patient takes, the more likely one or more of the medications in their regimen will be potentially inappropriate. The association between polypharmacy and the use of PIMs has been demonstrated with Beers 2012 Criteria [80], STOPP [83], and HEDIS DAE Criteria [84], which is consistent with results from older people without cancer [85]. Flood et al. [19], identified PIM use defined by Beers 2012 Criteria was associated with polypharmacy, while Nightingale et al. [25] found PIM use defined by Beers 2012 Criteria, STOPP and HEDIS DAE 2011 Criteria was associated with polypharmacy (5–9 medications) and excessive polypharmacy (≥ 10 medications). Likewise, in an American prescription database, Fahlman et al. found PIM use defined by Beers 1997 Criteria was associated with increasing prescription count [86]. Additionally patients with cancer had higher odds of receiving ≥ 2 PIMs compared to patients without cancer.

Not every study has demonstrated associations between use of PIMS and clinically important outcomes. Using Beers 2012 Criteria, Zhan Criteria and the HEDIS DAE 2011 Criteria, Maggiore et al. [24] were unable to detect significant associations between PIM use and chemotherapy toxicity or hospitalization in patients with solid tumors receiving chemotherapy. Likewise, Elliot et al. [18] were unable to find associations between use of Beers 2012 Criteria medication and 30 day mortality, complete remission, ICU admission or increased length of stay in a cohort of patients receiving induction therapy for acute myelogenous leukemia.

While Sect. 4.3 of this text book considers chronic conditions at end of life, it is worth mentioning that some medications may become potentially inappropriate for patients with reduced life expectancy. For example, many medications used in the treatment of chronic conditions are used to prevent future complications. These medications may become inappropriate when the time to benefit exceeds a patients predicted life expectancy [87, 88]. Statins are an example of medications used for primary or secondary prevention of cardiovascular events where the time to benefit may exceed predicted life expectancy [87]. Despite this, approximately 1-in-3 patients with terminal cancer were still using statins at the time of death [89, 90]. An Australian study found that statin use in older people was associated with a four-fold increase in pain for patients aged ≥ 80 years, which is the age group that has no evidence to support statins reducing mortality [91, 92]. Reviewing the benefit and harms for each medication will help clinicians and patients identify medications that are no longer required. Stopping unnecessary medications reduces polypharmacy, and reduces the potential for ADEs and drug-drug or drug-disease interactions. The process for reducing unnecessary medications is discussed below.

9.7 Drug-Drug Interactions

Polypharmacy increases the risk of drug-drug and drug-disease interactions [48, 49]. The potential for drug-drug interactions increases with each additional medication used [62]. The prevalence of drug-drug interactions in people with cancer ranges from 27–63 % and has been reported to be the cause of 4 % cancer related deaths in hospitalized patients [42, 49, 93]. Drug-drug interactions may occur between medications prescribed to manage chronic conditions and IV or oral chemotherapy or supportive treatments. Likewise, medication prescribed to treat cancer or provide symptomatic and supportive treatment may interact with medications prescribed to treat chronic conditions.

Oral cancer treatments are becoming increasingly common because they can provide patients with improved convenience and quality of life. However, the potential for drug-drug interactions, resulting in treatment toxicity or treatment failure is important to consider. For example, capecitabine is metabolized by cytochrome P450 3A4 (CYP3A4). Medications prescribed for the management of cardiovascular disease, including atorvastatin and diltiazem, are also metabolized by CYP3A4. When administered together, there is competition for the CYP3A4 enzyme, which can lead to irinotecan or capecitabine having reduced metabolism, leading to toxicity [94]. The reverse has also been demonstrated with the reduced efficacy of tamoxifen when co-administered with the CYP 2D6 inhibitor paroxetine. In one study, patients who used paroxetine for at least 75 % of the time they were being treated with tamoxifen had nearly an increase in the odds of death by almost 50 % compared to patients who did not use paroxetine (HR 1.46, 95 % CI 1.15–1.84) [95]. Drug-drug interactions are not limited to cytochrome mediated interactions. Erlotinib, dasatinib, gefitinib, nilotinib and ponatinib all require a low pH to be absorbed [96]. Therefore, when taken together with proton pump inhibitors, their absorption and efficacy is reduced. This clinical scenario can be quite common, with Todd et al. [97] identifying 55 % of patients prescribed erlotinib for the treatment of advanced non-small cell cancer were also prescribed proton-pump inhibitors.

Clinicians also need to be aware of medications that are prescribed as supportive therapy, particularly when prescribed as short term or cyclical use. For example anti-infective agents including trimethoprim/sulfamethoxazole, ciprofloxacin, clarithromycin and fluconazole may be commonly prescribed to patients with prolonged neutropenia to prevent Pneumocystis pneumonia [98]. Each of these anti-infective agents can interact with medications used in the management of diabetes (glipizide and glyburide), increasing the odds of hypoglycemia [99].

Intravenously administered chemotherapy is not susceptible to the pharmacodynamic drug absorption interactions that oral chemotherapy is susceptible to. However, as with oral chemotherapy, cytochrome mediated interactions are possible for injectable chemotherapy. Irinotecan is also metabolized by CYP3A4, and therefore can cause toxicity when co-administered with CYP3A4 inhibitors. Both doxorubicin and vinblastine are metabolized by CYP2D6 and, therefore, may interact with antidepressants including fluoxetine and paroxetine which are potent inhibitors of CYP2D6. Alternatively, interactions could occur via renal elimination. For example, methotrexate is predominantly renally cleared. Patients with cardiovascular disease may be prescribed angiotensin converting enzyme (ACE) inhibitors and diuretics, which can reduce renal function, causing methotrexate to accumulate. Likewise, nonsteroidal anti-inflammatory drugs (NSAIDs) can cause a rapid deterioration in renal function which has been observed to cause a lethal accumulation of both methotrexate and cisplatin when co-administered. Patients with chronic conditions such as rheumatoid arthritis may take NSAIDs on a regular or PRN basis, and therefore clinicians should take measures to prevent the co-administration of medications that reduce renal function for patients receiving renally cleared chemotherapy.

Unfortunately drug-drug interactions are common in people with cancer and chronic conditions and are associated with polypharmacy. On an inpatient hematology ward, Tavakoli-Ardakani et al. [100] reported 38 % of patients had potential drug-drug interactions with a significant correlation existing between the number of medications ordered and the number of potential drug-drug interactions identified. In 2005, Riechelmann et al. [42] identified 63 % of their cohort of inpatients diagnosed with cancer experienced drug-drug interactions, which was associated with an increased length of stay. Patients using ≥ 8 medications were at nearly 10 times higher odds of experiencing drug-drug interactions compared to those using <8 medications [42]. Riechelmann et al. also investigated outpatients with cancer in 2007 [49] and a palliative care setting in 2008 [48] and demonstrated that for each additional medication used the odds of drug-drug interactions rose by 40 and 30 % respectively. In the outpatient setting, they demonstrated that drug-drug interactions were associated with medications used to treat comorbid disease states, rather than supportive symptomatic treatment [49]. Therefore clinicians need to be mindful of all medications a patient is taking for their chronic diseases when choosing a cancer treatment regimen. Oncologists should also be vigilant in checking for new additions to the medication regimen by other prescribers, as specialists in other fields may be unaware of the potential for medications they prescribe to interact with cancer treatments.

While potential drug-drug interactions are common, not all interactions are clinically significant. Therefore, it can be difficult to determine which interactions should be avoided, and which interactions should be monitored. In a palliative care setting in the UK, 267 potential drug-drug interactions were observed in 132 patients. Over 40 % (n = 112) of the interactions were deemed clinically significant, with nearly a third of them (n = 31) deemed preventable by stopping medications that were no longer appropriate [101]. Where possible, clinicians can avoid drug-drug interactions by changing one of the interacting medications to an alternative that does not interact, for example, changing from atorvastatin to pravastatin if a statin is deemed to be necessary. If the statin is no longer required, ceasing statin treatment will also avoid the interaction and reduce polypharmacy.

9.8 Polypharmacy and Chronic Conditions as a Result of Cancer Treatment

The association between cancer treatments and the development of comorbidities is important to consider when caring for patients who are currently receiving, or have previously received, treatment for cancer. Thus far, this chapter has discussed polypharmacy due to patient's comorbidities, or as a result of symptomatic and supportive treatments. However, clinicians should be mindful of polypharmacy that may result from treating cancer, especially when treating younger patients. Older chemotherapies have well established associations with chronic diseases. For example, anthracyclines can damage myocardial tissue and, therefore, have detrimental effects on the cardiovascular system, with many guidelines recommending a lifetime limit on doxorubicin due to the potential to cause cardiotoxicity. Likewise alkylating agents, 5-fluorouracil and paclitaxel are associated with cardiotoxicity [102]. Therefore, treatment of younger patients may increase the prevalence of chronic conditions in later years, which will increase the likelihood of polypharmacy in the treatment of these chronic conditions [103]. It is important for clinicians to discuss these issues with younger patients before commencing and completing treatment.

In addition to the well-defined short-term ADEs and well-known long term ADEs from certain older chemotherapies, clinicians need to consider the less well known and less certain long-term ADEs of newer targeted therapies. Small molecule targeted therapies have only been used in clinical practice since the early 2000s. While they have dramatically changed the treatment course and survival outcomes of certain cancers, the long-term effects of these medications are largely unknown. Clinical trials with long term follow up for tyrosine kinase inhibitors have generally excluded patients with cardiovascular disease, thereby limiting the external generalizability of the results. Additionally, clinical trials of the second and third line tyrosine kinase inhibitors have had limited long-term follow up, generally confined to five years or less [104]. Larger, pharmacoepidemiological studies are required to adequately address the range of long term side effects associated with the wide use of these newer treatments. Despite the limited long-term follow up for many of the newer treatments, there is evidence to suggest that they are associated with the development of toxicities that include chronic conditions, such as congestive heart failure, cardiac arrhythmias, vascular events and pulmonary toxicity [104].

While there are well known and well established links between chronic diseases and some older therapies, these associations may be less obvious for newer therapies. For example, in a younger male who presents with symptoms of angina, it is difficult to distinguish between new development of cardiovascular disease, versus the presentation of ADEs such as coronary spasm, thrombus or vascular deficiency due to targeted therapy. Failure to differentiate symptoms of angina as an ADE as opposed to development of a chronic disease may lead to prescribing of guideline driven polypharmacy, rather than reassessment of the targeted treatment. Many doctors who are not familiar with cancer medications may be unaware of these potential ADEs, which highlights the importance of good communication and follow up with patients receiving long term oral therapies.

9.9 Methods to Address Polypharmacy

Addressing polypharmacy in patients with cancer and chronic conditions can be difficult, especially when one or more of the medications is a cancer treatment. This may cause a problem as prescribers who do not specialize in treating cancer may lack specialist knowledge relating to cancer medication, while clinicians who specialize in treating cancer may lack knowledge relating to the medications used in the treatment of chronic conditions [105]. Qualitative research has identified that prescribers often report reluctance to discontinue a medication initiated by another prescriber [105, 106]. Therefore without good communication between all clinicians, medications often accumulate.

Deprescribing refers to the reduction of medications after consideration of therapeutic goals, benefits and risks, and medical ethics [105]. While reducing inappropriate or unnecessary medication may provide benefits, it must be done with clear communication, to ensure the patient and their care-givers and families understand the reason. Often, in an effort to encourage compliance, patients are instructed that a medication for their chronic condition should be used "for life." Deprescribing such a medication can cause undue concern for patients including making them feel like they are not worthy of treatment, feeling like they have been abandoned by the health system, feeling concerned they are imminently about to die, or feeling confused with which prescriber they should believe [107]. For example, while statins may be inappropriate because they have a long time to benefit and their lack of mortality benefit in primary prevention for patients aged ≥ 80 years, stopping a statin may cause undue concern without good prescriber-patient communication.

Only one prospective study has investigated the outcomes of deprescribing medications in people with cancer and chronic diseases [108]. Unfortunately, this study might not be generalizable to the majority of people with cancer and comorbidities, as it was conducted in a palliative care setting. Patients with a life expectancy between 1 and 12 months were randomized to deprescribing their statin or control. No significant difference was observed in either survival rate at 60 days or new cardiovascular events, suggesting there is no immediate harm from deprescribing statins. Interestingly, patients who stopped their statins reported significantly higher quality of life scores which is an important outcome for patients with a limited life expectancy [108].

The process for deprescribing medications in people with cancer and chronic conditions should be patient focused and appreciate that a patient's health status is dynamic, thereby benefits and harms for each medication may change over time [109]. Various methodologies have been developed to guide clinicians in reducing inappropriate polypharmacy [88, 110, 111]. Figure 9.4 summarizes the steps required for patient focused deprescribing in patients with cancer and chronic conditions.

Firstly, clinicians should discuss with patients and their families and care-givers about the goals of treatment. Patients have dynamic health status, which may shift between states of being robust, vulnerable and frail. Additionally, as a patient's health status deteriorates, they may have a higher focus on quality of life, rather than on life extension. As these goals change, the appropriateness of each medication should be reviewed. One way to review the appropriateness is to consider the benefit-to-harm ratio of each medication [113]. If the harms from a medication (including exposure to ADEs or drug-drug and drug-disease interactions) are greater than the benefit provided by the medication, it should be considered for deprescribing. When considering the benefit of each medication, the time to benefit should also be taken into account. Some preventative medications require years of continuous use before a mortality benefit becomes apparent. A useful way for discussing the benefit-to-harms ratio with patients and their families and care-givers is through the use of number needed to treat (NNT) and number needed to harm (NNH) [111].

The second step requires a thorough review of each medication a patient is using including regular and when required medications. This requires clinicians to specifically enquire about oral and intravenous chemotherapy, cyclical medications used to provide supportive and symptomatic relief, prescription medications used in the management of chronic conditions, over-the-counter medications and complementary and alternative therapies. Adherence should also be checked at this time, to identify medications that remain on the medication list despite no longer being used by the patient.

Once a complete medication history has been obtained, each medication should be checked to ensure it aligns with the patients current goals of care. Medications which have no clinical indication, have a time-to-benefit longer than the patients' predicted life expectancy, or medications that no longer meet the patients' goals of care can be identified for deprescribing. Likewise, medications causing ADEs or drug-drug interactions should be considered for deprescribing. In addition, for patients aged 65 years and over, the medication list should be assessed to ensure it does not contain any potentially inappropriate medications. Lists such as Beers criteria and STOPP/START criteria are the most commonly used tools for evaluating medication appropriateness in older people with cancer [73, 83].

Deprescribing medications is best done one at a time when possible, to allow monitoring for return of symptoms or withdrawal effects [114, 115]. Once a list of medications to be deprescribed has been compiled, the order in which they should

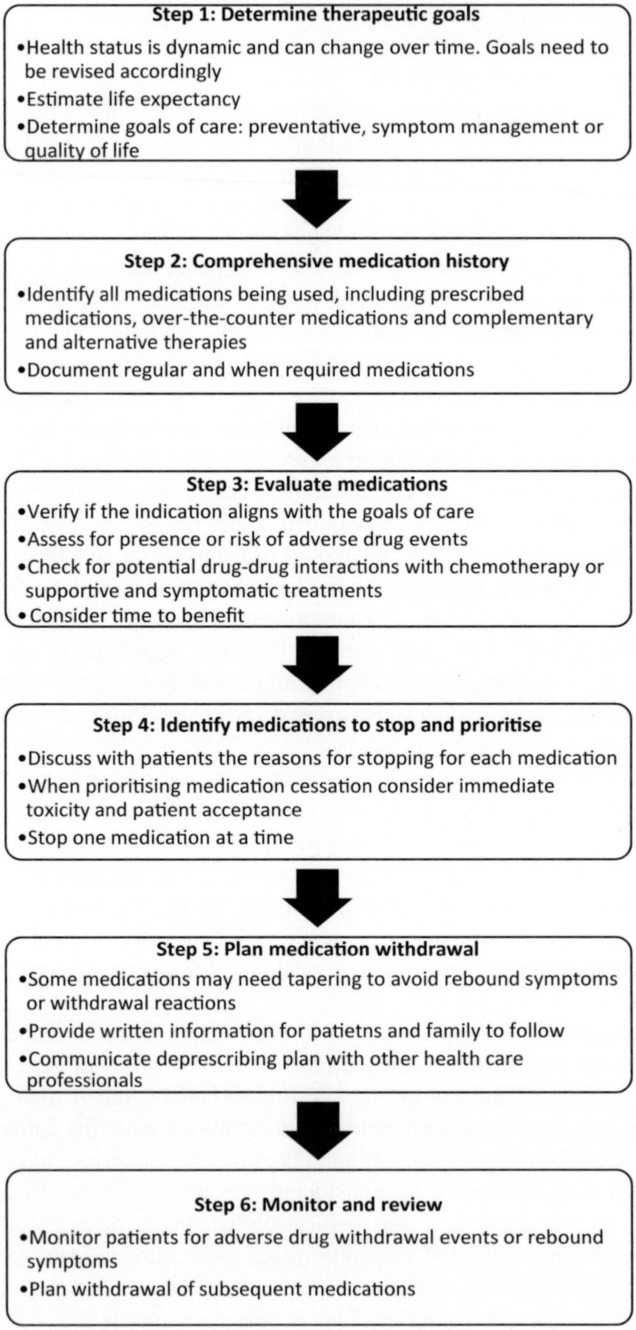

Fig. 9.4 Patient centered process for deprescribing. Adapted from Reeve et al. [112]

be discontinued needs to be determined. There are several factors to be considered when determining the order of deprescribing [88]. Firstly, deprescribing medications that are suspected of causing toxicity or serious drug-drug interactions may be a priority. Alternatively, deprescribing medications that patients prioritize for stopping may result in higher patient acceptance. Additionally, some clinicians choose to deprescribe medications that may potentially cause adverse drug withdrawal events last, as these may take longer to deprescribe, requiring a gradual tapering protocol.

The final steps in a patient focused deprescribing process involve patient monitoring and follow up. Depending on the patients' cancer treatments, they may have frequent appointments with their oncologist, making the oncologist an obvious choice for monitoring for withdrawal or rebound symptoms. However, if a patient is receiving outpatient therapy or oral chemotherapy and is not requiring regular visits with their oncologist, the role of follow up and monitoring might be performed more appropriately by another health care professional such as their family physician so long as each physician understands their role in the deprescribing process [116]. Regardless of who the follow up clinician is, the patient, their family, their caregiver and the whole health care team should be provided with documentation clearly stating what is occurring within the deprescribing process, and who the contact person is for follow up.

9.10 Future Directions for Research and Practice

Additional research is required into problems that can occur when treating people with chronic conditions and cancer. Firstly, longitudinal research is required to quantify the possible long-term ADEs associated with newer targeted therapies. This will be important to guide practice when choosing therapies for people with chronic conditions. For example, if a patient presents with cardiovascular disease, a physician may choose not to prescribe a targeted therapy that has been found to be associated with causing cardiovascular events. Similarly, research is required to understand the mechanism behind the possible long term ADEs of newer therapies, and to determine if switching medications can reverse the effects. This would inform practice and allow physicians to differentiate between symptoms being irreversible ADEs, reversible ADEs or development of chronic conditions. Being able to differentiate between the causes of symptoms will dramatically alter the way they are treated.

Further research is also required to determine the most effective ways to deprescribe for patients with chronic conditions and cancer. Discussing deprescribing of medications can cause undue concern for patients, as they may feel that they are being abandoned by their health care team, they are no longer deserving of treatment, their death is imminent, or they may lose hope [107, 117]. While qualitative research has been conducted in community dwelling people with chronic conditions and in long term care facilities to identify the barriers and enablers of deprescribing, there is a paucity of research investigating deprescribing on people with cancer and chronic conditions [105, 117, 118]. Future research needs to consider the barriers and enablers to deprescribing in people with cancer and chronic conditions because there is likely to be a number of important differences. Firstly, patients may be offered chemotherapy, along with supportive symptomatic treatments, each of which increases the medication burden, and increases the potential for ADEs, drug-drug interactions and drug-disease interactions, making the benefits of deprescribing greater [22, 42, 100, 101]. Additionally, the diagnosis of cancer is a sentinel event that may change the goals of care for people with chronic conditions. This may reduce the focus on preventative medications, to focusing on quality of life [107, 109]. Finally, access to specialist physicians and family physicians may be limited for residents of long term care facilities therefore making it difficult to discuss medication use and deprescribing [105]. This is in contrast to people with cancer and chronic conditions, who may visit doctors, and therefore need to actively manage the potential communication barriers between primary care and tertiary care [90, 94].

References

1. Jokanovic N, Tan EC, Dooley MJ, Kirkpatrick CM, Elliott RA, Bell JS (2016) Why is polypharmacy increasing in aged care facilities? The views of Australian health care professionals. J Eval Clin Pract
2. Boyd CM, Darer J, Boult C, Fried LP, Boult L, Wu AW (2005) Clinical practice guidelines and quality of care for older patients with multiple comorbid diseases: implications for pay for performance. JAMA 294:716–724
3. Nishtala PS, Salahudeen MS (2014) Temporal trends in polypharmacy and Hyperpolypharmacy in Older New Zealanders over a 9-year period: 2005–2013. Gerontology
4. American geriatrics society expert panel on the care of older adults with M. Patient-centered care for older adults with multiple chronic conditions: a stepwise approach from the American geriatrics society: American geriatrics society expert panel on the care of older adults with multimorbidity. J Am Geriatr Soc 60:1957–1968, 2012
5. Barnett K, Mercer SW, Norbury M, Watt G, Wyke S, Guthrie B (2012) Epidemiology of multimorbidity and implications for health care, research, and medical education: a cross-sectional study. Lancet 380:37–43
6. Hovstadius B, Astrand B, Petersson G (2009) Dispensed drugs and multiple medications in the Swedish population: an individual-based register study. BMC Clin Pharmacol 9:11
7. Hovstadius B, Hovstadius K, Åstrand B, Petersson G (2010) Increasing polypharmacy-an individual-based study of the Swedish population 2005–2008. BMC Clin Pharmacol 10:16
8. Onder G, Marengoni A, Russo P et al (2016) Advanced age and medication prescription: more years, less medications? A nationwide report from the Italian medicines agency. J Am Med Dir Assoc 17:168–172
9. Linjakumpu T, Hartikainen S, Klaukka T, Veijola J, Kivela SL, Isoaho R (2002) Use of medications and polypharmacy are increasing among the elderly. J Clin Epidemiol 55:809–817
10. Guthrie B, Makubate B, Hernandez-Santiago V, Dreischulte T (2015) The rising tide of polypharmacy and drug-drug interactions: population database analysis 1995-2010. BMC Med 13:74

11. Junius-Walker U, Theile G, Hummers-Pradier E (2007) Prevalence and predictors of polypharmacy among older primary care patients in Germany. Fam Pract 24:14–19
12. Slabaugh SL, Maio V, Templin M, Abouzaid S (2010) Prevalence and risk of polypharmacy among the elderly in an outpatient setting. Drugs Aging 27:1019–1028
13. Morgan TK, Williamson M, Pirotta M, Stewart K, Myers SP, Barnes J (2012) A national census of medicines use: a 24-hour snapshot of Australians aged 50 years and older. Med J Aust 196:50–53
14. Alexa T, Lavinia A, Luca A, Miron L, Alexa ID (2014) Incidence of chemotherapy discontinuation and characteristics of elderly patients with non-small cell lung cancer treated with platinum-based doublets. Contemp Oncol (Pozn) 18:340–343
15. Domingues D, Carneiro R, Costa I et al (2015) Therapeutic futility in cancer patients at the time of palliative care transition: an analysis with a modified version of the Medication Appropriateness Index. Palliat Med 29:643–651
16. Badgwell B, Stanley J, Chang GJ et al (2013) Comprehensive geriatric assessment of risk factors associated with adverse outcomes and resource utilization in cancer patients undergoing abdominal surgery. J Surg Oncol 108:182–186
17. Bylow K, Dale W, Mustian K et al (2008) Falls and physical performance deficits in older patients with prostate cancer undergoing androgen deprivation therapy. Urology 72:422–427
18. Elliot K, Tooze JA, Geller R et al (2014) The prognostic importance of polypharmacy in older adults treated for acute myelogenous leukemia (AML). Leuk Res 38:1184–1190
19. Flood KL, Carroll MB, Le CV, Brown CJ (2009) Polypharmacy in hospitalized older adult cancer patients: experience from a prospective, observational study of an oncology-acute care for elders unit. Am J Geriatr Pharmacother 7:151–158
20. Hamaker ME, Seynaeve C, Wymenga AN et al (2014) Baseline comprehensive geriatric assessment is associated with toxicity and survival in elderly metastatic breast cancer patients receiving single-agent chemotherapy: results from the OMEGA study of the Dutch breast cancer trialists' group. Breast 23:81–87
21. Huiart L, Bouhnik AD, Rey D et al (2013) Complementary or alternative medicine as possible determinant of decreased persistence to aromatase inhibitor therapy among older women with non-metastatic breast cancer. PLoS One 8:e81677
22. Iurlo A, Ubertis A, Artuso S et al (2014) Comorbidities and polypharmacy impact on complete cytogenetic response in chronic myeloid leukaemia elderly patients. Eur J Intern Med 25:63–66
23. Jorgensen T, Herrstedt J, Friis S, Hallas J (2012) Polypharmacy and drug use in elderly Danish cancer patients during 1996 to 2006. J Geriatr Oncol 3:33–40
24. Maggiore RJ, Dale W, Gross CP et al (2014) Polypharmacy and potentially inappropriate medication use in older adults with cancer undergoing chemotherapy: effect on chemotherapy-related toxicity and hospitalization during treatment. J Am Geriatr Soc 62:1505–1512
25. Nightingale G, Hajjar E, Swartz K, Andrel-Sendecki J, Chapman A (2015) Evaluation of a pharmacist-led medication assessment used to identify prevalence of and associations with polypharmacy and potentially inappropriate medication use among ambulatory senior adults with cancer. J Clin Oncol 33:1453–1459
26. Puts M, Costa-Lima B, Monette J et al (2009) Medication problems in older, newly diagnosed cancer patients in Canada: How Common are they? A prospective pilot study. Drugs Aging 26:519–536
27. Bourgeois FT, Shannon MW, Valim C, Mandl KD (2010) Adverse drug events in the outpatient setting: an 11-year national analysis. Pharmacoepidemiol Drug Saf 19:901–910
28. Marcum ZA, Amuan ME, Hanlon JT et al (2012) Prevalence of unplanned hospitalizations caused by adverse drug reactions in older veterans. J Am Geriatr Soc 60:34–41
29. Hohl CM, Dankoff J, Colacone A, Afilalo M (2001) Polypharmacy, adverse drug-related events, and potential adverse drug interactions in elderly patients presenting to an emergency department. Ann Emerg Med 38:666–671

30. Halvorsen KH, Granas AG, Engeland A, Ruths S (2012) Prescribing quality for older people in Norwegian nursing homes and home nursing services using multidose dispensed drugs. Pharmacoepidemiol Drug Saf 21:929–936
31. Maher RL, Hanlon J, Hajjar ER (2014) Clinical consequences of polypharmacy in elderly. Expert Opin Drug Saf 13:57–65
32. Kowatch RA, Youngstrom EA, Horwitz S et al (2013) Prescription of psychiatric medications and polypharmacy in the LAMS cohort. Psychiatr Serv 64:1026–1034
33. Baranzini F, Diurni M, Ceccon F et al (2009) Fall-related injuries in a nursing home setting: is polypharmacy a risk factor? BMC Health Serv Res 9:228
34. Turner JP, Shakib S, Singhal N et al (2014) Prevalence and factors associated with polypharmacy in older people with cancer. Support Care Cancer 22:1727–1734
35. Advinha AM, de Oliveira-Martins S, Mateus V, Pajote SG, Lopes MJ (2014) Medication regimen complexity in institutionalized elderly people in an aging society. Int J Clin Pharm 36:750–756
36. Cusack S, Rose Day M, Wills T, Coffey A (2012) Older people and laxative use: comparison between community and long-term care settings. Br J Nurs 21:711–714, 6–7
37. Honney K, Trepte NJ, Parker RA et al (2014) Characteristics and determinants of survival in oldest old nursing home residents admitted to hospital with an acute illness compared to their younger counterparts. Aging Clin Exp Res 26:153–160
38. Wimmer BC, Dent E, Visvanathan R et al (2014) Polypharmacy and medication regimen complexity as factors associated with hospital discharge destination among older people: a prospective cohort study. Drugs Aging 31:623–630
39. Jyrkka J, Vartiainen L, Hartikainen S, Sulkava R, Enlund H (2006) Increasing use of medicines in elderly persons: a five-year follow-up of the Kuopio 75 + Study. Eur J Clin Pharmacol 62:151–158
40. Gnjidic D, Hilmer SN, Blyth FM et al (2012) High-risk prescribing and incidence of frailty among older community-dwelling men. Clin Pharmacol Ther 91:521–528
41. Freyer G, Geay JF, Touzet S et al (2005) Comprehensive geriatric assessment predicts tolerance to chemotherapy and survival in elderly patients with advanced ovarian carcinoma: a GINECO study. Ann Oncol 16:1795–1800
42. Riechelmann RP, Moreira F, Smaletz O, Saad ED (2005) Potential for drug interactions in hospitalized cancer patients. Cancer Chemother Pharmacol 56:286–290
43. Turner JP, Jamsen KM, Shakib S, Singhal N, Prowse R, Bell JS (216) Polypharmacy cut-points in older people with cancer: how many medications are too many? Support Care Cancer 24:1831–1840
44. Karnofsky DA, Burchenal JH (1949) The clinical evaluation of chemotherapeutic agents in cancer. In: MacLeod CM (ed.) Evaluation of Chemotherapeutic Agents. Columbia University Press, pp. 1949:196
45. Kojima T, Akishita M, Nakamura T et al (2012) Polypharmacy as a risk for fall occurrence in geriatric outpatients. Geriatr Gerontol Int 12:425–430
46. Gnjidic D, Hilmer SN, Blyth FM et al (2012) Polypharmacy cutoff and outcomes: five or more medicines were used to identify community-dwelling older men at risk of different adverse outcomes. J Clin Epidemiol 65:989–995
47. Jokanovic N, Tan EC, Dooley MJ, Kirkpatrick CM, Bell JS (2015) Prevalence and factors associated with polypharmacy in long term care facilities: a systematic review. J Am Med Dir Assoc 16(535):e1–e12
48. Riechelmann RP, Zimmermann C, Chin SN et al (2008) Potential drug interactions in cancer patients receiving supportive care exclusively. J Pain Symptom Manage 35:535–543
49. Riechelmann RP, Tannock IF, Wang L, Saad ED, Taback NA, Krzyzanowska MK (2007) Potential drug interactions and duplicate prescriptions among cancer patients. J Natl Cancer Inst 99:592–600
50. Lees J, Chan A (2011) Polypharmacy in elderly patients with cancer: clinical implications and management. Lancet Oncol 12:1249–1257

51. Balducci L, Goetz-Parten D, Steinman MA (2013) Polypharmacy and the management of the older cancer patient. Ann Oncol 24(Suppl 7):vii36–vii40
52. Maggiore RJ, Gross CP, Hurria A (2010) Polypharmacy in older adults with cancer. Oncologist 15:507–522
53. Cope DG (2013) Polypharmacy in older adults: the role of the advanced practitioner in oncology. J Adv Pract Oncol 4:107–112
54. Hurria A, Browner IS, Cohen HJ et al (2012) Senior adult oncology. J Natl Compr Canc Netw 10:162–209
55. LeBlanc TW, McNeil MJ, Kamal AH, Currow DC, Abernethy AP (2015) Polypharmacy in patients with advanced cancer and the role of medication discontinuation. Lancet Oncol 16: e333–e341
56. Maddams J, Utley M, Moller H (2012) Projections of cancer prevalence in the United Kingdom, 2010–2040. Br J Cancer 107:1195–1202
57. Santos AP, da Silva DT, Dos Santos Junior GA et al (2015) Evaluation of the heterogeneity of studies estimating the association between risk factors and the use of potentially inappropriate drug therapy for the elderly: a systematic review with meta-analysis. Eur J Clin Pharmacol 71:1037–1050
58. Tinetti ME, Fried TR, Boyd CM (2012) Designing health care for the most common chronic condition–multimorbidity. JAMA 307:2493–2494
59. Nobili A, Marengoni A, Tettamanti M et al (2011) Association between clusters of diseases and polypharmacy in hospitalized elderly patients: results from the REPOSI study. Eur J Intern Med 22:597–602
60. Vyas A, Pan X, Sambamoorthi U (2012) Chronic condition clusters and polypharmacy among adults. Int J Family Med 2012:193168
61. Hughes CM, Cooper JA, Ryan C (2014) Going beyond the numbers—a call to redefine polypharmacy. Br J Clin Pharmacol 77:915–916
62. Johnell K, Klarin I (2007) The relationship between number of drugs and potential drug-drug interactions in the elderly: a study of over 600,000 elderly patients from the Swedish prescribed drug register. Drug Saf 30:911–918
63. Doan J, Zakrzewski-Jakubiak H, Roy J, Turgeon J, Tannenbaum C (2013) Prevalence and risk of potential cytochrome P450-mediated drug-drug interactions in older hospitalized patients with polypharmacy. Ann Pharmacother 47:324–332
64. Belfrage B, Koldestam A, Sjoberg C, Wallerstedt SM (2015) Number of drugs in the medication list as an indicator of prescribing quality: a validation study of polypharmacy indicators in older hip fracture patients. Eur J Clin Pharmacol 71:363–368
65. Payne RA, Abel GA, Avery AJ, Mercer SW, Roland MO (2014) Is polypharmacy always hazardous? A retrospective cohort analysis using linked electronic health records from primary and secondary care. Br J Clin Pharmacol 77:1073–1082
66. Loke YK, Somogyi AA, Ferro A, Ritter JM (2015) Editors' pick 2014. Br J Clin Pharmacol 79:354–356
67. Rocco N, Rispoli C, Pagano G et al (2013) Breast cancer surgery in elderly patients: postoperative complications and survival. BMC Surg 13(Suppl 2):S25
68. Tamura BK, Bell CL, Inaba M, Masaki KH (2012) Outcomes of polypharmacy in nursing home residents. Clin Geriatr Med 28:217–236
69. Jyrkka J, Enlund H, Korhonen MJ, Sulkava R, Hartikainen S (2009) Polypharmacy status as an indicator of mortality in an elderly population. Drugs Aging 26:1039–1048
70. Prithviraj GK, Koroukian S, Margevicius S, Berger NA, Bagai R, Owusu C (2012) Patient characteristics associated with polypharmacy and inappropriate prescribing of medications among older adults with cancer. J Geriatr Oncol 3:228–237
71. Decoster L, Kenis C, Van Puyvelde K et al (2013) The influence of clinical assessment (including age) and geriatric assessment on treatment decisions in older patients with cancer. J Geriatr Oncol 4:235–241
72. Patel D, Turner JP, Athreya V, Singhal N (2015) Outcomes of geriatric assessment for metastatic colorectal cancer patients from a dedicated geriatric oncology program. Poster

presentation: medical oncology group of Australia (MOGA) annual scientific meeting. Hobart, Australia
73. American Geriatrics Society Beers Criteria Update Expert P. American Geriatrics Society (2015) Updated beers criteria for potentially inappropriate medication use in older adults. J Am Geriatr Soc 2015(63):2227–2246
74. Beers M, Ouslander J, Rolingher J, Reuben D, Brooks J, Beck J (1991) Explicit criteria for determining inappropriate medication use in nursing home residents. UCLA Division of geriatric medicine. Arch Intern Med 151:1825–1832
75. Tjia J, Velten SJ, Parsons C, Valluri S, Briesacher BA (2013) Studies to reduce unnecessary medication use in frail older adults: a systematic review. Drugs Aging 30:285–307
76. Spinewine A, Schmader KE, Barber N et al (2007) Appropriate prescribing in elderly people: how well can it be measured and optimised? Lancet 2007 370:173–184
77. Anderson GM, Beers MH, Kerluke K (1997) Auditing prescription practice using explicit criteria and computerized drug benefit claims data. J Eval Clin Pract 3:283–294
78. Chang CB, Chan DC (2010) Comparison of published explicit criteria for potentially inappropriate medications in older adults. Drugs Aging 27:947–957
79. Santos AP, Silva DT, Alves-Conceicao V, Antoniolli AR, Lyra DP Jr (2015) Conceptualizing and measuring potentially inappropriate drug therapy. J Clin Pharm Ther 40:167–176
80. American geriatrics society beers criteria update expert P. American geriatrics society updated beers criteria for potentially inappropriate medication use in older adults. J Am Geriatr Soc 60:616–631, 2012
81. Milos V, Bondesson Å, Magnusson M, Jakobsson U, Westerlund T, Midlöv P (2014) Fall risk-increasing drugs and falls: a cross-sectional study among elderly patients in primary care. BMC Geriatr 14:40
82. Fede A, Miranda M, Antonangelo D et al (2011) Use of unnecessary medications by patients with advanced cancer: cross-sectional survey. Support Care Cancer 19:1313–1318
83. Gallagher P, Ryan C, Byrne S, Kennedy J, O'Mahony D (2008) STOPP (screening tool of older person's prescriptions) and START (screening tool to alert doctors to right treatment). Consensus validation. Int J Clin Pharmacol Ther 46:72–83
84. Healthcare Effectiveness Data and Information Set (HEDIS) (2015) Final NDC lists: use of high-risk medications in the elderly (DAE). National Committee on Quality Assurance, Washington DC
85. Guaraldo L, Cano F, Damasceno G, Rozenfeld S (2011) Inappropriate medication use among the elderly: a systematic review of administrative databases. BMC Geriatr 11:79
86. Fahlman C, Lynn J, Finch M, Doberman D, Gabel J (2007) Potentially inappropriate medication use by medicaid + choice beneficiaries in the last year of life. J Palliat Med 10:686–695
87. Riechelmann RP, Krzyzanowska MK, Zimmermann C (2009) Futile medication use in terminally ill cancer patients. Support Care Cancer 17:745–748
88. Scott IA, Hilmer SN, Reeve E et al (2015) Reducing inappropriate polypharmacy: the process of deprescribing. JAMA Intern Med 175:827–834
89. Stavrou EP, Buckley N, Olivier J, Pearson SA (2012) Discontinuation of statin therapy in older people: does a cancer diagnosis make a difference? An observational cohort study using data linkage. BMJ Open 2
90. Cashman J, Wright J, Ring A (2010) The treatment of co-morbidities in older patients with metastatic cancer. Support Care Cancer 18:651–655
91. Turner JP, Shakib S, Singhal N et al (2014) Statin use and pain in older people with cancer: a cross-sectional study. J Am Geriatr Soc 62:1900–1905
92. Chokshi NP, Messerli FH, Sutin D, Supariwala AA, Shah NR (2012) Appropriateness of statins in patients aged >/=80 years and comparison to other age groups. Am J Cardiol 110:1477–1481
93. Buajordet I, Ebbesen J, Erikssen J, Brors O, Hilberg T (2001) Fatal adverse drug events: the paradox of drug treatment. J Intern Med 250:327–341

94. Hall PS, Lord SR, El-Laboudi A, Seymour MT (2010) Non-cancer medications for patients with incurable cancer: time to stop and think? Br J Gen Pract 60:243–244
95. Kelly CM, Juurlink DN, Gomes T et al (2010) Selective serotonin reuptake inhibitors and breast cancer mortality in women receiving tamoxifen: a population based cohort study. BMJ 340:c693
96. Segal EM, Flood MR, Mancini RS et al (2014) Oral chemotherapy food and drug interactions: a comprehensive review of the literature. J Oncol Pract 10:e255–e268
97. Todd A, Williamson S, Husband A, Baqir W, Mahony M (2013) Patients with advanced lung cancer: is there scope to discontinue inappropriate medication? Int J Clin Pharm 35:181–184
98. Freifeld AG, Bow EJ, Sepkowitz KA et al (2011) Clinical practice guideline for the use of antimicrobial agents in neutropenic patients with cancer: 2010 update by the infectious diseases society of america. Clin Infect Dis 52:e56–e93
99. Schelleman H, Bilker WB, Brensinger CM, Wan F, Hennessy S (2010) Anti-infectives and the risk of severe hypoglycemia in users of glipizide or glyburide. Clin Pharmacol Ther 88:214–222
100. Tavakoli-Ardakani M, Kazemian K, Salamzadeh J, Mehdizadeh M (2013) Potential of drug interactions among hospitalized cancer patients in a developing country. Iran J Pharm Res 12:175–182
101. Todd A, Nazar H, Pearson H, Andrew L, Baker L, Husband A (2014) Inappropriate prescribing in patients accessing specialist palliative day care services. Int J Clin Pharm 36:535–543
102. Senkus E, Jassem J (2011) Cardiovascular effects of systemic cancer treatment. Cancer Treat Rev 37:300–311
103. Lipshultz SE, Franco VI, Miller TL, Colan SD, Sallan SE (2015) Cardiovascular disease in adult survivors of childhood cancer. Annu Rev Med 66:161–176
104. Caldemeyer L, Dugan M, Edwards J, Akard L (2016) Long-term side effects of tyrosine kinase inhibitors in chronic myeloid leukemia. Curr Hematol Malig Rep 11:71–79
105. Turner JP, Edwards S, Stanners M, Shakib S, Bell JS (2016) What factors are important for deprescribing in Australian long-term care facilities? Perspectives of residents and health professionals. BMJ Open 6:e009781
106. Anderson K, Stowasser D, Freeman C, Scott I (2014) Prescriber barriers and enablers to minimising potentially inappropriate medications in adults: a systematic review and thematic synthesis. BMJ Open 4:e006544
107. Stevenson J, Abernethy AP, Miller C, Currow DC (2004) Managing comorbidities in patients at the end of life. BMJ 329:909–912
108. Kutner JS, Blatchford PJ, Taylor DH Jr et al (2015) Safety and benefit of discontinuing statin therapy in the setting of advanced, life-limiting illness: a randomized clinical trial. JAMA Intern Med 175:691–700
109. Currow DC, To THM, Abernethy AP (2009) Prescribing at times of clinical transition in chronic or progressive diseases. Int J Gerontol 3:1–8
110. Reeve E, Wiese MD (2014) Benefits of deprescribing on patients' adherence to medications. Int J Clin Pharm 36:26–29
111. Hilmer SN, Gnjidic D, Le Couteur DG (2012) Thinking through the medication list—appropriate prescribing and deprescribing in robust and frail older patients. Aust Fam Physician 41:924–928
112. Reeve E, Shakib S, Hendrix I, Roberts MS, Wiese MD (2014) The benefits and harms of deprescribing. Med J Aust 201:386–389
113. Turner J, Singhal N, Bell JS (2013) Opportunities for deprescribing statins in patients with poor cancer prognosis. J Palliat Med 16:1328
114. Graves T, Hanlon JT, Schmader KE et al (1997) Adverse events after discontinuing medications in elderly outpatients. Arch Intern Med 157:2205–2210
115. Bain KT, Holmes HM, Beers MH, Maio V, Handler SM, Pauker SG (2008) Discontinuing medications: a novel approach for revising the prescribing stage of the medication-use process. J Am Geriatr Soc 56:1946–1952

116. Kouladjian L, Gnjidic D, Reeve E, Chen TF, Hilmer SN (2016) Passing the buck: Health care practitioners' perspectives on deprescribing anticholinergic and sedative medications in older adults. Ann. Pharmacother (ePub ahead of print)
117. Reeve E, To J, Hendrix I, Shakib S, Roberts MS, Wiese MD (2013) Patient barriers to and enablers of deprescribing: a systematic review. Drugs Aging 30:793–807
118. Schuling J, Gebben H, Veehof LJ, Haaijer-Ruskamp FM (2012) Deprescribing medication in very elderly patients with multimorbidity: the view of Dutch GPs. A qualitative study. BMC Fam Pract 13:56

Further Reading—Further information on de-prescribing medications can be found at:

119. Best Practice New Zealand "Stopping medicines" guide http://www.bpac.org.nz/BPJ/2010/April/docs/bpj_27_stop_guide_pages_10-23.pdf
120. Medstopper is an academic site for clinicians that provides an overview of number needed to treat and number needed to harm in elderly patients with comorbidities (not specific to cancer patients) medstopper.com
121. Deprescribing.org is a collaboration between clinicians, academics, researchers and patients, dedicated to the reduction of unnecessary and harmful medications in seniors (not specific to cancer patients) deprescribing.org
122. A summary of adverse drug withdrawal reactions can be found at: Bain KT, Holmes HM, Beers MH, Maio V, Handler SM, Pauker SG (2008) Discontinuing medications: a novel approach for revising the prescribing stage of the medication-use process. J Am Geriatr Soc 56:1946–1952

Further Reading—Further information on the definition of polypharmacy in people with cancer and chronic conditions:

123. Turner JP, Jamsen KM, Shakib S, Singhal N, Prowse R, Bell JS (2016) Polypharmacy cut-points in older people with cancer: how many medications are too many? Supp Care Cancer 24:1831–1840

Chapter 10
Breaking the Silos: Integrated Care for Cancer *and* Chronic Conditions

Lauren J. Cortis, Paul R. Ward, Ross A. McKinnon and Bogda Koczwara

Abstract People with cancer and a chronic condition have complex care needs that require input from multiple care providers in a variety of settings. Delivering these different aspects of care in isolation can give rise to fragmentations of care, experienced by patients as a disjointed and cumbersome care experience and by clinicians as gaps in communication and information flow. Fragmented care contributes to an ineffectiveness, inequality, inefficiency and higher cost of care. Reducing fragmentation through better care integration is thus a key health care priority for patients, health care providers and payers. This chapter reviews existing strategies to improve integration of care and reduce fragmentation and their respective strengths and limitations and argues further work is needed in developing novel models of care that support efficient and effective integration of care for patients with chronic conditions and cancer.

Keywords Integration · Team based care · Continuity of care · Health system design · Multidisciplinary care · Coordinated care

Key points

- Health care delivery in cancer and chronic conditions involves different health care providers, settings and health care systems. This increases likelihood of fragmentation which contributes to ineffectiveness, inequality, inefficiency and increased costs of care delivery.
- While a multidisciplinary care approach is designed to ensure input of multiple providers into cancer care planning, its application is frequently limited to cancer specific issues.

L.J. Cortis · R.A. McKinnon · B. Koczwara (✉)
Flinders Centre for Innovation in Cancer, Flinders University,
Flinders Drive, Bedford Park, SA 5042, Australia
e-mail: bogda.koczwara@flinders.edu.au

P.R. Ward
Discipline of Public Health, Flinders University, Flinders Drive,
Bedford Park, SA 5042, Australia

B. Koczwara (ed.), *Cancer and Chronic Conditions*,
DOI 10.1007/978-981-10-1844-2_10

- Integrated care offers an attractive conceptual model to deliver seamless care but there has been little empirical application of this approach in the cancer setting.
- There are multiple barriers to greater integration of care of cancer and chronic conditions, including lack of awareness of the problem, lack of common language and lack of system integration.

10.1 Introduction

Cancer is a complex condition which usually requires the input of multiple care providers in order to meet a patient's cancer-related needs. In cancer services, this team of provides is commonly known as the multidisciplinary team (MDT) (Fig. 10.1). People living with chronic conditions *and* cancer also have care needs that extend beyond cancer and its management, including concerns relating to management of non-cancer conditions and their interaction with cancer and its treatment. These needs are dynamic, varying in nature and intensity across time. Meeting these needs is unlikely to be achieved by the cancer MDT alone, rather it requires coordination across the healthcare workforce, incorporating of a broad collection of care providers spanning disciplines (medical, nursing, allied health), professional approaches (specialist and generalist) and settings of care (primary, secondary, tertiary) (Fig. 10.2). This type of multi-team system of care presents challenges to healthcare systems, care providers, and ultimately the patients themselves [1].

Despite the increasing recognition that contemporary healthcare systems need to enhance their capability for providing chronic care of complex conditions and multimorbidity, most health care systems are designed to meet the needs of people with single disease states in a short term or acute setting [3]. Within health care systems, services are often comprised of different teams, with separate information systems, performance indicators and payment models, contributing to the formation of organizational silos [4]. These silos exist at various levels, ranging from healthcare sectors and institutions to clinical units and individual disciplines. Within teams there is a tendency for attitudes and behaviors to be more homogenous and inwardly focused, giving rise to gaps between groups or teams and at the boundaries of care [5]. These holes may accentuate barriers to inter-professional relationships and information flow [6] which present as fragmentations in care. For the health care system this can result in inefficiency, ineffectiveness and inequality [7]. For clinicians, this can impede clinical decision making and workflow, affecting their ability to understand the patient as a whole and consider whether more aggressive or more conservative approach to management is warranted [8]. Most importantly for the patient, this can result in a disjointed care experience, feeling of "falling through the gaps" [9] and the need for a considerable effort to personally manage their overall care which may be beyond the capabilities of those more vulnerable on the grounds of poor health and/or limited health literacy [10].

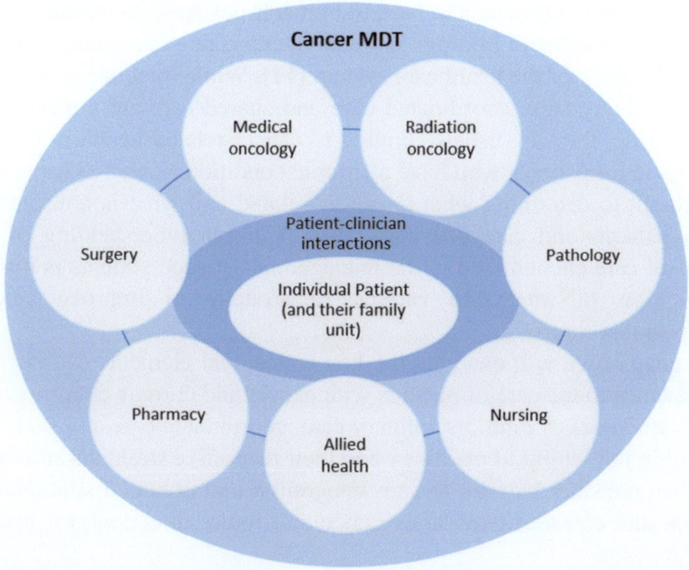

Fig. 10.1 An illustration of a cancer MDT, adapted from Levitt et al. [2] with permission from the National Academies Press, Copyright 2013, National Academy of Sciences

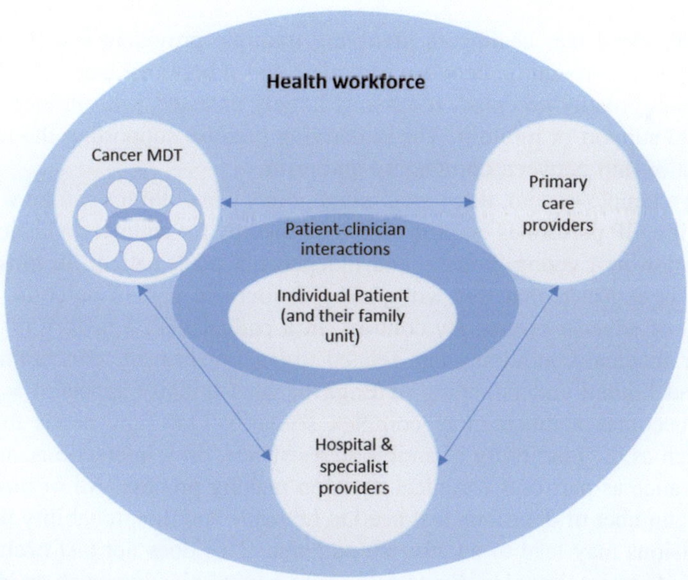

Fig. 10.2 An illustration of a coordinated healthcare workforce, adapted from Levitt et al. [2] with permission from the National Academies Press, Copyright 2013, National Academy of Sciences

Integrated care is an evidence based approach designed to overcome fragmentations of care, in order to improve patients' healthcare experience, care outcomes and to the efficiency of the healthcare system [11]. While integration strategies such as multidisciplinary care, coordinated care and shared care are utilized within the oncology setting, they are usually limited to cancer-related health needs. This can be problematic for patients who have a chronic condition as well as cancer, where it can be difficult to determine what is cancer-related and what is not, creating confusion for patients and care providers alike. Current understanding of the fragmentations of care encountered in the management of such patients is limited, as is the exploration of integrated care as a strategy to improve care at the primary-specialist interface.

In this chapter we will examine the key conceptual elements of integrated care and its relevance to the care of patients with cancer and chronic conditions, how the integration strategies of multidisciplinary care, coordinated care and shared care are applied within the setting of oncology and their respective strengths and limitations. We will then consider barriers to care integration and potential strategies to overcome them, and consider gaps in evidence and future directions for research and practice.

10.2 Increasing Complexity—Increasing Fragmentations in Care

It is hypothesized that healthcare involving multiple providers and organizations results in poor coordination between providers and suboptimal care [12]. While the hypothesis is broadly accepted, it remains largely untested, with limited empirical evidence to support or refute it. The underlying premise supporting the hypothesis is the relationship between complexity and error.

Within a simple system, there are limited points where things can go wrong. For example, if a GP prescribes empiric antibiotic therapy for an uncomplicated urinary tract infection in a young, healthy and independent adult patient, in most circumstances it is expected that this will yield a favourable patient outcome with low likelihood of adverse events. By contrast, in a patient with a history of antibiotic use, other medical conditions, age related organ impairment, concomitant medications and limited understanding of English, what initially appeared as a simple problem becomes a much more complex scenario. One now needs to consider factors such as the possibility of antibiotic resistance, drug interactions, and altered drug clearance as part of the clinical decision making process. All of these factors add to the number of decisions that need to be made and the probability that one of these decisions may lead to an adverse outcome. This does not just occur through errors in judgement, but also due to failures in communication, such as insufficient transfer of critical information between care providers, or patients obtaining insufficient or conflicting information from care providers. While the decisions that clinicians make are connected by a mutual individual patient, they are often made in isolation and reflect the care provider or team's focus on specific aspects of that individual's health.

Within a complex system of issues and providers, it may be unclear which provider is responsible for which aspect of care, such as the continued prescribing and ongoing monitoring of drug therapy. For the patient, not knowing who is responsible for what part of their treatment can create practical challenges as they attempt to coordinate their medication management across their conditions. Lack of clarity in roles and responsibilities can also lead to patient frustration and reduced trust in care providers [12] as well as the need to repetitively provide information to multiple clinicians, which is considered by patients to be disturbing and burdensome [12].

Management of medications can be a useful surrogate marker for the complexity of the health care needs of patients with coexisting cancer and chronic conditions. The total amount of medications used is increasing as the population ages and chronic conditions become more prevalent [13]. In addition to providing therapeutic benefit, multiple medications are important contributors to excessive healthcare costs and patient harm [14]. While it is possible for any patient using one or more medications to experience a preventable medication-related hospital admission, it has been shown to be more likely in patients taking multiple medications [15], as is the case in patients with multiple chronic conditions, including cancer. This issue is particularly challenging in cancer patients, as their cancer medications are often delivered intermittently and thus are not easily identified in their medication supply, and non-cancer health care providers are often unfamiliar with cancer drugs and their side effects.

This is not to say that polypharmacy is the only risk factor for care fragmentation —rather a simple example. In real life, a patient using multiple medications has multiple other care needs and multiple health care providers and information sources, creating a setting for a high risk of fragmentation and concomitant gaps in care.

When considering what fragmentations of care may be encountered, one can review the multiple layers of the environmental context that potentially influence the care of patients with cancer and chronic conditions (Fig. 10.3). Potential sources of fragmentation are present at all levels of the health system, including macro (system), meso (organizational) and micro (clinical). Trying to understand how disjointed healthcare experiences relate to contextual causes, rather than simply identifying that they exist, is necessary to þdevelop targeted integration strategies to improve care outcomes. If we return to the example of medication management, evidence suggests that in patients with breast cancer there is a reduced level of adherence to cardiovascular [16] and diabetes medications [17], beginning in the treatment phase and persisting into survivorship. While this indicates that medication management is not currently optimised across all conditions (i.e. fragmentation exists), it does not tell us how much this is associated with potentially changeable patient behaviour or clinical decision-making (i.e. targets for integration strategies).

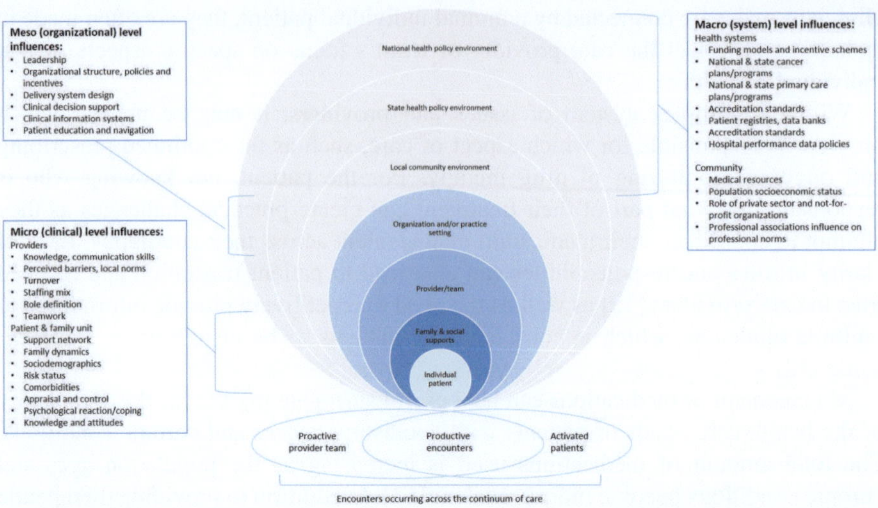

Fig. 10.3 The care of patients with cancer and a chronic condition is influenced by multiple layers. These represent potential sources of fragmentation, and opportunities for integration initiatives, adapted from Taplin and Rodgers [18] by permission of Oxford University Press

10.3 Care Integration—A Solution to Overcome Fragmentation

Integrated care is a conceptual term originating from organizational and systems theory that has been broadly applied in the healthcare literature. While there are in excess of 150 definitions of integrated care, most definitions agree that its key feature is the aim of improving outcomes for a target population through fostering coordination within and between healthcare organizations [11]. As such, integrated care refers to a broad concept that covers a range of approaches, which aim to improve the experience of patients, the outcomes of care and enhance overall efficiency. Integration is a nested concept within integrated care, used to describe the processes and methods that seek to bring about integrated care [11].

It is important to acknowledge that the understanding that an individual has of integrated care at a systems level is shaped by the health system context in which they reside. In the USA and countries with existing integrated care delivery systems, integrated care has come to be somewhat synonymous with full organizational integration and managed care. In this context, integrated care is seen as a structural or environmental concept, while coordination of care relates to practical implementation of interventions to improve patient care. In the UK and countries with a strong primary care system, like Australia, where the GP acts as the gatekeeper to other services and care providers, integrated care may be understood as a system that supports coordinating a patient's overall care, such as care networks and organizations that commission service providers. Across all health care systems, at an individual level, integrated care refers to the ease of addressing individual's diverse health care needs in a seamless fashion.

10.3.1 Dimensions of Integration

In designing an integration strategy, it is useful to consider it across five dimensions:

- Degree of integration (from informal working relationships of providers to coordinated networks, to full system integration)
- Level of the health system (health system, organization, clinical setting)
- Focus (target population)
- Direction (horizontal—affecting organizations at same level and, vertical—affecting organizations at different levels i.e. primary and secondary care)
- Type of intervention involved.

Interventions used to achieve integration may address any of the vast number of sources of fragmentation (Fig. 10.3). These include system redesign, including alignment of policies and governance and operational support systems to facilitate integrated management, building the culture of coordination and collaboration, facilitating professional relationships between care providers, designing integrated clinical care pathways. The design of an appropriate integration strategy should be determined by the objective of the overall integrated care initiative, the stakeholders involved and the health system environment in which it will be implemented [19]. No one type of integration is considered better than the other. It is generally felt preferable to use multiple types of integration strategies in conjunction with one another [19].

10.3.2 Measures of Integrated Care

There is no global measure of integration or integrated care available to evaluate it. There are tools that measure components of integration within existing systems and it is recommended that a comprehensive approach assessing multiple dimensions, components and perspectives is taken in order to reflect the complexity of the intervention [20]. Unfortunately, these tools do not necessarily translate across health jurisdictions or contexts. Most measurement tools evaluate integration from the perspective of health service providers within systems that are already integrated, little assess integration from patient perspective [21, 22].

10.4 Integration Approaches in Cancer

It may perhaps come as a surprise that integrated care is not a term commonly used in the cancer literature. There has only been a single systematic review assessing the efficacy of integrated care interventions in cancer [23]. Of the 33 studies included, none were found to address all components of integrated care. Rather, the cancer literature is comprised of research investigating aspects of integrated care through integration interventions or exploration of phenomena relating to integration. This includes multidisciplinary care, coordinated care and shared care.

10.4.1 Multidisciplinary Care

Multidisciplinary team (MDT) care, often considered the foundation of contemporary cancer care, encompasses a multitude of integration strategies that facilitate access to evidence based, holistic care through inclusion of multiple disciplines of providers, such as inclusion of other health professionals [24–36], care pathways [37–39] and multidisciplinary clinics [40, 41]. MDT care is care delivered by a group of health professionals whose scope of practice covers all the relevant expertise required to meet an individual patient's care needs and considers all relevant treatment options [42]. The desired outcome of the MDT is the development and maintenance of a single collaborative treatment plan for an individual patient.

For the past two decades, MDT care has been considered a key approach to promote the consistent delivery of evidence-based cancer care internationally, including many areas of Europe, Australia, USA, Canada, UK and New Zealand [43]. It has been adopted as an underlying principle of national cancer management policies and cancer guidelines since the late 1990s [44]. It is argued that the policy shift to MDT as the preferred method of cancer care delivery was not driven by newly available empiric evidence, but rather by political and public pressures to improve access to evidence based cancer care and improved patient outcomes [43, 44]. The key driving force behind the introduction of MDT care, has not been the desire to improve integration of care or delivery of patient centered, holistic care but rather, recognition that for many cancers, effective anticancer treatment is delivered through multiple treatment modalities i.e. chemotherapy, radiation therapy, surgery, some of which need to be delivered concurrently. Appropriate treatment decision making and planning, needs to involve representatives of multiple cancer related professions, like surgery, medical and radiation oncology. Indeed, these professions remain at the core of the multidisciplinary team today. MDT have now become ingrained into standard cancer care, and while there continues to be an absence of randomized controlled trials, there is a growing body of evidence to demonstrate that MDT care in cancer improves guideline compliant follow up and timeliness of follow up, positively impacts therapy planning and implementation and improves pain control and adherence to oral medications [1].

In the USA, MDTs evolved from tumor boards (or cancer conferences), which were originally designed as a formalized method to engage multiple medical specialists (e.g. radiology, surgery, pathology, medical oncology) into the collective review of patient cases for the purposes of audit and education [45]. These boards developed into a proactive opportunity to plan treatment for newly diagnosed patients and discuss complex cases. Such a consultative approach allows for consensus opinion on treatment to be reached, but it does not necessarily utilize a team approach, with the physician who is presenting the case ultimately responsible for treatment decisions and their implementation although many MDTs use a team structure to facilitate collaborative treatment planning. The focus of MDT may not solely be cancer pathology, but may be inclusive of the patient's psychosocial needs. Patient involvement is considered essential to ensuring patient-centered care, although it is not widely adopted.

Delivering effective MDT care does not organically result from simply gathering a group of healthcare providers around a common patient. Effective teamwork requires structure, leadership and work by all team members. Features common to effective MDTs include existence of a shared vision, defined membership with clear roles and responsibilities of team members in line with their scope of practice, and establishing a communications framework including meetings and documentation standards [1].

As a result, the performance of a MDT, and ultimately patient outcomes, can be variable depending on the quality of how well these elements are delivered, as demonstrated in the UK analysis of more than 1000 multidisciplinary teams working across six cancer types [44]. MDT performance is influenced by team structure, team processes, and the context in which care is being delivered, including institutional, technical and environmental factors [45]. While it is expected that there would be wide ranging variation in context of care, considerable diversity in MDT structure and processes may also exist.

10.4.1.1 MDT Focus/Scope

The focus or scope of the MDT may vary both in terms of clinical focus and place in the cancer trajectory.

Clinically, the MDT may focus solely on the cancer pathology or, as is becoming increasingly common, it may also include other aspects of care like psychosocial care. In most cases, anything that is not considered directly related to the effects of cancer or its treatment sits outside the scope of the cancer MDT, such as the management of non-cancer conditions. While this approach may seem relatively straightforward, it can present challenges in practice, where it is not uncommon for chronic conditions to present during the diagnosis and treatment phase, potentially triggered by the cancer or its treatment. This has implications when determining which care team is responsible for meeting these needs. For example, it is known that corticosteroids, commonly used in the management of cancer, are associated with numerous short and long term effects, including an increased risk of osteoporosis. Does the fact that it may be cancer treatment-related make prevention, monitoring and management of osteoporosis the responsibility of the cancer MDT? If such clinical responsibilities are left unclarified, they may result in duplication (tests, workload) or unmet need.

Many cancer MDTs confine their operations to the diagnosis and treatment phase. This presents similar issues in determining the roles and responsibilities of care providers, as patients move into survivorship or end of life care. Specific clinical responsibilities that may remain unclear as a patient moves from treatment to survivorship include the management of late-stage effects of cancer or its treatment (e.g. fatigue, cognitive impairment), non-primary cancer surveillance in cancer survivors and management of ongoing psychosocial effects and rehabilitation needs.

10.4.1.2 MDT Composition and Size

The composition and size of the MDT is determined by the defined scope of the MDT and the needs of the patient. The size of the MDT should allow for enough health professionals to ensure the patient's needs are met [45]. As the focus of clinical care broadens from cancer pathology to more holistic care, so does the number of health professionals involved, expanding beyond medical disciplines to include nursing, allied health and pharmacy (Fig. 10.1). Clinical roles and responsibilities of team members are expected to be in line with their professional scope of practice, while administrative and communication responsibilities, such as documentation of MDT meetings may be allocated to specific MDT members.

Bigger is not always better for MDTs. Expanding MDT size and diversity brings challenges in team coordination and communication. According to Fennell and colleagues, team effectiveness is impaired when size exceeds 10 members, when membership is not constant across the treatment process and when not all members are relevant to a given discussion [45]. One approach to facilitating consistent membership is to structure the MDT according to disease type, with core membership comprising the minimum disciplines required to provide quality routine care [42]. Membership is extended for individual cases according to patient needs, to include health professional who care for the individual patient (e.g. GP) and referred specialist providers (e.g. physiotherapist for a patient with lymphedema). Membership is therefore dynamic, expanding or contracting as needs change throughout the care continuum. It should be noted that this distinction between core and non-core members is made from the perspective of the oncology clinicians in relation to developing team processes, it does not imply a hierarchy of care providers, nor does it reflect the patient perspective.

Cancer MDTs function within a practice philosophy of evidence based medicine. While this aids in establishing team norms amongst healthcare professionals, it cannot be assumed that the patient shares these values. A strong foundation of evidence based medicine is essential to a high functioning MDT, but may be a potential source of conflict for patients who access external care providers and seek treatment options that are not supported by evidence.

There is evidence that patient-centered treatment plans are more likely to be implemented, clinically appropriate and acceptable to patients [46]. Indeed, it is considered by many that the inclusion of the patient or their advocate in the MDT decision-making process (e.g. involvement in the MDT meeting) is essential to achieve effective MDT care [45]. Clinicians have been shown to be generally poor at judging patient preferences [47] and studies suggesting that patients who do not attend MDT meetings have a limited opportunity to input to or influence the decision-making process of the MDT [48]. However, most MDTs do not allow for patient's attendance at the meeting and indeed, not all patients want to be included in the MDT. A Canadian study demonstrated that while nearly all patients want to be informed and presented with treatment options, half prefer to leave the decision to their doctor [49]. Clinicians acknowledge the need to keep the patient informed, but have expressed concerns that the presence of a patient in the high paced, explicit and technical MDT discussion may negatively impact the efficiency of the meetings and be potentially alarming to patients [44, 48].

Inclusion of the patient in the MDT is not the only method of providing them with greater involvement in their care, but as it stands, the best method for accurately representing patient views and ensuring they are appropriately informed remains unclear [44, 46]. Other strategies that have been shown to positively impact patient satisfaction by supporting greater patient involvement in their care include interventions involving provision of information to patients, decision aids and providing an audiotape of the consultation [23].

10.4.1.3 Multidisciplinary Team Processes

Regular MDT meetings are the key mechanism to achieving joint decision making and communicating actions, along with clear identification of MDT members and presence of a communications framework. An open and inclusive discussion is required to achieve consensual decision making.

In order to ensure sufficient attendance and participation of core team members, the conduct of MDT meetings tend to be centered on the needs of specialist providers. They are usually held within hospital or specialist locations and include discussion of an agenda of patients under the care of the oncology team, with case conferences about individual patients convened as necessary. Multiple analyses have demonstrated that the decision making that occurs within cancer MDTs relating to newly diagnosed patients tend to be medically dominated, maintaining a narrow focus on cancer pathology [46, 50, 51].

Methods to enhance MDT processes have been explored in the literature, including the use of integrated care pathways. An integrated care pathway is "*a complex intervention for the mutual decision-making and organization of care processes for a well-defined group of patients during a well-defined period*" [52]. Evidence that suggests care pathways reduce variation in outcomes for high-risk cancer within and between countries [53]. Integrated care pathways and programs of care have been explored relating to specific cancer types including breast cancer

[54] and head and neck cancer [39]. Pathways and programs to support the management of specific supportive care needs have also been explored, including post-operative management [37], febrile neutropenia in pediatrics [38], end of life care [55], depression care [56, 57] and pain management [58].

10.4.1.4 MDT Approach to Multimorbidity and Cancer

Cancer MDTs are designed to suit the needs of patients for whom cancer is the single clinical focus of care. They are generally based on the premise that care needs can be met by specialist providers in a hospital or similar specialist setting for a discrete period of acute need, usually the treatment phase. These are not the circumstances encountered in the management of patients with cancer and a chronic condition.

Failure to consider aspects such as the impact of patient preferences and comorbidities on treatment options in addition to cancer pathology has been shown to adversely impact the quality of MDT clinical decision making [46]. Despite this, those clinicians with the most comprehensive knowledge of the patient and responsibility for coordinating the management of non-cancer conditions (i.e. GPs) are often not in attendance. What results is that many MDTs do not benefit from the input of the primary care provider at the point of decision making, instead functioning reactively. If it becomes apparent that a non-cancer condition is going to impact the agreed treatment plan a number of consequences may arise: the plan may be amended by an individual clinician outside of usual clinical governance; treatment could be delayed to allow further discussion at the next MDT meeting, or; if the problem is recognized after the treatment plan has been implemented it could result in the administration of inappropriate treatment [50].

An alternative model that is yet to receive much attention is the proactive undertaking of holistic needs assessments at defined times along the continuum of care, and incorporation of this information into MDT meeting discussions [48]. There has been exploration of this in the care of frail elders, where incorporating holistic geriatric assessment that provides knowledge extending beyond that obtained by standard oncology assessment has been shown to positively influence cancer treatment planning and decision making [59–62]. Whatever the solutions may be, they must address the existing limitations in MDT scope, membership and processes that currently stand in the way of meeting the needs of patients with cancer and chronic conditions.

10.4.2 Coordinated Care

Coordinated cancer care refers to the orderly way in which patients with cancer receive their cancer care where there exists a designated primary point of contact within the MDT (a care coordinator). Cancer care coordinators/case managers/patient navigators are health professionals (nurse or other) with the specific role of supporting the MDT, including the patient and GP, in order to improve continuity of care and facilitate a patient-centered approach. There is also some exploration of the role of lay patient navigators, someone who undertakes a patient support role to help patients navigate the complex health system throughout the cancer care continuum and reduce barriers to access [63].

Care coordinators have been shown to play a critical role in patient education and in linking patients with support services [64]. They have also been demonstrated to improve patient experience and achieve greater adherence to therapy through a randomized trial investigating the use of a navigator early in the care trajectory of patients with newly diagnosed breast, colorectal and lung cancers [65]. As with the cancer MDT, the focus of coordinated care in cancer is organizing the provision of all elements of comprehensive cancer care including diagnosis, treatment and supportive care, within the paradigm of evidence based medicine, usually limited to the diagnosis and treatment phase. Anything that is not considered directly related to the effects of cancer or its treatment are out of scope. This has obvious implications for patients managing a chronic condition throughout their cancer care, particularly if they experience worsening of their condition or newly presenting conditions.

Acute cancer treatment causes a disruption to the usual care for patients who are managing a chronic condition prior to diagnosis with cancer. Literature suggests that patients who usually self-manage their chronic condition can be expected to need greater support during times of acute illness [12] yet they are known to have reduced contact with their GP and other care providers during acute cancer treatment [66]. When a patient experiences worsening of an existing condition or is diagnosed with a new chronic condition during acute cancer treatment there is further potential for role confusion between providers. If management of the chronic conditions is considered to be within the scope of cancer care coordination the management of the chronic condition would be facilitated through direct care provided through the cancer MDT or specialist provider via MDT referral. By contrast, if the management of the chronic condition is considered outside the scope of cancer care coordination this would imply the patient should seek care through standard channels of care, usually care provided directly from the GP or specialist via GP referral. What often results is the patient or their caregiver informally taking on the role of overall care coordination, acting as the conduit to ensure information transfer between all care providers [66].

10.4.3 Shared Care

Shared care refers to a joint participation of primary care physicians and specialty care physicians and other health care providers in the planned delivery of care [67]. It is a structured process with the aims of improving the level of communication and relationship between the MDT, the patient (and/or advocate) and their GP, and fostering the environment necessary for collaboration in provision of cancer care. Shared care between specialist and GP is receiving growing recognition as an integration strategy that offers potential to benefit patients by improving the structured transitions of care and promoting continuity of care with the GP.

There is a growing body of evidence exploring shared care between the GP and cancer services in treatment [68] and survivorship care [69–71]. It has been shown to increase contacts with the GP and improve patient satisfaction, with no effect on quality of life [72], improve clarity over roles and responsibilities of care providers relating to cancer care and provide facilitate information sharing [73]. Literature shows that, with simple guidelines, primary care providers are able to provide care to cancer survivors that is equivalent to that given by cancer specialists [73]. There is some concern however that an unintended consequence of GP sub-specialization is that GPs may function more as specialists than as primary care providers, resulting in unmet needs relating to chronic condition management and preventive care [74].

Collaborative care plans have been investigated in the setting of shared care in the diagnosis and treatment phase [68] and survivorship care [75] (where they are referred to as survivorship care plans) although they are yet to be utilized as part of routine clinical care. They are designed to provide clear documentation of responsibilities and outcomes relating to cancer treatment, its potential consequences, and recommendations for follow up cancer screening and diagnostic tests [72]. They have been shown to provide clarity in roles and responsibilities of care providers and enhance transfer of information between specialist and primary care relating to cancer care [73]. Collaborative care plans however, generally focus on a single disease state and are not designed to cater for the needs of patients with multimorbidity [76]. It is therefore unlikely that care plans alone will provide clarity regarding roles and responsibilities of care providers in areas of clinical ambiguity, such as interpreting if a generalized symptom relates to a late effect of treatment, is a manifestation of chronic disease, or a consequence of polypharmacy (the use of multiple medications) or others.

10.4.4 Novel Integration Strategies

What is considered to be a novel strategy to improve integration depends on the healthcare context in which you are situated. Many of the clinical models of care reported in the literature are being implemented within the integrated delivery systems of the US. Key features of these systems include discrete patient populations (often defined by enrollment), alignment of financial models and shared information systems [77]. In regions that do not have these integrated delivery systems in place, like Australia and Europe, initiatives that promote integration through the transfer of information such (e.g. patient held electronic health record), or assist in identifying vulnerable patient groups (e.g. hospital avoidance programs [77]) are increasingly being utilized.

A number of integration strategies are designed to overcome some of the recognized shortfalls of existing models of cancer care. One area of focus is promotion of information exchange. This includes initiatives that aid information flow between care providers such as decision-support systems and patient information systems [78], and strategies that improve information transfer between patients and providers, such as the patient held health record [79]. Another focus has been the way in which patients receive their multidisciplinary care, such as multidisciplinary 'one-stop' clinics and shared medical appointments.

Multidisciplinary one-stop clinics are not new in cancer where they have been utilized within specific clinical settings such as breast and prostate cancer. However, there has been little exploration of how they may potentially benefit patients with chronic conditions and cancer. One-stop clinics involve an individual patient consulting multiple care providers either as a single appointment or sequentially within a single clinic session. Evidence suggests that they reduce negative subjective health outcomes (anxiety and depression) [39], improve symptom control and patient satisfaction [80], improved practice patterns [40], improve quality of care, patient satisfaction and patient retention [41].

Shared medical appointments (SMAs) have been utilized in the USA, primarily in non-cancer chronic conditions, since the late 1990s. They are increasingly gaining recognition in other regions, such as Europe and Australia, as a potential model of care. An SMA is a medical consultation that is shared by a group of patients in a confidential setting. The consultation is generally led by a medical clinician or advanced practice nurse, with other disciplines included depending on the intent [81]. For example, a shared consultation for patients with steroid induced diabetes may include a dietician and pharmacist. In the general chronic condition setting, SMAs have been demonstrated to not only improve the availability of peer-education and support, but also improve access to specialist and multidisciplinary care, enhance therapeutic relationships, reduce waiting lists and promote self-management and psychosocial care [81]. There has been little exploration of SMAs within cancer. A Dutch study demonstrated that SMAs were a feasible method of enhancing breast cancer survivorship care, but did not find the same positive impact on psychosocial care, potentially increasing fear in some patients [82]. SMAs appear to be a promising model of care worthy of exploration in cancer, but further research is required to establish their cost-effectiveness and to determine the optimal criteria (e.g. professions involves, number of patients) [83].

It can be argued that within the context of general multimorbidity, clinical management needs to move away from clinical guidelines based upon individual disease states, and needs to transition towards models that incorporate clinical judgment and patient priorities into goal-oriented care that addresses overall health [8, 76, 84]. Reuben and Tinetti argue that an approach that aligns treatment goals across conditions enables patients to actively participate in identifying and achieving outcomes that improve overall health and prompts clinicians to have the difficult conversations with patients that are necessary when the desired goals are not attainable [84]. Such an approach is particularly relevant in the context of advanced or terminal cancer, and in caring for frail elders.

As it stands there is limited exploration of novel approaches to improve the interface of primary and specialist cancer care. What evidence does exist is primarily practice based reports, with few robust clinical trials [23, 56, 57, 85]. There is a need for investigation of initiatives that creatively utilize all aspects of the healthcare workforce, along with rigorous evaluation.

10.5 Integration Approaches and Multimorbidity

While patients with multimorbidity are expected to gain the most from integration initiatives, most evidence focuses on single disease states. There is limited empirical evidence investigating integrated care models of care, with little to guide models of care in the context of multimorbidity [86, 87].

There have been two published meta-analyses of systematic reviews exploring the literature regarding integrated care strategies applied within the context of general multimorbidity. Each review demonstrated that integrated care programs positively impact patient outcomes in chronic conditions [88, 89]. More recently, Mitchell and colleagues published a systematic review of integrated models of care delivered at the primary-secondary interface of care to improve outcomes for patients with chronic conditions. Their analysis of ten studies supported the findings of the meta-analyses, demonstrating that integrated care initiatives have a modest impact on clinical outcomes, substantial impact on process outcomes and mixed cost data in the context of general multimorbidity [90].

While these reviews were not specific to cancer populations, it has been shown that the principles relating to what make integrated care strategies successful transcend healthcare context and clinical setting [91]. Thus, the findings may not be immediately translatable to the oncology setting, but in an area where evidence is sparse, they do offer some valuable insight into what may work in a setting of multimorbidity.

10.6 Barriers to Achieving Integration for Cancer and Chronic Conditions

There are multiple barriers to overcoming the fragmentations of care encountered in the care of patients managing cancer and chronic conditions. Perhaps the most fundamental barrier relates to the limited evidence promoting awareness and understanding of the problem itself. Further to this, there is an absence of shared understanding across the health system of the strategies available to address recognized fragmentations in care (i.e. integrated care) presenting difficulties in developing effective collaborative solutions. Lack of system integration demonstrated by rigid funding models and absence of shared information systems present challenges when trying to implement integration initiatives in practice. Finally, effective collaboration and teamwork form the basis of all integration strategies; achieving this in practice is not necessarily an easy task.

The logical starting point for any integration initiative is establishing a shared understanding of the problem in order to design a solution to overcome it. With so little evidence available regarding the management of patients with chronic conditions and cancer, it cannot be assumed that the problem is recognized nor understood. Recognition of the issues across both primary and specialist care is a critical barrier to achieving integration at a system level. Similarly, there is no shared understanding across the health system of what integrated care entails and therefore no validated measures for assessing or benchmarking services. The lack of shared terminology has the potential to create challenges when attempting to put policy into practice, from intervention design through to implementation. Differing semantic understanding of integration may impede stakeholder buy in and collaboration. For example, 'integrated care' may be understood by a policy maker to result in a system that combines governance, administrative and financial structures, but by clinicians as a system that streamlines clinical processes and multidisciplinary teamwork. Inability to consistently measure integration initiatives may result in missed opportunities to identify variations in practice that could be addressed by specific interventions [78].

Another significant challenge to implementing integration strategies that cross the boundary of specialist and primary care is the way in which most health systems are designed. Different sectors and institutions often have separate IT infrastructure and funding models that prevent collaboration. For example, many community-based health services are designed to be accessed through primary care. For example, in Australia if a patient with cancer needs to access a publicly funded community based psychologist they cannot be referred by the cancer MDT under their cancer management plan. Rather, they must be referred by their GP under a GP Mental Health Treatment Plan, or by a psychiatrist under an appropriate assessment and management plan [92]. Thus any attempts to integrate care using these services can only occur through primary care and not acute cancer sector. Such barriers relating to system integration may be difficult to change at a grass roots level, potentially resulting in duplication of services or work around solutions.

Perhaps the most commonly encountered barrier to successful implementation of an integration initiative are the individual agents themselves (healthcare providers, managers, policy makers), regardless of clinical context or care setting. In an environment rich in professional tribalism, it can be difficult to establish normative integration. Similarly, convincing clinicians to participate in the collaborative approach necessary to put policy into practice, can present significant challenges [93]. Integration initiatives are fundamentally reliant on team collaboration. This brings with it a multitude of barriers including confusion or lack of role clarity, professional self-interest, competing ideologies and values, lack of mutual trust and conflicting views about client interests and role [91].

10.7 Overcoming the Barriers to Integration

Many of the systemic barriers to integration may not be able to be influenced at a grass roots level. It is possible however, to increase awareness and understanding of the problem, and to arm primary and specialist care providers with the knowledge and skills required to develop and implement clinically relevant solutions. Research that improves our understanding of the issues encountered in the management of cancer and chronic conditions is essential to achieving recognition of the problem across policy makers, managers, care providers and patients. Research that strengthens the knowledge base relating to integrated care is also needed to establish the shared taxonomy and conceptual application required to develop valid measures that enable benchmarking of services.

In order to effect change that results in improved patient care, research must be coupled with broad ranging education of patients and care providers. While it is not known what the most effective type of education intervention is, it has been suggested that education initiatives should be based on a shared curricula that span primary healthcare and oncology, and are inclusive of the full range of health professionals [78]. Ideally such education would be informed by a robust evidence base. In absence of this, education that demonstrates the conceptual basis of integrated care should be encouraged across professional groups and settings to ensure that effective collaboration is not blocked by divergent semantic meanings.

It is thought that a 'bottom up' rather than 'top down' approach to integration should be encouraged [94], with policymakers articulating the vision (and budget), and clinicians creating the workable solution. Ideally, the development of 'bottom up' clinical or service integration strategies occurs within well designed policy that supports them by ensuring the information systems, governance structures and financial management is in place. In reality, this may not be the case and it may not possible to overcome these system barriers for an individual project. In order to minimize the development of tedious mechanisms to work around systemic obstacles, it is recommended to develop strategies that target specific segments of the patient population, identified through population segmentation and risk stratification [19]. The idea being that clinicians are more willing to go to the effort to overcome systemic obstacles if they recognize it is meeting a need for a patient that would otherwise go unrealized.

Establishing normative integration is complex and presents one of the most challenging barriers to overcome. Teamwork can be facilitated by establishing explicit goals, establishing roles and managing interdependent work [95]. Building effective teams requires team members to have the appropriate knowledge and skills to participate in teamwork and may require specific training [95]. Methods that standardize the teams approach to care, such as guidelines and protocols have been found to be common elements of successful integrations initiatives [90]. Another recognized feature is the presence of organizational and cultural leadership [91].

Box 1: Recommendations to overcome the barriers to integration to improve the care for people with cancer and chronic conditions
Overcoming the barriers to integration requires:

- Research base that supports a shared understanding of the problem of multimorbidity and available solutions
- A framework of shared understanding
  - Clarity of definitions and language
  - Promotion a culture of integrated approach to care
- A policy environment that supports integration
  - Improved integration of systems (information systems, governance structures, financial management and incentives)
  - Encouragement of 'bottom up' approaches to integration
  - Availability of data to facilitate the identification of target groups through population segmentation, risk stratification and measurement of outcomes
- A practice environment that supports effective teamwork
  - Organizational and cultural leadership
  - Methods that standardize the teams approach to care
  - Clarified expectations within teams (goals, roles and responsibilities, interdependent work)
- Care providers that possess the appropriate knowledge and skills
  - Broad ranging education that spans primary healthcare and oncology, and includes the full range of health professionals
  - Education on the issues encountered in the management of cancer and chronic conditions
  - Education on the conceptual basis of integrated care, skills training regarding development and implementation of integration strategies
  - Education on the features of effective teamwork, teamwork skills training.

10.8 Recommendations for Research and Practice

There is a need for research to address the gaps in knowledge relating to our understanding of the fragmentations of care encountered in the management of patients with chronic conditions and cancer, particularly at the interface of primary and specialist care [66, 73, 90, 96]. Within the cancer literature, the examination of this interface appears to focus on the engagement of primary care providers to undertake specialist aspects of cancer care. There has been less exploration of the role of primary care providers in enhancing cancer care through their holistic knowledge of the patient, and how the healthcare delivery system, available decision support and clinical information systems may facilitate or impede this. There are indications that cancer diagnosis and treatment causes disruptions in the continuity of care with primary care providers and suggestions that this may result in a shift in focus of care away from chronic condition management and prevention activities, yet there has been little exploration of why this occurs and how it can be avoided. While it is generally accepted that fragmentations of care should be expected in the management of patients with chronic conditions and cancer, there is little research providing insight into what they are or why they occur.

Well-designed research is also required to provide the empirical evidence to support the integration initiatives that have been implemented in the oncology setting (multidisciplinary teams, coordinated care and shared care) in addition to novel models of care and strategies that promote patient involvement in their care.

Research that improves our understanding of effective approaches for involving patients in their care may be of particular relevance for patients who are managing a chronic condition as well as cancer, where self-management is considered a critical element of care [97]. Little is known about the impact of cancer on a person's capacity for self-management beyond broad indications that there is an adverse impact on medication adherence [16, 17]. Patients who are diagnosed with a chronic condition during the acute treatment phase may require additional self-management support [10]. Little is known about the self-management support patients receive when diagnosed with a chronic condition during the acute treatment phase. Similarly, little is known about the perceptions and understanding of cancer clinicians relating to self-management support, including awareness of community based chronic disease programs and services.

While there may not be evidence to provide in depth understanding of the fragmentations of care encountered in the management of patients with chronic conditions and cancer, it is likely that clinicians have an understanding of specific issues of concern within their practice. By developing an understanding of integrated care, clinicians can work toward developing collaborative solutions that affect change for their patient population. Importantly, the outcome of these strategies should be measured using approaches that allow flexibility and further improvements, such as Kolb's experiential learning model or the plan-do-study-act cycle of quality improvement [98]. Sharing the outcomes of these initiatives through publication is both a valuable contribution to the knowledge base, and important source of inspiration for colleagues in other practice settings.

10.9 Conclusions

In order to make improvements in the quality of care for patients with cancer and chronic conditions we must increase awareness and understanding of the fragmentations encountered across primary and secondary care. Research must flow in both directions. That is, to consider both how primary care providers can be utilized to enhance cancer care *and* how cancer clinicians can promote continuity of primary care throughout the cancer care continuum.

In addition to improving our understanding of the problems, we must also take steps to arm primary and specialist care providers with the knowledge and skills required to work collaboratively to develop and implement clinically relevant solutions. Integrated care offers the conceptual foundation and theoretical framework upon which this collaboration can be based.

References

1. Taplin SH, Weaver S, Salas E, Chollette V, Edwards HM, Bruinooge SS, Kosty MP (2015) Reviewing cancer care team effectiveness. J Oncol Pract Am Soc Clin Oncol 11(3):239–246. doi:10.1200/JOP.2014.003350
2. Levit L, Balogh E, Nass S, Ganz PA (eds) (2013). Delivering high-quality cancer care: charting a new course for a system in crisis. National Academies Press, Washington (DC). doi: 10.17226/18359
3. Britt HC, Harrison CM, Miller GC, Knox SA (2008) Prevalence and patterns of multimorbidity in Australia. Med J Aust 189(2):72–77
4. Plsek PE, Wilson T (2001) Complexity, leadership, and management in healthcare organisations. BMJ 323(7315):746–749
5. Burt RS (2004) Structural holes and good ideas. Am J Sociol 110(2):349–399
6. Braithwaite J (2010) Between-group behaviour in health care: gaps, edges, boundaries, disconnections, weak ties, spaces and holes. A systematic review. BMC Health Serv Res 10:330. doi:10.1186/1472-6963-10-330
7. Stange KC (2009) The problem of fragmentation and the need for integrative solutions. Ann Fam Med 7(2):100–103. doi:10.1370/afm.971
8. Roland M, Paddison C (2013) Better management of patients with multimorbidity. BMJ 346: f2510. doi:10.1136/bmj.f2510
9. Tarrant C, Windridge K, Baker R, Freeman G, Boulton M (2015) 'Falling through gaps': primary care patients' accounts of breakdowns in experienced continuity of care. Fam Pract 32(1):82–87. doi:10.1093/fampra/cmu077
10. Haggerty JL (2012) Ordering the chaos for patients with multimorbidity. BMJ 345:e5915. doi:10.1136/bmj.e5915
11. Kodner D (2009) All together now: a conceptual exploration of integrated care. Healthc Q 13 (Special Issue):S6–S15

12. Haggerty JL, Roberge D, Freeman GK, Beaulieu C (2013) Experienced continuity of care when patients see multiple clinicians: a qualitative metasummary. Ann Fam Med 11(3):262–271. doi:10.1370/afm.1499
13. Strand L, Cipolle R, Morley P (2012) Pharmaceutical care practice: the patient-centred approach to medication management services. McGraw-Hill Medical, USA
14. Roughead EE, Semple SJ (2009) Medication safety in acute care in Australia: where are we now? Part 1: a review of the extent and causes of medication problems 2002–2008. Aust NZ Health Policy 6(6):18. doi:10.1186/1743-8462-6-18
15. Roughead EE, Vitry AI, Caughey GE, Gilbert AL (2011) Multimorbidity, care complexity and prescribing for the elderly. Aging Health 7(5):695–705
16. Calip GS, Boudreau DM, Loggers ET (2013) Changes in adherence to statins and subsequent lipid profiles during and following breast cancer treatment. Breast Cancer Res Treat 138 (1):225–233. doi:10.1007/s10549-013-2424-2
17. Calip GS, Hubbard RA, Stergachis A, Malone KE, Gralow JR, Boudreau DM (2015) Adherence to oral diabetes medications and glycemic control during and following breast cancer treatment. Pharmacoepidemiol Drug Saf 24(1):75–85. doi:10.1002/pds.3660
18. Taplin SH, Rodgers AB (2010) Toward improving the quality of cancer care: addressing the interfaces of primary and oncology-related subspecialty care. JNCI Monogr 40:3–10. doi:10.1093/jncimonographs/lgq006
19. Shaw S, Rosen R, Rumbold B (2011) What is integrated care? An overview of integrated care in the NHS. Nuffield Trust, UK
20. Lynsgo AM, Godtfredsen NS, Host D, Frolich A (2014) Instruments to assess integrated care: a systematic review. Int J Integr Care, vol 14
21. Strandberg-Larsen M, Krasnik A (2009) Measurement of integrated healthcare delivery: a systematic review of methods and future research directions. Int J Integr Care 9:e01
22. Singer SJ, Friedberg MW, Kiang MV, Dunn T, Kuhn DM (2013) Development and preliminary validation of the patient perceptions of integrated care survey. Med Care Res Rev MCRR 70(2):143–164. doi:10.1177/1077558712465654
23. Ouwens M, Hulscher M, Hermens R, Faber M, Marres H, Wollersheim H, Grol R (2009) Implementation of integrated care for patients with cancer: a systematic review of interventions and effects. Int J Qual Health Care J Int Soc Qual Health Care ISQua 21 (2):137–144. doi:10.1093/intqhc/mzn061
24. Delaney L, Chambers C, Roldan G, De Robles P, Cairncross G, Forsyth P, Easaw J (2009) A feasibility study to assess the integration of a pharmacist into neurooncology clinic. J Oncol Pharm Pract 15(2):79–85. doi:10.1177/1078155208099281
25. Judge Santacroce S, Asmus K, Kadan-Lottick N, Grey M (2010) Feasibility and preliminary outcomes from a pilot study of coping skills training for adolescent–young adult survivors of childhood cancer and their parents. J Pediatr Oncol Nurs Off J Assoc Pediat Oncol Nurs 27 (1):10–20. doi:10.1177/1043454209340325
26. Pugliese P, Perrone M, Nisi E, Garufi C, Giannarelli D, Bottomley A, Terzoli E (2006) An integrated psychological strategy for advanced colorectal cancer patients. Health Qual Life Outcomes 4:9. doi:10.1186/1477-7525-4-9
27. Sharpe M, Walker J, Holm Hansen C, Martin P, Symeonides S, Gourley C, Wall L, Weller D, Murray G, Team SMO (2014) Integrated collaborative care for comorbid major depression in patients with cancer (SMaRT Oncology-2): a multicentre randomised controlled effectiveness trial. Lancet 384(9948):1099–1108. doi:10.1016/S0140-6736(14)61231-9
28. Walker J, Hansen CH, Martin P, Symeonides S, Gourley C, Wall L, Weller D, Murray G, Sharpe M, Team SMO (2014) Integrated collaborative care for major depression comorbid with a poor prognosis cancer (SMaRT Oncology-3): a multicentre randomised controlled trial in patients with lung cancer. Lancet Oncol 15(10):1168–1176. doi:10.1016/S1470-2045(14)70343-2
29. Walker S, Walker J, Richardson G, Palmer S, Wu Q, Gilbody S, Martin P, Hansen CH, Sawhney A, Murray G, Sculpher M, Sharpe M (2014) Cost-effectiveness of combining

systematic identification and treatment of co-morbid major depression for people with chronic diseases: the example of cancer. Psychol Med 44(7):1451–1460. doi:10.1017/S0033291713002079

30. Ben-Arye E, Schiff E, Raz OG, Samuels N, Lavie O (2014) Integrating a complementary medicine consultation for women undergoing chemotherapy. Int J Gynecol Obstet 124 (1):51–54. doi:10.1016/j.ijgo.2013.07.019
31. Ben-Arye E, Schiff E, Shapira C, Frenkel M, Shalom T, Steiner M (2012) Modeling an integrative oncology program within a community-centered oncology service in Israel. Patient Educ Couns 89(3):423–429. doi:10.1016/j.pec.2012.02.011
32. Brazier A, Cooke K, Moravan V (2008) Using mixed methods for evaluating an integrative approach to cancer care: a case study. Integ Cancer Ther 7(1):5–17. doi:10.1177/1534735407313395
33. Gage H, Storey L, McDowell C, Maguire G, Williams P, Faithfull S, Thomas H, Poole K (2009) Integrated care: utilisation of complementary and alternative medicine within a conventional cancer treatment centre. Complement Ther Med 17(2):84–91. doi:10.1016/j.ctim.2008.09.001
34. Kligler B, Homel P, Harrison LB, Levenson HD, Kenney JB, Merrell W (2011) Cost savings in inpatient oncology through an integrative medicine approach. Am J Manag Care 17 (12):779–784
35. Popper-Giveon A, Schiff E, Ben-Arye E (2013) We and they in the house of healing: debate among Arab complementary medicine practitioners on an integrative versus alternative approach to supportive cancer care. Integ Cancer Ther 12(6):488–495. doi:10.1177/1534735413485818
36. Popper-Giveon A, Schiff E, Hatem D, Samuels N, Ben-Arye E (2014) One hand cannot clap-a study of Arab practitioners of traditional and complementary medicine in Israel: identifying barriers to integrative oncology care. Explore (NY) 10(6):364–371. doi:10.1016/j.explore.2014.08.004
37. Letton C, Cheung C, Nordin A (2013) Does an enhanced recovery integrated care pathway (ICP) encourage adherence to prescribing guidelines, accelerate postoperative recovery and reduce the length of stay for gynaecological oncology patients? J Obstet Gynaecol J Inst Obstet Gynaecol 33(3):296–297. doi:10.3109/01443615.2012.758693
38. Selwood K (2000) Integrated care pathways: an audit tool in paediatric oncology. Br J Nurs 9 (1):34–38. doi:10.12968/bjon.2000.9.1.6410
39. Ouwens MM, Hermens RR, Hulscher MM, Merkx MA, van den Hoogen FJ, Grol RP, Wollersheim HC, Marres HA (2009) Impact of an integrated care program for patients with head and neck cancer on the quality of care. Head Neck 31(7):902–910. doi:10.1002/hed.21041
40. Bekelman JE, Suneja G, Guzzo T, Pollack CE, Armstrong K, Epstein AJ (2013) Effect of practice integration between urologists and radiation oncologists on prostate cancer treatment patterns. J Urol 190(1):97–101. doi:10.1016/j.juro.2013.01.103
41. Bjegovich-Weidman M, Haid M, Kumar S, Huibregtse C, McDonald J, Krishnan S (2010) Establishing a community-based lung cancer multidisciplinary clinic as part of a large integrated health care system: Aurora Health Care. J Oncol Pract 6(6):e27–e30. doi:10.1200/JOP.2010.000022
42. Cancer Australia (2016) All about multidisciplinary care. https://canceraustralia.gov.au/clinical-best-practice/multidisciplinary-care/all-about-multidisciplinary-care. Accessed on 13 Jan 2015
43. Patkar V, Acosta D, Davidson T, Jones A, Fox J, Keshtgar M (2011) Cancer multidisciplinary team meetings: evidence, challenges, and the role of clinical decision support technology. Int J Breast Cancer 2011:831605. doi:10.4061/2011/831605
44. Taylor C, Munro AJ, Glynne-Jones R, Griffith C, Trevatt P, Richards M, Ramirez AJ (2010) Multidisciplinary team working in cancer: what is the evidence? BMJ, vol 340

45. Fennell ML, Das IP, Clauser S, Petrelli N, Salner A (2010) (2010) The organization of multidisciplinary care teams: modeling internal and external influences on cancer care quality. J Natl Cancer Inst Monogr 40:72–80. doi:10.1093/jncimonographs/lgq010
46. Lamb BW, Taylor C, Lamb JN, Strickland SL, Vincent C, Green JS, Sevdalis N (2013) Facilitators and barriers to teamworking and patient centeredness in multidisciplinary cancer teams: findings of a national study. Ann Surg Oncol 20(5):1408–1416. doi:10.1245/s10434-012-2676-9
47. Mulley A, Trimble C, Elwyn G (2012) Patients' preferences matter. Stop the silent misdiagnosis. The King's Fund, London
48. Taylor C, Finnegan-John J, Green JSA (2014) "No decision about me without me" in the context of cancer multidisciplinary team meetings: a qualitative interview study. BMC Health Serv Res, vol 14
49. Levinson W, Kao A, Kuby A, Thisted RA (2005) Not all patients want to participate in decision making. a national study of public preferences. J Geriatr Intern Med 20:531–535. doi:10.1111/j.1525-1497.2005.0088.x
50. Bridges J, Hughes J, Farrington N, Richardson A (2015) Cancer treatment decision-making processes for older patients with complex needs: a qualitative study. BMJ Open 5(12): e009674. doi:10.1136/bmjopen-2015-009674
51. Hahlweg P, Hoffmann J, Harter M, Frosch DL, Elwyn G, Scholl I (2015) In absentia: an exploratory study of how patients are considered in multidisciplinary cancer team meetings. PLoS ONE 10(10):e0139921. doi:10.1371/journal.pone.0139921
52. Schrijvers G, van Hoorn A, Huiskes N (2012) The care pathway: concepts and theories: an introduction. Int J Integr, Care 12
53. Ellis PG (2013) Development and implementation of oncology care pathways in an integrated care network: the via oncology pathways experience. J Oncol Pract Am Soc Clin Oncol 9(3):171–173. doi:10.1200/JOP.2013.001020
54. Van Hoeve J, de Munck L, Otter R, de Vries J, Siesling S (2014) Quality improvement by implementing an integrated oncological care pathway for breast cancer patients. Breast 23 (4):364–370. doi:10.1016/j.breast.2014.01.008
55. Karthaus M, Weber U, Riesle-Keil J (2013) The implementation of an end-of-life integrated care pathway in cancer patients. Onkologie 36:6. doi:10.1159/000190043
56. Sharpe M (2014) Integrated collaborative care for major depression comorbid with a poor prognosis cancer (SMaRT Oncology-3): a multicentre randomised controlled trial in patients with lung cancer. Lancet Oncol 15(10):1168–1176. doi:10.1016/S1470-2045%2814%2970343-2
57. Walker J, Hansen CH, Martin P, Symeonides S, Gourley C, Wall L, Weller D, Murray G, Sharpe M (2014) Integrated collaborative care for major depression comorbid with a poor prognosis cancer (SMaRT Oncology-3): a multicentre randomised controlled trial in patients with lung cancer. Lancet Oncol 15(10):1168–1176. doi:10.1016/S1470-2045(14)70343-2
58. Cringles MC (2002) Developing an integrated care pathway to manage cancer pain across primary, secondary and tertiary care. Int J Palliat Nurs 8(5):247–255
59. Terret C, Zulian GB, Naiem A, Albrand G (2007) Multidisciplinary approach to the geriatric oncology patient. J Clin Oncol Off J Am Soc Clin Oncol 25(14):1876–1881. doi:10.1200/JCO.2006.10.3291
60. Caillet P, Canoui-Poitrine F, Vouriot J, Berle M, Reinald N, Krypciak S, Bastuji-Garin S, Culine S, Paillaud E (2011) Comprehensive geriatric assessment in the decision-making process in elderly patients with cancer: ELCAPA study. J Clin Oncol Off J Am Soc Clin Oncol 29(27):3636–3642. doi:10.1200/JCO.2010.31.0664
61. Wildiers H, Heeren P, Puts M, Topinkova E, Janssen-Heijnen ML, Extermann M, Falandry C, Artz A, Brain E, Colloca G, Flamaing J, Karnakis T, Kenis C, Audisio RA, Mohile S, Repetto L, Van Leeuwen B, Milisen K, Hurria A (2014) International society of geriatric oncology consensus on geriatric assessment in older patients with cancer. J Clin Oncol Off J Am Soc Clin Oncol 32(24):2595–2603. doi:10.1200/JCO.2013.54.8347

62. Tremblay D, Charlebois K, Terret C, Joannette S, Latreille J (2012) Integrated oncogeriatric approach: a systematic review of the literature using concept analysis. BMJ Open 2(6): e001483. doi:10.1136/bmjopen-2012-001483
63. Wells KJ, Battaglia TA, Dudley DJ, Garcia R, Greene A, Calhoun E, Mandelblatt JS, Paskett ED, Raich PC, Patient Navigation Research P (2008) Patient navigation: state of the art or is it science? Cancer 113(8):1999–2010. doi:10.1002/cncr.23815
64. NSW Cancer Institute (2011) Evaluation of the role of cancer care coordinator. Cancer Institute NSW, Australia
65. Wagner EH, Ludman EJ, Aiello Bowles EJ, Penfold R, Reid RJ, Rutter CM, Chubak J, McCorkle R (2014) Nurse navigators in early cancer care: a randomized, controlled trial. J Clin Oncol Off J Am Soc Clin Oncol 32(1):12–18. doi:10.1200/JCO.2013.51.7359
66. Sussman J, Baldwin LM (2010) The interface of primary and oncology specialty care: from diagnosis through primary treatment. J Natl Cancer Inst Monogr 40:18–24. doi:10.1093/jncimonographs/lgq007
67. Hickman M, Drummond N, Grimshaw J (1994) A taxonomy of shared care for chronic disease. J Pub Health 16(4):447–454
68. Johnson CE, Saunders CM, Phillips M, Emery JD, Nowak AK, Overheu K, Ward AM, Joske DJ (2015) Randomized controlled trial of shared care for patients with cancer involving general practitioners and cancer specialists. J Oncol Pract Am Soc Clin Oncol. doi:10.1200/JOP.2014.001569
69. Emery J, Doorey J, Jefford M, King M, Pirotta M, Hayne D, Martin A, Trevena L, Lim T, Constable R, Hawks C, Hyatt A, Hamid A, Violet J, Gill S, Frydenberg M, Schofield P (2014) Protocol for the ProCare Trial: a phase II randomised controlled trial of shared care for follow-up of men with prostate cancer. BMJ Open 4(3):e004972. doi:10.1136/bmjopen-2014-004972
70. Emery J (2014) Cancer survivorship—the role of the GP. MJA 43(8):521
71. Murchie P, Hannaford PC, Wyke S, Nicolson MC, Campbell NC (2007) Designing an integrated follow-up programme for people treated for cutaneous malignant melanoma: a practical application of the MRC framework for the design and evaluation of complex interventions to improve health. Fam Pract 24(3):283–292. doi:10.1093/fampra/cmm006
72. Medicine CoCSIo (2005) From cancer patient to cancer survivor: lost in transition. National Acadamies Press
73. Grunfeld E, Earle CC (2010) The interface between primary and oncology specialty care: treatment through survivorship. J Natl Cancer Inst Monogr 40:25–30. doi:10.1093/jncimonographs/lgq002
74. Starfield B, Gervas J (2007) Comprehensiveness v special interests. Family medicine should encourage its clinicians to specializa: negative. In: Kennealy T, Buetow S (eds) Idealogical debates in family medicine. Nova Publishing, New York
75. Howell P, Kinnane N, Whitfield K (2014) Supporting cancer survivors in Victoria: summary report. Department of Health, State Government of Victoria, Melbourne
76. Guthrie B, Payne K, Alderson P, McMurdo ME, Mercer SW (2012) Adapting clinical guidelines to take account of multimorbidity. BMJ 345:e6341. doi:10.1136/bmj.e6341
77. Nolte E, McKee M (2008) Caring for people with chronic conditions. A health system perspective. Open University Press, England
78. Rubin G, Berendsen A, Crawford SM, Dommett R, Earle C, Emery J, Fahey T, Grassi L, Grunfeld E, Gupta S, Hamilton W, Hiom S, Hunter D, Lyratzopoulos G, Macleod U, Mason R, Mitchell G, Neal RD, Peake M, Roland M, Seifert B, Sisler J, Sussman J, Taplin S, Vedsted P, Voruganti T, Walter F, Wardle J, Watson E, Weller D, Wender R, Whelan J, Whitlock J, Wilkinson C, de Wit N, Zimmermann C (2015) The expanding role of primary care in cancer control. Lancet Oncol 16(12):1231–1272. doi:10.1016/s1470-2045(15)00205-3
79. Gysels M, Richardson A, Higginson IJ (2007) Does the patient-held record improve continuity and related outcomes in cancer care: a systematic review. Health Expect Int J Pub Participation Health Care Health Policy 10(1):75–91. doi:10.1111/j.1369-7625.2006.00415.x

80. Bruera E, Michaud M, Vigano A, Neumann CM, Watanabe S, Hanson J (2001) Multidisciplinary symptom control clinic in a cancer center: a retrospective study. Support Care Cancer 9(3):162–168
81. Egger G, Binns A, Cole M, Ewald D, Daview L, Meldrum H, Stevens J, Noffsinger E (2014) Shared medical appointments: an adjunct for chronic disease management in Australia? Aust Fam Physician 43(3):151
82. Visser A, van Laarhoven HW, Govaert PH, Schlooz MS, Jansen L, van Dalen T, Prins JB (2015) Group medical consultations in the follow-up of breast cancer: a randomized feasibility study. J Cancer Surviv Res Pract 9(3):450–461. doi:10.1007/s11764-014-0421-z
83. Reed SC, Partridge AH, Nekhlyudov L (2014) Shared medical appointments in cancer survivorship care: a review of the literature. J Oncol Pract Am Soc Clin Oncol 11(1). doi:10.1200/JOP.2014.001411
84. Reuban DB, Tinetti ME (2012) Goal-oriented patient care—an alternative health outcomes paradigm. NEJM 366(9):777–779
85. Sharpe M, Walker J, Holm Hansen C, Martin P, Symeonides S, Gourley C, Wall L, Weller D, Murray G (2014) Integrated collaborative care for comorbid major depression in patients with cancer (SMaRT Oncology-2): a multicentre randomised controlled effectiveness trial. Lancet 384(9948):1099–1108. doi:10.1016/S0140-6736(14)61231-9
86. Marengoni A, Angleman S, Melis R, Mangialasche F, Karp A, Garmen A, Meinow B, Fratiglioni L (2011) Aging with multimorbidity: a systematic review of the literature. Ageing Res Rev 10(4):430–439. doi:10.1016/j.arr.2011.03.003
87. Smith SM, Soubhi H, Fortin M, Hudon C, O'Dowd T (2012) Managing patients with multimorbidity: systematic review of interventions in primary care and community settings. BMJ 345:e5205. doi:10.1136/bmj.e5205
88. Ouwens M, Wollersheim H, Hermens R, Hulscher M, Grol R (2005) Integrated care programmes for chronically ill patients: a review of systematic reviews. Int J for Qual Health Care 17(2):141–146
89. Martinez-Gonzalez NA, Berchtold P, Ullman K, Busato A, Egger M (2014) Integrated care programmes for adults with chronic conditions: a meta review. Int J for Qual Health Care 26 (5):561–570
90. Mitchell GK, Burridge L, Zhang J, Donald M, Scott IA, Dart J, Jackson CL (2015) Systematic review of integrated models of health care delivered at the primary? Secondary interface: how effective is it and what determines effectiveness? Aust J Prim Health. doi:10.1071/PY14172
91. Suter E, Oelke ND, Adair CE, Armitage GD (2009) Ten key priniples for suessful health systems integration. Healthcare Quart 13:16–23 (Toronto, Ont)
92. Department of Health (2015) Better access to psychiatrists, psychologists and general practitioners through the MBS (better access) initiatives. Commonwealth of Australia. http://www.health.gov.au/internet/main/publishing.nsf/Content/mental-ba. Accessed on 3 Mar 2016
93. Ahgren B, Axelsson SB, Axelsson R (2009) Evaluating intersectoral collaboration: a model for assessment by service users. Int J Integr Care 9:e03
94. Ahgren B (2003) Chain of care development in Sweden: results of a national study. Int J Integr Care 3(7)
95. Taplin SH, Weaver S, Chollette V, Marks LB, Jacobs A, Schiff G, Stricker CT, Bruinooge SS, Salas E (2015) Teams and teamwork during a cancer diagnosis: interdependency within and between teams. J Oncol Pract Am Soc Clin Oncol 11(3):231–238. doi:10.1200/JOP.2014.003376
96. Taplin SH, Clauser S, Rodgers AB, Breslau E, Rayson D (2010) Interfaces across the cancer continuum offer opportunities to improve the process of care. J Natl Cancer Inst Monogr 40:104–110. doi:10.1093/jncimonographs/lgq012

97. Wagner EH, Austin BT, Von Korff M (1996) Organizing care for patients with chronic illness. Millbank Quart 74(4):511–544
98. Plsek PE, Greenhalgh T (2001) Complexity science: the challenge of complexity in health care. BMJ 323(7313):625–628

Further Reading

99. Kodner D (2009) All together now: a conceptual exploration of integrated care. Healthc Q 13 (Special Issue):S6–S15
100. Suter E, Oelke ND, Adair CE, Armitage GD (2009) Ten key priniples for suessful health systems integration. Healthcare Quart 13:16–23 (Toronto, Ont)
101. Haggerty JL (2012) Ordering the chaos for patients with multimorbidity. BMJ 345:e5915. doi:10.1136/bmj.e5915
102. Taplin SH, Weaver S, Chollette V, Marks LB, Jacobs A, Schiff G, Stricker CT, Bruinooge SS, Salas E (2015) Teams and teamwork during a cancer diagnosis: interdependency within and between teams. J Oncol Pract Am Soc Clin Oncol 11(3):231–238. doi:10.1200/JOP.2014.003376
103. Reuban DB, Tinetti ME (2012) Goal-oriented patient care—an alternative health outcomes paradigm. NEJM 366(9):777–779

Chapter 11
Advocacy in Cancer and Chronic Conditions—Challenges and Opportunities

Paul Grogan and Sanchia Aranda

Abstract The WHO *World Cancer Report 2014* identified cancer as the leading global cause of death. The report was published at a time when multiple other reports showed an aggregate increase in the burden of prevalent chronic conditions, such as cardiovascular disease, diabetes and kidney disease. Whichever way the data are cut, significantly greater numbers of people are living with, and dying from, these conditions—many with multiple morbidities. The reasons include increased life expectancy and lifestyle risk factors, and a relative reduction in the infectious disease burden. While increased life expectancy is welcome, governments worldwide must develop evidence-based responses to the associated growth in chronic and co-morbid disease burden. Navigating through the evidence of population benefit will be a challenge, particularly at a time of increased patient expectations and expenditure on healthcare in most national economies. Although governments in many countries have reasonably good records in implementing health policy and delivering services, evidence is seldom the sole driver of decisions. Governments may favour political expediency, ideology and vested interests. Elected officials rarely invest optimal taxpayer funds into health and they are even less likely to invest when the returns take a long time to accrue. They may also protect powerful commercial groups whose interests are at odds with public health. For this reason, independent, evidence-based healthcare advocacy is a necessary and powerful driver for policy reform, either through a non-government organisation, a professional group or an individual. The potential for health professionals to drive the collection of evidence is another key reason why independent advocacy could be the key. This chapter summarises key challenges in health policy and advocacy for the management of cancer and chronic conditions. It explores the role of the healthcare professional as advocate. It analyses a case study in advocacy from the Australian experience and includes recommended principles and techniques for driving change.

P. Grogan (✉) · S. Aranda
Cancer Council Australia, Sydney, Australia
e-mail: paul.grogan@cancer.org.au

B. Koczwara (ed.), *Cancer and Chronic Conditions*,
DOI 10.1007/978-981-10-1844-2_11

Keywords Advocacy · Evidence · Policy · Healthcare · Professional · Consumers · Campaigning · Political · Lobbyist · Prevention · Integrated · Independent · Self-interest · Change · Reform · Systems · Outcome · Implementation

Key Points

- Independent health policy and advocacy must be guided by the evidence.
- Healthcare professionals have potential to be effective advocates, if they function without any perception of self-interest.
- There are a number of practical steps that advocates can take to help drive the translation of independent public policy recommendations into practice.
- Integrative health system advocacy across cancer and other chronic disease has barely extended beyond tobacco control, but there are key opportunities and a growing need for action and outcomes.

11.1 Introduction

Of all the topics in this book, advocacy is the least scientific in terms of evidence, literature and frameworks for professional practice. Advocacy can mean different things to different people. It varies widely in how it is defined and applied across settings.

By its broadest definition, "advocacy" describes the act or process of supporting a cause [1]. This is a useful starting point, and could explain why advocacy is so readily associated with politics, activism and campaigning.

Two of the most celebrated advocacy actions in recent history are the US civil rights movement and the abolition of apartheid in South Africa. Both involved an extraordinary amount of activity at multiple levels; both resulted in changes to constitutional law. Perhaps it is no coincidence that both movements were driven by a shared fundamental belief: that the same constitutional rights should be extended to all people irrespective of race or culture. In this sense, the broad definition of advocacy was easy to apply. The "cause"—racial equality under constitutional law—was clear, simple and supported by all advocates. The advocates then sought to work in varying alliances (with varying success rates) on actions and processes to support that cause.

There are a number of other geopolitical examples where the collective understanding and immediacy of a cause enabled advocates to come together. When it comes to health policy, however, it can be much more challenging to unify advocates behind a common cause. This is because the cause itself can be difficult to define, particularly if it involves working across multiple disciplines and disease groups.

Health system reform requires much more than amended constitutional law. The more complex the problem, the most complex the solution—and the advocacy. For example, we will assume that most readers of this book would support reforms that deliver improved outcomes in cancer and chronic conditions. That is a "cause" under the broad definition of advocacy. However, if a political leader asked for a five-minute pitch on what was required to support that cause, the responses from advocates would vary widely depending on settings, interpretations of the evidence, professional bias and in some cases self-interest.

If we as a healthcare community are to meet the growing challenges of cancer and chronic disease burden, we will have to unite behind evidence of benefit—as measured in epidemiology, clinical outcomes and overall equity. In some cases, collecting and disseminating that evidence will itself be a pillar of advocacy; indeed, when it comes to healthcare advocacy, cause, action and process become intertwined.

This is a theme that will recur—effective health advocacy is as much about healthcare professionals, consumer and other advocates working together to develop specific policy as it is about driving change to make things happen.

11.1.1 Does Advocacy Work?

There are multiple examples of successful health advocacy. Some of the most effective global and local advocacy to date has been focused on disease prevention, in particular the impact health professionals and their allies have had on changes to laws that have reduced smoking prevalence. As documented throughout this chapter, the anti-smoking movement is an (unfinished) advocacy success story and a cause that has mobilised and unified healthcare professionals everywhere. More recently, collaborative advocacy has also driven some (but little) policy change in nutrition, such as restrictions to junk food advertising (e.g. Quebec), government-sanctioned food labelling (Australia et al.) and a sugar levy on beverages introduced in the UK in March 2016.

It could be argued that one reason the anti-smoking advocacy movement was able to coordinate the efforts of multiple healthcare professionals and organisations is its relative simplicity and absence of potential turf wars between disciplines. During the formative days of the anti-smoking movement, the "cause" was straightforward: advocates sought restrictions to the way tobacco products were advertised (largely to protect children) and campaigned for health warnings to inform the population of the risks. Tailored interventions, such as price controls, smoke-free areas and sponsorship bans, and tailored strategies to compel reluctant governments to adopt them, evolved as required. Apart from rivalry over the research agenda, advocates, particularly those from the health sector, were not distracted by concerns about how policy reform to drive down smoking rates might affect their patch.

The same interdisciplinary and inter-sectoral collaboration will be required to develop and promote recommendations for improved management of cancer and chronic conditions. This in itself is an unprecedented challenge.

So we return to the "cause"—whether that cause is at the macro level (e.g. "a sustainable, equitable health system") or the micro level (e.g. "an enhanced billing system that reduces waiting times and accelerates referral pathways for patients with or at risk of multiple morbidities").

Essential to the challenge of driving health system reform to reduce cancer and chronic disease burden will be collecting the strongest evidence to define the "cause" at multiple levels.

By exploring challenges and policy opportunities across a range of topics, this book is contributing to the evidence base. The aim of this chapter is to provide context on how independent policy is supported, and some practical guidance for healthcare professionals who seek to drive change to improve outcomes in cancer and other chronic conditions.

11.2 The Challenge—Growing Burden of Cancer and Chronic Conditions

According to the WHO *World Cancer Report 2014*, cancer (as a single disease entity) is the biggest cause of mortality worldwide, with an estimated 8.2 million deaths from cancer in 2012. Cancer cases worldwide are forecast to rise by 75 % and reach close to 25 million over the next two decades [2].

Cancer death rates have increased in relation to heart disease and stroke, however, if the latter two are combined and aggregated as cardiovascular disease (as they are in some statistical frameworks) they continue to cause more deaths. Cancer (14 %) and cardiovascular diseases (31 %) combined caused an estimated 45 % of all the world's deaths in 2014. This percentage is higher in developed countries, which have lower relative rates of infectious disease. Yet in all countries combined, non-communicable diseases such as cancer and cardiovascular disease are on the rise. Around 68 % of all deaths in 2014 were attributed to non-communicable diseases, an 8 % increase from 2000 [3].

In developed countries such as Australia, cancer causes an even higher level of overall disease burden (years of healthy life lost). This is largely due to significant improvements in managing cardiovascular disease in recent decades, as well as the relatively low contribution of infectious disease deaths and unchanged trends in the impact of some cancers that cause death in younger people [4].

The impact of diabetes (types 1 and 2) on death rates continues to increase, with type 2 diabetes disease burden largely due to poor diet and high body mass [5]. Chronic obstructive lung disease and tobacco-related cancers are also increasing significantly, due to increased rates of smoking in developing countries and the time lag between exposure and disease in countries with relative reductions in smoking prevalence [6, 7]. In countries with longer life expectancy, dementia related illnesses are increasing at unprecedented rates [8] and having a major impact on health and aged care systems.

Whichever way these projections are cut, the message is simple: health systems and public policies will need to adapt to extraordinary growth in the rates of people with cancer and one or more other chronic conditions.

We cannot rely on governments alone to get the policy agenda right to ensure that optimal clinical and public health outcomes are delivered. The non-government healthcare professional as advocate can play an important role in working constructively with governments to help ensure that evidence is the primary driver of policy and practice. Indeed, motivated health professionals armed with the best available evidence and working with non-government organisations can be a powerful force for improving healthcare delivery and patient outcomes. Consumers can, and should, also be powerful advocates for change. Collaboration and coordination across disciplines, sectors and even nations will be required.

11.3 Global Non-communicable Disease Agenda

The World Health Organisation has formally recognised and seeks to address the growing global challenge of chronic disease burden with its *Global action plan for the prevention and control of non-communicable diseases* (*NCD*) 2013–2020. The global NCD agenda is an example of applying an international focus to a jointly recognised threat and providing a framework for acting globally and locally.

Observation shows that global alliances can help to take an issue forward and demonstrate that experts and leaders from a range of nations agree on problems and solutions. Collective advocacy across the global non-communicable disease agenda is one example. But working globally in pragmatic terms is limited by many factors. We are one world, but around 190 sovereign nations. (Even the number of sovereign nations is disputed, with the sovereignty of all who claim it not recognised by all nations.) It is almost impossible to establish a workable international mandate; governments will always prioritise domestic concerns. Translating in-principle agreements underpinned by treaties, conventions and declarations into implementation is seldom seamless. (The United Nations was established seventy-one years ago to maintain "international peace and security". An estimated 50 million people have died in armed conflicts since. Working globally is a challenge.)

There is, however, significant goodwill and collective purpose in improving global health outcomes. In the international setting, cancer is firmly located within a non-communicable framework for a variety of pragmatic and political reasons. Politically, the priority across the early 2000s was to problematize to the world the impact of non-communicable diseases on low and middle income countries in order to mobilise resources to address a growing problem. Up to that point NCDs were not mentioned within the United Nation's Millennium Development Goals (MDGs) and therefore were not able to access most international funds aimed at the global development agenda. Cancer NGOs and their counterparts in other chronic diseases reflected on the successful international effort against HIV/AIDS and believed that the problems facing LMICs in terms of NCDs were best approached, not as a health issue, but as a broad global development agenda. To this end in 2009 the CEO of the International Diabetes Federation, Ann Keeling, sought to convene a global NCD civil society movement to confront misconceptions that NCDs were of little importance in the developing world and to catalyse political action. The Union for International Cancer Control and the World Heart Federation, the International Union Against TB and Lung Disease joined IDF to form the NCD alliance.

The movement commenced by the NCD alliance led to a UN High-Level Meeting on the Prevention and Control of Non-Communicable Diseases in September 2011, only the second ever such meeting devoted to a health topic. This meeting subsequently led to a set of measurable targets and action plans to hold the world to account for this important issue.

Several factors were critical to the successful advocacy begun by Ann Keeling. First, the agenda for change was firmly located in an agenda that went beyond the health of individuals. NCDs were identified in a 2011 report by the World Economic Forum and Harvard Business School demonstrating the critical impact of NCDs on the economies of all countries with a cost in 2010 representing 48 % of global gross domestic product and rising. Critically NCDs were identified for their role in pushing millions of people into poverty and were linked to a complex interplay between health, economic growth and development and universal trends such as aging, urbanisation and unhealthy lifestyles. This report placed the issue of NCDs above the global economic crisis in terms of importance of impact on the global economy and suggested the solution lay beyond simply a health agenda.

Secondly, the formation of the NCDA strengthened the voice of the disease-based organisations. It did this by enabling a set of common messages, a clear ask for targets related to prevention of NCDs and provided a cohesive and clear path for communication and engagement between the NCDA and the UN and WHO in the lead up to the UN high-level meeting. In the follow-up period as targets and action plans were being formulated this single voice of interaction remained critical.

While the experience was positive there are downsides to any alliance. Alliances, while strengthening a common mission, reduce the ability of any one organisation to mobilise its own advocacy agenda. This may mean that members of the alliance require additional resources locally to enable a joint focus on working within the alliance and working on its core agenda.

Alliances also slow down decision-making processes as each organisation confers with its constituents about position statements and advocacy approaches. While this can be overcome to some extent with an empowered staff, the time needed to bring all parts of the alliance to one position cannot be under-estimated.

11.4 Advocacy and Health Policy

Drilling down past the dictionary definition in the Introduction, the World Health Organization (WHO) takes a specific approach to defining advocacy relating to health:

> A combination of individual and social actions designed to gain political commitment, policy support, social acceptance and systems support for a particular health goal or programme [9].

This is widely considered to be an appropriate (broad) definition in a health context, noting that the WHO's stakeholder base is global and highly diverse. From our experience, just about everything that occurs under an advocacy umbrella is picked up in the WHO definition. In relation to health system reforms for improved outcomes in cancer and other chronic conditions, the references to policy support and systems support are particularly important.

It should also be noted that, while the WHO definition might imply that advocacy is something done by non-government people to influence government people, this is not strictly the case. As explored later, government officials (political and non-political) can be among the most effective advocates for change.

So what does it all mean in practice? Are there agreed frameworks for action? Guiding principles that can be applied in practice? How can we target health advocacy to purpose, when systems of government, relative wealth and other variations prevail across settings? How do we even begin to drive change for more sustainable, equitable approaches to reducing cancer and chronic disease burden?

11.4.1 Frameworks for Health Advocacy

While there is no definitive framework for health advocacy, there is agreement among advocates on some key points. For example, Michael Moore (CEO of the Public Health Association of Australia) and co-authors have published a guiding framework for public health advocacy [10], based on the Kotter change model [11]. It contains 10 generic steps:

Step 1: Establishing a Sense of Urgency
Step 2: Creating the Guiding Coalition
Step 3: Developing and Maintaining Influential Relationships
Step 4: Developing a Change Vision
Step 5: Communicating the Vision for Buy-in
Step 6: Empowering Broad-based Action
Step 7: Be Opportunistic
Step 8: Generating Short-term Wins
Step 9: Never Letting Up
Step 10: Incorporating Changes into the Culture.

These are useful guiding principles, noting that they were developed for "public health advocacy"—i.e. political change to reduce risk factor prevalence in a population. They apply more readily to scenarios that might require a cultural shift and also involve adversarial interests (e.g. tobacco companies, whose commercial interests are at odds with public health). Seldom have the steps above played out in a linear fashion; yet most have been invoked at some point in achieving major policy reform.

To succeed in areas that require policy and systems change, however, requires even more nuanced, flexible and targeted approaches—particularly for driving reforms to reduce the combined burden of cancer and other chronic conditions, which will encompass prevention, early detection, integrated care and patient support. Some will be sweeping in scope, such as policies to improve population nutrition (poor diet is a risk factor for most chronic and co-morbid conditions); others will be highly specific, such as improved systems for integrated patient care.

Although our experience in advocacy relates primarily to cancer control policy, the core principles and effective strategies should just as readily apply to driving reforms in chronic disease control more broadly. The record shows that multiple stakeholders can collaboratively advocate to support a relatively simple cause such as tobacco control. But to do so in order to drive change in more complex policy areas such as integrated care is likely to require a more policy-focused and adaptive framework for advocacy.

11.4.2 Advocacy and Chronic Disease Management Reform

From our observation, effective advocacy in public health and disease control has tended to be built around a 10-part framework that is consistent with both the WHO definition of advocacy and the separate but intertwined 10 steps identified by Moore et al.

1. A scientific evidence base showing the population and individual health benefits of the policy recommendations being promoted.
2. Feasibility assessment.
3. Cost-effectiveness.
4. A framework for prioritisation—e.g. how do we weigh up relative benefits, short-term versus long-term goals, public acceptability etc.?
5. Maintaining political neutrality.
6. A focus on outcomes—not only those for individual patients but also for population health and the health system in terms of reduced cost and increased sustainability.
7. Running tight campaigns and strategies tailored to each objective.
8. Working locally, nationally and/or internationally, depending on circumstances.
9. Fostering and maintaining key personal relationships (trust, courtesy, mutual respect etc.).

10. Ensuring appropriate recognition and thanks are accorded those who make the decisions and allocate the funding (rather than to the non-government advocates).

These 10 points recognise the complexity of promoting highly specific and technical interventions that may require new and improved policy settings in a wide range of domains. On that basis, they might be a useful guide for healthcare advocates operating across disease groups and professions.

It should be noted that while the main focus of these principles and steps is a party-political audience, health advocacy at times will be targeted directly at businesses, communities and individuals. People from multiple walks of life all contribute to the way health policy is funded, developed, promoted and implemented. But the reality, in democratic countries with a mix of public and private health systems, is that political support will in most cases be required to embed policy reform in practice.

Box 1 summarises how these points were applied in practice in the establishment of a cancer screening program in Australia.

Box 1: Bowel Cancer Screening in Australia: A Study in Health Advocacy

Australia's National Bowel Cancer Screening Program (NBCSP) was phased in from 2006 and will be fully implemented in 2020. Its introduction was a pre-election policy recommendation from Cancer Council in 2004; its completion by 2020 was a 2013 Cancer Council election priority. The latest published data shows the program is a world-leading public health intervention; it is being held up as a model for international best practice [12].

Cancer Council Australia is the only non-government organisation that has been represented on all key multi-sectoral bodies formally tasked with the NBCSP's implementation. The program is an instructive study in inter-sectoral collaboration and public health advocacy. Following is a summary of how the 10 points identified at Sect. 11.4.2 were applied.

1. A scientific evidence base showing the population and individual health benefits of the policy recommendations being promoted

Evidence of benefit in Australia was first collected by independent researchers. Cancer Council (and allies) collated further evidence in representations to Government and Opposition in the lead-up to the 2004 election. Both sides of politics announced plans to introduce a program during the campaign.

As a non-government agency, we continued to collect and promote the evidence, to position it as the key rationale for our position. This included evidence-driven editorials in the *Medical Journal of Australia* [13], and the tactical use of mainstream media for wider dissemination.

In 2013, Cancer Council published estimates that showed, even on low participation rates, the NBCSP would prevent around 70,000 Australian deaths over the next 3–4 decades [14]. The then federal Opposition (and Government from September 2013) based its $100 million investment in completing the NBCSP according to this advice—and said so publicly [15].

2. Feasibility assessment
Government in Australia had run three successful pilot projects in diverse settings to test the feasibility of a program [16]. The subsequent reports helped to build the case and were key parts of our advocacy toolkit. However, feasibility in advocacy is about whether something will happen—not just if it will work. (We have not pushed for tobacco bans, for example, as it is unfeasible on current prevalence.)

Two things were clear from the NBCSP's introduction: it would be implemented incrementally (the Government in 2012 announced a 2034 program completion date); and an effective strategy would be required for acquiring funds to keep the program moving forward. Three years into the NBCSP's introduction, we did a feasibility assessment based on a scientifically acceptable timeframe and political realities. In 2011, we agreed that a 2020 program completion date would be feasible and acceptable.

3. Cost-effectiveness
Cancer Council advisers co-authored with US health economist Dr Michael Pignone the first-ever cost-effectiveness modelling of a full program in 2009 [17]. This was reported to the Government but did not enter the literature until 2011 [18]. Even pre-published, it became the standard for estimating cost-effectiveness, despite initial government resistance. As the evidence of clinical benefit grew, along with drug costs for treating late-stage disease, the estimates in Pignone et al. became more powerful.

We also brought in state government evidence, notably from the Cancer Institute NSW [19]. The cost of public hospital care in Australia is borne largely by state governments; thus the states have an economic stake in detecting disease early when treatment costs are lower.

Cancer Council Australia did its own cost estimates based on the available evidence; our costed pre-budget submissions to Treasury to expand and complete the NBCSP, in 2010 and 2013 respectively, were supported by government almost verbatim.

4. A framework for prioritisation—how do we weigh up relative benefits, short-term versus long-term goals, public acceptability?
The NBCSP is a good example of phasing and prioritising advocacy efforts. Evidence on public acceptability was collected in the pilot programs and strengthened by subsequent data on intention to rescreen. Prioritisation of our policy development and promotion, and government and community engagement, was based on feasibility assessment. For example, in 2011 we judged that a $50 million funding increase and age cohort expansion, and a

commitment to permanent recurrent funding, were the best outcomes we could feasibly strive for. Both were announced in the subsequent budget.

5. Maintaining political neutrality
This can be a challenge but it is a critical principle. There will be times when one side of politics will support your policy and the other will not. Both sides of politics in Australia's largely two-party state supported verbatim costed proposals published by Cancer Council Australia in the tens of millions.

6. A focus on outcomes—not just those for individual patients but also for the health system in terms of things like reduced cost and increased capacity
One of the challenges of a federated health system is seeking policy change that requires a response from multiple jurisdictions. In making a cost-effectiveness case for bowel cancer screening investment, we drew on potential savings at both the federal (subsidised pharmaceuticals, Medicare gap payments for unnecessary screening colonoscopy) and state (public hospital costs) level. We sought support from funders at both levels for our argument that detection at earlier stage was an economic benefit for multiple sectors. Ultimately, the cost-effectiveness arguments supported a compelling clinical case.

7. Running tight campaigns and strategies tailored to each objective
As documented, short and long-term outcomes based on the evidence and our assessments underpinned our representations, strategies and tactics. The co-opting of parliamentary Independents in a minority government is an example of tailoring strategies to objectives and circumstances. Collecting our own evidence, such as the "magic number" of 70,000 lives saved (deliberately timed to coincide with an election campaign) is another example.

8. Working locally, nationally and/or internationally, depending on circumstances
The establishment of the NBCSP, while specific to Australia, had an international dimension. The systematic reviews that drove the Australian pilot projects drew on international studies. Dr Pignone, an American, led the pivotal cost-effectiveness analysis; Cancer Council Australia had brought in other international experts to contribute to its advocacy agenda. These include Dr Roland Valori, clinical adviser to the UK's bowel screening program, and Dr Heather Bryant from the Canadian Partnership Against Cancer, a key driver of bowel cancer screening in Canada. Opportunities to share information and work globally continue.

9. Fostering key personal relationships (and maintaining trust, courtesy etc.)
Personal relationships are a vital component of advocacy. The valued relationships with cross-bench Independents was pivotal to a $50 million injection into the program in 2012. Trusted relationships with MPs in Opposition

also translated to major investments in the program when governments changed, without the advocates being drawn into the politics.

10. Ensuring appropriate recognition and kudos is given to those who make the decisions, allocate the funding etc. (rather than to the non-government advocates)
A good example of this is our proactive media statements in support of then Health Minister Peter Dutton's budget commitment to complete the program according to our plan in 2014. Australia's 2014–15 health budget was a contentious one for health, with a number of cost-cutting measures and criticisms. Media commentary from the non-government sector was negative. We were nonetheless determined to ensure the minister responsible received due recognition. The fact that he found almost $100 million in a budget focused on savings was, in one sense, even more reason to thank and acknowledge him.

Being adversarial and confrontational rarely works in health advocacy. And, when it does, it can be a Pyrrhic victory—a short-term gain that compromises the long game. There are, however, times when a bad government decision should be criticised—and loudly. This is a judgement call based on myriad circumstances. Sticking with the 10 points above should help to keep you on track.

11.4.3 Evidence and Recognition

The 10 points at Sect. 11.4.1 are inter-related. Points 1 and 10 require particular emphasis as they are sometimes overlooked.

Firstly, point 1. Evidence should underpin any health policy recommendations. This may seem obvious, but there have been numerous campaigns over the years that were not supported by the evidence. (Examples range from compensation for diseases not attributable to the claimed causes, to the impact of anti-vaccination campaigners.) Populism can be powerful, but health advocacy should be driven by evidence, based on a rigorous framework. Moreover, the strength of your evidence for change can:

- make it more difficult for opponents or resisters to reject your recommendations;
- remove or reduce the impact of opinion, bias, and politicisation;
- provide an unspoken position of moral authority;
- neutralise concerns around conflict of interest—which can be particularly important for the "clinician advocate"; and
- assist you in staying on-message in multiple contexts.

Collecting the evidence itself can be a powerful form of advocacy. Governments will not always gather information that requires them to fund interventions or change policies; in some cases they will evade or suppress the evidence. The work of Sir Richard Doll, whose epidemiology on lung cancer and smoking helped to drive the tobacco control movement, is a good example of how independent scientists can change the world with their research alone. As noted later, Doll did not see himself as an advocate; but his statistics were more powerful than many campaigns.

It is also important to further highlight point 10—recognition and kudos. No matter how effective the non-government advocate, accountability rests with a government official (usually an elected official). Governments, and in particular ministers, have to find the funds, make the decisions, work with their colleagues, balance the demands of multiple stakeholders and, ultimately, face the voters. Moreover, health ministers often have little time to make a long-term impact and are usually remembered for negative media rather than for their achievements.

It is therefore critical that the parliamentarians (usually ministers) receive most, if not all, the public recognition and kudos for their decisions—even if decisions were the result of your advocacy. It is important to resist the temptation to focus on your contribution.

Politics is a tough and thankless job, particularly in countries that have strong democracies and a cultural irreverence towards political leaders. There is also a sense of purpose in working with a government official (sometimes against their initial intention) to get a good health policy outcome and enabling them to enjoy the credit. In addition, your chances of succeeding as an advocate will increase if you ensure that ministers and others are duly acknowledged. Officials will want to work with you again if the end result of your advocacy reflects well on their administration.

11.4.4 Advocacy in the Context of a Western Health System

The observations and advice in this chapter are based on driving change in a relatively well-funded health and social services environment. Health advocacy in countries with significantly lower GDP and relative investment in healthcare will require different approaches. Countries that face greater challenges in areas such as tobacco control may also require more radical approaches that we explore here (apart from some historical references herein). We nonetheless hope readers from a range of socio-political environments will find our observations useful.

The increasing burden of chronic disease and multiple morbidities in Australia is reflected throughout the developed world. In Australia, in a population of just under 24 million (in 2016), more than 3.7 million people have at least one form of cardiovascular disease, 1 million have diabetes and 1.1 million are estimated to have had a cancer diagnosis and/or are in active treatment for cancer. Around 350,000 live with dementia; 310,000 have obstructive lung disease. One million Australians are estimated to be morbidly obese (arguably a risk factor rather than a disease). There are no integrated national datasets to indicate how many of these conditions coexist in the same people. We only know that the numbers are large and increasing.

Yet we have barely scratched the surface when it comes to integrating the multiple elements of a complex health system around the needs of the patient. And to date, most of the rhetoric has been about the problem rather than solutions. Identifying the problem is the easy part, particularly in a relatively well-resourced country with health-literate politicians and public servants. Few, if any, officials in countries like Australia, New Zealand and Canada would dispute the claim that a projected rise in chronic conditions is set to impose pressures on health systems. But developing workable solutions to meet that challenge, and pushing for improved outcomes and equity, are separate challenges altogether.

This is where the healthcare professional as advocate—acting with no sense (perceived or real) of professional self-interest—may be needed as never before.

11.4.5 The Healthcare Professional as Advocate

As discussed, "advocacy" has many interpretations and applications, and many potential agents. In Australia (and elsewhere) an increasing number of professional agencies and individuals are promoting services, usually on a consultancy basis, to assist non-government organisations in achieving a policy outcome. Services range from lobbying and campaigning to broad government relations, strategic engagement and grant applications.

In addition, a number of non-government organisations with a health policy focus (e.g. not-for-profit peak bodies) employ in-house specialists to drive public policy outcomes. Professionals involved in this sector, whether fee-for-service consultants or staff, tend to be former media and policy advisers with senior government experience. This makes sense, as professionals with this type of background understand how government policy is developed and implemented and how to engage with government at multiple levels. (These roles are explored under Sect. 11.4.5.)

What role, then, does the healthcare professional have as advocate? From our experience, the healthcare professional can be a highly effective advocate for change—particularly if the evidence to support the policy priority is strong.

The dedicated healthcare professional can be seen as mission-driven, with no personal stake in the policy outcomes being promoted other than seeking improved public health or clinical outcomes. However, a healthcare professional can also be seen to have self-interest, which is another key reason for the emphasis on points 1 and 10 above. (Concerns about conflict of interest in this respect will be explored later.) The mission-driven advocate is distinct from the "lobbyist"—a professional perceived as having a mercenary role to deliver results for a client. This perception played out in practical terms in Australia in 2008, when a lobbyist's register was introduced in the federal parliament—distinguishing professional lobbyists from community representatives. Mission-driven advocates are not required to register in order to access parliamentarians.

Again, we can return to the importance of the evidence and of recognition for policy makers (points 1 and 10 above) in framing this distinction. A professional consultancy will, in most cases, be driven by client aspirations rather than the evidence. Sometimes these align, but often they do not. The driver for a commercial consultancy is an outcome for their client. Governments know this and will be sceptical when dealing with professional lobbyists.

Professional lobbyists, campaigners and other consultants will also in many cases seek to claim *some* credit for an outcome. This is partly because professional lobbyists and campaigners are looking for the next client. Understandably, they need to tout (if not exaggerate) their achievements. This does not go down well with government officials.

What does this have to do with the healthcare professional as advocate? The effective advocate only promotes the policy and the evidence that supports it—not themselves (unless the latter is a well-judged tactic). The effective healthcare professional advocate will seek tactical advice from government relations professionals but never waver from the evidence, their sense of mission or their preparedness to put an outcome before all else.

11.4.5.1 Conservatives and 'Real Doctors'

There has been an observed tendency for some politicians, conservatives in particular, to value the opinion of a clinician over other health policy professionals. The question are they a "real" doctor (as distinct from doctoral researcher) has been asked in relation to health advocates—even if the policy issues are more relevant to non-medical fields (e.g. sociology, statistical analyses etc.). This bias towards medical expertise is likely to be shared within the community more broadly, given that few lay people understand the role of non-medical scientists in health policy yet almost everyone has consulted a GP. This perception may change, as people become more health literate. In any case, if a clinician makes an effective advocate for a health initiative developed by a non-clinician, so be it—provided the policy is evidence-based and the clinician understands the issues. The outcome is the key.

See box 2: Dr Nigel Gray, a case-study in the doctor-advocate.

Box 2: A Case-Study of the Doctor-Advocate

Dr Nigel Gray (1928–2014) is regarded as a pioneer of tobacco control, both in Australia and internationally. In an obituary published in *Cancer Forum* (the journal of Cancer Council Australia and the Clinical Oncology Society of Australia), it was suggested Dr Gray's work on tobacco alone "may have resulted in his preventing more disease than any other Australian" [20]. Either way, he is rightly regarded as a giant of tobacco control advocacy. Yet his medical career began in paediatrics and infection control.

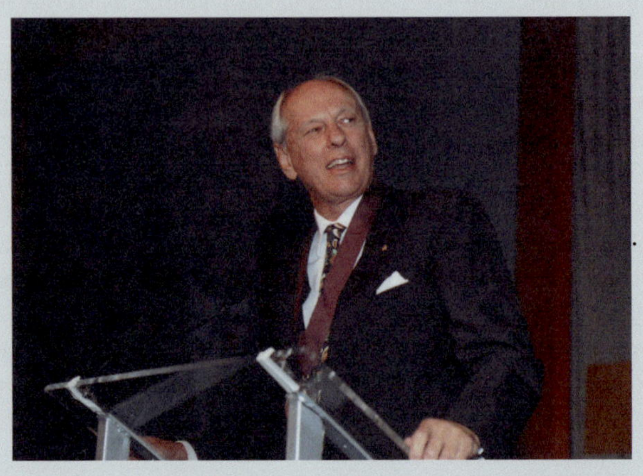

Director of Cancer Council Victoria from 1968 until 1995, and President of the Union for International Cancer Control from 1990 to 1994, Dr Gray also oversaw the introduction of Australia's first skin cancer awareness ads (the Slip, Slop Slap campaigns, now embedded in Australian culture). Dr Gray was at times a disrupter, took risks; tried things that had not been done before. Apathy towards tobacco control (and skin cancer) in Australia during the 1970s, and the substantially higher rates of tobacco prevalence, required different advocacy approaches than are needed today—at least in a country like Australia. Dr Gray challenged parliamentarians, instigated powerful anti-smoking ads, pushed for health warnings and helped establish robust behavioural research in both cancer and smoking, to build the evidence needed for policy change. He used the evidence to drive his agenda, and played a crucial role in the campaign to ban tobacco advertising. He went on to lead a global tobacco control movement, leveraging available international frameworks and helping to develop new ones (first with the Union for International Cancer Control then the World Health Organization).

Despite his radical tactics, those who worked closely with Dr Gray maintain he always presented as the gentlemen physician, the "good doctor"; even a political conservative. (He worked effectively with politicians from multiple backgrounds.) In that respect he is an instructive example of the medical professional as powerful advocate—his standing as a clinician, and his use of the evidence, transcended his disruptive methods.

To even be considered as the single health professional in Australia likely to have saved more lives than any other is an extraordinary achievement. Does the multi-morbidity disease control and integrated care agenda need a team of Dr Grays?

11.4.6 Consumer Advocates

Healthcare consumers are an integral part of advocacy, particularly in relation to treatment services. Non-government, not-for-profit organisations as a matter of course have formal consumer representation feeding into the policy process. (If they don't, they should.)

It can, however, be challenging to capture consumer input in a rigorous scientific framework. There is a key advantage in leveraging the emotional dimension of first-person health system experience, particular involving consumers with poignant stories. There is also a risk that emotion can trump evidence. (There are examples of knee-jerk reactions from government to powerful emotional stories that have not translated to best use of evidence or available funds.)

One powerful and poignant example of the consumer as advocate is the late Christina Fiddimore [21], whose personal intervention drove a change in superannuation policy in Australia. At the behest of the Breast Cancer Action Group, Ms Fiddimore, while receiving palliative care, wrote directly to the assistant treasurer seeking early access to superannuation for the terminally ill without a tax penalty. Cancer Council had made representations on the same issue. Our understanding is that the power of Ms Fiddimore's personal case was the catalyst for the policy change.

It should be noted that consumers can assist in prevention policy too. An instructive case is the late Clare Oliver [22], whose diagnosis with metastatic melanoma drove major policy change across all Australian jurisdictions on the regulation of sunbed (solarium) use. Cancer Council had long-held a core policy position on solarium regulation, but was unable to engage middle-ranking public servants on the issue. (Regulation was considered too complex, too niche; too difficult to enforce.) After Ms Oliver's story broke, the then Prime Minister John Howard stepped into say his government would lead a federal response to the problem. From 1 January 2016, commercial solariums were banned in all Australian jurisdictions except the Northern Territory (a tropical area with no commercial sunbeds). Cancer Council remains grateful to Clare and her family for taking a public position at a time of extraordinary duress and emotional distress which, by degrees, led to the eradication of commercial sunbeds in Australia.

A key to the success of these two examples was the integration of an extraordinarily powerful personal story with a well-developed public policy recommendation to get an outcome.

11.4.7 Non-government-Organisations

Non-government organisations by definition are a key to independent advocacy. Their level of independence, or how it is perceived, can however vary. Some industry associations will present as peak bodies but their priority may be the interests of their members, rather than the community. Even well-established medical professional groups, such as the Australian Medical Association (AMA), at times will be seen by government as acting out of member interests. The AMA has a good record of advocating for improved public health policy and is seen by Australian parliamentarians as a powerful advocacy group. However, as a professional body funded by member subscriptions, a perception of self-interest remains, whether fair or unfair.

Not-for-profit groups with recognised charitable status, on the other hand, are often perceived by government policy makers as prioritising the interests of their community stakeholders only. A problem with not-for-profit groups with a single disease focus can be that they are seen as "in competition" with other disease groups. This presents challenges, but also opportunities for collaboration that cut to the theme of this book. There is a case for single disease organisations to apply the (modest) collaboration they have utilised in joint prevention advocacy to health reform more broadly. In Australia, we are working towards this through alliances such as the Australian Chronic Disease Prevention Alliance (currently chaired by co-author Professor Aranda), which are exploring opportunities for collaboration beyond primary prevention. Similar groups are also emerging in other countries.

From our experience there is also value in collaborating with professional groups such as the AMA, while maintaining a separate level of independence and community focus as a charity organisation.

11.5 Examples of Effective Health Advocacy

Despite the lack of an accepted science, there are a growing number of agents who claim to know how advocacy is done. The advent of the internet and social marketing has facilitated new ways to advocate—including an unprecedented interest in digital or social media campaigning. Experience, however, shows that health advocacy is a specialised skill; technology and campaigning are only part of it. Generating noise, being populist and making an impact can be easy—or irrelevant.

(Check any snapshot of the week's trending YouTube clips.) But driving evidence-based, equitable and sustainable reform in health policy is seldom achieved by making noise. It usually requires multiple and nuanced approaches—sometimes as complex as a long-term multifaceted strategy; sometimes as simple as picking up the phone and talking to the right person.

Working in government provides a unique perspective on how to advocate as a non-government agent. Former government staff with policy and public affairs backgrounds (either within government agencies or parliamentarians' offices) are particularly well-placed to provide strategic and tactical advice. Experienced ex-government and ministerial staff have an understanding of the practicalities of how policy is developed and implemented. Moreover, former government staffers with public affairs experience have unique insights into what governments do to *avoid* adopting policies proposed by advocates.

As we have seen, the healthcare professional can be a powerful health policy advocate. That power will be better directed with the advice of a professional who understands how policy is developed and how to drive change.

11.5.1 Advocacy Toolkit

There are a number of tools and techniques that can be useful within the 10-point framework. As always, discretion, judgement and a detailed understanding of processes and personalities should be applied to their use. The basic components of an effective advocacy toolkit are as follows.

11.5.1.1 Evidence as a Tool

The evidence is not only a health advocate's most valuable tool and a core principle and enabler, it is also the most important lever, driver and justification for the cause. It is the most powerful tool in the kit.

We have elsewhere emphasised the importance of evidence—it is fundamental to mission and purpose. Different factors within an evidence base can also be emphasised for varying purposes (more on that below). Moreover, as highlighted in Sect. 11.4.2, professionals collecting the evidence can themselves be the most powerful advocates—without even trying. This is a call to epidemiologists and other researchers who might never see themselves as advocates, but whose work could be the most powerful advocacy tool.

Sir Richard Doll and Sir Austin Bradford Hill are two of the best examples. In the 1950s, Doll as medical epidemiologist and Hill as his statistician published the then most convincing evidence of an association between tobacco and both cancer and cardiovascular disease. Their research changed the world. Neither was an advocate; both were concerned that advocacy could compromise their impartiality as scientists [23]. Through their research alone (and similar studies in the US) they kick-started the global tobacco control movement. Their earliest studies did not even estimate mortality burden, but disease incidence—and attracted howls of scepticism from vested interests. Six decades later, the most robust Australia-specific study showed that two in three long-term smokers in Australia [24] would die of disease attributed to their smoking. The tobacco industry dared not question the findings.

Doll went on to be described as history's greatest epidemiologist and, arguably, Britain's most distinguished doctor. He is also an interesting study in how the "real doctor" is perceived. Some obituaries described him as the archetypal conservative Christian gentleman, yet he was a socialist and an atheist [25]. If the perception helps you to engage with a particular audience, go with it.

Applying the evidence to purpose

Evidence of mortality benefit is usually held up as the benchmark for driving health policy reform. There are, however, opportunities to apply different evidence for different purposes. For example, you might need a headline (see following) to take your agenda forward. If so, the big magic number might be useful. (As per box 1, our "70,000" lives saved from bowel cancer screening [26] is an example.)

Other big numbers, such as the Collins and Lapsley studies on the economic costs of tobacco and alcohol use [27], can also generate news and interest. It is important, however, to apply different data for different audiences. This might seem obvious, but emphasising dollar values weighted to disability adjusted life years (DALYs) for Treasury officials can miss the mark. Treasury economists seldom look at "dollarized" DALYs. At budget time, net revenue and expenditure in a timeframe of fewer than four years is the usual obsession. If your returns on investment take a long time to accrue, they need to be big. And they will be more compelling if they flow back into the budget that provides the outlay. Studies that show overall community costs for disease burden, inflated by myriad indirect expenses, won't turn the head of a Treasury official.

There will be other opportunities to match data with tactics. Some policy-makers, or influencers, take a particular interest in child health, indigenous health or some other specific area. Do your homework and find the most compelling data to fit your purpose—provided you stick within an evidence-based framework.

11.5.1.2 Media

Media and health advocacy go hand-in-hand. But they require high-level expertise and local intelligence to work effectively and without risk. Governments spend substantial taxpayer funds on media monitoring. It is an effective way for governments to gauge how their policy agenda plays out in the electorate and complements targeted party-political surveys and news-media polling. If your story plays well in media it will reach the attention of policy-makers. Timing and judgement are crucial.

It is also important to avoid being adversarial (in most cases). There are ways to apply pressure on governments though media without compromising valuable relationships. Finding third-party spokespeople, briefing trusted journalists without publicly involving your own organisation and leveraging relationships with local communities are among the recommended techniques. Rural and regional media can be particularly useful. Although audience numbers are lower in regional areas, local issues often gain prominence and local MPs take a strong interest in the media outlets that target "their" communities. Regional MPs can also be tactically valuable in getting national outcomes.

A media plan should be part of any coordinated advocacy strategy. If this is beyond your capacity, consider engaging with a not-for-profit organisation that supports your agenda.

11.5.1.3 Government Processes

Democratic governments share a number of conventions, practices and mechanisms to engage with their communities. Public consultations, parliamentary processes; budget and election cycles; questions on notice, speeches drafted for supportive MPs to read on your behalf in the parliament—there are a number of avenues to engage in the democratic process and to push a policy agenda along from outside government.

Even a letter to an MP can help. A well-crafted formal letter from an individual, or a number of individuals making similarly articulate representations, can have more impact that an online petition. MPs' advisers know how easy it is to generate a lot of noise with digital technology and social media; they know that this noise seldom reflects genuine voter intention. Data on voter intention is patchy and varies in different countries, depending on parliamentary and voting systems. In Australia, the most consistent driver of voter intention in recent decades has been the "time-for-change" factor. Between 1975 and 2016, government in Australia at the federal level only changed hands five times. The chances of your policy agenda being a voter issue are low. No one is going to "storm the bastille" over a recommended increase in tobacco tax or the expansion of a screening program's age cohort. Delude yourself into thinking you are part of a sweeping movement for change and you may miss opportunities to push for targeted reforms through direct engagement with policy makers.

Relationships (see following) with MPs, guided by experts in political advocacy, are essential for navigating these processes. MP support is vital. But extreme caution is required. A naïve or poorly timed public push can wedge an MP into going on record to rule out your proposal. If they do that, and there is no backlash, your reform agenda can be lost. Likewise, engaging with the "wrong" MP to support your cause can compromise your case. There is extraordinary vindictiveness in politics. "We are not supporting anything that *he* is backing …" Statements like this are often heard in minister's offices. Likewise, governments may be reluctant to "follow" oppositions into supporting a policy. You need good intel and relationships to get the detail right on these matters.

11.5.1.4 Relationships

Nothing ever occurs in a parliamentary democracy without the support of individuals in government. Effective parliamentary advocates exist inside and outside a minister's office. However, sooner or later your proposal will have to go to the relevant minister. Leaving aside ideological barriers, most ministers want to support their stakeholders and only say no because of budget constraints and the demands of managing multiple stakeholders. They are seldom the enemy.

Sooner or later your proposal will also go to the relevant government department. Ministers seldom do anything without advice from the people they pay to provide it. Even if a minister adopts your policy proposal from opposition, they will obtain departmental advice once in government. So it is important to have good relationships with professional public servants. If you or your organisation are well regarded by ministers, they will usually be comfortable with you engaging their departmental staff. Respect the officials. And remember, if your proposal is markedly out of step with departmental advice, it is unlikely to get up.

There might be times when you go to a higher level—e.g. the office of a prime minister. This can be effective; it can also fail badly. "Pulling rank" can close the door to future engagement with portfolio ministers and officials. Trusting relationships and good advice can help you to make a judgement call on these opportunities.

11.5.1.5 Toolkit Checklist

Items for inclusion in your advocacy toolkit might include:

- Lists of fast facts for a range of uses
- A clear statement of message (the elevator pitch)
- Published evidence specific to your policy agenda
- Pre-prepared proactive and reactive media statements and "grabs"
- Lists of important journalists and their contact details
- Lists of policy makers and areas of interest regarding your policy agenda
- Lists of potential supporters and allies
- Who's who in the parliament
- List of opponents
- List of key dates—e.g. elections, parliamentary sittings, budget timetable
- A learning list—what you did, when and why, and what you learned.

11.6 Summary

So what does all this mean for advancing healthcare policy to improve outcomes in the management of cancer and other chronic conditions? The principles and techniques articulated here should provide general guidance.

From experience, the policy and advocacy agenda on cancer and other chronic conditions has been most effective in disease prevention—taking forward a joint platform on reducing exposure to shared risk factors. While this has been challenged by vested commercial interests (e.g. tobacco, alcohol, unhealthy food) it has been easier to capture a collective position and collaborate on strategy. The global tobacco control agenda, for example, was driven to a large extent by cancer and cardiovascular disease groups, often working together. This approach has since extended to obesity and alcohol policy and involves other disease groups in multiple alliances, local and global.

But what about clinical and supportive care for people with multiple morbidities? These are challenges faced by the target audience for this book. Doctors, nurses, allied health workers, researchers, consumers and policy experts will need to find new ways to collaborate in order to drive an evidence-based policy agenda particularly when policy extends across state and federal domains and public and private settings. Collecting and synthesising that evidence and putting it into a framework that prioritises the points in Sect. 11.4.1 (feasibility, cost-effectiveness etc.) may facilitate a higher level of interdisciplinary collaboration than we have seen in independent healthcare reform. Now is the time to develop new networks.

A chronic disease policy agenda will also require healthcare professionals to step away from any perception of self-interest. Anyone working in health policy with a detailed understanding of how billing systems and health financing policies have been developed will be aware of examples where decisions were made on the basis of political pressure, not evidence, leading to overall higher healthcare costs and continued medical stranglehold on reimbursement systems. As a healthcare community, we will only be able to meet the challenges of cancer and chronic disease through a rigorous, evidence- and equity-driven approach to policy and advocacy that takes account of the changing shape of care delivery and the roles of many players. Supporting the interests of an individual professional group may yield a short-term win but compromise the long game. The first priority is to develop the evidence base, working down from mortality and morbidity benefit through to cost-effectiveness (for the taxpayer).

Leaving aside self-interest, observation also shows an inherent scientific discipline bias among professional groups. This is understandable when hardworking professionals spend countless hours immersed in a particular field of healthcare and see firsthand the benefits and lost opportunities. But a clear view of the big picture is necessary for the best outcomes.

There are also times when enthusiasm for a new intervention can get ahead of the evidence. The example of Herceptin in breast cancer treatment in Australia is instructive. It has been suggested that media pressure, rather than scientific rigour, forced early decisions on subsidisation in Australia [28]. (Subsidy arrangements were adjusted after the initial product listing.) By all accounts, the push was well-intentioned, but leveraging media and emotion in ways that go beyond the evidence is ethically questionable, can lead to unintended harms and can make government officials overly guarded against future claims.

One of the great strengths of the disease-prevention advocacy agenda is that it is free of perceived professional interest. No one ostensibly makes money from keeping people well. Yet everyone does. A population with increased life expectancy, life quality and reduced dependence on drugs like statins (economically disastrous in Australia) provides business opportunities for everyone, especially healthcare professionals. Greater equity in healthcare access is the key. This is critical in view of evidence showing the cyclical nature of health outcomes and prosperity. The principle of equity, and the evidence that underpins it, should be the driving force of independent advocacy.

The collection and publication of new evidence will be pivotal to a new collaborative agenda in managing cancer and chronic conditions. In our view, greater collaboration among health groups and individuals, and the application of advocacy principles and techniques that work, could be the drivers of effective reform.

References

1. Oxford Dictionary, Mirriam-Webster Dictionary; definitions of "advocacy"
2. World Health Organization (2014) World cancer report 2014. Available at: http://www.who.int/mediacentre/factsheets/fs297/en/
3. World Health Organization. http://www.who.int/gho/ncd/mortality_morbidity/en/
4. Australian Institute of Health and Welfare (2015) Australian burden of disease study series no. 1. Cat. no. BOD 1. In: Australian burden of disease study: fatal burden of disease 2010. AIHW, Canberra
5. World Health Organization, Fact sheet on diabetes. Available at: http://www.who.int/mediacentre/factsheets/fs312/en/
6. World Health Organization, Fact sheet on non-communicable disease. Available at: http://www.who.int/mediacentre/factsheets/fs355/en/
7. Australian Institute of Health and Welfare, Chronic disease in Australia. Available at: http://www.aihw.gov.au/chronic-diseases/
8. World Health Organization, Fact sheet on dementia. Available at: http://www.who.int/mediacentre/factsheets/fs362/en/
9. World Health Organisation (1998) Health promotion glossary, Geneva
10. Moore M, Yeatman H, Pollard C (2013) Evaluating success in public health advocacy strategies. Illawarra Health and Medical Research Institute, Faculty of Science, Medicine and Health. University of Wollongong, Research online. Available at: http://ro.uow.edu.au/cgi/viewcontent.cgi?article=1407&context=ihmri
11. Kotter J, Kotter International. http://www.kotterinternational.com/our-principles/changesteps
12. St John J, Grogan P (2015) Compelling new data on the effectiveness of Australia's national bowel cancer screening program: a model for best practice? Asia Pac J Clin Oncol
13. Olver I, Grogan P (2013) Early success for Australia's bowel screening program: let's move it along. Med J Aust 198(6):300–301

14. Cenin DR, St John DJB, Ledger MJN et al (2014) Optimising the expansion of the national bowel cancer screening program. Med J Aust 201:456–461
15. The Coalition's Policy to Support Australia's Health System (2013) Liberal national coalition of Australia. Available at: http://www.liberal.org.au/latest-news/2013/08/22/tony-abbott-coalitions-policy-support-australias-health-system
16. Australian Government Department of Health and Ageing (2005) Screening monograph 6/2005. The Australian bowel cancer screening pilot program and beyond: final evaluation report (Oct 2005)
17. Pignone M (2011) Costs and cost-effectiveness of full implementation of a biennial faecal occult blood test screening program for bowel cancer in Australia. Final report to the Australian Department of Health and Ageing
18. Pignone MP, Flitcroft KL, Howard K, Trevena LJ, Salkeld GP, St John JB (2011) Costs and cost-effectiveness of full implementation of a biennial faecal occult blood test screening program for bowel cancer in Australia, Med J Aust
19. Bishop J, Glass P, Tracey E, Hardy M, Warner K, Makino K, Gordois A, Wilson J, Guarnieri C, Feng J, Sartori L (2008) Health economics review of bowel cancer screening in Australia. Cancer Institute NSW
20. Harper T, Hill D, Daube M (2015) Dr Nigel Gray AO, 12 Sept 1928–20 Dec 2014. Cancer forum 2015. http://cancerforum.org.au/obituary/2015/march/dr-nigel-gray-ao/
21. Obituary of Christina Fiddimore in the Sydney Morning Herald (2008). Available at: http://www.smh.com.au/news/obituaries/fighter-drove-legal-change-to-aid-the-dying/2008/02/27/1203788436920.html
22. Obituary of Ms Clare Oliver in the Melbourne Age (2007). Available at: http://www.theage.com.au/articles/2007/09/13/1189276855381.html
23. Bulletin of the World Health Organization (2009). Available at: http://www.who.int/bulletin/volumes/88/7/09-075325/en/
24. Banks E, Joshy G, Weber M et al (2015) Tobacco smoking and all-cause mortality in a large Australian cohort study: findings from a mature epidemic with current low smoking prevalence. BMC Med. Available at: http://bmcmedicine.biomedcentral.com/articles/10.1186/s12916-015-0281-z
25. Bulletin of the World Health Organization (2009). Available at: http://www.who.int/bulletin/volumes/88/7/09-075325/en/
26. Cenin DR, St John DJB, Ledger MJN et al (2014) Optimising the expansion of the national bowel cancer screening program. Med J Aust 201:456–461
27. Collins D, Laspley H (2008) The costs of tobacco, alcohol and illicit drug abuse to Australian society in 2004/05. Commonwealth of Australia
28. Mackenzie R, Chapman S, Salkeld G, Holding S (2008) Media influence on herceptin subsidization in Australia: application of the rule of rescue? J R Soc Med. Available at: http://www.ncbi.nlm.nih.gov/pmc/articles/PMC2408635/

Further Reading

29. Moore M, Yeatman H, Pollard C (2013) Evaluating success in public health advocacy strategies. Illawarra Health and Medical Research Institute, Faculty of Science, Medicine and Health. University of Wollongong, Research online. Available at: http://ro.uow.edu.au/cgi/viewcontent.cgi?article=1407&context=ihmri

Chapter 12
Research Considerations in Patients with Cancer and Comorbidity

Marjan van den Akker, Laura Deckx, Rein Vos and Christiane Muth

Abstract Research in patients with cancer and comorbidity poses methodological challenges due to heterogeneous study populations, difficulties with recruitment and a variety of relevant outcome measures. This chapter discusses methodological choices regarding study design to ensure best fit with the research questions regarding cancer and comorbidity, the most appropriate study populations and potential strategies to recruit patients, the availability and fit of data sources, methods to measure comorbidity, and relevant outcomes and strategies for statistical analyses with a particular focus on the handling of longitudinal data.

Keywords Research methods · Study population · Outcomes · Comorbidity index · Statistical analysis

---

M. van den Akker (✉)
Department of Family Medicine, CAPHRI School for Public Health and Primary Care, Maastricht University, Maastricht, The Netherlands
e-mail: marjan.vandenakker@maastrichtuniversity.nl

M. van den Akker · L. Deckx
Discipline of General Practice, School of Medicine University of Queensland, Brisbane, Australia

L. Deckx
Department of Public Health and Primary Care, Academic Center of General Practice, KU Leuven, Louvain, Belgium

R. Vos
Department of Methodology and Statistics, CAPHRI School for Public Health and Primary Care, Maastricht University, Maastricht, The Netherlands

R. Vos
Department of Medical Informatics, Erasmus University Rotterdam, Rotterdam, The Netherlands

C. Muth
Institute of General Practice, Johann Wolfgang Goethe University, Frankfurt/Main, Germany

B. Koczwara (ed.), *Cancer and Chronic Conditions*,
DOI 10.1007/978-981-10-1844-2_12

Key Points

- Similarly to other areas of research, choosing a study design should be primarily guided by the research question one aims to answer (e.g. to describe a problem or to reject a hypothesis) taking into account the pros and cons of the design (such as the influence of recall bias and selection bias).
- Cancer patients with comorbidity form an older and very heterogeneous study population and their recruitment is a major challenge. Strategies to improve recruitment come at considerable costs, because they require a substantial increase in time and efforts.
- There is no single comorbidity measure available that satisfies all needs. A measure should be selected taking into account the research question, the available data sources, and the context of the study (e.g. community setting, nursing home, hospital).
- Statistical analyses of studies involving cancer patients with comorbidity should take into account the skewedness and non-normality of data, dependence between longitudinal clinical data and cancer related outcomes, competing causes of death and individual illness trajectories.

12.1 Introduction

Comorbidity of cancer—the co-occurrence of cancer with one or more diseases within one person—is a phenomenon with consequences for the patient, his or her family and friends, the health care system and society at large. Similarly, clinical research in this patient population is associated with complex methodological considerations and decisions.

In a primary care based study Deckx et al. [1] reported that only 22 % of newly diagnosed cancer patients did not have any co-occurring chronic disease; the vast majority were suffering from diabetes, lipid disorders, ischemic heart disease, myocardial infarction, and/or chronic obstructive pulmonary disease (COPD). In addition to comorbidities present pre cancer diagnosis, Deckx et al. also found that in the period following a cancer diagnosis other new chronic diseases develop, sometimes as a result of cancer and/or its treatment (e.g. thrombosis), but overall in a similar pattern to people from a similar age without a cancer diagnosis. Other studies report slightly higher occurrence of comorbidity in cancer patients [2, 3], or report an increased incidence of specific disease, for example deep venous thrombosis [1, 4]. The presence of co-occurring conditions in cancer patients increases patients' complexity at many levels. Interactions between diseases and their treatments may attenuate benefits and increase harms of any kind of diagnostic or therapeutic intervention. Patients may be overwhelmed by treatment burden resulting from multiple disorders and prioritization is needed. Therefore, a single-disease perspective on cancer falls short when managing real world patients. Research in this patient population has to take into account these clinical necessities but major challenges arise from this approach. In the following paragraphs we will focus on challenges related to research in cancer and comorbidity and some strategies to address these challenges will be provided.

Below, we summarize the key considerations that inform research in this field.

1. Comorbidity and multimorbidity are related but distinct concepts (see also Chap. 1). Comorbidity is the presence of other chronic diseases in addition to cancer; hence the index disease is cancer. Multimorbidity on the other hand does not focus on an index disease but looks at the co-occurrence of multiple diseases and conditions as a whole. Both concepts are helpful in research (and practice) and should not be used interchangeably. For example, life expectancy of patients with chronic heart failure is comparable to that of patients with colon, prostate and breast cancer [5, 6]. Depending on the research question the condition identified as the index disease may vary (heart failure with comorbid cancer or cancer with comorbid heart failure) or should not follow a pre-specified hierarchy at all. The choice of the appropriate concept—comorbidity or multimorbidity—provides a framework for the study and its further operationalization supports the selection of outcome measures and procedures to control for potential confounders.
   Many research considerations for comorbidity and multimorbidity are similar, given the overlap between both concepts. However, because this chapter focuses on research challenges in patients *with cancer and chronic diseases*, we will predominantly use the term '*comorbidity*'. We will only use the term '*multimorbidity*' if the studies that are being discussed clearly focus on multimorbidity.
2. The choice of the appropriate **study design** is of crucial importance. Although, the randomized controlled trial (RCT) design is the experimental gold standard in intervention research, it is often not possible to test the effectiveness of interventions such as a drug treatment in varying patterns of multimorbidity in cancer patients. RCTs may be conducted for the most important cancer-comorbidity combinations and observational studies may generate further evidence whether an intervention has comparable or attenuated benefits in cancer patients with and without comorbidity. Further, observational study designs are helpful to estimate harm in patients with cancer and comorbidity, e.g. arising from drug-disease and drug-drug interactions.
3. Older and more vulnerable patients will have to be included in the **study population** to take comorbidity into account. This population has been generally excluded from randomized controlled trials [7], and in many other aspects of cancer research [8, 9]. Although, more research in this population is needed, research including an older and sicker population raises important methodological and ethical challenges relating to recruitment, survival of the fittest, and hence requires special attention of researchers in this area.
4. Research in comorbidity of cancer cannot be limited to studies collecting primary data, given the enormous research needs and complexity. Other **available data sources** collected for different purposes (e.g. claims data), data from registries or research practice networks come to play. However, the use of these data is frequently hampered by their variable validity and difficulties arising

from combining different data sources. Combining available data sources with additionally collected primary data may be preferable, but might not always be feasible.

5. **Comorbidity operationalization and measurement** is needed to describe the morbidity of the included population, to adjust for confounding, and to be applied as an outcome in itself. With more than 10,000 known diseases the number of potential combinations is vast. However, existing measures reflect some ongoing discussion about definitions resulting in a multiplicity of operationalizations and instruments. Also, some of these instruments have been developed and validated in certain populations and are applied in others. Their use may be further complicated by limitations of available data sources.
6. The choice of appropriate **outcome measures** may be difficult and has to go beyond the classical "hard outcomes", such as survival and hospitalization. In particular in older patients with cancer and comorbidity, quality of life often outweighs length of survival [10]. In patient-centered care, the ultimate outcome measure would include those preferred by the patients. However, goal attainment scaling instruments have been restricted to rehabilitation medicine and have been rarely applied in cancer until now [11, 12]. Appropriate (age-adapted) measures of health related quality of life and functionality—including all domains of social, cognitive, mental, and physical functioning—should be applied to provide evidence to support decisions for or against certain treatments adequately. The choice of outcomes may also be challenging in epidemiological studies where research on the relationship between cancer, comorbidity, and other potential determinants goes beyond mere correlation.
7. **Statistical analyses** in cancer research in general are not trivial, as they should often include time-dependent analyses to take into consideration that neoplasms have their specific natural course and that treatment at times is highly toxic. Often, cancer status is unclear, disease may be progressive despite aggressive treatment, and patients may develop serious toxicity as a consequence of the treatment. This has led to the development of oncology-specific outcomes such as disease free survival, prediction of toxicity, and tolerance to treatment, which may not reflect the interaction with comorbidity. Interferences from comorbidity or multimorbidity enhance the complexity of the statistical models and may hamper the transparency of analyses as well as the interpretation of the results.

Box 1: Research challenges in studying the comorbidity of cancer

- Study design
- Study population
- Data sources
- Measures and operationalization of comorbidity
- Outcomes
- Statistical analyses of longitudinal data.

12.2 Study Design—Design to Fit the Question

The choice of the appropriate study design is of crucial importance. The randomized controlled design is the gold standard when it comes to testing the effectiveness of an intervention. However, the possible combinations of cancer and different comorbid diseases are endless, which pushes us to explore other avenues. Generally, study designs can be subdivided in descriptive studies versus analytic studies, although there may be some overlap between both as well (see Fig. 12.1).

Descriptive studies generally focus on describing the characteristics of a study population, i.e. the population of patients with cancer. The aim is to provide a picture of what is happening in a population, for example the prevalence and incidence of comorbidity in a population of cancer patients. This information is often gathered using cross-sectional observational studies (e.g. population surveys). Descriptive studies can also include qualitative studies. Qualitative studies generally aim to understand the experience of a certain problem. For example, a qualitative study design can be used to understand the impact of comorbidity on daily life in cancer patients or the impact of comorbidity on top of cancer [13]. They can also be used to understand the views of primary care physicians in the management of comorbidity in cancer patients, since primary care physicians are seen as experts in dealing with multimorbidity [14]. Other applications of a qualitative study designs are to generate hypotheses or to provide in-depth understanding of quantitative studies. For example, a qualitative study design can be used as part of a process evaluation of a new model of care that especially targets cancer patients with extra needs, such as other chronic health problems.

Analytic studies generally attempt to quantify a relationship between two or more factors. For example, analytic designs can be used to quantify the relation

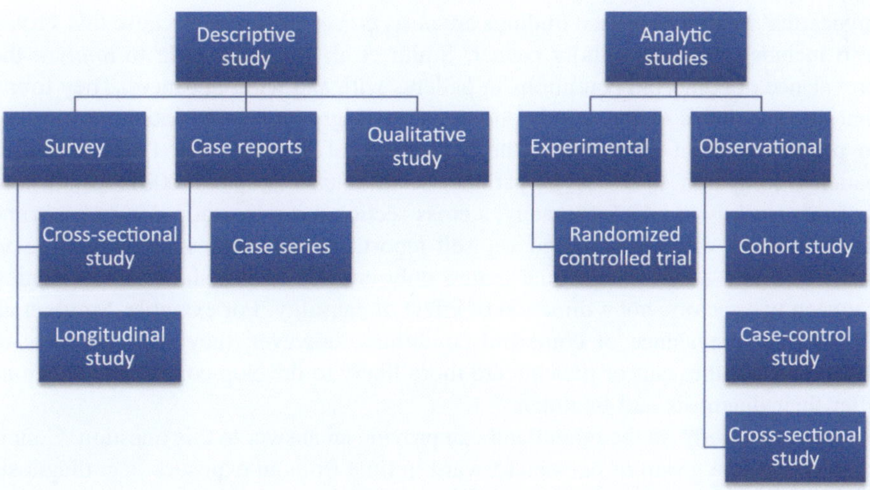

Fig. 12.1 Study designs. *Source* [16]: adapted from http://www.cebm.net/study-designs/

between comorbidity in cancer patients and different outcomes, such as treatment toxicity, disease-free survival, and overall survival. The best-known analytical study design is the randomized controlled trial, which is designed to test the effect of an intervention. In this respect, the effect of a new drug can be tested in the presence of comorbidity (e.g. compare a treatment group with and without comorbidity to standard care). These studies are often referred to as trials or experimental designs. Another type of analytic study design is the observational study. This includes cohort studies, and case control studies, and they are often used to evaluate the effect of an exposure on an outcome, for example, to investigate the effect of comorbidity (exposure) on cancer survival (outcome). However, there might be some overlap between descriptive and analytic study designs as well. Cross-sectional studies can be both descriptive and analytic. A population survey can be used to *describe* the prevalence of comorbidity in cancer patients (e.g. describe prevalence of comorbidity across different types of cancer and stage at diagnosis). However, it can also be used to *analyze* the relationship between two factors or groups (e.g. quantify the relation between presence or absence of comorbidity and cancer stage at diagnosis).

Depending on the research question one aims to answer, a descriptive or more analytic design might be more appropriate. Below we will discuss some examples of different study designs that were used to study cancer and comorbidity. This is not a comprehensive overview of study design. For such an overview we refer to one of the many epidemiological handbooks, like the one from Rothman et al. [15].

As a first example, we will discuss the **cross-sectional** study design, which can be both descriptive and analytic. Using a Medicare Health Outcomes **Survey**, Smith et al. [2] illustrated the prevalence of the most common comorbid conditions in cancer patients. The sample of cancer patients that participated had a mean age of 75 years and 48 % of them were female. For this sample, they showed that 54 % of cancer patients had hypertension, 17 % had diabetes, and 10 % has had a myocardial infarction. These findings are *descriptive*. However, because this survey also included patients without cancer, Smith et al. were also able to *analyze* the prevalence of comorbid conditions in patients with and without cancer. They found that the prevalence of comorbid conditions was higher in cancer patients compared to patients without cancer (e.g. the prevalence of diabetes was 17 % in cancer patients compared to 16 % in patients without cancer, $p < 0.0001$) [2]. These findings are *analytic*. Unfortunately, a cross-sectional survey study-design has some limitations as well; it is based on self-reports, which makes it susceptible to recall-bias and its cross-sectional nature only enables one to show an association between two factors, not a direction of effect or causality. For example, Smith et al. showed the prevalence of comorbid conditions, however, they were not able to determine whether cancer patients are more likely to develop comorbid conditions after their diagnosis and treatment.

A **cohort study** on the other hand can provide an answer to this question. Cohort studies follow a group of persons forward in time from an exposure (e.g. diagnosis of cancer) to one or more outcomes (e.g. new chronic conditions). Deckx et al. [1] used a cohort study to assess the incidence of new comorbid conditions in cancer patients compared to patients without cancer, using data from a large primary care based cohort study. This cohort study includes approximately 135,000 people, participants are registered with a general practitioner (GP), and all their relevant health problems are recorded continuously in time. All patients with cancer were selected from this cohort and the incidence of new comorbid conditions—after the diagnosis of cancer—was assessed and compared to the patients without a diagnosis of cancer. They found that the incidence of new comorbid conditions was largely similar for patients with and without cancer. Although a cohort study is the best design to study the incidence and natural history of a problem, the disadvantages of this design are that it is very time-consuming and labor-intensive, it relies strongly on long-term and substantial commitments of the participants, and it is not feasible in rare disorders.

Case-control studies are much more efficient from this perspective. In case-control studies, patients with and without a disease (e.g. cancer) are recruited and information on the exposure is then gathered retrospectively (e.g. evaluate exposure to cigarettes in patients with and without lung cancer). For example, Hang et al. [17] conducted a large case-control study to investigate the effects of lifestyle factors and comorbidities on the risk for colorectal cancer. They recruited 1144 patients who were diagnosed with colorectal cancer and 60,549 community controls. Both groups were interviewed using structured questionnaires that included questions on comorbidity history and lifestyle factors. They found that four comorbid conditions (diabetes, hyperlipidemia, inflammatory bowel disease and polyps) and some lifestyle factors (e.g. reduced physical activity and eating red meat) were associated with an increased risk for colorectal cancer. Nevertheless, case-control studies have some limitations as well. For example, case-controls studies are prone to recall bias; patients with the disease are more (or less) likely to remember exposure compared to people without the disease. Also the selection of an appropriate control group might be difficult (selection bias); it is important that patients and controls are similar in all factors that could influence the relationship under study (e.g. selection of controls could have been inappropriate if they were generally younger and therefore had less or less severe comorbid conditions).

The latter is not an issue in **a randomized controlled trial** design. The random allocation of participants to the treatment or the placebo group should ensure that the two groups are balanced in terms of confounding factors (e.g. age and comorbid conditions are balanced across both groups). Klepin et al. [18] reported the results of a randomized controlled trial that focused on the influence of age and comorbidity. In the parent trial, women aged 65 years or older with stages I–III breast cancer were randomly allocated to standard adjuvant chemotherapy or capecitabine [19]. They found that women who were treated with standard chemotherapy had a lower risk of breast cancer recurrence and death than those treated with capecitabine. In the companion study it was explored if women with a greater number of comorbid conditions would experience more treatment toxicity during adjuvant chemotherapy, if they would have a shorter time to relapse, and reduced overall survival. It was shown that self-reported comorbidity was not associated with toxicity, or breast cancer relapse, regardless of treatment (standard/capecitabine).

However, having four or more comorbid conditions was associated with shorter overall survival. Although this study was based on a randomized controlled trial design—which is considered to be the gold standard for clinical trials—even this study was not without limitations. For example, the authors acknowledged that the analyses were restricted to a selected population of women healthy enough to receive chemotherapy, which might contribute to a lower comorbidity burden at baseline. In unselected real world patients, some adjustments of chemotherapy regimen may be necessary to reduce toxicity. Here, an additional observational cohort study might provide insight in the treatment outcomes of women who are not fit enough to receive standard regimen.

In conclusion, no study design is perfect. Choosing a study design should be primarily guided by the research question one aims to answer, taking into account the pros and cons of the design.

12.3 Study Population—Tensions Between Homogeneity, Reproducibility and Recruitment

In studies evaluating an intervention, like randomized controlled trials, **homogeneous** study populations are often recruited, to enable more specific effect estimates and narrower confidence intervals. Historically, older patients have been underrepresented in clinical trials, as have been patients with (severe) comorbidity [7]. This is also true for trials evaluating cancer treatments [8, 9]. This approach, however, comes at the cost of a decreased possibility to generalize study results. As a result, there is a serious lack of information on both the efficacy and the effectiveness of cancer treatment in patients with comorbidity, as well as a lack of information regarding safety and adverse events of cancer treatment in this population. But also, other questions regarding burden of treatment, quality of survival, and acceptability of treatment in a vulnerable (older) population of cancer patients with comorbidity remain largely unanswered.

Trying to find answers to important research questions relating to the effectiveness of treatment, safety, and acceptability of treatment in more heterogeneous study populations is often jeopardized by the difficult **recruitment** of cancer patients with comorbidity. This has been identified as a major challenge in research with older cancer patients [20, 21]. Low inclusion rates have been attributed to limited physical and cognitive capacity of the patient, and insufficient awareness of the study by the treating physicians [21]. From the patients' perspective, barriers to participation included feeling too anxious (40 %) or being not interested (25 %) [22]. In this respect, it is important to carefully plan the moment of recruitment, e.g. after the treatment plan is explained to the patient, when the first wave of anxiety has decreased. A number of other strategies have been recommended to help overcome age- and health-related barriers to participation [21–23]:

- Providing information about the study in a written form, but always ensuring it is explained face-to-face as well
- Including family members in the recruitment process; often they are concerned about the burden it will place on the patient
- Informing and regularly reminding the entire hospital staff of the study
- Researchers being present in the clinics as much as possible to reinforce the reminders when the physicians see their patients
- Performing data collection face-to-face while the patient is hospitalized, during ambulatory care, or at home visits, ensuring no extra burden for the patients. If this is not feasible, ensure at least one face-to-face contact at the start of the study, so that the patient knows who is going to call them
- Keeping the length of the interview acceptable (less than one hour)
- Being flexible to reschedule interviews if the patient is not feeling well or if hospital appointments are postponed
- Using the same interviewer as much as possible, also for follow-up data collection
- Only providing a self-administered questionnaire if it is agreed with the patient that this is feasible.

Unfortunately, these strategies require considerable time and effort, which makes these types of studies even more expensive [21, 22].

12.4 Data Sources—Overcoming Silos

Although older people with comorbid conditions have been underrepresented in clinical cancer trials [8, 9], it is virtually impossible to do all cancer trials again given the heterogeneity of the population. Countless combinations of age cohorts with different combinations of comorbidity types and stages of cancer are possible. Therefore, the necessity arises to broaden the scope of research in comorbidity of cancer beyond studies collecting mere primary data.

Other available data sources collected for different purposes come to play as well. Information on diseases and other relevant measures can be collected using different methods and different resources, each with their own strengths and limitations.

1. **Patient self-reported**. Methods to collect data directly from the patients are written or digital questionnaires, telephone or face-to-face interviews, using either closed or open-ended questions. This method of data collection is gathering information directly from the person under study, but the validity of information has to be taken into account. For clearly defined and more serious diseases, such as diabetes, myocardial infarction and also cancer, patient self-reports have high levels of agreement compared to physician-registered morbidity. However, for other diseases like rheumatoid arthritis, migraine, and

chronic back problems, the agreement between patients and primary care physicians is limited [24]. This general problem may arise from the distinct representation of medical problems in patients and health professionals: physicians' representation is mostly (data) driven, by biomedical knowledge underlying the disease (disease model), whereas patients' representation is frequently based on narrative structures, the social and moral meaning attached to the dysfunction of the body which involves the disruption of the patient's normal life (illness model) [25, 26]. Patients with cancer might overestimate or underestimate the presence of other diseases unconsciously, because of presumed associations between cancer and e.g. cardiovascular disease or certain life styles. Also, mental illness might cause patients to be more prone to recall or reporter bias than other somatic disease, due to cognitive or emotional dysfunction, experiences of taboo, shame or social desirability. Also, the accuracy of recall may be an important source of bias, depending on the time frame and subject and should be considered in the selection of data sources, the choice of measurement and the interpretation of results.

2. **Clinician reported**, usually written/digital. Clinical reports are likely to be accurate about treatments and issues related to the condition of interest, but clinicians may not be aware of, or may under-report, other health issues [27].
3. **Electronic medical records** are valuable data sources and are often considered 'gold standard'. A major advantage of medical records is that they are a good representation of daily practice, assuming that physicians keep written or digital track of their patient population. In case of longitudinal studies covering a large time-window, retrospective information going back into the 20th century might be less comprehensive, but increasingly electronic patient records are the norm and minimal data sets are increasingly required, also for refunding purposes. An important pitfall of medical records is that the quality of documentation may vary and that the information included is often strongly related to the reason for encounter. Further, the primary consideration of medical specialists is naturally related to the subjects of their discipline, whereas documentation of information on conditions that are out of scope might be lacking. In some countries, such as the UK and the Netherlands, where the general practitioner acts as a gate keeper in health care, the use of medical records from general practice might therefore provide the most comprehensive medical information.
4. **Research practice networks** are increasingly common. In various Western countries, like the Netherlands, Belgium and the UK, where the vast majority of individuals are registered with a single general practice, *registration* networks continuously collect data about routine consultations such as the General Practice Research Database in UK. Data are extracted directly from the clinical record utilizing a combination of clinical codes and free text comments. Their strengths include large population sizes, longitudinal follow up, and cost avoiding the need to contact patients directly [28–31]. In some registration networks, hybrid data from medical records and annual questionnaires for research purposes are collected such as the Study into Medical Information and Lifestyle (SMILE) in Eindhoven attached to the Maastricht University [32].

5. **Cancer registries** or extensive cohorts of patients diagnosed with cancer are available and often contain sufficient medical information to analyze the influence of comorbidity on cancer related outcomes [33, 34] and can be linked to hospitalization data [35] but facilities may vary widely between countries. Some cohorts specifically focus on other domains, such as sociodemographic and psychosocial evolutions [36]. Taking into account privacy legislation, possibilities to link databases are increasingly common [37] sometimes even encompassing several databases [38].
6. **Administrative databases**, such as claims data from health care insurers usually cover large numbers of patients and contain very structured information. These databases are convenient for surveillance of survival and mortality [39], morbidity [40], recurrence rates [41], and treatment effects [42]. The main limitation of this type of databases is the lack of clinical, lifestyle and demographic data [42]. Also, it is recognized that routinely collected databases may underestimate the prevalence and incidence of comorbidity, because databases were not originally designed for research purposes and may suffer from incomplete coding, especially in the earlier years [37]. Additionally, information collected for reimbursement purposes may be distorted—in particular, where financial incentives may have unintended consequences such as fraudulence coding [43].

Given the enormous resources and costs which are spent to collect primary data and given the pitfalls in data documented for other than research purposes, activities to provide and share data sets of completed studies for secondary analyses should be a core research consideration in patients with cancer and chronic comorbidity [44]. Patients with comorbidity are frequently (but not always) excluded in cancer trials and under-reporting of comorbidity may pretend a distorted picture that no evidence is available for this patient group. However, individual patient data meta-analyses in large data sets may identify subgroups of sufficient sample size to answer questions of comparative effectiveness and harms in patients with cancer and high prevalent comorbidity, such as cardiovascular disease. Similarly, data exchange between cancer registries or administrative data bases may support research in patients with cancer and comorbidity of low prevalence in future but safety concerns of patients and stakeholders as well as technical challenges of the connection of data bases differing in structure have to be overcome [45–47].

12.5 Measures of Comorbidity—From Simple Count to Cancer Specific Index

There are many comorbidity measures available, developed for different purposes, each with their own flaws and benefits. Some list diseases separately, with or without weighing of the diseases, some present aggregate measures, and in the case of comorbidity of cancer many studies describe specific combinations (i.e. cancer plus specific chronic condition). Conditions taken into account in an index may be psychological or somatic, complaints or diagnoses, chronic or acute, including or excluding social aspects and functional status. Finally, there are proxy based indices, e.g. counting the number of chronic medications [48] or scoring of selected patterns of prescriptions such as the Chronic Disease Score (CDS) [49].

In many observational studies **comorbidity** can act as a serious **confounder**. When a large number of comorbid diseases may be relevant to take into account, controlling for individual comorbid diseases may not be practical for methodological reasons, including loss of power. Furthermore, it may be more appropriate to control for the overall burden of comorbidity, rather than the individual effect of each comorbid disease. In their systematic review Yurkovich et al. [42] showed that for specific applications (e.g. with cancer patients) often new indices were developed or existing indices were adapted for the use in specific patient groups.

Many different comorbidity indices have been **validated for various outcomes**, most often mortality or hospitalization, but only few have been tested in a population of (older) cancer patients. Lee et al. [34] evaluated the impact on management and prediction of outcomes in patients with oral squamous cell carcinoma (OSCC) using ECIS and CCIS. Mayr et al. [50] evaluated five comorbidity indices assessed preoperatively in patients with bladder cancer, scheduled to have a radical cystectomy. All five appeared to be predictive for cancer-independent mortality, but none of them predicted cancer specific mortality, when adjusting for other relevant characteristics (age, sex and cancer severity indicators).

Fröhner and Wirth [51] described the impact of comorbidity in patients with early prostate cancer and suggested a classification of relevant comorbidity for this patient group; comorbid diseases have **prognostic and clinical relevance, i.e. be associated with an increased mortality risk**. Furthermore, in order to be clinically relevant, these diseases should have a considerable impact on survival time and should occur rather frequently. Also Briganti et al. [52] studied the survival of patients with prostate cancer, taking into account type and severity of comorbidity.

Furthermore, definitions of comorbidity should both inform and reflect clinical practice. This objective may be difficult to achieve when epidemiology oriented definitions are less inclusive and aim at a limited set of clear-cut criteria. For 'diseases' with varying latency or a chronic course, developing a definition depends on decisions regarding the phase to monitor—asymptomatic, early disease, late disease—and the circumscription of the spectrum of morbidity [15]. Each of these definitions as Rothman et al. argue, would measure different segments of the population, each would have strengths and limitations, and each would require a unique approach, data source and monitoring system.

Moreover, it is important to distinguish comorbidity from **complications of cancer**. When complications are not considered separately, the total comorbidity burden will be overestimated [53]. This distinction is, however, not always evident: cancer and its treatments are well-recognized risk factors for venous thromboembolism (VTE), but not all VTEs in cancer patients are due to cancer treatment [54]. This underlines the relevance to distinguish between general susceptibility and disease related susceptibility/complications when analyzing comorbidity [55].

There are a number of studies to describe the **co-occurrence of diseases known to share risk factors**. Gottlieb et al. describe the prevalence of pulmonary comorbidity among patients with lung and head and neck cancer [56]. Knowing comorbidity that is pathophysiologically related to the index disease (such as COPD and lung cancer) and optimizing the treatment of comorbid diseases could influence interventions tested.

Below, some examples of indices and other measurements of comorbidity are specified and commented:

The **Charlson comorbidity index** (CCI) [57] is probably the most commonly used and cited comorbidity index. The National Cancer Institute comorbidity index was developed as an adaptation of the CCI [58]. However, the validation of the CCI was based on a relatively small cohort of general medical patients and was executed nearly 30 years ago. The CCI includes conditions that may not have an impact on survival among patients with cancer nowadays, because of substantial improvements in management (e.g. peptic ulcer disease), and it does not incorporate some that evidently have such impact (e.g. noncerebrovascular neurological conditions) [40]. Another limitation of the CCI is that it does not take into account some disorders that might affect prognosis or evolution of quality of life in cancer patients, like Parkinsonism, blood transfusions, transplantations, thromboses, lung embolisms, and angina pectoris [59]. Furthermore, Streiner and Norman [60] state that for a valid comorbidity index inclusion of as many relevant items (diseases) as possible, is more important than the weighting of individual conditions.

Also, **cancer specific** indices have been developed. The **C3 Index** [40] was developed as a cancer specific index using data from over 14,000 cancer patients, aiming to include all conditions that were likely to have an impact on functional status or length of life among cancer patients. They include conditions from other indices and conditions that were mentioned as relevant by clinical experts. The C3 index assesses the presence of 42 chronic conditions in five years previous to the diagnosis of cancer. Conditions are weighted to their impact on non-cancer mortality among cancer patients and then summed to arrive at an aggregated score. The C3 Index outperformed the CCI for the combined cancer types. The C3 Index was also used to evaluate of the impact of comorbidity on the stage of cancer at diagnosis [35]. Results indicated that (1) the presence of comorbidity increased the odds of a patient being diagnosed with distant metastases, (2) did not lead to earlier diagnosis, and (3) increased the likelihood of a patient receiving no staging of disease at diagnosis. The latter finding might be related to the fact that in case of severe comorbidity and hence poor prognosis, the clinician might decide not to extend diagnostics.

Guo et al. [61] assessed the prognostic value of the **Adult Comorbidity Evaluation-27** (ACE-27), which was also developed for patients with cancer, on the course and prognosis of nasopharyngeal carcinoma. They found increasing levels of accurateness in patients with higher stages of cancer.

Apart from prognostic indices which predict hospitalization or death, other indices have been developed which differ in the selection of included diseases. For example, prognostic indices usually include asymptomatic but prognosis limiting diseases, such as hypertension but frequently exclude diseases without a short-term impact on mortality, such as osteoarthritis or mental illnesses other than dementia [57]. On the other hand, osteoarthritis may have a severe impact on physical functioning and mental illnesses on emotional or social well-being and all together may significantly reduce quality of life. Therefore, indices to predict other outcomes than mortality or health services utilization are needed. Recently, the **health-related quality of life comorbidity index** (HRQL-CI) has been developed and validated by Mukherjee et al. [62], using diseases that have the strongest association with health-related quality of life. Furthermore, Lorem et al. developed a comorbidity index named the health impact index, using **self-rated health** (SRH) as an outcome [63].

Bender et al. [64] evaluated the presence of **symptom clusters** in patients who have cancer as a comorbid disease to other chronic conditions. Their **Comorbidity Questionnaire** is a self-reported measure based on the CCI and modeled to assess conditions and symptoms.

The diversity of available measures reflects the fact that there is no single measure which satisfies all needs. Depending on the available data sources and the purpose for which the measure is intended, in research, comorbidity measure should be careful selected. Moreover, indices are often context-dependent from the characteristics of the population where they were derived from and underlie a change over time due to improved survival in conditions, changed (drug) treatments, and the overall demographic change. Therefore, indices such as the CDS have been adapted to certain populations and over time [65, 66] and others, such as the CCI may be outperformed by newer indices. However, it is increasingly popular to develop prognostic models and caution is needed about their methodological appropriateness in development and validation [67, 68].

12.6 Outcomes—Disease Related and Patient Related

The choice of appropriate outcome measures depends on a variety of factors, primarily on the main research question, feasibility, and methodological issues, such as study design and setting. Outcome measures shall be sensitive to changes, e.g. to detect pre- and post-intervention differences. These general requirements meet a number of challenges in patients with comorbidity such as confounding. Moreover, certain comorbidity may preclude the application of outcome measures such as the application of a questionnaire on cancer specific quality of life in patients with cognitive dysfunction. Apart from methodological issues, the key question is about the relevance of the outcome for patients. In patients with co- and multimorbidity, health outcomes shift from disease-specific to generic and patient's values often swing from life expectancy to quality of life. Desired outcomes, such as symptom relief, preservation of physical, mental, and social functioning, or disease prevention are often of equal importance as the avoidance of undesired outcomes such as nausea, drowsiness, dizziness, lethargy, or confusion [69–71]. Considering this, research should provide effect estimates on efficacy/effectiveness with respect to a full range of holistic, cross-disease outcomes and should also provide sufficient information on potential harms. This evidence would support weighing of potential benefits and harms in decision making with patients with cancer and co-occurring conditions.

Studies that focus on comorbidity as the outcome have often investigated the association between cancer and susceptibility to subsequent comorbidity. In this respect, cancer has been suggested as an indicator of aging, showing through an increased susceptibility to comorbidity, also for young cancer survivors [72]. Studies that focus on comorbidity as a confounding factor generally focused on the effect of comorbidity on treatment decisions (e.g. treatment choices and adherence to clinical guidelines) and cancer-related outcomes (e.g. treatment tolerance, 5-year survival) [73].

Survival/mortality. When analyzing mortality after a certain treatment, comorbidity is an essential patient characteristic which has to be taken into account [37]. Moreover, attention should be paid to different time windows and specific comorbid conditions. Tovikkai et al. [37] showed changes in prevalence of comorbid conditions dependent on the study era, but also showed different effects in different time windows after liver transplantation, where chronic renal disease tended to be related to a short term (first 90 days) increase of mortality, whereas dementia seemed to be associated with an increased mortality after 5 years.

When different patient populations or clinical settings are considered the survival probabilities may differ significantly between patients with apparently identical levels of comorbidities [51].

Delay of the diagnosis of cancer/stage of cancer at diagnosis. Comorbidity has an impact on cancer stage at diagnosis, but until now findings regarding this subject are ambiguous, and there are explanations for both positive and negative relations. People with comorbidity in general have an increased number of contacts to health services, which may result in a so-called surveillance effect, leading to earlier diagnosis. On the other hand, comorbidity may also distract both the physician and the patient from early signs and symptoms of cancer, resulting in a diagnostic delay [35]. In case of severe comorbidity that causes a serious limitation of life expectancy, diagnostics do not always appear warranted. Finally, specific conditions or their treatments can have a direct influence on cancer growth [74]. When further analyzing this, also other characteristics have to be taken into account, because patients with more comorbid diseases are in general also older, more often female, and tend to have lower socio-economic status. Also, when relating summary measures of comorbidity to staging colorectal cancer at diagnosis, results are conflicting [75].

Treatment decisions/prognosis/recurrence of cancer. Comorbidity can have an important impact on the treatment decision making process for patients with cancer [76], e.g. in the administration of radiotherapy and chemotherapy [77]. Even though this is relevant and frequently applied in clinical practice, it is not common practice in oncology research.

Patient related outcome measures (PROMs). Of the PROMs, the most commonly applied are quality of life, functional status, and disease burden/treatment burden [78]. Quality of life measurement tools can be divided into generic tools and disease specific instruments. Generic quality of life tools can be used for all patient groups, irrespective the absence of presence of e.g. cancer. An important advantage of generic instruments is the generalizability of the results, allowing the comparison of quality of life in patients with different diseases, or diseases in different stages. Generic quality of life instruments usually cover multiple domains, possibly including less relevant domains when applied to patients with cancer. At the same time those general instruments are potentially lacking details on other relevant domains, such as side effects of e.g. chemotherapy. A subgroup of the generic quality of life instruments are the utility generating tools, to assess cost-effectiveness from a societal perspective, expressed quality adjusted life years (QALYs) [79]. Disease-specific quality of life measures contain domains relevant to that disease. In oncology the most commonly applied disease-specific quality of life tools are the EORTC QLQ-C30 [80] and the FACT-scale [81]. However, these instruments have been mainly designed for patients with advanced disease stages and may have limitations when applied to patients with localized disease [82]. For use in patients with localized prostate cancer, Schmidt and co-workers identified eight instruments, but only three out of eight instruments showed a good performance regarding development process, metric properties, and administrative issues [82]. To assist the selection of instruments, Valderas et al. developed a tool for the standardized assessment of patient-reported outcomes (EMPRO) [83].

12.7 Statistical Analyses of Longitudinal Data

Statistical analysis of cancer research data encompasses an extensive spectrum of methods and software tools for analysis and reporting. These methods and analyses also apply to oncological studies encompassing comorbidity:

- Measures of cancer burden (incidence, prevalence, mortality, and survival);
- Therapeutic endpoints in the various phases of oncology clinical trials, from phase I, phase II, up to phase III trials;
- Validation of biomarkers in diagnosis and prognosis of cancer;
- Overall and net survival, relative survival ratio, excess mortality hazard;
- Survival of cancer with the relative survival design, including cohort, complete, period, and hybrid approaches;
- Methods of handling missing data and data quality; and
- Estimation of avoidable deaths and personal or population "cure".

Examples of resources on cancer statistics include the National Cancer Institute's (NCI) overview of SEER tools (SEER stands for Surveillance, Epidemiology, and End Results Program) [84] the International Agency for Research on Cancer

(IARC) [85] and handbooks of statistics in oncology, such as Crowley and Hoering [85]. These resources provide overview of and insight in the tools and methods to analyze incidence, mortality, survival, prevalence, and other related cancer statistics. If no follow-up data are available, linear and logistic regression analysis of outcomes are standard techniques for describing the relationship between an exposure variable and an outcome variable. Comorbidity can be used both as input and output to such modelling, for which the reader is referred to the literature.

The emphasis here is on cancer and comorbidity from a **longitudinal** perspective. On the one hand, attention is paid to studies with the availability of short-term and long-term follow-up information on cancer patients. On the other hand, when cancer and comorbidities are considered from a chronic disease perspective, whence there is a need to monitor the late effects of the disease and the treatment as well as the potentially negative neurocognitive, somatic and psychosocial outcomes of cancer survivors [86]. It is, perhaps, overstated to claim that statistics in oncology research is more complex and time consuming compared to other therapeutic areas. However, it is true that the analysis of longitudinal data, and especially survival data (time to event), is inherently difficult. Nonetheless, taking cancer and comorbidity into account significantly complicates statistical analyses through:

- Skewed and non-normal distributed data;
- Dependence between longitudinal clinical data and cancer outcomes;
- Competing causes of death;
- Different illness trajectories.

Skewed and non-normal distributed data: survival analysis is in many ways like conventional statistical analyses: information is gathered on the outcome or response variable on the one hand and covariates of interest on the other hand. It differs, however, in a very intricate aspect: the event of interest may not occur for each subject under study. Not all subjects will experience the outcome during the course of observation, resulting in the absence of a time-to-event for that particular individual. This situation is referred to as censoring in the analysis of survival data, and a study subject for whom no time-to-event is available is called censored. A typical situation is one in which a survival study has to end due to, for example, time constraints or resource limitations. In this case, for subjects whose survival events have not occurred at the end of the study, their survival times are not observed exactly but are known to be greater than the end of the study end time i.e., they are right-censored. For subjects who have already had the event at the end of the study, the time-to-event is known exactly. In essence, censoring implicates that an observation on a survival time of interest is incomplete; the survival time is observed only to fall into a certain range instead of being known exactly. Censored data are different from missing data as censored observations still provide partial information, whereas missing observations provide no information about the variable of interest. Different types of censoring arise in practice, but the one that receives most of the attention in the literature is right censoring [87].

Censored data analysis requires special methods to compensate for the information lost by not knowing the time of failure of all subjects. In addition, survival data analysis must account for skewed data [88]. Some individuals will experience the event of interest much sooner or later than the majority of individuals under study, giving the overall distribution of failure times a skewed appearance and preventing the use of the normal distribution in the analysis. Mostly, logarithmic transformations are used to stabilize the variance and allow for non-symmetric confidence intervals. Thus, the analysis of survival data requires techniques that are able to incorporate the possibility of skewed and censored observations. The reader is referred to the many excellent books and reviews of the major approaches in survival analysis: the parametric approach (e.g. exponential model, the Weibull model, the log-normal and logistic models), the non-parametric approach (e.g. the log-rank test), and the semi-parametric approach, e.g. the Cox proportional hazard model, perhaps the most widely used model in in clinical survival analysis [88, 89].

Dependence between longitudinal clinical data and cancer outcomes: Complicating it even more, standard statistical tools for the analysis of censored observations assume random censoring: event time and censoring time should be **independent**. However, in reality this might not be the case. A negative association between censoring and event time could occur when patients who are entering the study later have a better prognosis due to increased experience of surgeons. A positive association between censoring and event time occurs when patients are leaving the study because their health status is getting worse.

When event time and censoring time are not independent, the proportional hazards assumption of the commonly used Cox proportional hazard model does not hold. Several approaches exist to overcome this problem by extending the Cox proportional hazard model. One possible approach is to stratify a patient group, according to the values of some variable, mostly a variable which is considered a confounder rather than the main exposure of interest, e.g. comorbidity. The effect of the confounder is not estimated, but its effects are controlled for. An example is a study evaluating the therapeutic effects of intraperitoneal chemotherapy in which comorbidity is used as confounder variable [90]. A second approach is to include an exposure-time interaction term; that is to model the dynamic behavior of time-dependent variables. The third approach is to split the follow-up time into different periods. The latter puts emphasis on an important aspect of survival analysis: the choice of the time axis, because risks sets of patients will correspond to the choices made. The fourth approach is to model the complex changes over time itself, for example, by choosing one of the many available parametric models. Such models may be of particular use when the aim is to predict survival probabilities in different groups. If multiple pathologies are considered, which may have a distinct time scale, then such an approach might be conceivable. This is a technical and complex issue, for which the reader is referred to the specialized literature [91]. Van Houwelingen and Putter [92] show that within a short-term scope of the study the violations of the survival models are limited and small, whereas the effects will show up in large studies with long follow up.

This becomes more intricate, when addressing issues of variability in treatment response and chances of complete remission in patients with cancer, particularly when addressing **heterogeneous** patient populations, such as patients with comorbidity.

Competing causes of death: The literature on these combined or joint models is extensive and good examples are described by Fieuws et al. [93] and Brant et al. [94]. Studies including comorbidity or multimorbidity in such models are scarce. A notable exception is a study by Bayliss et al. [33] who analyzed a cohort of 6500 adults with initial cancer diagnosis between 2001 and 2008, SEER 5-year survival probability equal to or greater than 26 %, and a range of cardiovascular comorbidities. They modeled the competing risks by comparing different, cause-specific Cox proportional hazard models. Following cancer diagnosis, it was shown that 15.3 % of causes of death were attributed to cancer deaths, 5.1 % to serious cardiovascular deaths and 8.3 % of death from other causes. Thus, it was shown that in oncology populations, comorbidities interact to affect the competing risks of different outcomes. Another example is the nationwide, cohort study by Erichsen et al. [95], with 56,963 colorectal cancer (CRC) patients and five times as many patients from the general population (N = 271,670) matched by age, gender, and specific comorbidities. Among CRC patients with low comorbidity scores the 0-1 year mortality rate was 415 out of 1000-person-years (95 % CI: 401;430) and the interaction estimating the excess mortality rate in patients with both CRC and comorbidity accounts for 9.3 % of this rate. For patients with a severe comorbidity score the interaction consists of 34 % of the mortality. The interaction between CRC and comorbidity limited influence on mortality beyond 1 year after diagnosis, except again for the interaction between colorectal cancer and a high comorbidity burden accounting for 14 % of mortality 2-5 year after diagnosis. In sum, the authors showed that comorbidity interacts with colorectal cancer to increase the rate of mortality beyond that explained by the independent effects of CRC and comorbid conditions.

This shows that when taking comorbidity into account one often faces the problem of **competing causes of death**; the patient group under study may be more likely to die from complications due to the comorbid condition rather than due to the cancer [96–98]. Binbing et al. described a method to estimate the **personal cure rate** of cancer patients using population-based grouped cancer survival data [99]. Cancer patients are subject to multiple competing risks of death and may die from causes other than the cancer diagnosed. The probability of not dying from the cancer diagnosed, which is one of the patients' main concerns, is sometimes called the "personal cure" rate. Binbing et al. [99] used two approaches of modelling competing-risk survival data, namely cause-specific hazards approach, and the mixture model approach. The authors used the colorectal survival data from the SEER Programme of the NCI (N = 199,715 colorectal cancer patients diagnosed between 1975 and 2002), with a maximum follow-up time of 28 years. They applied the models in particular, because comorbidity for cancer patients may limit treatments and increases the risk of death from other causes. Usually comorbidity from competing causes increases with advancing age and is greater for patients in poor health.

The above shows that statistical analysis of cancer survival data is a delicate issue by itself. The study of the intricate relationships between cancer—occurrence as well as recurrence—and comorbidity, complicates statistical analysis in various ways. The integration of comorbidity in the statistical analysis in cancer research emphasizes the need for:

- The multi-adjustment of cancer survival not only for age, stage, and other cancer-related factors, but also for the co-occurring diseases
- Multi-variable modelling of the excess hazard of death (due to comorbidity)
- The comparison with different statistical tools, e.g. with Cox and Poisson approaches. The analysis of heterogeneity, variability and chance of health risks in various subgroups (stratified according to age, sex, and comorbidity). Some subjects might be more prone or more likely to experience an event. Normally, in most clinical applications, survival analysis implicitly assumes a homogeneous population to be studied. This means that all individuals sampled in that study are subject, in principle, to the same risk (e.g., risk of death and risk of disease recurrence). In many applications, the study population cannot be assumed to be homogeneous but must be considered as a heterogeneous sample, i.e., a mixture of individuals with different hazards. For example, in many cases, it is impossible to measure all relevant covariates related to the disease of interest [98, 100, 101] and special approaches are required to include heterogeneity in the analysis, e.g. different forms of frailty models [100, 102].

Taking into account the illness trajectory: In longitudinal study approaches data on patient characteristics, clinical data, and survival data are frequently collected simultaneously. For example, in many medical studies, clinical researchers collect patients' information (e.g. blood pressures, X-ray measures) repeatedly over time and they are also interested in the time to recovery, recurrence of a disease (i.e. cancer) or death.

As such, **longitudinal approaches** are becoming increasingly important. Longitudinal approaches can be subdivided in:

1. Adaptive designs
2. Reciprocal designs: randomized clinical trial methodologies, e.g. potential clinical outcome model, causal modelling, propensity stratification integrated within observational studies; observational methodologies integrated within oncology trials [103]
3. Trajectories: population-based and personalized trajectories.

Longitudinal clinical data and survival data are often associated in several ways, with the time to event (death) being associated with the longitudinal trajectories of clinical characteristics. Separate analyses of longitudinal clinical data and survival data may lead to inefficient and biased results as they do not take the underlying relationship between one another into account. In these settings, the multivariate longitudinal profiles and the event information need to be combined. Several methods have been proposed to combine longitudinal clinical data with event history data (e.g. survival, recurrence) [104, 105]. Most statistical methods, such as linear regression models, logistic regression models and survival models, are based on the assumption that the observations in a sample are independent of each other and that is the value of one observation is not influenced by the value of another. This **assumption of independence** will be violated if the data are clustered. **Clustering or correlation** is at hand, if observations in one cluster tend to be more similar to each other than in the rest of the sample. Clustered data usually arise when subjects are grouped, e.g. in cluster randomized trials of general practices or hospitals, family studies or cluster sampled surveys. Also when subjects are repeatedly measured as in longitudinal studies there are often clustered data (within subjects, e.g. the repeated measurement of blood pressure). In analyzing clustered data, connectedness of data has to be taken into account by aggregating data, or applying advanced statistical methods such as Generalized Estimating Equations or random effect models [106]. More information on these advanced statistical methods can, for example, be found in Hox [107] or Hox and Roberts [108].

Patients with comorbidity may face different **illness trajectories**, an important aspect of disease that is often neglected in current research. While a great deal of literature concerns the prediction of risk and the prognosis of co-occurring diseases in patients with multimorbidity, relatively little research is concerned with the course or "**trajectory**" of the illness of patients with multimorbidity [109]. Most multimorbidity studies focus on the identification of specific disease combinations in patient populations, based on one index disease and additional diseases, either in general or specific population-based studies or in administrative databases. In recent years a few studies investigated **multimorbidity patterns**, using data mining techniques, e.g. factor analysis methods, to investigate clusters of diseases. However, these studies are cross-sectional and investigate prevalence patterns in specific age groups, and restrict comorbidities to lists of common chronic conditions [110, 111].

Few studies have analyzed such multimorbidity patterns integrated with cancer as one of the health conditions. Islam et al. [112], reported three important multimorbidity patterns, one of which included cancer, coronary heart disease and stroke. Vos et al. [109] showed that 49 % of patients with more than ten chronic health conditions had at least one diagnosis of cancer during the course of their life. Jensen et al. [113], investigated a population-wide registry data, covering 6.2 million cancer patients of Denmark, and showed distinct disease development patterns for different types of cancer. For example, they showed a clustering of malignant neoplasms of the prostate and secondary malignant neoplasms of other sites. However, research on disease trajectories is rather limited and more research into the patterns and relating characteristics for different types of cancer as well different age and gender groups is needed.

With the growing population of patients with cancer together with other chronic health conditions [114], **integrative analysis** of cancer and multimorbidity is urgent. Two major challenges are open. One is to connect multimorbidity research with the rapid developments in integrative cancer data analysis; cancer informatics; and high-dimensional data analysis [115]. The other challenge is to elaborate and implement a longitudinal approach, from a clinical and a family practice perspective. Studies of multimorbidity patterns over long time periods are scarce [109, 116].

The concept of distinct trajectories of illness over time is well established in other advanced diseases [117, 118]. Longitudinal analysis of multimorbidity, however, is complex. Varying definitions of multimorbidity exist and different scopes of time windows are abound. If a research time-frame is short, a point in time (time independent, cross-sectional) comorbidity measure is sufficient. Many studies are longitudinal, raising questions how best to measure comorbidity over time [39]. Different approaches are available to model and analyze the multiple events and multiple pathways in these trajectories [87, 105].

The new developments include time-dependent covariates, recurrent events, quantile regression in identifying important prognostic factors for patient subpopulations and joint modelling such as quality of life and time to event data. Similarly, there is an explosion in new areas of statistics, such as space and time modelling, which might help to track an individual's lifetime exposure while taking into account other clinically relevant histories, or track an individual's access to cancer screening or treatment services. There is a rather large literature on Bayesian methods for survival data [89, 119]. It is not possible to do justice here to Bayesian methods and the many computational advances of recent years.

12.8 Recommendations for Future Research

- Hospitals and research institutes should actively seek collaboration to join expertise and facilitate large epidemiological studies that include patients with different comorbid diseases, or disease patterns. This can also facilitate more efficient recruitment of patients.
- Evidence on comparative effectiveness and safety of treatment in patients with cancer and comorbidity is needed and serious efforts should be made to share data of completed trials to conduct individual patient data meta-analyses and investigate subpopulations of sufficient sample size.
- More input from patients in research is required, e.g. involvement in writing patient information or in developing strategies to recruit patients.
- Research should further elicit the construction of patient's preferences and the process of prioritization of conditions and treatments in patients with cancer and multiple disorders.
- Comorbidity should always be taken into account, because of the proven impact on diagnostics, therapeutic decisions, psychosocial needs, and other needs during follow-up care. Furthermore, comorbidity as well as cancer are related to aging, and both are increasingly considered chronic health status, underlining the importance of studying the two as combined concepts.

- When studying cancer and comorbidity, it is relevant to distinguish between complications of cancer regimen (long-term and late effects of treatments) and comorbidity.

12.9 Conclusions

Comorbidity is frequent in clinical practice amongst patients with cancer, but in scientific research too often comorbidity is ignored or methods are applied that insufficiently take into account comorbidity. It is, however, of vital importance to recognize the impact of comorbidity on a broad spectrum of outcomes when studying patients with cancer and comorbidity. Though complex to handle, ignoring or avoiding comorbidity in research is not an option.

The population of patients with cancer and comorbid conditions is a heterogeneous group. If it is decided to focus on a more homogeneous subgroup, results are more specific, but lack external validity and generalizability to the heterogeneous group of cancer patients.

Recruitment of (older) patients with cancer and comorbidity is a major challenge. Strategies to improve recruitment come at considerable costs because they require a substantial increase in time and efforts.

There is no single comorbidity measure available that satisfies all needs. A measure should be selected taking into account the research question, the available data sources, and the context of the study (e.g. community setting, nursing home, hospital).

Statistical analyses of studies encompassing oncological patients with comorbidity should reckon with complexity due to skewedness and non-normality of data, dependence between longitudinal clinical data and cancer related outcomes, competing causes of death and individual illness trajectories.

References

1. Deckx L, van den Akker M, Metsemakers J, Knottnerus A, Schellevis F, Buntinx F (2012) Chronic diseases among older cancer survivors. J Cancer Epidemiol 2012:206414
2. Smith AW, Reeve BB, Bellizzi KM, Harlan LC, Klabunde CN, Amsellem M, Bierman AS, Hays RD (2008) Cancer, comorbidities, and health-related quality of life of older adults. Health Care Financ Rev 29(4):41–56
3. Khan NF, Mant D, Carpenter L, Forman D, Rose PW (2011) Long-term health outcomes in a British cohort of breast, colorectal and prostate cancer survivors: a database study. Br J Cancer 105(Suppl 1):S29–S37
4. Ording AG, Horvath-Puho E, Lash TL, Ehrenstein V, Borre M, Vyberg M, Sorensen HT (2015) Prostate cancer, comorbidity, and the risk of venous thromboembolism: a cohort study of 44,035 Danish prostate cancer patients, 1995–2011. Cancer 121(20):3692–3699

5. Stewart S, Ekman I, Ekman T, Oden A, Rosengren A (2010) Population impact of heart failure and the most common forms of cancer: a study of 1 162 309 hospital cases in Sweden (1988 to 2004). Circ Cardiovasc Qual Outcomes 3(6):573–580
6. Quinn M, Babb P, Brock A (2001) Chronic heart failure: management of chronic heart failure in adults in primary and secondary care (CG108). In: Cancer trends in England and Wales 1950–1999. NICE National Institute for Health + Clinical Excellence, AHRQ Agency for Healthcare Research + Quality, The Stationary Office, London. Available from http://guidance.nice.org.uk/CG108
7. Shenoy P, Harugeri A (2015) Elderly patients' participation in clinical trials. Perspect Clin Res 6(4):184–189
8. Hutchins LF, Unger JM, Crowley JJ, Coltman CA Jr, Albain KS (1999) Underrepresentation of patients 65 years of age or older in cancer-treatment trials. N Engl J Med 341 (27):2061–2067
9. Mohile S, Dale W, Magnuson A, Kamath N, Hurria A (2013) Research priorities in geriatric oncology for 2013 and beyond. Cancer Forum 37(3):216–221
10. Balducci L, Fossa SD (2013) Rehabilitation of older cancer patients. Acta Oncol 52 (2):233–238
11. Reuben D, Tinetti M (2012) Goal-oriented patient care—an alternative health outcomes paradigm. N Engl J Med 366(9):777–779
12. Blom JW, El Azzi M, Wopereis DM, Glynn L, Muth C, van Driel ML (2015) Reporting of patient-centred outcomes in heart failure trials: are patient preferences being ignored? Heart Fail Rev 20(4):385–392
13. Millman J, Galway K, Santin O, Reid J (2016) Cancer and serious mental illness—patient, caregiver and professional perspectives: study protocol. J Adv Nurs 72(1):217–226
14. Sada YH, Street RL Jr, Singh H, Shada RE, Naik AD (2011) Primary care and communication in shared cancer care: a qualitative study. Am J Manag Care 17(4):259–265
15. Rothman K, Greenland S, Lash T (2008) Modern Epidemiology, 3rd ed. Lippincot Williams & Wilkins, Philadelphia (Wolters Kluwer Health)
16. CEBM. Study Designs. Available from http://www.cebm.net/study-designs/. Cited 16 Mar 2016
17. Hang J, Cai B, Xue P, Wang L, Hu H, Zhou Y, Ren S, Wu J, Zhu M, Chen D, Yang H, Wang L (2015) The joint effects of lifestyle factors and comorbidities on the risk of colorectal cancer: a large chinese retrospective case-control study. PLoS ONE 10(12):e0143696
18. Klepin HD, Pitcher BN, Ballman KV, Kornblith AB, Hurria A, Winer EP, Hudis C, Cohen HJ, Muss HB, Kimmick GG (2014) Comorbidity, chemotherapy toxicity, and outcomes among older women receiving adjuvant chemotherapy for breast cancer on a clinical trial: CALGB 49907 and CALGB 361004 (alliance). J Oncol Pract 10(5):e285–e292
19. Muss HB, Berry DA, Cirrincione CT, Theodoulou M, Mauer AM, Kornblith AB, Partridge AH, Dressler LG, Cohen HJ, Becker HP, Kartcheske PA, Wheeler JD, Perez EA, Wolff AC, Gralow JR, Burstein HJ, Mahmood AA, Magrinat G, Parker BA, Hart RD, Grenier D, Norton L, Hudis CA, Winer EP (2009) Adjuvant chemotherapy in older women with early-stage breast cancer. N Engl J Med 360(20):2055–2065
20. Gridelli C (2001) The ELVIS trial: a phase III study of single-agent vinorelbine as first-line treatment in elderly patients with advanced non-small cell lung cancer. Elderly lung cancer vinorelbine Italian study. Oncologist 6(Suppl 1):4–7
21. Hempenius L, Slaets JP, Boelens MA, van Asselt DZ, de Bock GH, Wiggers T, van Leeuwen BL (2013) Inclusion of frail elderly patients in clinical trials: solutions to the problems. J Geriatr Oncol 4(1):26–31
22. Puts MT, Monette J, Girre V, Wolfson C, Monette M, Batist G, Bergman H (2009) Participation of older newly-diagnosed cancer patients in an observational prospective pilot study: an example of recruitment and retention. BMC Cancer 9:277
23. Deckx L (2015) The older cancer patient. Consequences of cancer and ageing, in Biomedical Sciences Group, Faculty of Medicine, Department of Public Health and Primary Care. KU Leuven: Leuven

24. van den Akker M, van Steenkiste B, Krutwagen E, Metsemakers JF (2015) Disease or no disease? Disagreement on diagnoses between self-reports and medical records of adult patients. Eur J Gen Pract 21(1):45–51
25. Emson HE (1987) Health, disease and illness: matters for definition. CMAJ 136(8):811–813
26. Patel VL, Arocha JF, Kushniruk AW (2002) Patients' and physicians' understanding of health and biomedical concepts: relationship to the design of EMR systems. J Biomed Inform 35(1):8–16
27. De-loyde KJ, Harrison JD, Durcinoska I, Shepherd HL, Solomon MJ, Young JM (2015) Which information source is best? Concordance between patient report, clinician report and medical records of patient co-morbidity and adjuvant therapy health information. J Eval Clin Pract 21(2):339–346
28. Garcia Rodriguez LA, Perez Gutthann S (1998) Use of the UK general practice research database for pharmacoepidemiology. Br J Clin Pharmacol 45(5):419–425
29. Truyers C, Goderis G, Dewitte H, van den Akker M, Buntinx F (2014) The Intego database: background, methods and basic results of a Flemish general practice-based continuous morbidity registration project. BMC Med Inform Decis Mak 14:48
30. Walley T, Mantgani A (1997) The UK general practice research database. Lancet 350(9084):1097–1099
31. Van den Akker M, Metsemakers J, Limonard C, Knottnerus J (2004) General practice: a gold mine for research. Data and scientific use of the registration network family practices. Maastricht: Unigraphic
32. van den Akker M, Spigt MG, de Raeve L, van Steenkiste B, Metsemakers J, van Voorst E, de Vries H (2008) The SMILE study: a study of medical information and lifestyles in Eindhoven, the rationale and contents of a large prospective, dynamic cohort study. BMC Publ Health 8:19
33. Bayliss E, Reifler L, Zeng C, McQuillan D, Ellis J, Steiner J (2014) Competing risks of cancer mortality and cardiovascular events in individuals with multimorbidity. J Comorbidity 4:29–36
34. Lee CC, Ho HC, Su YC, Chen PC, Yu CH, Yang CC (2015) Comparison of different comorbidity measures for oral cancer patients with surgical intervention: a longitudinal study from a single cancer center. Auris Nasus Larynx
35. Gurney J, Sarfati D, Stanley J (2015) The impact of patient comorbidity on cancer stage at diagnosis. Br J Cancer 113(9):1375–1380
36. Dunn J, Ng SK, Holland J, Aitken J, Youl P, Baade PD, Chambers SK (2013) Trajectories of psychological distress after colorectal cancer. Psychooncology 22(8):1759–1765
37. Tovikkai C, Charman SC, Praseedom RK, Gimson AE, van der Meulen J (2015) Time-varying impact of comorbidities on mortality after liver transplantation: a national cohort study using linked clinical and administrative data. BMJ Open 5(5):e006971
38. Beckmann KR, Bennett A, Young GP, Cole SR, Joshi R, Adams J, Singhal N, Karapetis C, Wattchow D, Roder D (2016) Sociodemographic disparities in survival from colorectal cancer in South Australia: a population-wide data linkage study. BMC Health Serv Res 16 (1):24
39. Wang CY, Baldwin LM, Saver BG, Dobie SA, Green PK, Cai Y, Klabunde CN (2009) The contribution of longitudinal comorbidity measurements to survival analysis. Med Care 47 (7):813–821
40. Sarfati D, Gurney J, Stanley J, Salmond C, Crampton P, Dennett E, Koea J, Pearce N (2014) Cancer-specific administrative data-based comorbidity indices provided valid alternative to Charlson and National Cancer Institute Indices. J Clin Epidemiol 67(5):586–595
41. Deshpande AD, Schootman M, Mayer A (2015) Development of a claims-based algorithm to identify colorectal cancer recurrence. Ann Epidemiol 25(4):297–300
42. Yurkovich M, Avina-Zubieta JA, Thomas J, Gorenchtein M, Lacaille D (2015) A systematic review identifies valid comorbidity indices derived from administrative health data. J Clin Epidemiol 68(1):3–14

43. Glasziou PP, Buchan H, Del Mar C, Doust J, Harris M, Knight R, Scott A, Scott IA, Stockwell A (2012) When financial incentives do more good than harm: a checklist. BMJ 345:e5047
44. Taichman DB, Backus J, Baethge C, Bauchner H, de Leeuw PW, Drazen JM, Fletcher J, Frizelle FA, Groves T, Haileamlak A, James A, Laine C, Peiperl L, Pinborg A, Sahni P, Wu S (2016) Sharing clinical trial data: a proposal from the international committee of medical journal editors. Lancet 387(10016):e9–e11
45. Weitzman ER, Kaci L, Mandl KD (2010) Sharing medical data for health research: the early personal health record experience. J Med Internet Res 12(2):e14
46. Weitzman ER, Kelemen S, Kaci L, Mandl KD (2012) Willingness to share personal health record data for care improvement and public health: a survey of experienced personal health record users. BMC Med Inform Decis Mak 12:39
47. Wen KY, Kreps G, Zhu F, Miller S (2010) Consumers' perceptions about and use of the internet for personal health records and health information exchange: analysis of the 2007 health information national trends survey. J Med Internet Res 12(4):e73
48. Perkins AJ, Kroenke K, Unutzer J, Katon W, Williams JW Jr, Hope C, Callahan CM (2004) Common comorbidity scales were similar in their ability to predict health care costs and mortality. J Clin Epidemiol 57(10):1040–1048
49. von Korff M, Wagner E, Saunders K (1992) A chronic disease score from automated pharmacy data. J Clin Epidemiol 45(2):197–203
50. Mayr R, May M, Martini T, Lodde M, Comploj E, Pycha A, Strobel J, Denzinger S, Otto W, Wieland W, Burger M, Fritsche HM (2012) Comorbidity and performance indices as predictors of cancer-independent mortality but not of cancer-specific mortality after radical cystectomy for urothelial carcinoma of the bladder. Eur Urol 62(4):662–670
51. Frohner M, Wirth MP (2012) Age and comorbidity in early prostate cancer. Urologe A 51 (10):1356–1361
52. Briganti A, Spahn M, Joniau S, Gontero P, Bianchi M, Kneitz B, Chun FK, Sun M, Graefen M, Abdollah F, Marchioro G, Frohenberg D, Giona S, Frea B, Karakiewicz PI, Montorsi F, Van Poppel H, Jeffrey Karnes R (2013) Impact of age and comorbidities on long-term survival of patients with high-risk prostate cancer treated with radical prostatectomy: a multi-institutional competing-risks analysis. Eur Urol 63(4):693–701
53. Ording AG, Sorensen HT (2013) Concepts of comorbidities, multiple morbidities, complications, and their clinical epidemiologic analogs. Clin Epidemiol 5:199–203
54. Lee A, Levine M (2003) Four topics in venous thromboembolism. venous thromboembolism and cancer: risks and outcomes. Circulation 107(1):17–21
55. Van den Akker M, Vos R, Knottnerus J (2006) In an exploratory prospective study on multimorbidity general and disease related susceptibility could be distinguished. J Clin Epidemiol 59(9):934–939
56. Gottlieb M, Marsaa K, Godtfredsen NS, Mellemgaard A (2015) Prevalence and management of pulmonary comorbidity in patients with lung and head and neck cancer. Acta Oncol 54 (5):767–771
57. Charlson M, Pompei P, Ales K, MacKenzie C (1987) A new method of classifying prognostic comorbidity in longitudinal studies: development and validation. J Chron Dis 40 (5):373–383
58. Klabunde CN, Legler JM, Warren JL, Baldwin LM, Schrag D (2007) A refined comorbidity measurement algorithm for claims-based studies of breast, prostate, colorectal, and lung cancer patients. Ann Epidemiol 17(8):584–590
59. Deckx L, van Abbema D, Nelissen K, Daniels L, Stinissen P, Bulens P, Linsen L, Rummens JL, Robaeys G, de Jonge ET, Houben B, Pat K, Walgraeve D, Spaas L, Verheezen J, Verniest T, Goegebuer A, Wildiers H, van den Berkmortel F, Tjan-Heijnen VC, Buntinx F, van den Akker M (2011) Study protocol of KLIMOP: a cohort study on the wellbeing of older cancer patients in Belgium and the Netherlands. BMC Publ Health 11:825
60. Streiner D, Norman GR (2008) Health measurement scales. Oxford University Press, Oxford/New York/Tokyo

61. Guo R, Chen XZ, Chen L, Jiang F, Tang LL, Mao YP, Zhou GQ, Li WF, Liu LZ, Tian L, Lin AH, Ma J (2015) Comorbidity predicts poor prognosis in nasopharyngeal carcinoma: development and validation of a predictive score model. Radiother Oncol 114(2):249–256
62. Mukherjee B, Ou HT, Wang F, Erickson SR (2011) A new comorbidity index: the health-related quality of life comorbidity index. J Clin Epidemiol 64(3):309–319
63. Lorem GF, Schirmer H, Emaus N (2016) Health impact index. Development and validation of a method for classifying comorbid disease measured against self-reported health. PLoS ONE 11(2):e0148830
64. Bender CM, Engberg SJ, Donovan HS, Cohen SM, Houze MP, Rosenzweig MQ, Mallory GA, Dunbar-Jacob J, Sereika SM (2008) Symptom clusters in adults with chronic health problems and cancer as a comorbidity. Oncol Nurs Forum 35(1):E1–E11
65. Johnson ML, El-Serag HB, Tran TT, Hartman C, Richardson P, Abraham NS (2006) Adapting the Rx-Risk-V for mortality prediction in outpatient populations. Med Care 44 (8):793–797
66. Vitry A, Wong SA, Roughead EE, Ramsay E, Barratt J (2009) Validity of medication-based co-morbidity indices in the Australian elderly population. Aust NZ J Publ Health 33 (2):126–130
67. Collins GS, Reitsma JB, Altman DG, Moons KG (2015) Transparent reporting of a multivariable prediction model for individual prognosis or diagnosis (TRIPOD). Ann Intern Med 162(10):735–736
68. Hemingway H, Croft P, Perel P, Hayden JA, Abrams K, Timmis A, Briggs A, Udumyan R, Moons KG, Steyerberg EW, Roberts I, Schroter S, Altman DG, Riley RD (2013) Prognosis research strategy (PROGRESS) 1: a framework for researching clinical outcomes. BMJ 346: e5595
69. Fried T, McGraw S, Agostini J, Tinette M (2008) Views of older persons with multiple morbidities on competing outcomes and clinical decision-making. JAGS 56:1839–1844
70. Fried TR, Tinetti M, Agostini J, Iannone L, Towle V (2011) Health outcome prioritization to elicit preferences of older persons with multiple health conditions. Patient Educ Couns 83 (2):278–282
71. Muth C, van den Akker M, Blom JW, Mallen CD, Rochon J, Schellevis FG, Becker A, Beyer M, Gensichen J, Kirchner H, Perera R, Prados-Torres A, Scherer M, Thiem U, van den Bussche H, Glasziou PP (2014) The Ariadne principles: how to handle multimorbidity in primary care consultations. BMC Med 12:223
72. Henderson TO, Ness KK, Cohen HJ (2004) Accelerated aging among cancer survivors: from pediatrics to geriatrics. Am Soc Clin Oncol Educ Book, pp e423–e430
73. Meneses K, Benz R, Azuero A, Jablonski-Jaudon R, McNees P (2015) Multimorbidity and breast cancer. Semin Oncol Nurs 31(2):163–169
74. Giovanucci E, Harlan D, Archer M, Bergenstal R, Gaprstur S, Habel LA, Pollak M, Regensteiner J, Yee D (2010) Diabetes and cancer: a consensus report. Diab Care 33 (7):1674–1685
75. Corkum M, Urquhart R, Kendell C, Burge F, Porter G, Johnston G (2012) Impact of comorbidity and healthcare utilization on colorectal cancer stage at diagnosis: literature review. Cancer Causes Control 23(2):213–220
76. Stairmand J, Signal L, Sarfati D, Jackson C, Batten L, Holdaway M, Cunningham C (2015) Consideration of comorbidity in treatment decision making in multidisciplinary cancer team meetings: a systematic review. Ann Oncol 26(7):1325–1332
77. Rodrigues G, Sanatani M (2012) Age and comorbidity considerations related to radiotherapy and chemotherapy administration. Semin Radiat Oncol 22(4):277–283
78. Wister AV, Levasseur M, Griffith LE, Fyffe I (2015) Estimating multiple morbidity disease burden among older persons: a convergent construct validity study to discriminate among six chronic illness measures, CCHS 2008/09. BMC Geriatr 15:12
79. Schölzel-Dorenbos C (2012) Quality of life [Kwaliteit van leven], in cancer in older patients [Kanker bij ouderen]. In: Wymenga A et al. (ed). De Tijdstroom, Utrecht

80. Aaronson NK, Ahmedzai S, Bergman B, Bullinger M, Cull A, Duez NJ, Filiberti A, Flechtner H, Fleishman SB, de Haes JC et al (1993) The European Organization for research and treatment of cancer QLQ-C30: a quality-of-life instrument for use in international clinical trials in oncology. J Natl Cancer Inst 85(5):365–376
81. Cella DF, Tulsky DS, Gray G, Sarafian B, Linn E, Bonomi A, Silberman M, Yellen SB, Winicour P, Brannon J et al (1993) The functional assessment of cancer therapy scale: development and validation of the general measure. J Clin Oncol 11(3):570–579
82. Schmidt S, Garin O, Pardo Y, Valderas JM, Alonso J, Rebollo P, Rajmil L, Garcia-Forero C, Ferrer M (2014) Assessing quality of life in patients with prostate cancer: a systematic and standardized comparison of available instruments. Qual Life Res 23(8):2169–2181
83. Valderas JM, Ferrer M, Mendivil J, Garin O, Rajmil L, Herdman M, Alonso J (2008) Development of EMPRO: a tool for the standardized assessment of patient-reported outcome measures. Value Health 11(4):700–708
84. National Cancer Institute (2015) Surveillance, epidemiology, and end results program. Available from: http://seer.cancer.gov/seerstat/. Cited on 16 Mar 2016
85. Crowley R, Hoering A (2012) Handbook of statistics in clinical oncology, 3rd ed. CRC Press, Seattle
86. Rubin G, Berendsen A, Crawford SM, Dommett R, Earle C, Emery J, Fahey T, Grassi L, Grunfeld E, Gupta S, Hamilton W, Hiom S, Hunter D, Lyratzopoulos G, Macleod U, Mason R, Mitchell G, Neal RD, Peake M, Roland M, Seifert B, Sisler J, Sussman J, Taplin S, Vedsted P, Voruganti T, Walter F, Wardle J, Watson E, Weller D, Wender R, Whelan J, Whitlock J, Wilkinson C, de Wit N, Zimmermann C (2015) The expanding role of primary care in cancer control. Lancet Oncol 16(12):1231–1272
87. Kleinbaum D, Klein M (2012) Survival analysis. A self-learning text, 3rd ed. Springer, New York
88. Verbeke G (2009) Biostatistics in oncology trials: survival analysis. "why clinicians hope for survivors and statisticians for deaths". Available from: https://perswww.kuleuven.be/~u0018341/documents/oncology.pdf. Cited on 8 Mar 2016
89. Kalbfleisch J, Prentice R (2002) The statistical analysis of failure time data, 2nd ed. John Wiley, New York
90. Chang YH, Li WH, Chang Y, Peng CW, Cheng CH, Chang WP, Chuang CM (2016) Front-line intraperitoneal versus intravenous chemotherapy in stage III–IV epithelial ovarian, tubal, and peritoneal cancer with minimal residual disease: a competing risk analysis. BMC Cancer 16(1):235
91. Perperoglou A, Keramopoullos A, van Houwelingen HC (2007) Approaches in modelling long-term survival: an application to breast cancer. Stat Med 26(13):2666–2685
92. van Houwelingen H, Putter H (2012) Dynamic prediction in clinical survival analysis. CRC Press, Boca Raton
93. Fieuws S, Verbeke G, Maes B, Vanrenterghem Y (2008) Predicting renal graft failure using multivariate longitudinal profiles. Biostatistics 9(3):419–431
94. Brant L, Sheng S, Morrell C, Verbeke G, Lesaffre E, Carter H (2003) Screening for prostate cancer by using random-effects models. J Roy Stat Soc Ser A 166:51–62
95. Erichsen R, Horvath-Puho E, Iversen LH, Lash TL, Sorensen HT (2013) Does comorbidity interact with colorectal cancer to increase mortality? A nationwide population-based cohort study. Br J Cancer 109(7):2005–2013
96. Fine J, Gray R (1999) A proportional hazards model for the subdistribution of a competing risk. J Am Stat Assoc 94(446):496–509
97. Putter H, Fiocco M, Geskus RB (2007) Tutorial in biostatistics: competing risks and multi-state models. Stat Med 26(11):2389–2430
98. Scrucca L, Santucci A, Aversa F (2010) Regression modeling of competing risk using R: an in depth guide for clinicians. Bone Marrow Transplant 45(9):1388–1395
99. Binbing Y, Tiwari RC, Feuer EJ (2011) Estimating the personal cure rate of cancer patients using population-based grouped cancer survival data. Stat Methods Med Res 20(3):261–274

100. Haller B, Schmidt G, Ulm K (2013) Applying competing risks regression models: an overview. Lifetime Data Anal 19(1):33–58
101. Satagopan JM, Ben-Porat L, Berwick M, Robson M, Kutler D, Auerbach AD (2004) A note on competing risks in survival data analysis. Br J Cancer 91(7):1229–1235
102. Cox D (1972) Regression models and life tables (with discussion). J R Statist Soc B 34:187–220
103. Hernan MA (2010) The hazards of hazard ratios. Epidemiology 21(1):13–15
104. Singer J, Willett J (2003) Applied longitudinal data analysis. Modeling change and event occurrence. University Press, Oxford
105. Diggle P, Heagerty P, Liang K, Zeger S (2013) Analysis of longitudinal data. In: Oxford statistical science series, 2nd ed. Oxford University Press, Oxford
106. Kirkwood B, Sterne J (2003) Essential medical statistics, 2nd ed. Blackwell Science, Oxford
107. Hox J (2010) Multilevel analysis: techniques and applications, 2nd ed. Routledge, New York
108. Hox J, Roberts K (2011) Handbook of advanced multilevel analysis. Routledge, New York
109. Vos R, van den Akker M, Boesten J, Robertson C, Metsemakers J (2015) Trajectories of multimorbidity: exploring patterns of multimorbidity in patients with more than ten chronic health problems in life course. BMC Fam Pract 16:2
110. van den Bussche H, Koller D, Kolonko T, Hansen H, Wegscheider K, Glaeske G, von Leitner EC, Schäfer I, Schön G (2011) Which chronic diseases and disease combinations are specific to multimorbidity in the elderly? Results of a claims data based cross-sectional study in Germany. BMC Publ Health 11:101
111. Newcomer S, Steiner J, Bayliss E (2011) Identifying subgroups of complex patients with cluster analysis. Am J Manag Care 17(8):e324–e332
112. Islam MM, Valderas JM, Yen L, Dawda P, Jowsey T, McRae IS (2014) Multimorbidity and comorbidity of chronic diseases among the senior Australians: prevalence and patterns. PLoS ONE 9(1):e83783
113. Jensen AB, Moseley PL, Oprea TI, Ellesoe SG, Eriksson R, Schmock H, Jensen PB, Jensen LJ, Brunak S (2014) Temporal disease trajectories condensed from population-wide registry data covering 6.2 million patients. Nat Commun 5:4022
114. Sorensen HT (2013) Multimorbidity and cancer outcomes: a need for more research. Clin Epidemiol 5(Suppl 1):1–2
115. Wei Y (2015) Integrative analyses of cancer data: a review from a statistical perspective. Cancer Inform 14(Suppl 2):173–181
116. Hsu HC (2015) Trajectories of multimorbidity and impacts on successful aging. Exp Gerontol 66:32–38
117. Wong A, Boshuizen HC, Schellevis FG, Kommer GJ, Polder JJ (2011) Longitudinal administrative data can be used to examine multimorbidity, provided false discoveries are controlled for. J Clin Epidemiol 64(10):1109–1117
118. Huntley A, Johnson R, Purdy S, Valderas J, Salisbury C (2012) Measures of multimorbidity and morbidity burden for use in primary care and community settings: a systematic review and guide. Ann Fam Med 10(2):134–141
119. Ibrahim J, Chen M, Sinha D (2001) *Bayesian* Survival Analysis. Springer series in statistics. Springer, New York

Chapter 13
The Cost of Cure: Chronic Conditions in Survivors of Child, Adolescent, and Young Adult Cancers

Christina Signorelli, Joanna E. Fardell, Claire E. Wakefield, Kate Webber and Richard J. Cohn

Abstract Few children and young adults with cancer have a pre-existing chronic condition which contributes to their cancer risk, highlighting the unique aetiology of most cancers in this age group. Children and adolescents often tolerate acute cancer treatments well, however, the majority will experience life-altering, and some even life-threatening, conditions as a result of the cancer treatments they received. Young people face particular challenges, due to significant disruptions to a developmentally important time of life, placing them at higher risk of physical and psychological conditions. Many chronic conditions related to cancer treatment do not appear until children and adolescents mature, years to decades after completion of treatment. Available data highlights the high prevalence and severe nature of treatment-related conditions, supporting the need for continuing management through long-term follow-up care well into adult life. Both survivors and health care professionals must be knowledgeable about the risk of chronic conditions in survivors of child, adolescent and young adult cancers and must be aware of the appropriate follow-up care aimed at their prevention and management. Knowledge of late complications also informs modification of new treatment, helping to avoid chronic conditions in future survivors. Researchers' efforts should be focused on the development of strategies to reduce the potential burden of chronic conditions in this vulnerable population.

C. Signorelli · J.E. Fardell · C.E. Wakefield · R.J. Cohn (✉)
Discipline of Paediatrics, School of Women's and Children's Health, UNSW Medicine, University of New South Wales, Kensington, NSW, Australia
e-mail: richard.cohn@health.nsw.gov.au

C. Signorelli · J.E. Fardell · C.E. Wakefield · R.J. Cohn
Kids Cancer Centre, Sydney Children's Hospital (SCH), Randwick, NSW, Australia

K. Webber
Department of Medical Oncology, Prince of Wales Hospital, Randwick, NSW, Australia

K. Webber · R.J. Cohn
National Centre for Cancer Survivorship, University of New South Wales, Kensington, NSW, Australia

B. Koczwara (ed.), *Cancer and Chronic Conditions*,
DOI 10.1007/978-981-10-1844-2_13

Keywords Chronic illness · Childhood cancer · Adolescent · Young adults · Survivorship

Key Points

- Over 80 % of children and young people diagnosed with cancer will survive, adding to the growing population of survivors
- Survivors of child, adolescent and young adult cancers face unique challenges, due to the crucial developmental stage during which they are treated, placing them at higher risk of medical and psychological treatment-related conditions
- Childhood and adolescent cancer survivors experience a range of physical (e.g. cardiovascular) and emotional (e.g. lower quality of life) treatment-related complications, often severe and more characteristic of people much older
- Young survivors are also more likely to die prematurely, due to recurrence of the primary malignancy, subsequent neoplasms, or other treatment-related conditions
- Long term follow-up care is therefore critical, but practices are inconsistent and face many patient and system-related challenges
- Exposure-based, risk-stratified models of care allow best use of limited resources for this population

13.1 Introduction

"Looking forward … ever more refined and precisely targeted methods of treatment (*are needed*), so that increasing numbers of successfully treated children of today do not become the chronically ill adults of tomorrow" [1].

The words of D'Angio were written in 1975, when there were few survivors of cancer diagnosed in children and young people aged under 25. He anticipated the late consequences of childhood cancer therapy which threaten survival and detract from the quality of survival. Decades on, and with a growing population of young cancer survivors, due to vastly improved treatment outcomes and survival rates, significant numbers of chronic conditions appearing in this population reinforce D'Angio's message. Given high survival rates for most cancers in young people, and the number of years of life ahead for young survivors, there is a significant need to be mindful of possible late effects or chronic conditions that may emerge during survivorship.

Until the 1970s, cancer treatment relied almost exclusively upon surgery and radiation. Receiving a cancer diagnosis in childhood or adolescence was almost universally fatal [2]. With the introduction of multimodal therapy and combination chemotherapy (i.e. administering multiple drugs with different mechanisms of action) and improvements in supportive care, the number of children surviving most types of cancer has steadily increased [3]. Today over 80 % of children with cancer will survive at least five years post-diagnosis and the majority will be cured of their cancer (see Fig. 13.1) [4]. More than 400,000 young people who are currently alive worldwide have survived childhood cancer and 1 in every 530 young person aged between 20 and 39 years old is now a cancer survivor [4, 5]. With potentially six decades of life ahead after treatment for cancer in childhood, it is important to consider the ongoing impact of cancer and its treatment on children and young adults [6].

Fig. 13.1 Five-year survival rates (%) for selected childhood (aged 0–14 years) and adolescents and young adult (AYA, 15–24) cancers [203]

Diagnosis	Childhood %	AYA %
Thyroid carcinomas	98.8	99.5
Retinoblastoma[a]	97.5	-
Germ cell: testis	96.8	96.9
Germ cell: ovary	95.3	98.4
Hodgkin lymphomas	95.2	93.1
Melanoma of the skin	-	92.2
Malignant Melanoma	88.1	-
Lymphoid leukaemias	85.4	49.5
Non-Hodgkin lymphomas	82.3	74.4
Ovarian carcinoma	70	89.5
Acute myeloid leukaemias	66.8	59.1
Astrocytomas	62.9	55.8
Osteosarcoma[b]	77.3	59.8
Bone	-	61.8
Ewing tumour	66.5	48
Soft tissue sarcomas	-	67.5
CNS tumours	62.8	61.7
Cervix	-	85.7
Ovarian carcinoma	70	83.3
Renal carcinomas	78.8	-
Colon	-	80.2
Breast	-	85.5
Lung	-	72.1

Abbreviations: CNS = central nervous system

[a]Children aged 0-4 years only

[b]Children aged 10-14 years only

Cancer presenting during childhood and the adolescent years represents 1 % of the annual incidence of cancer in most developed countries, but differs from adult cancer with respect to cancer type, biological features, response to treatment and long-term prognosis [7]. It is the commonest cause of disease-related death among children and adolescents in developed countries, second only to accidental deaths [8]. The cancer types found in children and adolescents differ from that of adult cancers, with leukaemias, lymphomas and cancers of the brain and nervous system representing the majority [9]. Children with cancer rarely have pre-existing chronic conditions that contribute to their cancer risk, although there is a growing appreciation that some carry germline mutations in cancer-predisposing genes [10, 11]. The differences between most adult and paediatric cancers necessitate different treatments and supportive care approaches to that used in adult oncology [12, 13].

While children and adolescents often tolerate acute cancer treatment well, they can be more affected in the long term by the intensive treatments administered to their developing organs, putting them at significantly higher risk of developing late toxicities from cancer treatment [14]. Chronic conditions in childhood cancers are not likely to be the result of pre-existing or environmental exposures, but rather are a direct or indirect effect of cancer and its treatment. Young people diagnosed with cancer during the teenage and young adult years face particular challenges, due to significant disruptions to a developmentally important time of life. The adolescent and young adult (AYA) years are a peak time for psychosocial, sexual, educational, and career development [15–17]. Diagnosis and treatment during such a time places them at higher risk of ongoing treatment related complications, for instance second cancers, depression or anxiety [18, 19]. Long term follow-up of young people treated during these critical years has allowed study of the time course for development of such chronic conditions and identification of individuals at greatest risk. Large cohort studies of childhood cancer survivors, following survivors for decades post-treatment, have not been matched in survivors of adult cancers [20]. Despite these unique challenges, which is much of what has been learnt from child and adolescent survivorship research and clinical practice is of relevance to adult oncology, bringing attention to the importance of surveillance for late treatment-related morbidities in models of care for adult cancer survivors.

Surveillance of young survivors has highlighted the need for risk-based, exposure-related follow-up, using evidence-based survivorship guidelines. For example, the International Late Effects of Childhood Cancer Guideline Harmonization Group has developed evidence-based recommendations for breast cancer surveillance in childhood cancer survivors (see Fig. 13.2). Recommendations are categorized according to a 4-level colour system based on existing levels of evidence; green (strong recommendation, high quality evidence), yellow and orange (intermediate level recommendations, moderate quality evidence), and red (recommend against a particular intervention). The guidelines are designed to improve health outcomes and facilitate care for young cancer survivors, with similar evidence-based recommendations developed for the surveillance of cardiac disease, metabolic syndrome, and other chronic conditions [21–24].

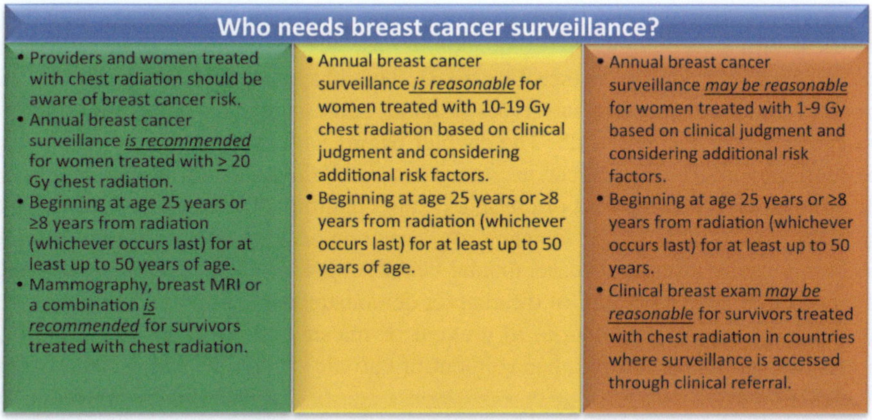

Fig. 13.2 Breast cancer screening recommendations for childhood cancer survivors, as advised by the International Late Effects of Childhood Cancer Guideline Harmonization Group; *green* indicates a strong recommendation, *yellow* a moderate recommendation, and *orange* a weak recommendation [204]

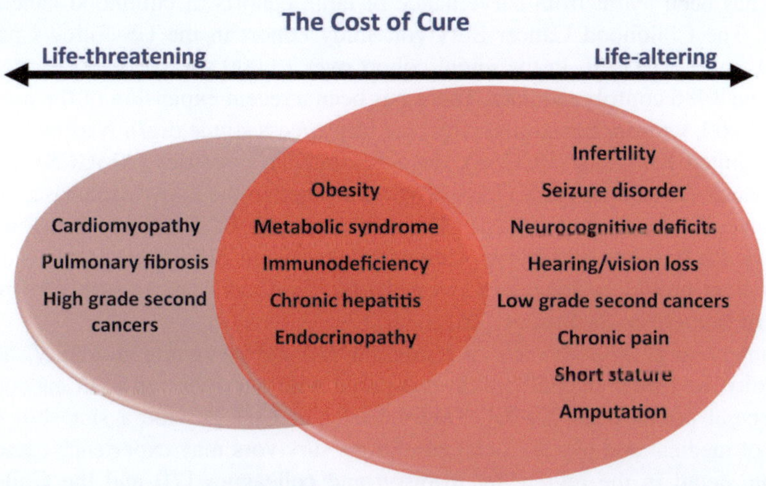

Fig. 13.3 Some of the life threatening/life altering chronic complications at which survivors are at risk of following treatment for childhood cancer

Surveillance must continue indefinitely as many of the late effects may only manifest many years, and even decades after therapy is completed. Survivors should be prepared for transition from patient focused acute cancer care to risk-stratified community-based holistic follow-up through education, provision of treatment summaries and survivorship care plans which allow them to be their own advocates. Lifestyle education is important in minimising the number and severity of many late chronic complications.

Survivors experience a range of morbidities after cancer treatment, including physical and psychological chronic conditions, which begin to emerge during adolescence and adulthood (see Fig. 13.3). This chapter summarises some of the chronic conditions faced by survivors of child, adolescent and young adult cancers diagnosed under the age of 25. The chapter begins with an overview of the unique biology associated with cancer in young people. Following this is a summary of illustrative data on long-term or chronic health conditions facing CCS (summarised in Tables 13.1 and 13.2), focusing on common examples of chronic disease including cardiovascular disease, mental health, cognition, and education and other life outcomes. The latter half of the chapter demonstrates the importance of ongoing surveillance for this population, to prevent or manage such conditions, including presenting guidelines for the management of chronic conditions and recommended models of care.

13.2 Long-Term Health Outcomes in Young Survivors

Much has been learnt from surveillance of large cohorts of childhood cancer survivors. The Childhood Cancer Survivor Study cohort in the US follows patients treated from 1970 [25]. In the initial cohort over 12,000 survivors treated between 1970 and 1986 contributed data. There has been a recent expansion of the cohort to over 24,000, with increased diversity (see https://ccss.stjude.org/). National cohorts in the United Kingdom (BCCSS), the Scandinavian countries (ALiCCS), and the Netherlands (DCOG LATER) have also contributed to the knowledge base, as have many single centre studies [26]. The establishment of PanCare (Pan-European Network for the Care of Survivors after Childhood and Adolescent Cancer) has the potential to provide a cohort of over 80,000 childhood cancer survivors for the study of late effects in Europe [26].

Many young survivors are at increased risk of premature mortality, serious morbidity, and poor mental health, compared with survivors of adult cancers and the general population [27–30]. Tables 13.1 and 13.2 provide a snapshot of the range of medical and psychosocial conditions survivors may experience (described in more detail in the review by Robison and colleagues [7]) and the Children's Oncology Group (COG) Survivorship Guidelines [31].

Many chronic conditions do not become evident until many years or decades after treatment, and become more clinically significant as child and adolescent cancer survivors continue to age [32, 33]. Due to the time lapse between the cessation of cancer treatment and their late emergence, chronic conditions are commonly referred to as 'late morbidity', 'late effects' or 'late sequelae'. In the decades that follow 'cure', disabling or life altering chronic health conditions will affect three out of four young survivors [34]. A further 37 % experience severe and possibly fatal conditions [34]. Prolonged follow-up data from the St Jude Lifetime Follow-up Study suggests even higher cumulative rates over time. The study

Table 13.1 Selected examples of established radiation-associated conditions

Radiation exposure	Toxicity/late effects	High risk groups	Available prevalence data	Exposure based screening recommendations[a]
Cardiovascular	• Cardiomyopathy • Carotid and subclavian artery disease • Coronary artery disease • Dysrhythmias and conduction disorders • Heart valve abnormalities • Pericardial fibrosis and pericarditis	• Chest and spinal irradiation • Mediastinal irradiation	23.2 % of HL survivors report cardiac events 25 years later [205] Cardiac disease in 1.2 % of CNS survivors by age 40, compared with 32.6 % in HL survivors [206]	• Echocardiogram every 1–5 years (depending on age at treatment, see COG guidelines) [31] • Electrocardiogram upon entry to LTFU and repeated as clinically indicated • Annual blood pressure check and biannual blood test to check for cholesterol levels, glucose, and Hemogobin A1c
Central nervous system	• Neurocognitive deficits, including learning deficits and diminished intelligence quotient, executive function, sustained attention, memory processing speed and visual-motor integration • Cerebrovascular disease, including stroke, moyamoya and occlusive cerebral vasculopathy • Clinical leukoencephalopathy, which causes spasticity, ataxia, dysarthia, dysphagia, hemiparesis and seizures • Neurological and neurosensory deficits including hearing loss	Cranial irradiation • Auditory deficits • Neurocognitive deficits	Stroke reported in 6.3 % of CNS tumour survivors [207] Impairments in intellectual (67 %) and motor functioning (69 %), verbal memory and languages (each 50 %), and problem solving (79 %) in Medulloblastoma survivors [112] Bilateral hearing loss in 61 % of survivors [208]	Neurocognitive deficits • Yearly review of education and/or vocational progress • Neuropsychological evaluation upon entry to LTFU and repeated as clinically indicated Auditory • Complete audiologic evaluation yearly until age 10, then five yearly if no hearing loss detected
Endocrine	• Pituitary dysfunction, including altered pubertal timing; growth hormone, TSH, ACTH, LH and FSH deficiency; altered body composition (reduced lean muscle mass, overweight and obesity); and metabolic syndrome • Thyroid abnormalities, including hypothyroid, hyperthyroid and thyroid nodules • Diabetes mellitus	Cranial Irradiation • Precocious puberty • Growth hormone deficiency • Obesity Radiation to thyroid gland (neck, mantle, spinal scatter) • Hypothyroidism	34 % of HL survivors report at least one thyroid abnormality [209] Obesity present in 16–56 % of ALL survivors [210] In survivors treated with CRT, 47.8 % overweight/obese [211]	Precocious puberty • Check height, weight, Tanner staging yearly until sexually mature Growth hormone deficiency • Biannual until growth is completed, then yearly targeted history and physical examination including height, weight, BMI and Tanner staging Obesity • Check height, weight and BMI yearly Hypothyroidism • Free thyroxine and thyroid stimulating hormone yearly

(continued)

Table 13.1 (continued)

Radiation exposure	Toxicity/late effects	High risk groups	Available prevalence data	Exposure based screening recommendations[a]
Gastrointestinal	• Bowel obstruction • Chronic enterocolitis • Colorectal cancer • Esophageal stricture • Gallstones • Gastrointestinal fistula or stricture • Hepatic fibrosis • Cholelithiasis	Radiation • Doses higher than 30Gr • To the neck, chest, abdomen, or pelvis	37.6 % cumulative incidence of any gastronintestinal condition 20 years later [212]	• Annual physical examination • X-rays, blood tests, guaiac testing, colonoscopy, or endoscopies as needed • Ultrasounds for suspected gallstones or other gallbladder problems
Reproductive system (females)	• Uterine vascular insufficiency that predisposes to spontaneous abortion, neonatal death, infants who have low birthweights, foetal malposition and premature labour • Ovarian dysfunction that results in delayed or arrested puberty, premature menopause and infertility • Ovarian failure (hypogonadism)	TBI, craniospinal, abdomino-pelvic irradiation, or irradiation • Ovarian failure • Infertility Treatment during peripubertal or postpubertal period • Infertility	Overall primary (4.5 %) and acute (6.3 %) ovarian failure [23]	Ovarian failure • Yearly pubertal onset, tempo and Tanner staging until sexually mature • In females at 13 years and repeated as clinically indicated: Serum follicle-stimulating hormone, luteinizing hormone, and oestradiol Infertility • Yearly targeted history and physical examination
Reproductive system (males)	• Leydig cell dysfunction that results in delayed or arrested puberty and androgen insufficiency • Germ cell failure, oligospermia, azoospermia and infertility • Hypogonadism • Infertility	Craniospinal, abdomino-pelvic irradiation, or irradiation • Hypogonadism • Infertility	Overall 4.3 % hypogonadism in male survivors 30 years later [213]	Hypogonadism • In males at 14 years and repeated as clinically indicated: Serum testosterone, ideally in the morning Infertility • Annual check-up including careful analysis of hormone and puberty status • Semen analysis upon patient request and follicle-stimulating hormone if unable to obtain semen analysis

(continued)

Table 13.1 (continued)

Radiation exposure	Toxicity/late effects	High risk groups	Available prevalence data	Exposure based screening recommendations[a]
Musculoskeletal	• Hypoplasia and fibrosis • Reduced or uneven growth (resulting in shortened trunk height, limb length discrepancy and kyphoscoliosis) • Reduced bone mineral density	Short stature/growth problems: • Cranial irradiation dose > 18 Gy • TBI (unfractioned 10 Gy) Scoliosis/kyphosis • Radiation to chest, abdomen, trunk, or spine • Higher radiation doses • Thoracic or abdominal surgery or neurosurgery (spine) Reduced bone mineral density Craniospinal or gonadal irradiation, or TBI • Hypothyroidism • Hypogonadism • Growth hormone deficiency	Growth hormone deficiency present in 24 % of ALL survivors [214]	Short stature/growth problems • Yearly standing and sitting height measured until growth completed Scoliosis/kyphosis • Yearly spine exam until growth completed; may need to be more frequent assessment during puberty Reduced bone mineral density • Bone density evaluation (DEXA or quantitative CT), upon entry to LTFU and repeated as clinically indicated
Pulmonary	• Pulmonary fibrosis • Interstitial pneumonitis • Restrictive or obstructive lung disease	Pulmonary fibrosis/Interstitial pneumonitis • Bleomycin, chest or whole lung irradiation • Bleomycin dose >400 U/m^2	3.5 % cumulative incidence of lung fibrosis 20 years later [215]	Pulmonary fibrosis/Interstitial pneumonitis • Pulmonary function tests upon entry to LTFU and repeated as clinically indicated
Urinary tract	• Bladder fibrosis • Dysfunctional voiding • Vesicoureteral reflux • Hydronephrosis • Renal insufficiency • Hypertension	Abdominal irradiation • Renal dysfunction • Bladder complications	Renal insufficiency in 11 %, of Lymphoma survivors 10 years later [216]	Renal dysfunction • Yearly blood pressure and urinalysis • Serum blood urea nitrogen, creatinine and electrolytes (including calcium, phosphorus, magnesium) upon entry to LTFU and repeated as clinically indicated Bladder complications • Yearly targeted history and urinalysis

(continued)

Table 13.1 (continued)

Radiation exposure	Toxicity/late effects	High risk groups	Available prevalence data	Exposure based screening recommendations[a]
Subsequent neoplasms (see Sect. 13.2.3)	• Including those of the skin (predominantly basal cell carcinoma), breast, thyroid, bone and brain • Increasing amounts of data indicate a risk of radiation-associated colorectal cancers	Cranial radiation under 6 years • Brain tumours Cranial and neck radiation under 5 years • Thyroid cancer General field radiation • Bone or soft-tissue sarcoma	Overall 3.2 % 20 years after primary diagnosis. In HL survivors 12.9 % cumulative incidence of breast cancer at 40 years of age [209]	Subsequent neoplasms • Regular examinations to screen for potential subsequent neoplasms (e.g. yearly mammogram for breast cancer, yearly physical examination for skin or thyroid cancers, or 5 yearly colonoscopy for colorectal cancer) Myelodysplasia/therapy-related acute myeloid leukaemia • Yearly targeted history/physical examination
Psychosocial impact (see Sect. 13.2.3)	• Adverse psychosocial effects (mental health disorders, risky behaviours)		Psychological problems (maladjustment, mood disorders etc.) in up to 20 % of survivors [217]	Yearly psychosocial assessment with attention to educational and/or vocational progress, social withdrawal, anxiety, depression, posttraumatic stress, suicidal ideation, health care and insurance access
Teeth	Teeth abnormalities (caries, stunted development, sensitivity, dry mouth, alterations in taste)	Cranial irradiation • Younger age at treatment, or before teeth are fully formed	Teeth decay in 52.2 % of survivors, and 49.7 % with teeth affected with demarcated opacities [218]	Biannual dental examination (including oral cancer screening) and cleaning
Eyes	Cataracts	• Cranial irradiation • TBI • Mix of steroids and radiation	Ocular late effects in 5.7 % of survivors 5 years post-diagnosis [219]	• Annual eye exam focusing (visual acuity, fundoscopic exam) • Ophthalmologist evaluations yearly (if radiation was >30 Gy) or every 3 years (if <30 Gy)

(continued)

Table 13.1 (continued)

Radiation exposure	Toxicity/late effects	High risk groups	Available prevalence data	Exposure based screening recommendations[a]
Life threatening infections		Life threatening infection • Splenectomy • Radiation impacting the spleen (>40 Gy) • Chronic active graft-versus-host disease • Anatomic asplenia • Ongoing immunosuppression • Hypogammaglobulinemia		Life threatening infection • Blood culture when febrile (temperature >38.3 ° C) • Advice about antibiotic prophylaxis

Abbreviations: *CNS* Central Nervous System; *ACTH* adrenocorticotropic hormone; *FSH* follicle-stimulating hormone; *HL* Hodgkin's Lymphoma; *BMI* Body Mass Index; *LH* leutinizing hormone; *CRT* cranial radiotherapy; *TBI* Total body irradiation; *TSH* thryoid-stimulating hormone; *ALL* Acute Lymphocytic Leukaemia

[a]Exposure based screening recommendations are based on the *Children's Oncology GroupLong Term Follow-Up Guidelines*, available at www.survivorshipguidelines.org

Table 13.2 Selected examples of established chemotherapy-associated conditions

Chemotherapy class (agents)	Toxicity/late effects	High risk groups	Available prevalence data	Exposure based screening recommendations
Cardiovascular	• Left ventricular dysfunction • Cardiomyopathy • Dysrhythmias • Dyslipidemia	Anthracyclines (dose-related) • Left ventricular dysfunction • Cardiomyopathy • Dysrhythmias Alkylating agents (Cisplatin) • Dyslipidemia	Congestive heart failure in up to 16 % and subclinical cardiomyopathy in up to 57 % of Ewing-, soft tissue-, and osteosarcoma survivors [220]	Cardiovascular conditions • Echocardiogram every 1–5 years (depending on age at treatment; see COG guidelines) [31] • Electrocardiogram upon entry to LTFU and repeated as clinically indicated
Central nervous system	• Peripheral sensory and motor neuropathy (tingling hands/feet, numbness, sensitivity, pain, poor balance/coordination and reflexes, muscle weakness) • Neurocognitive impairment • Neurological and neurosensory deficits including hearing loss • Leukoencephalopathy • Ototoxicity	Higher doses or combinations of vinca alkaloids and platinum-based therapies containing alkylating agents (cisplatin or carboplatin) • Peripheral neuropathy Vinca alkaloids, Antimetabolites Intrathecal methotrexate, or high dose methotrexate and cytarabine • Sensory/motor and neurocognitive impairments Platinum-base chemotherapy or high dose chemotherapy (especially cisplatin or high doses of carboplatin) • Auditory impairments • Ototoxicity Corticosteroids • Leukoencephalopathy	Sensory and motor impairments detected in 20 and 17.5 % of solid tumours survivors respectively [221]	Peripheral sensory and motor neuropathy • Symptom management only Neurocognitive deficits • Yearly review of education and/or vocational progress • Neuropsychological evaluation upon entry to LTFU and repeated as clinically indicated Auditory impairments • Complete audiologic evaluation upon entry to LTFU and repeated as clinically indicated for patients who received platinum-based chemotherapy
Eye	• Cataracts	Corticosteroids especially combined with radiation • Cataracts		Cataracts • Yearly eye exam focusing (visual acuity, fundoscopic exam)
Hepatobiliary	• Hepatic fibrosis	Methotrexate, mercaptopurine, thioguanine • Hepatic fibrosis		Hepatic fibrosis • Alanine aminotransferase, aspartate aminotransferase, total bilirubin upon entry to LTFU and repeated as clinically indicated

(continued)

Table 13.2 (continued)

Chemotherapy class (agents)	Toxicity/late effects	High risk groups	Available prevalence data	Exposure based screening recommendations
Musculoskeletal	• Decreased bone mineral density • Reduced or uneven growth (resulting in shortened trunk height, limb length discrepancy and kyphoscoliosis) • Osteonecrosis	Antimetabolites • Decreased bone mineral density Corticosteroids • Reduced or uneven growth • Decreased bone mineral density • Osteonecrosis Dexamethasone • Osteonecrosis	Growth hormone deficiency in 48 % of survivors treated with chemotherapy [214] Reduced bone mineral density in 68 % of ALL survivors [222]	Reduced bone mineral density • Bone density evaluation (DEXA or quantitative CT), upon entry to LTFU and repeated as clinically indicated Reduced or uneven growth • Yearly standing and sitting height measured until growth completed Osteonecrosis • Yearly targeted history and physical examination • Bone density evaluation (DEXA or quantitative CT), upon entry to LTFU and repeated as clinically indicated
Reproductive system (females)	• Ovarian failure (hypogonadism) • Gonadal dysfunction and infertility • Ovarian dysfunction that results in delayed or arrested puberty, premature menopause and infertility	Alkylating agents (busulfan, nitrogen mustard, carboplatin, cisplatin or cyclophosphamide) especially combined with radiation Anthracyclines (to lesser extent) • Ovarian failure • Hypogonadism • Infertility	Pubertal abnormalities observed in 32 % of survivors treated with chemotherapy [214]	Ovarian failure • Yearly pubertal onset, tempo and Tanner staging until sexually mature • In females at 13 years and repeated as clinically indicated: Serum follicle-stimulating hormone, luteinizing hormone, and oestradiol Infertility • In females: yearly targeted history and physical examination
Reproductive system (males)	• Hypogonadism • Infertility	Alkylating agents (procarbazine, nitrogen mustard, carboplatin, cisplatin or cyclophosphamide) especially combined with radiation Anthracyclines (to lesser extent) • Hypogonadism • Infertility	Fertility deficit in about 60 % of males [223] 58.8 % azoospermia, 29.4 % oligospermia, and 88.2 % low sperm count in male survivors [224]	Hypogonadism • In males at 14 years and repeated as clinically indicated: Serum testosterone, ideally in the morning Infertility • In males: semen analysis upon patient request and follicle-stimulating hormone if unable to obtain semen analysis

(continued)

Table 13.2 (continued)

Chemotherapy class (agents)	Toxicity/late effects	High risk groups	Available prevalence data	Exposure based screening recommendations
Pulmonary	• Pulmonary fibrosis	Alkylating agents (carmustine, lomustine, busulfan) especially combined with radiation • Pulmonary fibrosis	Pulmonary fibrosis rates vary depending on dose of bleomycin (450 mg, 3–5 %; 500 mg, 20) or carmustine (cumulative dose >700 mg, up to 30 %) [183, 225]	Pulmonary fibrosis • Pulmonary function tests upon entry to LTFU and repeated as clinically indicated
Teeth	• Teeth abnormalities (shortening/thinning of roots, cavities, absence of teeth or roots, easy staining of teeth)	Exposure to any chemotherapy at a younger age • Dental abnormalities	At least one tooth abnormality in 82.9 % ALL survivors [226]	Dental abnormalities • Biannual dental examination (including oral cancer screening) and cleaning
Urinary tract	• Urinary tract abnormalities • Renal dysfunction • Renal toxicity • Liver dysfunction	Alkylating agents (especially cyclophosphamide, ifosfamide) • Urinary tract abnormalities • Bladder complications (especially high-dose without bladder uroprophylaxis) High dose chemotherapy (cisplatin, carboplatin, methotrexate, ifosfamide) • Renal dysfunction • Liver dysfunction Platinum-based therapy • Renal dysfunction	Renal dysfunction in 25 % of patients treated with high dose ifosfamide (14 g/m^2) [227]	Bladder complications • Yearly targeted history and urinalysis Renal dysfunction • Yearly blood pressure and urinalysis • Serum blood urea nitrogen, creatinine and electrolytes (including calcium, phosphorus, magnesium) upon entry to LTFU and repeated as clinically indicated
Any organ system	• Subsequent neoplasms	Anthracyclines • Secondary myelodysplasia Alkylating agents • Myeloid leukaemia • Non-Hodgkin's lymphoma • Hodgkin's disease Epipodophyllotoxins • Myeloid leukaemia		Subsequent neoplasms Regular examinations to screen for potential subsequent neoplasms (e.g. yearly mammogram for breast cancer, yearly physical examination for skin or thyroid cancers, or 5 yearly colonoscopy for colorectal cancer)

Abbreviations: *LTFU* Long Term Follow-Up; *DEXA* Dual Energy X-Ray Absorptiometry; *CT* computed tomography

[a]Exposure based screening recommendations are based on the *Children's Oncology GroupLong Term Follow-Up Guidelines*, available at www.survivorshipguidelines.org

reported that 95.5 % of survivors have a chronic health condition, 80.5 % of which are life threatening by age 45 years [30, 35].

In contrast to survivors of adult cancers, where pre-morbid lifestyle factors such as obesity, physical inactivity and smoking predispose to both the cancer diagnosis and a range of chronic conditions, a young survivor's risk of a particular chronic condition can be linked primarily to the treatment they received. For many chronic conditions, what is seen in young survivors mirrors chronic conditions seen in older, healthy, adults with aging, but occurs at a younger age. Many morbidities may remain undiagnosed and therefore unmanaged due to a lack of awareness about such risks amongst health care providers. Premature atherosclerosis, early onset metabolic syndrome and young age at development of breast cancer highlight this point [36, 37].

13.2.1 Late Mortality in Survivors

Late mortality in child and adolescent cancer survivors is defined as a death five or more years from diagnosis [38]. Survivors' long-term health trajectory differs from that of their age-matched peers, with survivors' risk of late mortality remaining at least 3-fold higher three decades post-diagnosis [38, 39]. Overall risk of mortality is most prominent in the first decade post-diagnosis, steadily decreasing in the subsequent 10 years [40]. However, survivors' risk of death does not ever decrease to a point which mirrors population norms [38]. Of those survivors alive and disease free at 5 years, 88.1 % are alive at 20 years after diagnosis (see Fig. 13.4) [38]. The commonest cause of death is recurrence of the primary cancer (55–75 %), followed by complications arising from the treatment (most commonly cardiac and pulmonary problems, 6–18 %), and new second cancers (12–16 %) (see Fig. 13.5) [38, 40–42]. With further follow-up, deaths from recurrence of the primary cancer plateau, while deaths from second cancers and non-cancer causes become more prevalent [43, 44].

Survivors who are younger at diagnosis (especially <5 years) and those who experience a relapse and are re-treated have a notably higher risk of late mortality [40, 45, 46]. Female sex may increase survivors' risk of late mortality by 1.3–2.1 times compared with males [41, 47], however not all studies demonstrate this, with the effect potentially depending on the specific cause of death (e.g. due to second cancers or non-cancer causes) [19].

Second malignant neoplasms (SMN), defined as histologically distinct malignancies developing at least two months after completion of the treatment of the primary malignancy, are the most serious late toxicities of child and adolescent cancer treatment and over time become the greatest cause of late mortality [48]. In the United States, SEER data suggests that 16 % of all cancers (approximately one in six cases) represent SMNs in all cancer survivors [49]. The cumulative incidence of second neoplasms among survivors treated between 1970 and 1986 and followed in the Childhood Cancer Survivor Study (CCSS) was 20.5 % at 30 years after the

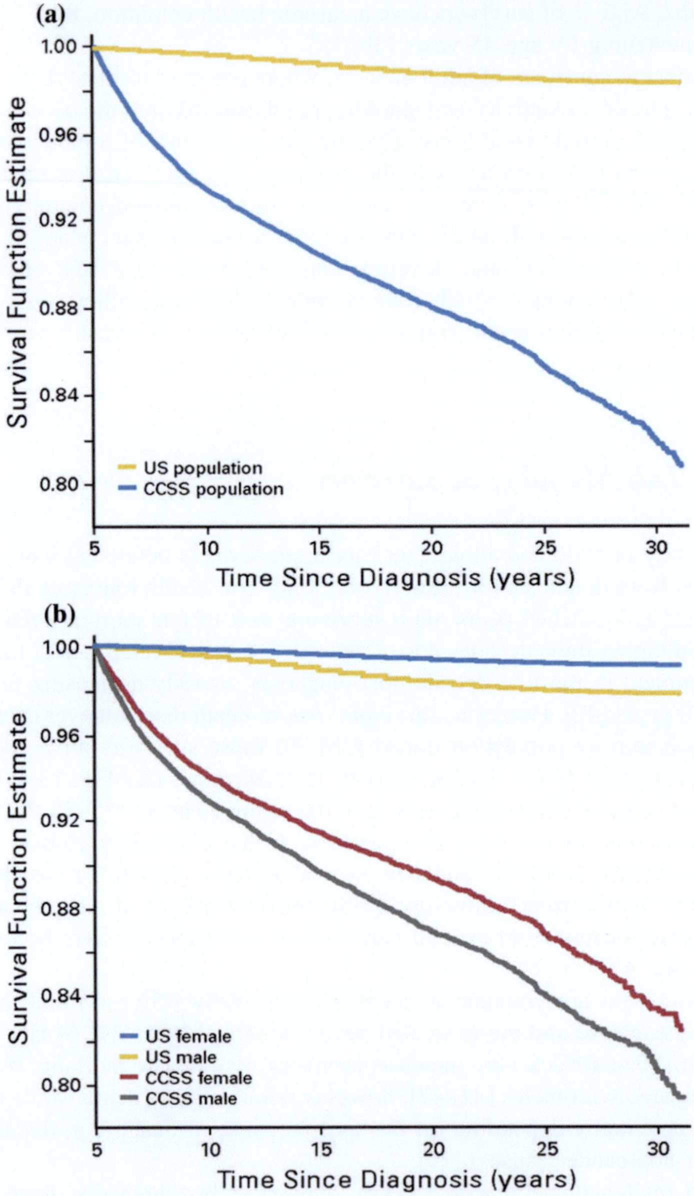

Fig. 13.4 All-cause mortality (survival function estimate) in the general US population and CCSS sample (**a**), and by sex (**b**) [38]

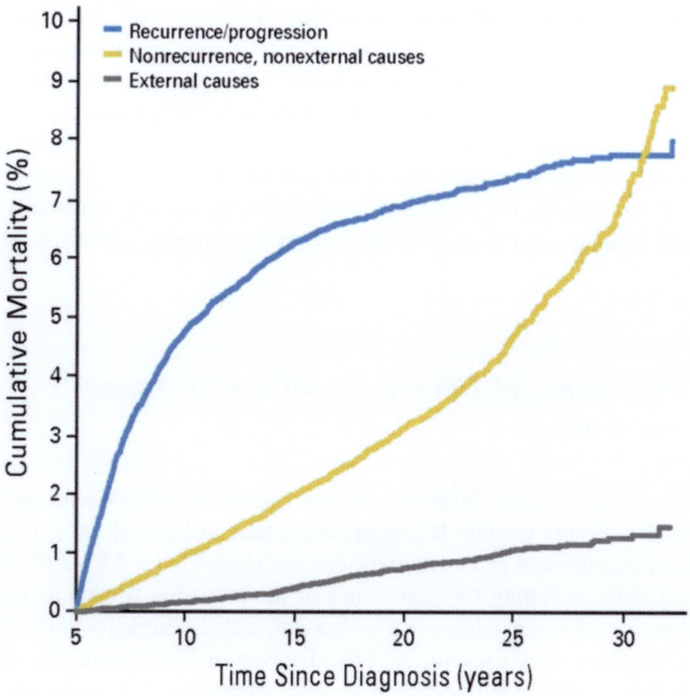

Fig. 13.5 Cumulative cause-specific mortality in the CCSS sample: proportion of deaths attributable to recurrence/progression, non-recurrence/non-external and external causes [38]

childhood cancer diagnosis, 7.9 % for second malignant neoplasms, 9.1 % for non-melanoma skin cancer and 3.1 % for meningioma [50]. Relative to the general population, the risk of SMNs is higher after all primary diagnoses, with the highest risk being following Hodgkin Lymphoma (more common in adolescents and young adults) which is 8.7 fold [50].

The primary cancer diagnosis and the specific therapy received influence the incidence and type of SMNs [51, 52]. Chemotherapy-related myelodysplasia and acute myeloid leukaemia are associated with alkylating agents and topoisomerase inhibitors, and occur after a short latent period with the risk plateauing after 10–15 years [53]. Radiation-related solid SMNs have a latency that exceeds 10 years and does not plateau and include cancer of the breast, thyroid, sarcoma, lung, melanoma and the brain. With increasing age, many survivors experience multiple SMNs. The incidence of solid SMNs does not plateau with time. Even in the 5th and 6th decades of life, survivors have an increased risk of SMNs, highlighting the need for life-long monitoring [53]. In addition to treatment exposures as a cause for SMNs in survivors, the latency suggests potential genetic susceptibility [52].

Genetic cancer syndromes in adult cancer survivors are well described (e.g. the hereditary breast and ovarian cancer syndromes). Genetic syndromes predisposing to cancers occurring in childhood and in young adults are less well described, but appear to occur in 5–10 % of young cancer survivors [11], making up to 29 % of young survivors suitable for genetics assessment [54]. Adult cancer survivors carry additional risks for second cancer which are seldom seen in younger survivors, such as occupational carcinogen exposures and lifestyle factors, especially tobacco smoking and obesity, which add to the multifactorial risk of SMNs after adult cancer [55].

13.2.2 The Nature of Chronic Conditions in Young Survivors

Chronic late conditions may relate to surgery, radiation and/or chemotherapy used to treat cancer in young people. It is beyond the scope of this chapter to address all potential treatment-related chronic conditions in detail. Tables 13.1 and 13.2 offer a detailed overview, including the prevalence of the particular organs and systems at risk of chronic conditions, organised by the anti-cancer therapies a child receives (for comprehensive reviews see [7, 33, 56]). By way of illustration, this section will address cardiovascular complications as one example of a prevalent medical chronic condition, as well as summarising mental health and psychosocial outcomes as examples of non-medical chronic conditions.

13.2.2.1 Long Latent Period Before Chronic Conditions Manifest

Cancer has become a chronic disease in many young people. On average, young people who survive cancer live an additional six decades [6], meaning that their survivorship care must traverse puberty, through to menopause, and old age. While some side effects, such as ototoxicity, develop on treatment or soon afterwards and persist, many conditions due to cancer treatment do not appear until many years after completion of therapy [48]. Figure 13.6 demonstrates ageing survivors' gap in knowledge about chronic conditions due to their cancer treatment, despite their incidence continuing to rise as they age [32, 33]. In AYA cancer survivors, 15 % report 2 or more comorbidities up to 14 months post-treatment, which is associated with higher mental health service needs and poorer self-reported health status [57].

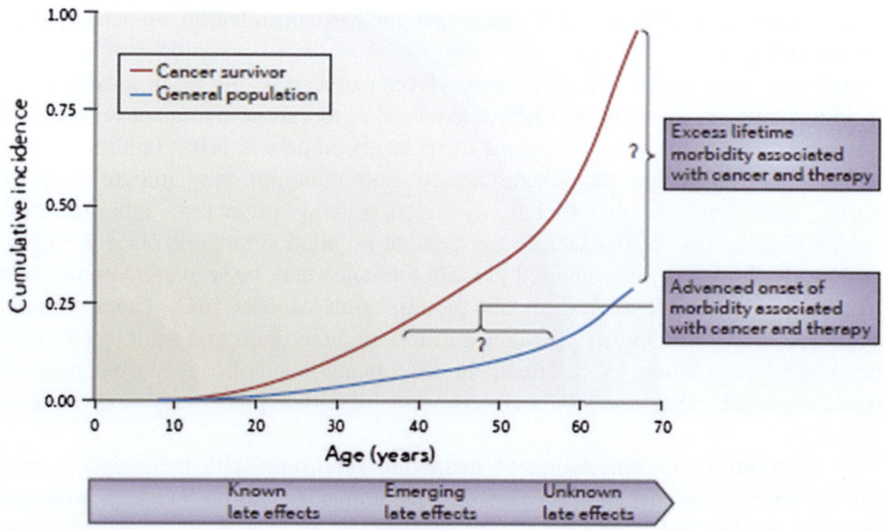

Fig. 13.6 Young cancer survivors increasing gaps in knowledge related to long-term outcomes and late morbidities, with increasing time since treatment [7]

13.2.2.2 Multifactorial Causes of Late Arising Chronic Conditions

While treatment received is incriminated in the development of late effects, the cause of many chronic conditions may be multifactorial. Even before diagnosis and commencement of therapy, the primary malignancy may predispose to late complications, such as hydrocephalus in association with brain tumours causing cognitive dysfunction and possible deafness [58].

13.2.2.3 Cardiometabolic Disorders as One Example of a Chronic Medical Condition

Cardiometabolic disorders exemplify the multifactorial nature of some chronic disorders in young survivors and further consideration is needed in the approach to managing chronic conditions in survivors. Cardiovascular disease (CVD) is the leading non-cancer cause of death in adult survivors of childhood cancer and the cause of significant morbidity [41, 59]. CVD can be the result of direct cardiovascular (CV) damage caused by chemotherapy and/or by radiation to the heart [59]. Although Anthracyclines are the best studied cause of cardiomyopathy and congestive heart failure, nearly all chemotherapeutics have some acute or chronic cardiotoxicity, including therapeutic antibodies and tyrosine kinase inhibitors. Cardiomyopathy can occur early in treatment or can have its onset many years after completion of therapy. The risk is dose dependent, with female gender, age less than 5 years at treatment and concomitant mediatinalirradiation associated with highest risk [59].

It is now appreciated that CVD in survivors can also be the result indirectly of, or aggravated by, accelerated atherosclerosis due to cancer treatment-related cardiovascular risk factors [60]. Previous focus has been on end organ failure, but it is increasingly recognised that chemotherapy and radiation may initiate vascular injury, and lead to endothelial dysfunction and premature atherogenesis. Cardiovascular risk factors seen in the general population such as obesity, hypertension, dyslipidemia and impaired glucose tolerance may be seen at a younger age in survivors of child, adolescent and young adult cancers [61]. The metabolic syndrome occurs at a higher prevalence following both child and adult cancer than the general population [62]. Treatment associated metabolic syndrome may be associated with cardio-metabolic disease and increased predisposition to second cancers.

In adult survivors, correlation of metabolic syndrome with treatment is complicated by the fact that the prevalence of metabolic syndrome increases with age and may predate colon and breast cancer [63]. In adult patients, metabolic syndrome has been documented following haematopoietic stem cell transplant and in association with hypogonadism in testicular, prostate and ovarian cancer [63]. A prospective, cross-sectional study of 248 survivors attending the long-term follow-up clinic at Sydney Children's Hospital, Australia reported a prevalence of insulin resistance of 18 % in pubertal and adult survivors of childhood cancer, at a median follow up of 13 years, double that of controls [64]. None of the prepubertal children met the criteria. Fifty-eight percent of those with insulin resistance had undergone bone marrow transplantation. The most prominent risk factor for development of hyperinsulinism, impaired glucose tolerance and diabetes mellitus was Total Body Irradaition (TBI). However, untreated hypogonadism and abdominal obesity also emerged as important. The finding of hypogonadism as an independent metabolic risk factor is consistent with other studies assessing bone marrow transplantation patients and adults after testicular cancer and underlines the need for screening of patients and appropriate replacement therapy [63]. The pathogenesis of the metabolic syndrome in survivors is largely unknown but may differ from the general population and help researchers to identify effective preventive and therapeutic measures.

In children treated for cancer, interactions between lifestyle, treatment and environmental factors all probably contribute to the clustering of metabolic abnormalities [62] Endocrine dysfunction (usually but not exclusively radiation induced) is a frequent common factor. Additionally, chemotherapy induced electrolyte deficiencies or direct toxicity to muscle, adipose tissue and the endothelium might also contribute to metabolic syndrome in childhood cancer survivors [63]. Emerging literature is suggesting a role for visceral adipose tissue as an endocrine organ capable of causing dyslipidemia.

In the absence of understanding a central aetiological factor, therapeutic interventions for metabolic syndrome are directed toward individual components of the syndrome and cardiovascular risk factors. Screening to identify at-risk survivors and provide directed health counselling is recommended [62]. COG and other Childhood Survivorship guidelines have developed risk based, exposure related recommendations for follow-up of cardiovascular risk factors [21, 31]. Lifestyle interventions include advice against smoking and an increasing amount of literature supports the benefits of dietary and exercise interventions [65]. Other ongoing interventions aim to address maladaptive feeding behaviours established during cancer treatment and a persisting taste and smell dysfunction in survivors which may influence their food choices [66, 67]. The correction of hormone deficiencies may also reduce the risk of developing the metabolic syndrome. When reduction of metabolic risk factors is insufficient, drug interventions to treat hyperglycaemia may be necessary [63]. The longitudinal effect of the treatment of metabolic syndrome on the development of cardiovascular disease in survivors is unknown and should be the focus of future research.

13.2.3 Chronic Psychosocial Conditions and Life Outcomes in Survivors

13.2.3.1 Mental Health

Child and adolescent cancer can have a profound impact on young survivors and their families [68]. Early psychosocial research focussed primarily on identifying possible deleterious effects of cancer affecting young people (including depression, anxiety, generalised distress, suicidal ideation, and posttraumatic stress disorder). Newer evidence however, suggests that young survivors can also experience concomitant positive outcomes, including posttraumatic growth, benefit finding, and improved interpersonal maturity [68, 69]. Identifying survivors most at risk of developing poor mental health, and intervening early with effective interventions, appear to be key to planning best practice supportive care for survivors in the long term.

As a group, childhood cancer survivors generally have psychosocial outcomes that are on a par with their siblings and peers without cancer [68]. Many young survivors demonstrate considerable resilience in their recovery from a highly disruptive and often frightening life event. Many re-integrate well into school, social life, and their early careers [69]. Some survivors also describe finding benefits in their cancer experience [70], often conceptualised as posttraumatic growth [68, 71]. Early work suggests that survivors of leukaemia, and those diagnosed in middle childhood (i.e. over 5 years of age) may experience more benefit finding than younger and older patients [68, 72].

There are, however, particular subgroups at significant risk of developing substantial mental health problems, particularly in the early years post-treatment [73]. For some survivors, mental health problems and poor adjustment can be experienced simultaneously with aspects of posttraumatic growth [68, 69]. Young survivors of central nervous system tumours are particularly at risk of both poor psychosocial and neurocognitive outcomes, as are those who have had cranial radiation or a stem cell transplant. Other medical factors, such as experiencing chronic pain and other health conditions after cancer treatment are also associated with poorer mental health outcomes [68]. Data on the impact of other potential clinical/medical predictors of poor mental health are more mixed, although some research suggests that young people who experienced more intense treatment may be more likely to develop posttraumatic stress symptoms and distress [74, 75].

There is growing evidence to suggest that survivors diagnosed during adolescence may experience more disruption to their mental health than survivors diagnosed in early childhood or adulthood [75]. Other key risk factors for experiencing worse mental health for children and AYAs include female sex, and social factors (such as having a lower household income, lower educational achievement, and being unmarried). A recent review also highlighted the importance of health beliefs in young cancer survivors, demonstrating that survivors with poor perceived physical health also had poorer mental health [68].

In keeping with the notion that families, rather than patients, should the unit of care, young survivors' families appear particularly important in influencing their mental health. Young adults with a family history of mental illness are more likely to experience psychosocial distress themselves [76]. Several studies conducted across different cultural groups have also demonstrated that family functioning during and after cancer treatment is a significant predictor of young survivors' mental health outcomes [77, 78]. One US study, for example, reported that 75 % of adolescent cancer survivors with PTSD had families categorised as functioning poorly [78]. Considering, and treating, the mental health concerns of parents of young cancer survivors might be a fruitful area for future interventions to improve outcomes for the whole family [73].

13.2.3.2 Cognitive Outcomes

Children and young people treated for cancer are at risk of neurocognitive difficulties during survivorship. Deficits are most typically seen in the core areas of cognition: attention, working memory, processing speed, executive function and visual motor integration [24, 79, 80]. However, difficulties with learning and memory are also prevalent, and can be secondary to problems with attention, working memory and executive function [24, 81]. On an individual level, the profile and severity of difficulties observed in any single survivor will be unique and dependent on factors such as age at diagnosis, developmental stage, premorbid intellectual ability and the interaction with diagnosis and treatment received. For example, adolescents and young adults (AYAs) experience cancer at an age which is typified by rapid neurocognitive development in higher level thinking skills and executive functions, as well as social and emotional function which is crucial for identity formation [82]. As such, AYAs are at increased risk of difficulties with executive functions including task efficiency, inhibition (or emotion regulation), and memory [16].

Many young survivors initially demonstrate age appropriate cognitive skills after treatment. However neurocognitive problems, deficits in thinking skills, learning and memory, can appear in the years following treatment [24, 79]. Problems with cognitive skills can become apparent when a child enters high school and learning requires more higher level skills, such as self-implemented organisation and planning [16]. This distinction is important to make: children do not lose cognitive skills, rather, cancer and its treatment can to interrupt normal neurodevelopmental processes such that children fail to acquire crucial cognitive skills and age appropriate neurocognitive milestones [83]. Cognitive difficulties can be lasting and experienced long into adulthood, with up to 48 % of survivors experiencing neurocognitive impairment more than 25 years after treatment [20]. Verbal intellectual skills may initially appear within the normal range relative to that of their peers shortly after treatment, however well after treatment ceases, survivors may experience difficulties with verbal intellectual skills potentially related to ongoing difficulties with attention [84].

Modern treatment regimens, where exposure to CNS radiotherapy is reduced, have led to a reduction in the occurrence of cognitive difficulties for survivors. Despite these treatment improvements, 40–60 % of children with ALL experience cognitive impairment during survivorship [85, 86]. Chemotherapy alone can cause difficulties with cognitive function [87]. Survivors who received high dose methotrexate and cytarabine (commonly used in ALL treatment), are at increased risk of cognitive impairment [85]. Survivors at particular risk of cognitive difficulties after treatment are those with Central Nervous System (CNS) cancer, and those who have received CNS directed therapy (including surgery, radiotherapy and chemotherapy). Approximately 40–100 % of children with brain cancers experience cognitive impairment [79]. New molecularly targeted biological therapies also have the potential to impact developing cognitive abilities, but are yet to be followed up longitudinally [88]. Individual risk factors associated with poor cognitive outcomes include younger age at diagnosis (particularly <3 years at diagnosis and treatment), being female, and a longer time since treatment [24]. In addition, some genetic polymorphisms related to oxidative stress and/or neuroinflammation may confer additional risk of neurocognitive conditions [89, 90]. Environmental risk factors include family or parents who do not prioritise education [91].

13.2.3.3 Educational Outcomes

Compared with the general population, childhood cancer survivors have reduced academic achievement [92, 93], are more likely to repeat a school grade [94, 95], and require educational support [94, 96]. Children who had CNS tumours are at particular risk and have poorer educational and employment outcomes than survivors of non-CNS cancer and the general population [93, 97]. Poor educational attainment among childhood cancer survivors is likely due to multiple factors. Children can struggle to re-integrate into the school environment after cancer treatment is complete [98]. This may be due in part to prolonged absences from the classroom and learning environment during treatment which can continue long into survivorship. Even 10 years after diagnosis survivors of childhood cancer may miss almost twice as many school days compared with their peers [99].

AYA cancer survivors are especially vulnerable to the negative effects of absence from school. Re-integration with education is particularly important in AYAs and cancer treatment causes significant disruption to normal school attendance (when compared with the majority of childhood diagnoses occurring under 5 years of age). Poor reintegration to school is associated with reduced emotional well-being and global self-esteem [82]. Many AYAs also report social difficulties together with academic difficulties on return to school [82, 100]. Treatment-related side effects, such as loss of hair, can negatively impact self-esteem, and AYAs with body image concerns can withdraw from usual social activities including engagement with school [82, 101]. Other barriers to school attendance for AYAs include ongoing fatigue and treatment related side-effects as well as lack of support or understanding from teachers [82, 100, 102].

In addition to time spent away from formal learning, impairment in cognitive skills due to cancer and its treatment impact educational outcomes [15, 83]. Difficulties with reading, spelling, and mathematics have been consistently demonstrated among young survivors [103–106]. A good understanding of an individual survivors' neurocognitive profile after cancer allows appropriate school and higher education support to be identified. Students placed in special support classes or given additional educational support perform better than those not offered the same support [94, 96].

Box 1: What do neurocognitive deficits look like?
Attention and concentration difficulties impact a child's ability to learn and remember new information in the classroom and at home, and can result in inconsistent academic performance, careless errors, and incomplete assignments. Difficulties with processing speed can mean children take longer to complete schoolwork or assignments, and may miss instruction details. Their work may therefore be incomplete or missing some aspects. Children with weaknesses in executive functions may struggle to correctly sequence or order their responses, so that their work appears haphazard and unorganised or poorly considered. They may also have difficulty moving between tasks and become flustered or upset when task demands change.

13.2.3.4 Life Milestones

Children surviving all cancer types experience social difficulties after cancer to some degree [107]. Survivors of CNS cancers, or those who have received CNS directed therapy, may be particularly vulnerable to negative social outcomes

[108–110]. They can also be more socially isolated and less likely to be rated as a close friend than their classroom peers [108]. As adults, survivors who experience social difficulties are less likely to form lasting romantic relationships, and experience reduced quality of life and emotional well-being as a result [107, 111–113].

Life milestones such as living independently and achieving career promotions are achieved at lower rates among survivors of childhood brain cancer [93, 97, 111, 114]. For survivors of other childhood and adolescent cancers, vocational outcomes are variable. Some studies report no difference in rates of current employment between survivors and the general population [15, 16, 94, 115], though not all have found this [15, 114]. Young survivors may be older when starting their first occupation [15]. Key risk factors for unemployment include poor cognitive or educational outcomes after cancer, younger age at diagnosis, and being female [15, 114].

13.3 Managing Chronic Conditions in Young Survivors

13.3.1 Modifying Treatment Regimens to Reduce Risk of Treatment-Related Chronic Conditions

The decade in which patients were diagnosed influences survivors' risk of short and long term mortality, reflecting medical advances in detection and treatment. Evidence for a decline in cumulative late mortality due to cancer treatment in more recent decades of primary diagnosis and treatment is strong [38, 116, 117]. The modification of current therapy approaches is driven by knowledge gained from early survivors and has led to significant reductions in some of the ongoing treatment-related illnesses observed in this cohort.

13.3.1.1 Surgical Changes to Reduce the Risk of Chronic Conditions in Survivors

Early successes in treating cancer in young people were achieved by disfiguring surgery, including limb amputation and bladder exenteration which caused life-long functional disability. With advances in imaging and effective chemotherapy regimens, the aim of surgery today is to avoid disfigurement and impaired function. Limb sparing procedures for bone tumours have largely replaced amputation and reduced functional deformity [118]. With modern imaging, splenectomy for staging is avoided, averting the risk of overwhelming infection [119]. Cystectomy is rarely performed for tumours involving the bladder [120]. Nephron sparing surgery is now commonly performed for Wilms' tumour, conserving renal function and avoiding chronic renal issues [121].

13.3.1.2 Radiation Changes to Reduce the Risk of Chronic Conditions in Survivors

Radiation therapy has been a mainstay of management of childhood malignancy, but has resulted in many chronic conditions. The risk associated with radiation relates to the radiation source, total dose administered, and volume and fractionation, as well as sex, age at time of treatment and the organ irradiated (see Table 13.1). Invasive and non-invasive second cancers are seen in survivors treated with radiation, after a relatively long latent period. Second Neoplasms are discussed below.

Knowledge of late adverse effects of radiation has driven attempts to eliminate or reduce radiation where possible. The radiation technique used for Wilms' tumour patients has also changed. Patients with Wilms' tumour who previously received radiation to the flank developed severe scoliosis, while the new technique (including the whole vertebral body) still causes height loss but no functional deformity due to wedging of the vertebrae (see Fig. 13.7) [122].

Except in very high risk leukaemia patients, cranial radiation therapy is now avoided in children due to the long-term sequelae and every effort is made to avoid its use in brain tumour patients less than 3 years of age because of the devastating effects on cognitive function REF [123, 124]. Total Body Irradiation (TBI) has been eliminated in the treatment of neuroblastoma. Patients who received TBI as part of their conditioning were reported to have growth (100 %) and pubertal failure (83 %), hearing impairment (73 %), orthopaedic complications (63 %), renal impairment (47 %) and thyroid dysfunction (36 %) [125].

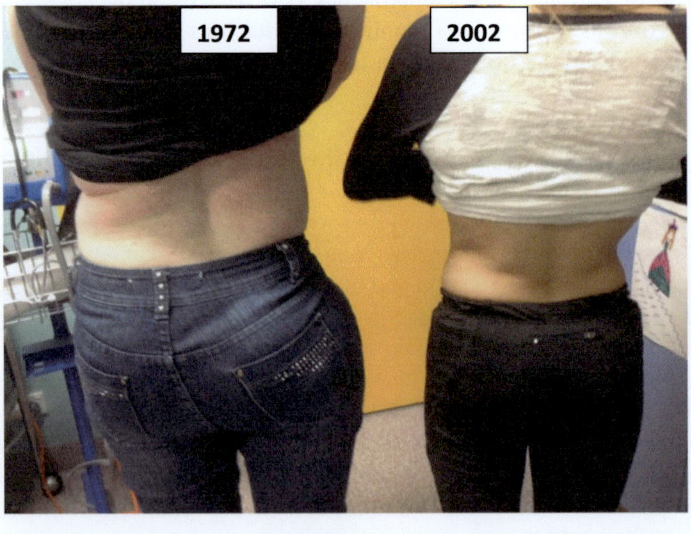

Fig. 13.7 Cancer survivors treated with radiation in 1972 (*left*) and 2002 (*right*). The patient treated earlier displays noticeable Kyphoscoliosis, whilst the patient treated more recently, using new radiation techniques, is spared this late effect

There is a current randomised trial investigating whether relapsed Acute Lymphoblastic Leukaemia can be successfully treated without TBI in view of the multiple chronic effects documented (see Table 13.1).

13.3.1.3 Chemotherapy Changes to Reduce Risk of Chronic Conditions in Survivors

A number of chronic conditions have been attributed to chemotherapy used in successful treatment protocols for childhood cancer (see Table 13.2). Late or chronic toxicities of chemotherapy are related to cumulative dose received, scheduling, as well as the sex and age of the patient at the time of treatment. Higher risk of such conditions is associated with certain classes of chemotherapeutic agents, including alkylating agents, anthracycline antibiotics, antimetabolites, corticosteroids, epipodophylotoxins, and vinca alkaloids [7]. Newer agents such as the therapeutic antibodies and tyrosine kinase inhibitors have also been implicated [59]. With the accumulation of knowledge of late effects, newer treatment protocols attempt to limit the total dose of anthracyclines to reduce the risk of cardiovascular disease, and avoid alkylating agents where possible to decrease the risk of second cancers [126, 127].

13.3.2 Importance of Surveillance

Ongoing surveillance is vital for young cancer survivors as demonstrated by the seriousness, scope and prevalence of chronic conditions in this population. Without early intervention, these conditions can shorten survivors' lives and can severely impact quality of life [41]. Fortunately, many of these conditions are modifiable through prevention, or early detection and intervention (see Sect. 13.3 for examples) [128]. It is crucial that all young survivors receive on-going follow-up care well into adulthood, to continue monitoring for potential physical and psychosocial conditions. Young cancer survivors represent an especially unique cohort: during the six or more decades after they are 'cured' [129], they will function mostly outside the tertiary health care system; yet their health risks are significantly higher than their peers as reviewed above [130].

Clinicians now widely recognise that risk-based long-term follow-up (LTFU) care for young survivors is essential [131] and long term follow-up centres have been established in most major cities worldwide. In Australia, all paediatric tertiary centres run LTFU clinics to provide anticipatory medical and psychosocial care to young survivors. The potential benefit of these centres is two-fold. Clinically, they provide surveillance for this high risk group, to ensure the highest possible level of well-being of all long-term survivors. They also assist in improving our understanding of chronic illness in this population, thereby leading to the refinement of future treatment protocols to minimise treatment toxicity in the next generation of young people affected by cancer. If survivors do not participate in appropriate follow-up, they forgo optimal management of chronic conditions and opportunities for prevention, early detection and risk reduction, as well as not contributing to the benefits of longitudinal research in this patient population.

13.3.3 Chronic Condition Management and Survivorship Guidelines

In the landmark 2003 publication, "Lost in transition", the Institute of Medicine recommended that all survivors receive follow-up care from a practitioner knowledgeable about the survivor's cancer history, their long-term risks and their recommended health care and surveillance, to minimise the impact of potential late effects of cancer therapy [132]. A number of national groups in the USA (see sample Fig. 13.8), Scotland, Sweden and the Netherlands have developed surveillance guidelines which incorporate risks based on therapeutic exposures and allow prediction of chronic illness based on treatment received [22, 133, 134]. In an attempt to ensure concordance of guidelines, the International Late Effects of Childhood Cancer Guideline Harmonization Group (IGHG) is reviewing available literature to develop standardised recommendations for follow-up of childhood cancer survivors [135].

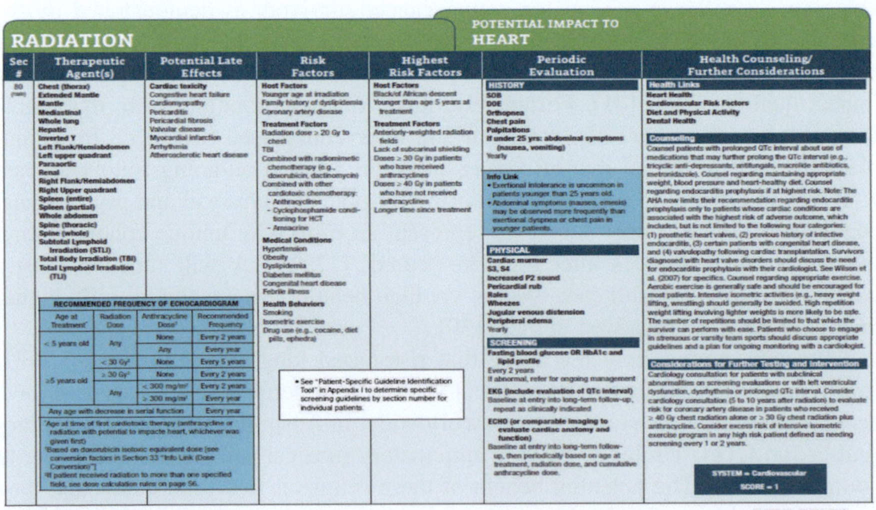

Fig. 13.8 A sample from the children's oncology group (COG) Guidelines for health living after treatment for childhood cancer, specifically the potential impact to male survivors' hearts as a result of radiation [31]

The development of comprehensive, harmonised, guidelines for young survivors, based on treatment received, stand in contrast to the approach traditionally taken in adult survivorship guidelines, which tend to be tumour specific. Recommendations for follow-up care of adult survivors now feature in a number of tumour-specific guidelines [136–138], however such guidance is not available for all adult tumour types, especially rare cancers, nor is the advice necessarily consistent across guidelines for common treatment exposures (for example, the NCCN adult breast cancer guidelines do not comment on monitoring for cardiac toxicity after anthracyclines and chest radiotherapy, whereas the guidelines for Hodgkin's lymphoma by the same group provides a suggested approach). General survivorship guidelines are emerging for adults [139], however these are not as comprehensive as the guidelines available for childhood cancer survivors. It is arguable that the exposure-based approach taken by the childhood groups provides a rational approach which is applicable to all survivors, and adoption of such an approach for adults may help to address some of the short-comings with the tumour-based approach (Fig. 13.9).

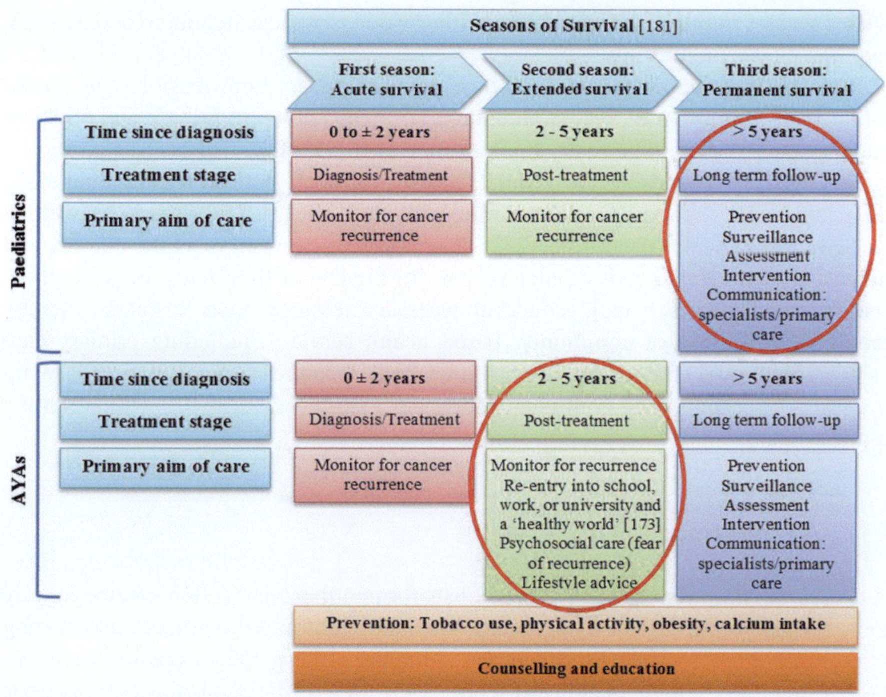

Fig. 13.9 Trajectory of risk-based long-term follow-up care of paediatric cancer survivors and adolescent and young adult cancer survivors (AYAs), highlighting the importance of the third season in paediatrics as opposed to the second season in AYA survivors

13.3.3.1 Risk Stratification

Individual, ongoing multidisciplinary follow-up for every young survivor, whilst ideal, is both financially unviable and difficult to maintain given the escalating number of young people surviving cancer every year [140]. Follow-up practices often vary both within and between centres, often revealing an unnecessary dependence on hospitals and in older survivors, an age-inappropriate setting [141, 142]. This emphasises the need for more manageable, systematic, and evidence-based models of long term follow-up care. In recognising that not all survivors require hospital-based long term follow-up care [143], a possible solution is to offer individually tailored care by stratifying survivors by their risk of developing chronic illnesses.

Risk-based models of care are founded upon the notion that survivors' risk of developing long-term adverse health outcomes can be predicted by their underlying malignancy, including its site, as well as the nature and intensity of cancer therapy received [140]. Evidence-based guidelines incorporating this approach (as reviewed above) categorise patients into therapy-based groups, usually consisting of three levels of risk (low, moderate and high) [144, 145]. A high level of risk is associated with a greater number and more severe illness due to cancer treatment and as such, requires closer monitoring.

The stratification of survivors in this manner appears both feasible and appropriate [140]. Importantly, risk stratification has been shown to be safe and effective and reported by staff to be easily implemented [146]. Ideally, risk-based care should be anticipatory and proactive, whilst addressing each patient's individual risks associated with their diagnosis, treatment received, health behaviours, as well as any co-morbid health conditions [27]. This model of care can meet the unique, and potentially changing, needs of each patient for the rest of their lives. Importantly, a risk-stratified approach may reduce unnecessary reliance upon hospitals, thereby maximising the use of community based health services, including primary care [140]. This model enables already resource-limited centres to focus their follow-up programs on maintaining continued follow-up with those survivors who are at the highest risk.

13.3.3.2 Survivorship Care Plans

As survivors may visit a range of specialists for treatment and follow-up, they rarely have a single integrated medical record when they return to the primary care setting [147]. Survivorship Care Plans (SCPs) summarise the patient's profile for themselves and their future healthcare team [145, 148–150]. Typically they include details about survivors' diagnosis, treatment, an ongoing follow-up care plan including personalised recommendations, and sometimes include lifestyle and health behaviour advice or support [145, 148]. SCPs have the potential to improve post-treatment care for childhood cancer survivors, by facilitating communication between members of a survivor's health care team (e.g. oncologist, GP and specialists) or between health settings (e.g. between primary and tertiary, or between hospitals if a patient relocates) [145]. Additional benefits include the promotion of survivor independence and continuity of care, especially as they transition to adult services [151]. Given that most SCPs are populated by oncology teams, the significant time taken for their preparation is a noteworthy barrier to their implementation [152]. Additional research is necessary to establish their utility in clinical practice, including measures for maximising their efficacy [148].

In childhood cancer survivors, a small single arm study found that provision of a care plan was associated with uptake of recommended screening for second cancers and cardiac toxicity [153]; whether this will translate to a reduction in chronic disease remains unproven. In the adult cancer setting, a number of qualitative studies have demonstrated that both cancer survivors and clinicians view receipt of a care plan document favourably [154–156], but establishing evidence of clinically meaningful benefits has proven challenging and to date SCP trials have largely proven negative. A number of methodological issues cloud interpretation of these findings however, including the nature and timing of delivery of the intervention, targeting of the appropriate patient population, selection of clinically relevant endpoints, and the duration of follow-up required.

Such challenges are exemplified in a randomised trial of survivorship care plans in breast cancer survivors, which proved negative for its primary endpoint of cancer-related distress and other self-reported quality of life outcomes [157]. However, this study has been criticised for the patient population selected, being several years after treatment completion, and the failure to report on clinically important outcomes such as adherence to recommended follow-up, lifestyle behaviours, tumour recurrence and survival. It is also likely that the control arm in this study received an intervention in the form of a survivorship-focussed discharge visit (without SCP provision), which is not part of routine care. A study of SCPs in endometrial cancer similarly found no difference in satisfaction with information provision or care, but an increase in patients' concerns, symptoms and cancer related health care utilisation [158]. It is conceivable that this may translate into appropriate health surveillance and promotion activities; however this remains unproven. Given these challenges with the evidence-base, it would be premature to overlook the important function that SCPs can serve in information transfer between health settings and at care transitions. Efforts to establish their long term impact on chronic disease management should therefore continue.

They are particularly important tools for the management of chronic conditions stemming from childhood and adolescence (refer to Sect. 3.2 for further detail on the use of SCPs in the management of adult chronic conditions). The use of SCPs spans many life stages, requiring ongoing management and updating of information to ensure that the information remains relevant. Furthermore, SCPs may be particularly important for accompanying patients upon their transition to adulthood, particularly as their care shifts from family/parent-focused to more patient-centred care in the adult setting.

13.3.4 Transition and Engagement with Primary Care

The purpose of transition is to ensure that survivors receive age-appropriate follow-up care. Facilitating more formal transition from paediatric care to adult survivorship services may help to better meet young survivors' unique and changing medical, developmental, and psychosocial needs. Ideally, transition should be a 'purposeful' and 'planned' process rather than a single event [159]. That is, it should be discussed early with the patient and family to more effectively prepare them, and to encourage greater health-related responsibility in the young person [160]. This ensures that movement towards adult care is not unexpected and therefore undesired, whilst also maintaining continuity of care.

The transition from paediatric to adult-centred care is complex. Unfortunately, many patients are lost to active follow-up at this stage [161]. Many young survivors have insufficient knowledge of their cancer-related medical history and the recommended health promotion and screening practices that could improve their long-term outcomes [162]. Even in survivors who are engaged in follow-up care, much of the chronic illness education is often directed at their parents and may not be transferred formally to the child. This contributes to young survivors' lack of knowledge about their risk of such illnesses, and may be partly responsible for the declining participation in survivorship programs with age.

There are several, widely documented, barriers which prevent formal and effective transition to age-appropriate care [160, 161, 163]. Hospital processes (such as poor supervision during the transition stage) or staff attitudes, usually a reluctance to pass care onto adult units, are common obstacles [161]. A lack of parent/caregiver knowledge, including a lack of familiarity with chronic treatment-related conditions and risks, or patient factors such as a dependency on oncologists or other members of the treating team, or over-protective families may also prevent effective transition [161]. Providers of care in adult health settings may also inhibit the successful transition of patients, due to lack of experience/knowledge of the issues unique to young survivors, or a lack of experience building patient rapport in this age group [163]. Even among oncologists, substantial gaps exist in knowledge about the late effects likely to affect young cancer survivors [164].

Most paediatric oncology clinics discharge survivors between ages 18–25, and there is a lack of services to which to transition discharged survivors [165]. Increasing acknowledgement of the unsuitability of paediatric follow-up centres, especially for AYAs, has encouraged the creation of some age-appropriate centres [142]. However many of these are still situated within paediatric units. Adolescence is characterised by increasing independence, self-awareness, understanding of abstract and complex information, and changing relationships, identity, roles and responsibilities [166]. A formal transition process from family to adult-focused health care services is therefore essential to alleviate the detrimental impact of these changes on AYA survivors' engagement with follow-up care.

Not all young survivors need specialist tertiary care. Some survivors with lower risk cancers (e.g. Wilms' tumour) and those who received less intense treatment may receive adequate follow-up care through their general practitioner (GP) [167]. LTFU clinics at paediatric centres commonly discharge, mainly low-risk, survivors to a GP. However, GPs report lack of confidence in caring for this cohort and prefer not to be primarily responsible for young survivors' care [167, 168]. GPs typically care for few young cancer patients in their career and have limited knowledge of chronic illness in this population [169]. This can be compounded by a perceived lack of information and communication regarding their patient's medical history and care plan from the treating hospital [170–172].

Despite these barriers, GPs may be willing to provide care to this population with appropriate tertiary support [173]. GPs are already involved in some aspect of survivors' follow-up care in almost 60 % of childhood cancer survivors [174]. However unfortunately, LTFU clinic limitations and GPs; lack of confidence compels many survivors to become disengaged with their cancer care and therefore deprived of appropriate surveillance [167, 168].

13.3.5 Survivors' Engagement in Follow-up Care for Chronic Conditions

Despite health-risks escalating over time, engagement in follow-up care actually decreases with the passage of time, resulting in a significant gap in care [22, 130, 175–177]. As many as 1 in 2 survivors do not attend any form of cancer-related follow-up care [178]. Yet a large proportion of these disengaged survivors are at high risk of adverse health outcomes, or unknowingly experience them [179], and are therefore in need of ongoing surveillance and early intervention [178].

To encourage appropriate follow-up care, survivors should be educated about their medical history, including their diagnosis and treatment, as well as the significance of regular survivorship care. Disengaged survivors are compelled to become their own 'care integrator', single-handedly managing multiple, non-cancer specialist appointments (e.g. cardiologist, neurologist, etc.), multiple screening schedules (e.g. breast exams after chest irradiation, etc.), significant costs and time off work/study, in order to adhere to survivorship guidelines which are revised regularly [167, 168].

Young survivors experience many barriers to remaining engaged in follow-up services. These are commonly classified as survivor-related barriers (such as lack of awareness about their treatment history or resulting risk of chronic illness, or being unaware of long term follow up services), provider-related barriers (for instance, a lack of appointment reminders/prompts, poor communication with the survivor and/or specialists, lack of knowledge or relevant experience), health care environment-related barriers (including financial costs, or distance to the centre/clinic), and insurance/policy-related barriers [7, 180]. Many survivors also choose not to engage in follow-up care due to a desire to leave their past behind, or due to a perceived lack of control over developing/preventing chronic illness. They may also experience heightened distress when returning to their treating hospital, another disincentive to remaining engaged with their follow up care [180].

13.3.6 Ideal Models of Ongoing Surveillance for Chronic Conditions in Survivors

Physician and cancer survivor, Fitzhugh Mullan, brings attention to the inadequacy of the binary description of the cancer trajectory as 'sickness' followed by 'cure' [181]. His own experience of acute illness following treatment and 'cure' informed the development of three "seasons" of survival: acute, extended and permanent survival. The first is rather medical and describes the diagnosis stage, characterised by anxiety, pain and confrontation with death. The second, extended survival describes the remission phase and is usually a period of reduced strength (from treatment), healing, and fear of recurrence. Finally, permanent survival roughly aligns with "cure", whereby the patient becomes a survivor coping with the after-effects of the cancer experience. In this latter phase of permanent survival, young survivors may be faced with discrimination, vocational and insurance restrictions, and other difficulties reintegrating back to 'normal' life. The benefit of understanding these seasons extends beyond beating the cancer itself, to address the specific needs of survivors and minimise the lasting medical and psychosocial effects of cancer often experienced well into survivorship.

Children and adolescents are generally well cared for at their oncology centre during the first and second seasons. However, adult and AYA survivors often experience a sense of abandonment upon entering the second season, permanent survival, particularly after such close observation during and following treatment [69]. Given the family-centred care approach of most paediatric oncology units, parents (and even siblings) are usually intimately involved with the child's initial treatment, and therefore often remain involved in survivorship care planning for young survivors. When children are diagnosed very young, survivors can have limited recall and understanding about their cancer and the treatment they received [48, 182], increasing their reliance on parents and making their transition to independent adult healthcare settings more complex.

An ideal approach to survivorship care for young survivors is characterised as being risk-based, involving routine health care and a personalised care plan, aimed at the management and prevention of chronic conditions that arise due to cancer and its treatment, while at the same time ensuring their normal, holistic care is met [183]. This is best achieved using a 'hybrid approach' [7] which encompasses evidence-based guidelines, developed by and agreed upon by the multidisciplinary team involved in the long-term follow–up care of childhood cancer survivors and involving, primary care physicians who can offer more holistic care to survivors following transition and well into adulthood, addressing both their survivorship and general health needs [184]. There is little about such an approach which is not equally applicable to survivors of adult cancers.

13.4 Directions for Future Research and Practice

Many treatment-related conditions do not become apparent for years or decades after treatment completion. The prevalence and severity of such conditions highlight the need for improved ongoing surveillance and comprehensive follow-up care following treatment, well into adulthood. It is also imperative that survivors and health care professionals are educated about survivors' increasing risk of late treatment-related conditions as well as about the appropriate follow-up care for their prevention or management. Available data and knowledge about late complications arising from childhood cancer treatment are important for the modification of new protocols, and to reduce further chronic conditions in future generations. Researchers' efforts should be focused on surveillance studies, interventions and prevention to reduce the potential burden of these chronic conditions and to ensure the years of life saved are of the highest possible quality.

The need for effective interventions to reduce the burden of chronic physical and mental health conditions in young survivors and their families is urgent [32, 185, 186]. Fortunately, many chronic conditions following childhood cancer treatment are preventable or treatable with appropriate medical care, emphasising the importance of proactive care [128]. Treatment related risks may be modified by health-related behaviours (smoking, alcohol, exercise and obesity). It is now possible to reduce the incidence of chronic conditions in survivors with focused prevention strategies [35, 187]. Behavioural medicine interventions can help to address osteoporosis [188], obesity and metabolic syndrome [62], and cardiovascular disease [187]. Mental health interventions can effectively reduce anxiety/depression, and poor social skills [189, 190]. Parent-targeted interventions can create 'whole family' change [191–196]. There is however, a serious gap in the availability of age-appropriate evidence-based interventions.

Survivors of adult cancer may enter their cancer journey from a very different place in their lives, but these recommendations are equally applicable to survivors of adult cancer. Providers of adult cancer survivorship care may benefit from considering the experience of their paediatric colleagues. By contrast with the childhood cancer model, there are relatively few specialised survivorship services or long term follow-up clinics for survivors of adult cancer in Australia. The majority of adult survivors are followed by their treating oncologist for a variable period of time, typically somewhat proportional to their risk of relapse, before being discharged to care in the community with their general practitioner. This model of care has provided little opportunity to accurately capture the late morbidity burden experienced by these survivors, or to implement appropriate early intervention or preventive care. Much could be learned from the childhood cancer experience in this regard.

Adult cancer survivors report poorer physical and psychological well-being, are at increased risk of a range of co-morbid medical conditions and are approximately 50 % more likely to die of non-cancer causes compared to their peers [197, 198]. They too carry an excess chronic disease burden related to their cancer and its treatment which is not solely explained by pre-morbid lifestyle factors. The adverse lifestyle risk factors of many adult cancer survivors should not be underestimated however, with population data suggesting that fewer than 5 % are meeting recommendations for all three of diet, exercise and smoking [199], yet less than 10 % will have a discussion with a health care provider about all three lifestyle behaviours [200]. Just as in considering the needs of young survivors, a holistic approach to follow-up is essential for adults too, to monitor and manage chronic illness following cancer treatment, which may include the treating oncologist but must acknowledge the central role of the general practitioner in health promotion, chronic disease management and psychosocial care.

Current research in the field is promising, as are efforts to create unified and grounded models of care to manage chronic illness in young cancer survivors. However, additional resources should be allocated to the more systematic evaluation and real-world application of such research. Ideally, these should be in the form of randomised controlled trials (RCTs) and translation-focused, which evaluate the efficacy of interventions promoting healthy behaviours, targeting modifiable risk factors for treatment-related chronic illness.

Greater attention must also be given to developing and accessing comprehensive models of care, incorporating more appropriate risk-stratification, facilitating communication between patients and health providers as well as between health professionals, whilst promoting continuity of care with careful transition approaches. In conjunction with these efforts, further resources should be prioritised in practice for those who are at highest risk of developing conditions due to their treatment. Overall, we recommend a model of care which prepares patients from their diagnosis, for appropriate long term follow-up required to prevent and manage ongoing treatment-related conditions.

13.5 Conclusion: The 'Cost of Cure'

While the majority of children diagnosed with cancer will survive, the impact of their cancer and treatment may continue to affect survivors and their families in the long-term. Unsurprisingly, survivors with the largest number of treatment-related chronic conditions have the poorest quality of life [201]. Given the lifetime that is lived beyond a diagnosis of cancer in childhood [129], it is essential to ensure that the life years saved are of good quality and do not continue to burden the individual, family unit, society and the healthcare system.

Ongoing surveillance for chronic illness arising following cancer increases detection and thus the possibility of prevention or treatment [27]. In comparison to the costs of providing healthcare for survivors who do not engage in follow-up care, ongoing follow-up care aimed at prevention and early detection may be highly cost effective [202]. To date, there is no data quantifying the financial burden of managing treatment-related chronic conditions in young cancer survivors. The range and severity of late toxicities provides some insight into the significant costs that a survivor might face for the rest of their lives. Respectively, 62.3, 37.6, and 23.8 % of survivors experience 1, 2 or 3 late effects, each one entailing visits to health professionals, tests, treatment, and possibly ongoing management or screening for future related complications [35]. For example, a young survivor at risk of cardiovascular complications may require ongoing screening and, in the event of positive results, may be encouraged to make significant lifestyle changes (e.g. diet and exercise) or undergo costly treatment and possibly additional measures to manage further complications. Moreover, these late effects impose a considerable logistical and economic burden on society and the healthcare system [142].

However, long term follow-up, particularly screening and other testing, may be problematic for some patients, especially those without health insurance, or with limited insurance. Further assessment of the benefits of surveillance and the ongoing financial consequences, including cost of managing chronic illness in survivors of childhood cancer, is an important area of focus for future research.

Acknowledgments The Behavioural Sciences Unit (BSU) is proudly supported by the Kids with Cancer Foundation. The BSU's survivorship research program is funded by the Kids Cancer Project and a Cancer Council NSW Program Grant PG16-02 with the support of the Estate of the Late Harry McPaul. Claire Wakefield is supported by a Career Development Fellowship from the National Health and Medical Research Council of Australia (APP1067501). Christina Signorelli is supported by a PhD scholarship from The Kids Cancer Project.

References

1. D'Angio GJ (1975) Pediatric cancer in perspective. cure is not enough. Cancer 35(S3):866–870
2. Ganz PA (2014) Cancer survivors: a look backward and forward. Journal of Oncology Practice:JOP. 2014:001552
3. Balis FM (1997) The challenge of developing new therapies for childhood cancers. Oncologist 2(1):1–1
4. Ward E, DeSantis C, Robbins A, Kohler B, Jemal A (2014) Childhood and adolescent cancer statistics, 2014. CA Cancer J Clin 64(2):83–103
5. Youlden D, Baade P, Ward L, Valery P, Hassall T, Green A, Aitken J (2010) Childhood cancer survival in Australia, 1995–2004. Viertel Centre for Research in Cancer Control, Cancer Council Queensland and the Australian Paediatric Cancer Registry, Brisbane, Queensland
6. Smith MA, Seibel NL, Altekruse SF, Ries LA, Melbert DL, O'Leary M, Smith FO, Reaman GH (2010) Outcomes for children and adolescents with cancer: challenges for the twenty-first century. J Clin Oncol 28(15):2625–2634
7. Robison LL, Hudson MM (2014) Survivors of childhood and adolescent cancer: life-long risks and responsibilities. Nat Rev Cancer 14(1):61–70

8. International Agency for Research on Cancer (2014) World cancer report 2014. WHO, Geneva
9. Siegel R, Naishadham D, Jemal A (2012) Cancer statistics, 2012. CA Cancer J Clin 62 (1):10–29
10. Pizzo PA, Poplack DG, Adamson PC, Blaney SM, Helman LJ (2006) Principles and practice of pediatric oncology. Lippincott Williams & Wilkins Philadelphia, PA
11. Zhang J, Walsh MF, Wu G, Edmonson MN, Gruber TA, Easton J, Hedges D, Ma X, Zhou X, Yergeau DA (2015) Germline mutations in predisposition genes in pediatric cancer. N Engl J Med 373(24):2336–2346
12. Simone JV, Weiner SL, Hewitt M (2003) Childhood cancer survivorship: improving care and quality of Life. National Academies Press
13. Bleyer A, Barr R, Hayes-Lattin B, Thomas D, Ellis C, Anderson B (2008) The distinctive biology of cancer in adolescents and young adults. Nat Rev Cancer 8(4):288–298
14. Pizzo PA, Poplack DG (2015) Principles and practice of pediatric oncology. Wolters Kluwer Health
15. Dieluweit U, Debatin K-M, Grabow D, Kaatsch P, Peter R, Seitz DCM, Goldbeck L (2011) Educational and vocational achievement among long-term survivors of adolescent cancer in Germany. Pediatr Blood Cancer 56(3):432–438. doi:10.1002/pbc.22806
16. Prasad PK, Hardy KK, Zhang N, Edelstein K, Srivastava D, Zeltzer L, Stovall M, Seibel NL, Leisenring W, Armstrong GT, Robison LL, Krull K (2015) Psychosocial and neurocognitive outcomes in adult survivors of adolescent and early young adult cancer: a report from the childhood cancer survivor study. J Clin Oncol 33(23):2545–2552
17. Stinson JN, Jibb LA, Greenberg M, Barrera M, Luca S, White ME, Gupta A (2015) A qualitative study of the impact of cancer on romantic relationships, sexual relationships, and fertility: perspectives of canadian adolescents and parents during and after treatment. J Adolesc Young Adult Oncol 4(2):84–90
18. Schultz KAP, Ness KK, Whitton J, Recklitis C, Zebrack B, Robison LL, Zeltzer L, Mertens AC (2007) Behavioral and social outcomes in adolescent survivors of childhood cancer: a report from the childhood cancer survivor study. J Clin Oncol 25(24):3649–3656
19. Zhang Y, Goddard K, Spinelli JJ, Gotay C, McBride ML (2012) Risk of late mortality and second malignant neoplasms among 5-year survivors of young adult cancer: a report of the childhood, adolescent, and young adult cancer survivors research program. J Cancer Epidemiol
20. Hudson MM, Ness KK, Gurney JG et al (2013) Clinical ascertainment of health outcomes among adults treated for childhood cancer. JAMA 309(22):2371–2381. doi:10.1001/jama.2013.6296
21. Armenian SH, Hudson MM, Mulder RL, Chen MH, Constine LS, Dwyer M, Nathan PC, Tissing WJ, Shankar S, Sieswerda E (2015) Recommendations for cardiomyopathy surveillance for survivors of childhood cancer: a report from the international late effects of childhood cancer guideline harmonization group. Lancet Oncol 16(3):e123–e136
22. Landier W, Bhatia S, Eshelman DA, Forte KJ, Sweeney T, Hester AL, Darling J, Armstrong FD, Blatt J, Constine LS (2004) Development of risk-based guidelines for pediatric cancer survivors: the children's oncology group long-term follow-up guidelines from the children's oncology group late effects committee and nursing discipline. J Clin Oncol 22(24):4979–4990
23. Metzger ML, Meacham LR, Patterson B, Casillas JS, Constine LS, Hijiya N, Kenney LB, Leonard M, Lockart BA, Likes W (2013) Female reproductive health after childhood, adolescent, and young adult cancers: guidelines for the assessment and management of female reproductive complications. J Clin Oncol 31(9):1239–1247
24. Nathan PC, Patel SK, Dilley K et al (2007) Guidelines for identification of, advocacy for, and intervention in neurocognitive problems in survivors of childhood cancer: a report from the children's oncology group. Arch Pediatr Adolesc Med 161(8):798–806. doi:10.1001/archpedi.161.8.798

25. Robison LL, Mertens AC, Boice JD, Breslow NE, Donaldson SS, Green DM, Li FP, Meadows AT, Mulvihill JJ, Neglia JP (2002) Study design and cohort characteristics of the childhood cancer survivor study: a multi-institutional collaborative project. Med Pediatr Oncol 38(4):229–239
26. Winther JF, Kenborg L, Byrne J, Hjorth L, Kaatsch P, Kremer LC, Kuehni CE, Auquier P, Michel G, de Vathaire F (2015) Childhood cancer survivor cohorts in Europe. Acta Oncol 54 (5):655–668
27. Oeffinger KC, McCabe MS (2006) Models for delivering survivorship care. J Clin Oncol 24 (32):5117–5124
28. Siegel R, DeSantis C, Virgo K, Stein K, Mariotto A, Smith T, Cooper D, Gansler T, Lerro C, Fedewa S (2012) Cancer treatment and survivorship statistics. CA Cancer J Clin 62(4):220–241
29. Stein KD, Syrjala KL, Andrykowski MA (2008) Physical and psychological long-term and late effects of cancer. Cancer 112(S11):2577–2592
30. Hudson MM, Ness KK, Gurney JG, Mulrooney DA, Chemaitilly W, Krull KR, Green DM, Armstrong GT, Nottage KA, Jones KE (2013) Clinical ascertainment of health outcomes among adults treated for childhood cancer. JAMA 309(22):2371–2381
31. Children's Oncology Group (2013) Long-term follow-up guidelines for survivors of childhood, adolescent and young adult cancers, version 4.0 Monrovia. Children's Oncology Group, CA, Oct 2013; Available online: www.survivorshipguidelines.org
32. Oeffinger KC, Hudson MM, Landier W (2009) Survivorship: childhood cancer survivors. Prim Care 36(4):743–780
33. Diller L, Chow EJ, Gurney JG, Hudson MM, Kadin-Lottick NS, Kawashima TI, Leisenring WM, Meacham LR, Mertens AC, Mulrooney DA (2009) Chronic disease in the childhood cancer survivor study cohort: a review of published findings. J Clin Oncol 27 (14):2339–2355
34. Geenen MM, Cardous-Ubbink MC, Kremer LC, van den Bos C, van der Pal HJ, Heinen RC, Jaspers MW, Koning CC, Oldenburger F, Langeveld NE (2007) Medical assessment of adverse health outcomes in long-term survivors of childhood cancer. JAMA 297(24):2705–2715
35. Oeffinger KC, Mertens AC, Sklar CA, Kawashima T, Hudson MM, Meadows AT, Friedman DL, Marina N, Hobbie W, Kadan-Lottick NS, Schwartz CL, Leisenring W, Robison LL, Childhood Cancer Survivor S (2006) Chronic health conditions in adult survivors of childhood cancer. N Engl J Med 355(15):1572–1582
36. Bowers DC, McNeil DE, Liu Y, Yasui Y, Stovall M, Gurney JG, Hudson MM, Donaldson SS, Packer RJ, Mitby PA (2005) Stroke as a late treatment effect of Hodgkin's disease: a report from the childhood cancer survivor study. J Clin Oncol 23(27):6508–6515
37. Landier W, Bhatia S (2008) Cancer survivorship: a pediatric perspective. Oncologist 13 (11):1181–1192
38. Armstrong GT, Liu Q, Yasui Y, Neglia JP, Leisenring W, Robison LL, Mertens AC (2009) Late mortality among 5-year survivors of childhood cancer: a summary from the childhood cancer survivor study. J Clin Oncol 27(14):2328–2338
39. Lawless SC, Verma P, Green DM, Mahoney MC (2007) Mortality experiences among 15+ year survivors of childhood and adolescent cancers. Pediatr Blood Cancer 48(3):333–338
40. Cardous-Ubbink M, Heinen R, Langeveld N, Bakker P, Voute P, Caron H, Van Leeuwen F (2004) Long-term cause-specific mortality among five-year survivors of childhood cancer. Pediatr Blood Cancer 42(7):563–573
41. Wilson CL, Cohn RJ, Johnston KA, Ashton LJ (2010) Late mortality and second cancers in an Australian cohort of childhood cancer survivors. Med J Aust 193(5):258–261
42. Mertens AC (2007) Cause of mortality in 5-year survivors of childhood cancer. Pediatr Blood Cancer 48(7):723–726. doi:10.1002/pbc.21114
43. Garwicz S, Anderson H, Olsen JH, Falck Winther J, Sankila R, Langmark F, Tryggvadóttir L, Möller TR, for the Association of the Nordic Cancer R, the Nordic Society for Pediatric Hematology O (2012) Late and very late mortality in 5-year survivors of childhood cancer:

changing pattern over four decades—experience from the nordic countries. Int J Cancer 131 (7):1659–1666. doi:10.1002/ijc.27393
44. Mertens AC, Liu Q, Neglia JP, Wasilewski K, Leisenring W, Armstrong GT, Robison LL, Yasui Y (2008) Cause-specific late mortality among 5-year survivors of childhood cancer: the childhood cancer survivor study. J Natl Cancer Inst 100(19):1368–1379
45. Li FP, Myers MH, Heise HW, Jaffe N (1978) The course of five-year survivors of cancer in childhood. The Journal of pediatrics 93(2):185–187
46. Green DM, Zevon MA, Reese PA, Lowrie GS, Michalek AM (1994) Factors that influence the further survival of patients who survive for five years after the diagnosis of cancer in childhood or adolescence. Med Pediatr Oncol 22(2):91–96
47. Mertens AC, Yasui Y, Neglia JP, Potter JD, Nesbit ME, Ruccione K, Smithson WA, Robison LL (2001) Late mortality experience in five-year survivors of childhood and adolescent cancer: the childhood cancer survivor study. J Clin Oncol 19(13):3163–3172
48. Landier W, Armenian S, Bhatia S (2015) Late effects of childhood cancer and its treatment. Pediatr Clin North Am 62(1):275–300. doi:10.1016/j.pcl.2014.09.017
49. Fromer M (2007) New SEER report documents high risk of second cancers in cancer survivors. Oncol Times 29(5):8
50. Friedman DL, Whitton J, Leisenring W, Mertens AC, Hammond S, Stovall M, Donaldson SS, Meadows AT, Robison LL, Neglia JP (2010) Subsequent neoplasms in 5-year survivors of childhood cancer: the childhood cancer survivor study. J Natl Cancer Inst 102(14):1083–1095
51. Bluhm EC, Ronckers C, Hayashi RJ, Neglia JP, Mertens AC, Stovall M, Meadows AT, Mitby PA, Whitton JA, Hammond S (2008) Cause-specific mortality and second cancer incidence after non-Hodgkin lymphoma: a report from the childhood cancer survivor study. Blood 111(8):4014–4021
52. Best T, Li D, Skol AD, Kirchhoff T, Jackson SA, Yasui Y, Bhatia S, Strong LC, Domchek SM, Nathanson KL (2011) Variants at 6q21 implicate PRDM1 in the etiology of therapy-induced second malignancies after Hodgkin's lymphoma. Nat Med 17(8):941–943
53. Bhatia S, Sklar C (2002) Second cancers in survivors of childhood cancer. Nat Rev Cancer 2 (2):124–132
54. Knapke S, Nagarajan R, Correll J, Kent D, Burns K (2012) Hereditary cancer risk assessment in a pediatric oncology follow-up clinic. Pediatr Blood Cancer 58(1):85–89
55. Wood ME, Vogel V, Ng A, Foxhall L, Goodwin P, Travis LB (2012) Second malignant neoplasms: assessment and strategies for risk reduction. J Clin Oncol 30(30):3734–3745
56. Dickerman JD (2007) The late effects of childhood cancer therapy. Pediatrics 119(3):554–568
57. Wu X-C, Prasad PK, Landry I, Harlan LC, Parsons HM, Lynch CF, Smith AW, Hamilton AS, Keegan TH (2015) Impact of the AYA HOPE comorbidity index on assessing health care service needs and health status among adolescents and young adults with cancer. Cancer Epidemiol Biomark Prev 24(12):1844–1849
58. Aarsen FK, Arts WF, Van Veelen-Vincent ML, Lequin MH, Catsman-Berrevoets CE (2014) Long-term outcome in children with low grade tectal tumours and obstructive hydrocephalus. Eur J Paediatr Neurol 18(4):469–474
59. Lipshultz SE, Franco VI, Miller TL, Colan SD, Sallan SE (2015) Cardiovascular disease in adult survivors of childhood cancer. Annu Rev Med 66:161–176
60. Mulrooney DA, Blaes AH, Duprez D (2012) Vascular injury in cancer survivors. J Cardiovasc Transl Res 5(3):287–295
61. Lipshultz S, Adams M, Colan S, Constine L, Herman E, Hsu D, Hudson M, Kremer L, Landy D, Miller T (2013) American heart association congenital heart defects committee of the council on cardiovascular disease in the young CoBCSCoC, Stroke Nursing CoCR. Long Term Cardiovasc Toxicity Child Adolescents Young Adults Who Receive Cancer Ther Pathophysiol Course Monit Manage Prev Res Dir Sci Statement Am Heart Assoc Circ 128:1927–1995

62. Ehrhardt MJ, Mulrooney DA (2015) Metabolic syndrome in adult survivors of childhood cancer: the intersection of oncology, endocrinology, and cardiology. Lancet Diab Endocrinol. doi:10.1016/S2213-8587(15)00031-5
63. De Haas EC, Oosting SF, Lefrandt JD, Wolffenbuttel BH, Sleijfer DT, Gietema JA (2010) The metabolic syndrome in cancer survivors. Lancet Oncol 11(2):193–203
64. Neville KA, Cohn RJ, Steinbeck KS, Johnston K, Walker JL (2006) Hyperinsulinemia, impaired glucose tolerance, and diabetes mellitus in survivors of childhood cancer: prevalence and risk factors. J Clin Endocrinol Metab 91(11):4401–4407
65. Cohen J, Wakefield CE, Fleming CA, Gawthorne R, Tapsell LC, Cohn RJ (2012) Dietary intake after treatment in child cancer survivors. Pediatr Blood Cancer 58(5):752–757
66. Cohen J, Laing DG, Wilkes FJ, Chan A, Gabriel M, Cohn RJ (2014) Taste and smell dysfunction in childhood cancer survivors. Appetite 75:135–140
67. Fleming CA, Cohen J, Murphy A, Wakefield CE, Cohn RJ, Naumann FL (2015) Parent feeding interactions and practices during childhood cancer treatment. A qualitative investigation. Appetite 89:219–225
68. Bitsko MJ, Cohen D, Dillon R, Harvey J, Krull K, Klosky JL (2015) Psychosocial late effects in pediatric cancer survivors: a report from the children's oncology group. Pediatric Blood & Cancer
69. Wakefield CE, McLoone J, Goodenough B, Lenthen K, Cairns DR, Cohn RJ (2010) The psychosocial impact of completing childhood cancer treatment: a systematic review of the literature. J Pediatr Psychol 35(3):262–274
70. Zebrack BJ, Chesler MA (2002) Quality of life in childhood cancer survivors. Psycho-Oncology 11(2):132–141
71. Barakat LP, Alderfer MA, Kazak AE (2005) Posttraumatic growth in adolescent survivors of cancer and their mothers and fathers. J Pediatr Psychol
72. Michel G, Taylor N, Absolom K, Eiser C (2010) Benefit finding in survivors of childhood cancer and their parents: further empirical support for the benefit finding scale for children. Child Care Health Dev 36(1):123–129
73. Wakefield CE, McLoone JK, Butow P, Lenthen K, Cohn RJ (2011) Parental adjustment to the completion of their child's cancer treatment. Pediatr Blood Cancer 56(4):524–531
74. Zeltzer LK, Recklitis C, Buchbinder D, Zebrack B, Casillas J, Tsao JC, Lu Q, Krull K (2009) Psychological status in childhood cancer survivors: a report from the childhood cancer survivor study. J Clin Oncol 27(14):2396–2404
75. Kazak AE, DeRosa BW, Schwartz LA, Hobbie W, Carlson C, Ittenbach RF, Mao JJ, Ginsberg JP (2010) Psychological outcomes and health beliefs in adolescent and young adult survivors of childhood cancer and controls. J Clin Oncol 28(12):2002–2007
76. Davidson J, Swartz M, Storck M, Krishnan RR, Hammett E (1985) A diagnostic and family study of posttraumatic stress disorder. Am J Psychiatry 142(1):90–93
77. Ozono S, Saeki T, Mantani T, Ogata A, Okamura H, Si Nakagawa, Ueda K, Inada H, Yamawaki S (2010) Psychological distress related to patterns of family functioning among Japanese childhood cancer survivors and their parents. Psycho Oncol 19(5):545–552
78. Alderfer MA, Navsaria N, Kazak AE (2009) Family functioning and posttraumatic stress disorder in adolescent survivors of childhood cancer. J Fam Psychol 23(5):717
79. Mulhern RK, Palmer SL (2003) Neurocognitive late effects in pediatric cancer. Curr Probl Cancer 27(4):177–197. doi:10.1016/S0147-0272(03)00026-6
80. Castellino SM, Ullrich NJ, Whelen MJ, Lange BJ (2014) Developing Interventions for Cancer-Related Cognitive Dysfunction in Childhood Cancer Survivors. Journal of the National Cancer Institute 106(8). doi:10.1093/jnci/dju186
81. Mulhern RK, Merchant TE, Gajjar A, Reddick WE, Kun LE (2004) Late neurocognitive sequelae in survivors of brain tumours in childhood. Lancet Oncol 5(7):399–408. doi:10.1016/s1470-2045(04)01507-4
82. Pini S, Hugh-Jones S, Gardner PH (2012) What effect does a cancer diagnosis have on the educational engagement and school life of teenagers? A Syst Rev. Psycho Oncol 21(7):685–694

83. Mabbott DJ, Spiegler BJ, Greenberg ML, Rutka JT, Hyder DJ, Bouffet E (2005) Serial evaluation of academic and behavioral outcome after treatment with cranial radiation in childhood. J Clin Oncol 23(10):2256–2263. doi:10.1200/jco.2005.01.158
84. Krull KR, Zhang N, Santucci A, Srivastava DK, Krasin MJ, Kun LE, Pui C-H, Robison LL, Hudson MM, Armstrong GT (2013) Long-term decline in intelligence among adult survivors of childhood acute lymphoblastic leukemia treated with cranial radiation. Blood 122(4):550–553. doi:10.1182/blood-2013-03-487744
85. Conklin HM, Krull KR, Reddick WE, Pei D, Cheng C, Pui CH (2012) Cognitive outcomes following contemporary treatment without cranial irradiation for childhood acute lymphoblastic leukemia. J Natl Cancer Inst 104(18):1386–1395. doi:10.1093/jnci/djs344
86. Moleski M (2000) Neuropsychological, neuroanatomical, and neurophysiological consequences of CNS chemotherapy for acute lymphoblastic leukemia. Arch Clin Neuropsychol 15(7):603–630. doi:10.1093/arclin/15.7.603
87. Iyer NS, Balsamo LM, Bracken MB, Kadan-Lottick NS (2015) Chemotherapy-only treatment effects on long-term neurocognitive functioning in childhood ALL survivors: a review and meta-analysis. Blood 126(3):346–353. doi:10.1182/blood-2015-02-627414
88. Wells EM, Nageswara Rao AA, Scafidi J, Packer RJ (2012) Neurotoxicity of biologically targeted agents in pediatric cancer trials. Pediatr Neurol 46(4):212–221. doi:10.1016/j.pediatrneurol.2012.02.006
89. Cole PD, Finkelstein Y, Stevenson KE, Blonquist TM, Vijayanathan V, Silverman LB, Neuberg DS, Sallan SE, Robaey P, Waber DP (2015) Polymorphisms in genes related to oxidative stress are associated with inferior cognitive function after therapy for childhood acute lymphoblastic leukemia. J Clin Oncol. doi:10.1200/jco.2014.59.0273
90. Krull KR, Bhojwani D, Conklin HM, Pei D, Cheng C, Reddick WE, Sandlund JT, Pui C-H (2013) Genetic mediators of neurocognitive outcomes in survivors of childhood acute lymphoblastic leukemia. J Clin Oncol 31(17):2182–2188. doi:10.1200/jco.2012.46.7944
91. Patel SK, Peters BB, Bell T, Verner J, Katz ER, Baron MN, Buckwalter JG (2014) Parent involvement and neurocognitive functioning in childhood cancer survivors. J Behav Health 3 (1):43–52
92. Lancashire ER, Frobisher C, Reulen RC, Winter DL, Glaser A, Hawkins MM (2010) Educational attainment among adult survivors of childhood cancer in great britain: a population-based cohort study. J Natl Cancer Inst 102(4):254–270. doi:10.1093/jnci/djp498
93. Ghaderi S, Engeland A, Gunnes M, Moster D, Ruud E, Syse A, Wesenberg F, Bjørge T (2015) Educational attainment among long-term survivors of cancer in childhood and adolescence: a Norwegian population-based cohort study. J Cancer Surviv 1–9. doi:10.1007/s11764-015-0453-z
94. Gerhardt CA, Dixon M, Miller K, Vannatta K, Valerius KS, Correll J, Noll RB (2007) Educational and occupational outcomes among survivors of childhood cancer during the transition to emerging adulthood. J Dev Behav Pediatr 28(6):448–455. doi:10.1097/DBP.0b013e31811ff8e1
95. Kuehni CE, Strippoli M-PF, Rueegg CS, Rebholz CE, Bergstraesser E, Grotzer M, von der Weid NX, Michel G, for the Swiss Pediatric Oncology G (2012) Educational achievement in Swiss childhood cancer survivors compared with the general population. Cancer 118 (5):1439–1449. doi:10.1002/cncr.26418
96. Haupt R, Fears TR, Robison LL, Mills JL, Nicholson HS, Zeltzer LK, Meadows AT, Byrne J (1994) Educational attainment in long-term survivors of childhood acute lymphoblastic leukemia. JAMA 272(18):1427–1432
97. Boman KK, Lindblad F, Hjern A (2010) Long-term outcomes of childhood cancer survivors in Sweden: a population-based study of education, employment, and income. Cancer 116 (5):1385–1391. doi:10.1002/cncr.24840
98. McLoone JK, Wakefield CE, Cohn RJ (2013) Childhood cancer survivors' school (re)entry: Australian parents' perceptions. Eur J Cancer Care 22(4):484–492. doi:10.1111/ecc.12054

99. French AE, Tsangaris E, Barrera M, Guger S, Brown R, Urbach S, Stephens D, Nathan PC (2013) School attendance in childhood cancer survivors and their siblings. The Journal of Pediatrics 162(1):160–165. doi:10.1016/j.jpeds.2012.06.066
100. McLoone JK, Wakefield CE, Butow P, Fleming C, Cohn RJ (2011) Returning to school after adolescent cancer: a qualitative examination of australian survivors' and their families' perspectives. J Adolesc Young Adult Oncol 1(2):87–94
101. Pini S, Gardner P, Hugh-Jones S (2013) The impact of a cancer diagnosis on the education engagement of teenagers—patient and staff perspective. Eur J Oncol Nurs 17(3):317–323
102. Donnan B (2009) What about schol …? Educational pathways to a successful future for children and adolescents with cancer. Asia Pac J Clin Oncol 5:A212
103. Hinds PS, Nuss SL, Ruccione KS, Withycombe JS, Jacobs S, DeLuca H, Faulkner C, Liu Y, Cheng YI, Gross HE (2012) PROMIS pediatric measures in pediatric oncology: Valid and clinically feasible indicators of patient-reported outcomes. Pediatr Blood Cancer
104. Garcia SF, Cella D, Clauser SB, Flynn KE, Lad T, Lai JS, Reeve BB, Smith AW, Stone AA, Weinfurt K (2007) Standardizing patient-reported outcomes assessment in cancer clinical trials: a patient-reported outcomes measurement information system initiative. J Clin Oncol Official J Am Soc Clin Oncol 25(32):5106–5112. doi:10.1200/jco.2007.12.2341
105. Harshman LA, Barron S, Button AM, Smith BJ, Link BK, Lynch CF, Denburg NL (2012) Population-based exploration of academic achievement outcomes in pediatric acute lymphoblastic leukemia survivors. J Pediatr Psychol. doi:10.1093/jpepsy/jsr119
106. Simard SB, Savard JE (2015) Screening and comorbidity of clinical levels of fear of cancer recurrence. J Cancer Surviv 1–11. doi:10.1007/s11764-015-0424-4
107. Zebrack BJ, Gurney JG, Oeffinger K, Whitton J, Packer RJ, Mertens A, Turk N, Castleberry R, Dreyer Z, Robison LL, Zeltzer LK (2004) Psychological outcomes in long-term survivors of childhood brain cancer: a report from the childhood cancer survivor study. J Clin Oncol 22(6):999–1006. doi:10.1200/jco.2004.06.148
108. Vannatta K, Gartstein MA, Short A, Noll RB (1998) A controlled study of peer relationships of children surviving brain tumors: teacher, peer, and self ratings. J Pediatr Psychol 23 (5):279–287. doi:10.1093/jpepsy/23.5.279
109. Moyer KH, Willard VW, Gross AM, Netson KL, Ashford JM, Kahalley LS, Wu S, Xiong X, Conklin HM (2012) The impact of attention on social functioning in survivors of pediatric acute lymphoblastic leukemia and brain tumors. Pediatr Blood Cancer 59(7):1290–1295. doi:10.1002/pbc.24256
110. Willard VW, Conklin HM, Boop FA, Wu S, Merchant TE (2014) Emotional and behavioral functioning after conformal radiation therapy for pediatric ependymoma. Int J Radiat Oncol Biol Phys 88(4):814–821. doi:http://dx.doi.org/10.1016/j.ijrobp.2013.12.006
111. Hocking MC, McCurdy M, Turner E, Kazak AE, Noll RB, Phillips P, Barakat LP (2014) Social competence in pediatric brain tumor survivors: Application of a model from social neuroscience and developmental psychology. Pediatr Blood Cancer 62(3):375–384. doi:10.1002/pbc.25300
112. Maddrey A, Bergeron J, Lombardo E, McDonald N, Mulne A, Barenberg P, Bowers D (2005) Neuropsychological performance and quality of life of 10+ year survivors of childhood medulloblastoma. J Neurooncol 72(3):245–253. doi:10.1007/s11060-004-3009-z
113. Crom D, Lensing S, Rai S, Snider M, Cash D, Hudson M (2007) Marriage, employment, and health insurance in adult survivors of childhood cancer. J Cancer Surviv 1(3):237–245. doi:10.1007/s11764-007-0026-x
114. de Boer AGEM, Verbeek JHAM, van Dijk FJH (2006) Adult survivors of childhood cancer and unemployment. Cancer 107(1):1–11. doi:10.1002/cncr.21974
115. Boman KK, Bodegård G (2004) Life after cancer in childhood: social adjustment and educational and vocational status of young-adult survivors. J Pediatr Hematol Oncol 26 (6):354–362
116. Möller TR, Garwicz S, Barlow L, Winther JF, Glattre E, Olafsdottir G, Olsen JH, Perfekt R, Ritvanen A, Sankila R (2001) Decreasing late mortality among five-year survivors of cancer

in childhood and adolescence: a population-based study in the Nordic countries. J Clin Oncol 19(13):3173–3181

117. Armstrong GT, Chen Y, Yasui Y, Leisenring W, Gibson TM, Mertens AC, Stovall M, Oeffinger KC, Bhatia S, Krull KR (2016) Reduction in late mortality among 5-year survivors of childhood cancer. N Engl J Med
118. Anderson ME (2016) Update on survival in osteosarcoma. Orthop Clin North Am 47 (1):283–292
119. Jockovich M, Mendenhall NP, Sombeck MD, Talbert JL, Copeland E 3rd, Bland KI (1994) Long-term complications of laparotomy in Hodgkin's disease. Ann Surg 219(6):615
120. Rodeberg DA, Anderson JR, Arndt CA, Ferrer FA, Raney RB, Jenney ME, Brecht IB, Koscielniak E, Carli M, Bisogno G (2011) Comparison of outcomes based on treatment algorithms for rhabdomyosarcoma of the bladder/prostate: combined results from the children's oncology group, German cooperative soft tissue sarcoma study, Italian cooperative group, and International society of pediatric oncology malignant mesenchymal tumors committee. Int J Cancer 128(5):1232–1239
121. Davidoff AM, Interiano RB, Wynn L, Santos ND, Dome JS, Green DM, Brennan RC, McCarville MB, Krasin MJ, Kieran K (2015) Overall survival and renal function of patients with synchronous bilateral wilms tumor undergoing surgery at a single institution. Ann Surg 262(4):570–576
122. Wilson CL, Gawade PL, Ness KK (2015) Impairments that influence physical function among survivors of childhood cancer. Children 2(1):1–36
123. Wilejto M, Giuseppe GD, Hitzler J, Gupta S, Abla O (2015) Treatment of young children with CNS-positive acute lymphoblastic leukemia without cranial radiotherapy. Pediatr Blood Cancer 62(11):1881–1885
124. Cohen BH, Geyer JR, Miller DC, Curran JG, Zhou T, Holmes E, Ingles SA, Dunkel IJ, Hilden J, Packer RJ (2015) Pilot study of intensive chemotherapy with peripheral hematopoietic cell support for children less than 3 years of age with malignant brain tumors, the CCG-99703 phase I/II study. A report from the children's oncology group. Pediatric neurology
125. Trahair T, Vowels M, Johnston K, Cohn R, Russell S, Neville K, Carroll S, Marshall G (2007) Long-term outcomes in children with high-risk neuroblastoma treated with autologous stem cell transplantation. Bone Marrow Transplant 40(8):741–746
126. Green DM, Grigoriev YA, Nan B, Takashima JR, Norkool PA, D'Angio GJ, Breslow NE (2001) Congestive heart failure after treatment for Wilms' tumor: a report from the National Wilms' tumor study group. J Clin Oncol 19(7):1926–1934
127. Kollmannsberger C, Beyer J, Droz J, Harstrick A, Hartmann J, Biron P, Flechon A, Schöffski P, Kuczyk M, Schmoll H (1998) Secondary leukemia following high cumulative doses of etoposide in patients treated for advanced germ cell tumors. J Clin Oncol 16(10):3386–3391
128. Schwartz CL (1999) Long-term survivors of childhood cancer: the late effects of therapy. Oncologist 4(1):45–54
129. Goldsby RE, Ablin AR (2004) Surviving childhood cancer; now what? controversies regarding long-term follow-up. Pediatr Blood Cancer 43(3):211–214
130. Freyer DR (2010) Transition of care for young adult survivors of childhood and adolescent cancer: rationale and approaches. J Clin Oncol 28(32):4810–4818
131. Oeffinger KC, Argenbright KE, Levitt GE, McCabe MS, Anderson PR, Berry E, Maher J, Merrill J, Wollins DS (2014) Models of cancer survivorship health care: moving forward. In: ASCO survivorship care compendium. American Society of Clinical Oncology
132. Hewitt M (2003) In: Greenfield S, Stovall E (eds) From cancer patient to cancer survivor: lost in transition (Report of the Institute of Medicine & National Research Council). National Academy Press, Washington, DC
133. Wallace W, Thompson L, Anderson R (2013) Long term follow-up of survivors of childhood cancer: summary of updated SIGN guidance. BMJ 346
134. Sieswerda E, Postma A, van Dalen EC, van der Pal HJ, Tissing WJ, Rammeloo LA, Kok WE, van Leeuwen FE, Caron H, Kremer L (2012) The Dutch childhood oncology group

guideline for follow-up of asymptomatic cardiac dysfunction in childhood cancer survivors. Ann Oncol 23(8):2191–2198
135. Kremer L, Mulder RL, Oeffinger KC, Bhatia S, Landier W, Levitt G, Constine LS, Wallace WH, Caron HN, Armenian SH (2013) A worldwide collaboration to harmonize guidelines for the long-term follow-up of childhood and young adult cancer survivors: a report from the international late effects of childhood cancer guideline harmonization group. Pediatr Blood Cancer 60(4):543–549
136. National Breast and Ovarian Cancer Centre (Australia) (2010) Recommendations for follow-up of women with early breast cancer. National Breast and Ovarian Cancer Centre, Strawberry Hills N.S.W.
137. Skolarus TA, Wolf A, Erb NL, Brooks DD, Rivers BM, Underwood W, Salner AL, Zelefsky MJ, Aragon-Ching JB, Slovin SF (2014) American cancer society prostate cancer survivorship care guidelines. CA Cancer J Clin 64(4):225–249
138. Runowicz CD, Leach CR, Henry NL, Henry KS, Mackey HT, Cowens-Alvarado RL, Cannady RS, Pratt-Chapman ML, Edge SB, Jacobs LA (2016) American cancer society/american society of clinical oncology breast cancer survivorship care guideline. CA Cancer J Clin 66(1):43–73
139. Ligibel JA, Denlinger CS (2013) New NCCN guidelines® for survivorship care. J Natl Compr Canc Netw 11(5S):640–644
140. Edgar A, Duffin K, Borthwick S, Marciniak-Stepak P, Wallace W (2013) Can intensity of long-term follow-up for survivors of childhood and teenage cancer be determined by therapy-based risk stratification? BMJ open 3 (8):e002451
141. Taylor A, Hawkins M, Griffiths A, Davies H, Douglas C, Jenney M, Wallace WHB, Levitt G (2004) Long-term follow-up of survivors of childhood cancer in the UK. Pediatr Blood Cancer 42(2):161–168
142. Skinner R, Wallace WHB, Levitt GA, LEG LEG, Group UCsCS (2006) Long-term follow-up of people who have survived cancer during childhood. Lancet oncol 7(6):489–498
143. Jenney M, Levitt G (2008) Follow-up of children who survive cancer. BMJ. Br Med J 336 (7647):732
144. Wallace WHB, Blacklay A, Eiser C, Davies H, Hawkins M, Levitt GA, Jenney ME (2001) Developing strategies for long term follow up of survivors of childhood cancer. BMJ 323 (7307):271–274
145. Hewitt M, Greenfield S, Stovall E (2006) From cancer patient to cancer survivor: lost in transition. Committee on cancer survivorship: improving care and quality of life, institute of medicine and national research council. The National Academies Press, Washington, DC
146. Eiser C, Absolom K, Greenfield D, Glaser A, Horne B, Waite H, Urquhart T, Wallace WHB, Ross R, Davies H (2006) Follow-up after childhood cancer: evaluation of a three-level model. Eur J Cancer 42(18):3186–3190
147. Ganz PA, Casillas J, Hahn EE (2008) Ensuring quality care for cancer survivors: implementing the survivorship care plan. In: Seminars in oncology nursing, vol 3. Elsevier, pp 208–217
148. Salz T, Oeffinger KC, McCabe MS, Layne TM, Bach PB (2012) Survivorship care plans in research and practice. CA Cancer J Clin 62(2):101–117. doi:10.3322/caac.20142
149. Hahn EE, Ganz PA (2011) Survivorship programs and care plans in practice: variations on a theme. J Oncol Pract Am Soc Clin Oncol 7(2):70–75. doi:10.1200/JOP.2010.000115
150. Makari-Judson G, Hubbard S, Wrenn T (2013) Use of survivorship care plans to re-engineer breast cancer follow-up. Open Breast Cancer J 5(1):23–26
151. Jackson C, Cheater FM, Reid I (2008) A systematic review of decision support needs of parents making child health decisions. Health Expect Int J Publ Participation Health Care Health Policy 11(3):232–251. doi:10.1111/j.1369-7625.2008.00496.x
152. Burg MA, Lopez ED, Dailey A, Keller ME, Prendergast B (2009) The potential of survivorship care plans in primary care follow-up of minority breast cancer patients. J Gen Intern Med 24(Suppl 2):S467–S471. doi:10.1007/s11606-009-1012-y

153. Oeffinger KC, Hudson MM, Mertens AC, Smith SM, Mitby PA, Eshelman-Kent DA, Ford JS, Jones JK, Kamani S, Robison LL (2011) Increasing rates of breast cancer and cardiac surveillance among high-risk survivors of childhood Hodgkin lymphoma following a mailed, one-page survivorship care plan. Pediatr Blood Cancer 56(5):818–824
154. Baravelli C, Krishnasamy M, Pezaro C, Schofield P, Lotfi-Jam K, Rogers M, Milne D, Aranda S, King D, Shaw B (2009) The views of bowel cancer survivors and health care professionals regarding survivorship care plans and post treatment follow up. J Cancer Surviv 3(2):99–108
155. Brennan ME, Butow P, Spillane AJ, Boyle FM (2010) Survivorship care after breast cancer: follow-up practices of Australian health professionals and attitudes to a survivorship care plan. Asia Pac J Clin Oncol 6(2):116–125
156. Mayer DK, Gerstel A, Leak AN, Smith SK (2012) Patient and provider preferences for survivorship care plans. J Oncol Pract 8(4):e80–e86
157. Grunfeld E, Julian JA, Pond G, Maunsell E, Coyle D, Folkes A, Joy AA, Provencher L, Rayson D, Rheaume DE (2011) Evaluating survivorship care plans: results of a randomized, clinical trial of patients with breast cancer. J Clin Oncol 29(36):4755–4762
158. Nicolaije KA, Ezendam NP, Vos MC, Pijnenborg JM, Boll D, Boss EA, Hermans RH, Engelhart KC, Haartsen JE, Pijlman BM (2015) Impact of an automatically generated cancer survivorship care plan on patient-reported outcomes in routine clinical practice: longitudinal outcomes of a pragmatic, cluster randomized trial. J Clin Oncol 33(31):3550–3559
159. Blum RW, Garell D, Hodgman CH, Jorissen TW, Okinow NA, Orr DP, Slap GB (1993) Transition from child-centered to adult health-care systems for adolescents with chronic conditions: a position paper of the Society for Adolescent Medicine. J Adolesc Health 14 (7):570–576
160. Reiss J, Gibson R (2002) Health care transition: destinations unknown. Pediatrics 110 (Supplement 3):1307–1314
161. Ginsberg JP, Hobbie WL, Carlson CA, Meadows AT (2006) Delivering long-term follow-up care to pediatric cancer survivors: transitional care issues. Pediatr Blood Cancer 46(2):169–173
162. Bashore L (2004) Childhood and adolescent cancer survivors' knowledge of their disease and effects of treatment. J Pediatr Oncol Nurs 21(2):98–102
163. Fox A (2002) Physicians as barriers to successful transitional care. Int J Adolesc Med Health 14(1):3–8
164. Henderson TO, Hlubocky FJ, Wroblewski KE, Diller L, Daugherty CK (2010) Physician preferences and knowledge gaps regarding the care of childhood cancer survivors: a mailed survey of pediatric oncologists. J Clin Oncol 28(5):878–883
165. Eshelman-Kent D, Kinahan KE, Hobbie W, Landier W, Teal S, Friedman D, Nagarajan R, Freyer DR (2011) Cancer survivorship practices, services, and delivery: a report from the children's oncology group (COG) nursing discipline, adolescent/young adult, and late effects committees. J Cancer Surviv 5(4):345–357
166. Taylor PJ, McClanahan KK (2010) Essential adolescent medicine. Elsevier
167. Cowens-Alvarado R, Sharpe K, Pratt-Chapman M, Willis A, Gansler T, Ganz PA, Edge SB, McCabe MS, Stein K (2013) Advancing survivorship care through the national cancer survivorship resource center. CA Cancer J Clin 63(3):147–150
168. Kaur JS (2014) How should we "empower" cancer patients? Cancer 120(20):3108–3110
169. Grunfeld E (2005) Cancer survivorship: a challenge for primary care physicians. Br J Gen Pract 55(519):741–742
170. Nissen MJ, Beran MS, Lee MW, Mehta SR, Pine DA, Swenson KK (2007) Views of primary care providers on follow-up care of cancer patients. Fam Med 39(7):477–482
171. Mitchell GK, Burridge LH, Colquist SP, Love A (2012) General practitioners' perceptions of their role in cancer care and factors which influence this role. Health Soc Care Community 20 (6):607–616. doi:10.1111/j.1365-2524.2012.01075.x

172. Johnson CE, Lizama N, Garg N, Ghosh M, Emery J, Saunders C (2014) Australian general practitioners' preferences for managing the care of people diagnosed with cancer. Asia Pac J Clin Oncol 10(2):e90–e98. doi:10.1111/ajco.12047
173. CanTeen (2015) Exploring survivorship care for adolescent and young adult cancer survivors in australia. CanTeen, Australia (unpublished)
174. Nathan PC, Greenberg ML, Ness KK, Hudson MM, Mertens AC, Mahoney MC, Gurney JG, Donaldson SS, Leisenring WM, Robison LL (2008) Medical care in long-term survivors of childhood cancer: a report from the childhood cancer survivor study. J Clin Oncol 26 (27):4401–4409
175. Mulrooney RC, Singh N, Kaur N, Callan JF (2009) An "off-on" sensor for fluoride using luminescent CdSe/ZnS quantum dots. Chem Commun 6:686–688. doi:10.1039/b817569a
176. Oeffinger KC, Mertens AC, Hudson MM, Gurney JG, Casillas J, Chen H, Whitton J, Yeazel M, Yasui Y, Robison LL (2004) Health care of young adult survivors of childhood cancer: a report from the childhood cancer survivor study. The Annals of Family Medicine 2 (1):61–70
177. Casillas J, Oeffinger KC, Hudson MM, Greenberg ML, Yeazel MW, Ness KK, Henderson TO, Robison LL, Armstrong GT, Liu Q, Leisenring W, Yasui Y, Nathan PC (2015) Identifying predictors of longitudinal decline in the level of medical care received by adult survivors of childhood cancer: a report from the childhood cancer survivor study. Health Serv Res. doi:10.1111/1475-6773.12282
178. Edgar A, Borthwick S, Duffin K, Marciniak-Stepak P, Wallace W (2012) Survivors of childhood cancer lost to follow-up can be re-engaged into active long-term follow-up by a postal health questionnaire intervention. Eur J Cancer 48(7):1066–1073
179. Blaauwbroek R, Groenier K, Kamps W, Meyboom-de Jong B, Postma A (2007) Late effects in adult survivors of childhood cancer: the need for life-long follow-up. Ann Oncol
180. Earle EA, Davies H, Greenfield D, Ross R, Eiser C (2005) Follow-up care for childhood cancer survivors: a focus group analysis. Eur J Cancer 41(18):2882–2886
181. Mullan F (1985) Seasons of survival: reflections of a physician with cancer. N Engl J Med 313(4):270–273
182. Syed IA, Klassen AF, Barr R, Wang R, Dix D, Nelson M, Rosenberg-Yunger ZR, Nathan PC (2015) Factors associated with childhood cancer survivors' knowledge about their diagnosis, treatment, and risk for late effects. J Cancer Surviv 1–12
183. Oeffinger KC, Hudson MM (2004) Long-term complications following childhood and adolescent cancer: foundations for providing risk-based health care for survivors. CA Cancer J Clin 54(4):208–236
184. Group CsO, Group CsO (2008) Long-term follow-up guidelines for survivors of childhood, adolescent, and young adult cancers. Children's Oncology Group, Arcadia, CA
185. Steinberger J, Sinaiko AR, Kelly AS, Leisenring WM, Steffen LM, Goodman P, Mulrooney DA, Dietz AC, Moran A, Perkins JL, Baker KS (2012) Cardiovascular risk and insulin resistance in childhood cancer survivors. J Pediatr 160(3):494–499. doi:10.1016/j.jpeds.2011.08.018
186. Stolley MR, Restrepo J, Sharp LK (2010) Diet and physical activity in childhood cancer survivors: a review of the literature. Ann Behav Med 39(3):232–249. doi:10.1007/s12160-010-9192-6
187. Nathan PC, Ford JS, Henderson TO, Hudson MM, Emmons KM, Casillas JN, Lown EA, Ness KK, Oeffinger KC, Nathan PC, Ford JS, Henderson TO, Hudson MM, Emmons KM, Casillas JN, Lown EA, Ness KK, Oeffinger KC (2009) Health behaviors, medical care, and interventions to promote healthy living in the childhood cancer survivor study cohort. J Clin Oncol 27(14):2363–2373
188. Neville KA, Cohn RJ (2015) Bone health in survivors of childhood cancer. Lancet Diabetes & Endocrinology. doi:10.1016/S2213-8587(15)00029-7
189. Durlak JA, Wells AM (1998) Evaluation of indicated preventive intervention (secondary prevention) mental health programs for children and adolescents. Am J Commun Psychol 26 (5):775–802

190. Butler AC, Chapman JE, Forman EM, Beck AT (2006) The empirical status of cognitive-behavioral therapy: a review of meta-analyses. Clin Psychol Rev 26(1):17–31
191. Greening L, Stoppelbein L (2007) Brief report: pediatric cancer, parental coping style, and risk for depressive, posttraumatic stress, and anxiety symptoms. J Pediatr Psychol 32 (10):1272–1277
192. Overholser JC, Fritz GK (1991) The impact of childhood cancer on the family. J Psychosoc Oncol 8(4):71–85
193. Drotar D (1997) Relating parent and family functioning to the psychological adjustment of children with chronic health conditions: what have we learned? What do we need to know? J Pediatr Psychol 22(2):149–165
194. Frank NC, Blount RL, Brown RT (1997) Attributions, coping, and adjustment in children with cancer. J Pediatr Psychol 22(4):563–576
195. Canning EH, Hanser SB, Shade KA, Boyce WT (1993) Maternal distress and discrepancy in reports of psychopathology in chronically ill children. Psychosom J Consultation Liaison Psychiatry 34:506–511
196. Mulhern RK, Fairclough DL, Smith B, Douglas SM (1992) Maternal depression, assessment methods, and physical symptoms affect estimates of depressive symptomatology among children with cancer. J Pediatr Psychol 17(3):313–326
197. Eakin EG, Youlden DR, Baade PD, Lawler SP, Reeves MM, Heyworth JS, Fritschi L (2006) Health status of long-term cancer survivors: results from an Australian population-based sample. Cancer Epidemiol Biomark Prev 15(10):1969–1976
198. Baade PD, Fritschi L, Eakin EG (2006) Non-cancer mortality among people diagnosed with cancer (Australia). Cancer Causes Control 17(3):287–297
199. Blanchard CM, Courneya KS, Stein K (2008) Cancer survivors' adherence to lifestyle behavior recommendations and associations with health-related quality of life: results from the American Cancer Society's SCS-II. J Clin Oncol 26(13):2198–2204
200. Sabatino SA, Coates RJ, Uhler RJ, Pollack LA, Alley LG, Zauderer LJ (2007) Provider counseling about health behaviors among cancer survivors in the United States. J Clin Oncol 25(15):2100–2106
201. Zebrack BJ, Yi J, Petersen L, Ganz PA (2008) The impact of cancer and quality of life for long-term survivors. Psycho Oncol 17(9):891–900
202. Glaser A, Levitt G, Morris P, Tapp J, Gibson F (2013) Enhanced quality and productivity of long-term aftercare of cancer in young people. Arch Dis Child archdischild-2013-304348
203. Gatta G, Zigon G, Capocaccia R, Coebergh JW, Desandes E, Kaatsch P, Pastore G, Peris-Bonet R, Stiller CA, Group EW (2009) Survival of European children and young adults with cancer diagnosed 1995–2002. Eur J Cancer 45(6):992–1005
204. Mulder RL, Kremer LC, Hudson MM, Bhatia S, Landier W, Levitt G, Constine LS, Wallace WH, van Leeuwen FE, Ronckers CM (2013) Recommendations for breast cancer surveillance for female survivors of childhood, adolescent, and young adult cancer given chest radiation: a report from the international late effects of childhood cancer guideline harmonization group. Lancet Oncol 14(13):e621–e629
205. Galper SL, James BY, Mauch PM, Strasser JF, Silver B, LaCasce A, Marcus KJ, Stevenson MA, Chen MH, Ng AK (2011) Clinically significant cardiac disease in patients with Hodgkin lymphoma treated with mediastinal irradiation. Blood 117(2):412–418
206. Haddy N, Diallo S, El-Fayech C, Schwartz B, Pein F, Hawkins M, Veres C, Oberlin O, Guibout C, Pacquement H (2015) Cardiac diseases following childhood cancer treatment: cohort study. Circulation CIRCULATIONAHA–115.016686
207. Bowers DC, Liu Y, Leisenring W, McNeil E, Stovall M, Gurney JG, Robison LL, Packer RJ, Oeffinger KC (2006) Late-occurring stroke among long-term survivors of childhood leukemia and brain tumors: a report from the childhood cancer survivor study. J Clin Oncol 24(33):5277–5282
208. Knight KRG, Kraemer DF, Neuwelt EA (2005) Ototoxicity in children receiving platinum chemotherapy: underestimating a commonly occurring toxicity that may influence academic and social development. J Clin Oncol 23(34):8588–8596

209. Armstrong GT, Stovall M, Robison LL (2010) Long-term effects of radiation exposure among adult survivors of childhood cancer: results from the childhood cancer survivor study. Radiat Res 174(6b):840–850
210. Gregory JW, Reilly JJ (2004) Body composition and obesity. In: Wallace WH, Green DM (eds) Late effects of childhood cancer. Arnold, London, United Kingdom, pp 147–161
211. Gunn HM, Emilsson H, Gabriel M, Maguire AM, Steinbeck KS (2015) Metabolic health in childhood cancer survivors: a longitudinal study in a long-term follow-up clinic. J Adolesc Young Adult Oncol
212. Goldsby R, Chen Y, Raber S, Li L, Diefenbach K, Shnorhavorian M, Kadan–Lottick N, Kastrinos F, Yasui Y, Stovall M (2011) Survivors of childhood cancer have increased risk of gastrointestinal complications later in life. Gastroenterology 140(5):1464–1471. e1461
213. Romerius P, Ståhl O, Moëll C, Relander T, Cavallin-Stahl E, Wiebe T, Giwercman YL, Giwercman A (2009) Hypogonadism risk in men treated for childhood cancer. J Clin Endocrinol Metab 94(11):4180–4186
214. Rose SR, Schreiber RE, Kearney NS, Lustig RH, Danish RK, Burghen GA, Hudson MM (2004) Hypothalamic dysfunction after chemotherapy. J Pediatr Endocrinol Metab 17(1):55–66
215. Mertens AC, Yasui Y, Liu Y, Stovall M, Hutchinson R, Ginsberg J, Sklar C, Robison LL (2002) Pulmonary complications in survivors of childhood and adolescent cancer. Cancer 95 (11):2431–2441
216. Moser EC, Noordijk EM, Carde P, Tirelli U, Baars JW, Thomas J, Bron D, Meerwaldt JH, van Glabbeke M, Raemaekers JM (2005) Late non-neoplastic events in patients with aggressive non-Hodgkin's lymphoma in four randomized European organisation for research and treatment of cancer trials. Clin Lymphoma Myeloma 6(2):122–130
217. Hudson MM, Mertens AC, Yasui Y, Hobbie W, Chen H, Gurney JG, Yeazel M, Recklitis CJ, Marina N, Robison LR (2003) Health status of adult long-term survivors of childhood cancer: a report from the childhood cancer survivor study. JAMA 290(12):1583–1592
218. Duggal M, Curzon M, Bailey C, Lewis I, Prendergast M (1997) Dental parameters in the long term survivors of childhood cancer compared with siblings. Oral Oncol 33(5):348–353
219. Whelan KF, Stratton K, Kawashima T, Waterbor JW, Castleberry RP, Stovall M, Sklar CA, Packer RJ, Mitby P, Aitken CL (2010) Ocular late effects in childhood and adolescent cancer survivors: a report from the childhood cancer survivor study. Pediatr Blood Cancer 54 (1):103–109
220. Paulides M, Kremers A, Stöhr W, Bielack S, Jürgens H, Treuner J, Beck J, Langer T (2006) Prospective longitudinal evaluation of doxorubicin-induced cardiomyopathy in sarcoma patients: a report of the late effects surveillance system (LESS). Pediatr Blood Cancer 46 (4):489–495
221. Ness KK, Jones KE, Smith WA, Spunt SL, Wilson CL, Armstrong GT, Srivastava DK, Robison LL, Hudson MM, Gurney JG (2013) Chemotherapy-related neuropathic symptoms and functional impairment in adult survivors of extracranial solid tumors of childhood: results from the St. Jude Lifetime Cohort Study. Arch Phys Med Rehabil 94(8):1451–1457
222. Kaste S, Jones-Wallace D, Rose S, Boyett J, Lustig R, Rivera G, Pui C, Hudson M (2001) Bone mineral decrements in survivors of childhood acute lymphoblastic leukemia: frequency of occurrence and risk factors for their development. Leukemia 15(5):728–734
223. Byrne J, Mulvihill JJ, Myers MH, Connelly RR, Naughton MD, Krauss MR, Steinhorn SC, Hassinger DD, Austin DF, Bragg K (1987) Effects of treatment on fertility in long-term survivors of childhood or adolescent cancer. N Engl J Med 317(21):1315–1321
224. Kenney LB, Laufer MR, Grant FD, Grier H, Diller L (2001) High risk of infertility and long term gonadal damage in males treated with high dose cyclophosphamide for sarcoma during childhood. Cancer 91(3):613–621
225. Weiner DJ, Maity A, Carlson CA, Ginsberg JP (2006) Pulmonary function abnormalities in children treated with whole lung irradiation. Pediatr Blood Cancer 46(2):222–227

226. Minicucci EM, Lopes LF, Crocci AJ (2003) Dental abnormalities in children after chemotherapy treatment for acute lymphoid leukemia. Leuk Res 27(1):45–50
227. Jones DP, Spunt SL, Green D, Springate JE (2008) Renal late effects in patients treated for cancer in childhood: a report from the children's oncology group. Pediatr Blood Cancer 51 (6):724–731

Further Reading

228. Alderfer MA, Navsaria N, Kazak AE (2009) Family functioning and posttraumatic stress disorder in adolescent survivors of childhood cancer. J Fam Psychol 23(5):717
229. Armenian SH, Bhatia S (2016) Looking back to inform the future: Lesson learned from survivors of childhood cancer. Cancer
230. Armenian SH, Hudson MM, Mulder RL, Chen MH, Constine LS, Dwyer M, Nathan PC, Tissing WJ, Shankar S, Sieswerda E (2015) Recommendations for cardiomyopathy surveillance for survivors of childhood cancer: a report from the international late effects of childhood cancer guideline harmonization group. Lancet Oncol 16(3):e123–e136
231. Bleyer A, Barr R, Hayes-Lattin B, Thomas D, Ellis C, Anderson B (2008) The distinctive biology of cancer in adolescents and young adults. Nat Rev Cancer 8(4):288–298
232. Bitsko MJ, Cohen D, Dillon R, Harvey J, Krull K, Klosky JL (2015) Psychosocial late effects in pediatric cancer survivors: a report from the children's oncology group. Pediatric blood & cancer
233. Children's Oncology Group (2013) Long-term follow-up guidelines for survivors of childhood, adolescent and young adult cancers, version 4.0 Monrovia. Children's Oncology Group, CA, Oct 2013; Available online: www.survivorshipguidelines.org
234. D'Angio GJ (1975) Pediatric cancer in perspective: cure is not enough. Cancer 35(S3):866–870
235. Diller L, Chow EJ, Gurney JG, Hudson MM, Kadin-Lottick NS, Kawashima TI, Leisenring WM, Meacham LR, Mertens AC, Mulrooney DA (2009) Chronic disease in the childhood cancer survivor study cohort: a review of published findings. J Clin Oncol 27 (14):2339–2355
236. Kazak AE, DeRosa BW, Schwartz LA, Hobbie W, Carlson C, Ittenbach RF, Mao JJ, Ginsberg JP (2010) Psychological outcomes and health beliefs in adolescent and young adult survivors of childhood cancer and controls. J Clin Oncol 28(12):2002–2007
237. Landier W et al (2015) Late effects of childhood cancer and its treatment. In: Pizzo PA, Poplack DG (eds.) Principles and practice of pediatric oncology. Wolters Kluwer Health
238. Mulder RL, Kremer LC, Hudson MM, Bhatia S, Landier W, Levitt G, Constine LS, Wallace WH, van Leeuwen FE, Ronckers CM (2013) Recommendations for breast cancer surveillance for female survivors of childhood, adolescent, and young adult cancer given chest radiation: a report from the international late effects of childhood cancer guideline harmonization group. Lancet Oncol 14(13):e621–e629
239. Oeffinger KC, Mertens Sklar CA (2007) Chronic health conditions in adult survivors of childhood cancer. Oncol Times 29(1):26
240. Oeffinger KC, Nathan PC, Kremer LC (2010) Challenges after curative treatment for childhood cancer and long-term follow up of survivors. Hematol Oncol Clin N Am 24 (1):129–149
241. Robison LL, Hudson MM (2014) Survivors of childhood and adolescent cancer: life-long risks and responsibilities. Nat Rev Cancer 14(1):61–70
242. Zebrack BJ, Chesler MA (2002) Quality of life in childhood cancer survivors. Psycho-Oncology 11(2):132–141

Chapter 14
Chronic Conditions and Cancer in Older Adults

Arduino A. Mangoni, Kimberley Ruxton, Anna Rachelle Mislang and Laura Biganzoli

Abstract As a result of the progressive ageing of the population worldwide, an increasing number of older adults suffer from the sequelae of acute and chronic disease states. The latter are not confined to structural or functional impairments of individual organs or systems. Rather, they often impact on global domains of physical and cognitive function, leading to loss of independence, disability and frailty. An increasing number of older adults either suffer or have suffered, from cancer. Older cancer patients often have distinctive clinical features warranting consideration by healthcare practitioners, including significant co-morbidity burden, polypharmacy, and high inter-individual variability in homeostatic capacity, functional status and social circumstances. Although these factors are likely to influence cancer treatment options and follow-up, relatively little information is available on how to best screen, diagnose and manage this complex patient group. With the expected increase in the prevalence of older cancer patients, development and validation of dedicated care pathways, tailored to specific healthcare settings, are increasingly recognized issues in modern clinical practice. This chapter discusses general epidemiological principles of human ageing in the context of co-morbidity burden and cancer, the available information on the prevalence and outcomes of specific types of cancer in older adults, the interplay between cancer and other common disease conditions, the available tools to assess functional status and frailty in older cancer patients, and their role in clinical decision making in common cancer types in this group, namely prostate and breast cancer.

Keywords Ageing · Older patients · Frailty · Co-morbidity · Cancer · Breast cancer · Prostate cancer · Functional status · Management · Outcomes

A.A. Mangoni (✉) · K. Ruxton
Department of Clinical Pharmacology, School of Medicine, Flinders Medical Centre, Flinders University, Bedford Park, Adelaide, SA 5042, Australia
e-mail: arduino.mangoni@flinders.edu.au

A.R. Mislang · L. Biganzoli
Medical Oncology Department, Nuovo Ospedale-Santo Stefano, Instituto Toscano Tumori, Prato, Italy

B. Koczwara (ed.), *Cancer and Chronic Conditions*,
DOI 10.1007/978-981-10-1844-2_14

Key Points

- An ever-increasing number of older adults with various degrees of frailty and functional status suffer, or has suffered, from cancer
- Older cancer patients often have co-morbidities influencing treatment options and treatment-related toxicity
- Assessment of health status in older cancer patients should include the presence and severity of co-morbidities as well as patient-centered end-points such as self-rated health and functional status
- Newer, easy to use, tools to routinely assess traditional and patient-centered end-points have the potential to facilitate treatment decisions and follow-up in older cancer patients

14.1 Introduction

The world population is ageing, primarily as a result of reduced fertility rates and increased life expectancy [1]. The increase in global life expectancy, from 46.5 years in the period 1950–1955 to 66.0 years in the period 2000–2005, can be explained by a number of factors, such as better economic conditions and access to health services, political and social stability, introduction of population screening programs and improved management of disease states [2]. In the United Kingdom, the older population, defined as adults aged ≥ 65 years, was 2.2 million (5 %) in 1911 and 10.4 million (16 %) in 2011 [3]. In Australia, the proportion of people ≥ 65 years has grown from 8 % in 1970–71 to 13 % in 2001–02, and is projected to almost double (25 %) in 40 years [4]. The sub-group composition within the older population is also changing. For example, subjects ≥ 80 years are growing particularly fast because of their increased gain in life expectancy versus subjects <80 years [2].

An increasing number of older adults survive acute disease states, e.g. acute coronary syndrome, severe infection, or stroke, but also suffer from their long-term sequelae. These may adversely affect global measures of wellbeing and functional status, often leading to disability, reduced independence and frailty [5–8]. Although there is no universal consensus, frailty can be defined as a clinical syndrome in old age, with various causes, that is associated with an increased risk of adverse clinical outcomes, such as falls, disability, hospital admission and mortality [9].

Disease management in old age requires specific clinical skills in view of the co-existence of different medical conditions presenting with similar signs and symptoms, the different clinical presentation of the same disease versus younger patients, the possibility that presentations mimicking disease states are the result of adverse effects of medications, and the involvement of different healthcare professionals, as a result of co-morbid states, in formulating individual care plans. In this context, an important issue is the increasing age-related inter-individual variability in organ function and homeostasis, disease burden, type and number of medications, functional status and social support.

An increasing proportion of older patients either survives cancer diagnosed earlier in life or develops it, often after surviving other disease states. The increasing representation of older adults in the cancer patient population brings a number of issues, such as:

1. Optimal management and coordination of long-term care of cancer survivors in regards to the identification and management of co-morbidities as well as cancer follow-up
2. The potential role of baseline functional status, as well as co-morbidity burden, in decisions pertaining to cancer diagnosis and treatment options
3. The impact of frailty on cancer treatment-related toxicity and outcomes.

This chapter discusses the current information regarding the incidence, prevalence and outcomes of common cancer types and other common chronic disease conditions in older adults, the interaction between cancer and other disease states, and the importance of assessing key clinical and functional patient characteristics in order to formulate appropriate management and follow-up plans in this group. The available considerations will focus, when possible, on common cancer types in the older population, namely prostate and breast cancer.

14.2 Ageing and Cancer—Epidemiology and Outcomes

Data on the incidence and prevalence of cancer in older adults derive from a number of sources, including investigator-driven epidemiological studies, governmental datasets, insurance claim databases, surveys and clinical trials. Therefore, the quality of the information is inevitably influenced by the methods used to establish the presence, severity or history of cancer, e.g. patient reporting, biomarkers, administrative databases, imaging, or clinical notes. Therefore, variability in the results can be explained, at least partly, by differences in data collection.

In the United Kingdom, 64 % of all cancers, barring non-melanoma skin cancer, are diagnosed in patients ≥ 65 years [10]. In the United States, patients ≥ 65 years account for 54 % of all patients diagnosed with the four main types of cancer [11]. The overall incidence of cancer in patients >75 years has significantly increased over time in the United Kingdom, from 1,669 cases per 100,000 people in 1975 to 2,404 cases per 100,000 people in 2011 [10]. Similar trends have been reported in Australia and in the United States. In Australia, in the older subgroup 75–79 years the incidence was 1,926 cases per 100,000 people in 1982 and 2,379 cases per 100,000 people in 2011 [12]. In the United States, the incidence of cancer in subjects >75 years has increased from 2,096 cases per 100,000 people in 1975 to 2,217 cases per 100,000 people in 2012 [11]. The reported increased incidence of cancer in older adults over time could be secondary to better screening programs, increased longevity as well as a genuine increased risk of specific cancer types in this patient group.

In the United Kingdom, prostate cancer is the main cancer type in older males (25 %), followed by lung (17 %) and bowel cancer (15 %). By contrast, breast cancer is the main cancer type in older females (21 %), followed by bowel (15 %) and lung cancer (15 %) [10]. Similar figures have been reported in the United States, with prostate cancer being the most common type of cancer in older males (28 %), followed by lung (16 %) and bowel cancer (9 %), and breast cancer being the main cancer type in older females (24 %), followed by lung (18 %) and bowel cancer (10 %) [11].

More than 50 % of cancer-related deaths occur in patients >75 years [10]. In the United Kingdom, during the period 2007–2011, the five-year overall survival rate in women with breast cancer was 91 % in those 50–59 years old, 91 % in those 60–69 years old, 81 % in those 70–79 years old, and 61 % in those 80–89 years old. During the same period, the five-year overall survival rate in males with prostate cancer was 92 % in those 50–59 years old, 93 % in those 60–69 years old, 88 % in those 70–79 years old, and 59 % in those 80–89 years old [10]. Trends indicating a relatively lower overall survival rate in patients 80–89 years have also been observed with cancers affecting both sexes. For example, the five-year overall survival rate in lung cancer patients was 12–17 % in patients 50–59 years old versus 5 % in those 80–89 years old, and 61–64 % in bowel cancer patients 50–59 years old versus 43 % in those 80–89 years old [10].

Therefore, the available data for common cancer types in different geographical areas consistently demonstrate the significant burden of cancer in the older population. Notably, the five-year survival figures for the two most common cancer types in males and females, prostate and breast cancer, respectively, show overall survival rates well above 50 % in the old-old subgroups, 80–89 years [10].

14.3 Cancer and Chronic Conditions in Old Age

14.3.1 Epidemiology

Early studies investigated co-morbidity burden in older cancer patients by accessing epidemiological datasets. Coebergh et al. [13] studied ~34,000 newly diagnosed cancer patients from a Dutch cancer registry. The prevalence of significant co-morbidities increased with age, 12 % in patients <45 years, 28 % in patients 45–59 years, 53 % in patients 60–74 years and 60 % in patients $\geq$75 years. The most common co-morbidities included heart disease, cerebrovascular and peripheral vascular disease, hypertension, pulmonary disease and diabetes [13]. Holmes et al. [14] studied the prevalence of chronic disease conditions in 18,133 cancer survivors and 94,407 controls $\geq$65 years participating in the Behavioural Risk Factor Surveillance System 2009 telephone survey. When compared to controls, cancer survivors reported a slightly higher age-adjusted prevalence of ≥ 2 chronic conditions (67 % vs. 64 %) as well as individual conditions (hypertension, 60 % vs. 59 %; cardiovascular disease, 24 % vs. 23 %; hypercholesterolemia, 55 % vs. 53 %; diabetes, 21 % vs. 20 %; and arthritis, 57 % vs. 53 %) [14]. Berry et al. [15] investigated the prevalence of self-reported chronic disease conditions in patients with a history of cancer and age- and sex-matched controls with no history of cancer by conducting a telephone survey in South Australia. The mean age of the study population was 70 years in males and 68 years in females. When compared to controls, male patients with a history of cancer reported more frequently cardiovascular disease (OR 1.48, 95 % CI 1.15–1.90), hypercholesterolemia (OR 1.43, 95 % CI 1.16–1.76) and diabetes (OR 1.47, 95 % CI 1.11–1.94), with a non-significant trend for increased prevalence of hypertension (OR 1.19, 95 % CI 0.97–1.47). No significant differences were observed with osteoporosis (OR 1.11, 95 % CI 0.67–1.85) [15]. By contrast, women with a history of cancer reported similar prevalence of cardiovascular disease, hypertension, hypercholesterolemia, diabetes and osteoporosis compared to women without history of cancer [15]. Keating et al. [16] assessed the prevalence of several disease conditions in a population-based sample of community-dwelling Americans ≥ 55 years surviving cancer for more than four years and a control group with no history of cancer. Cancer patients reported higher rates of lung disease (13.9 % vs. 9.6 %, $P = 0.001$), heart disease (29.3 % vs. 22.9 %, $P < 0.001$), diabetes (18.2 % vs. 16.0 %, $P = 0.05$) and arthritis (69.4 % vs. 59.4 %, $P < 0.001$), but similar rates of hypertension, stroke and mental health problems [16].

A recent study by Leach et al. [17] assessed the prevalence of chronic disease conditions before and after a cancer diagnosis in 1,527 young, middle-age and older cancer survivors from two California cancer registries. In the whole population, patients reported on average 5 conditions ever diagnosed, and 1.9 conditions diagnosed after cancer. Notably, the number of chronic disease conditions was highest in breast cancer (5.8 ever, 2.9 after cancer diagnosis) and lowest in prostate cancer (4.0 ever, 1.0 after cancer diagnosis) patients. The most common chronic disease conditions ever diagnosed included hypertension (54 %), eye and ear problems (48 %), arthritis (46 %), heart disease (35 %) and lung disease (31 %) [17]. By contrast, the most common chronic disease conditions specifically diagnosed after cancer diagnosis included eye and ear problems (27 %), hypertension (17 %), heart disease (16 %), arthritis (16 %) and bone-related problems (12 %). Although data were collected from a population including older adults as well as young and middle-age patients, in multivariate analysis age >65 years was independently associated with a higher number of total conditions ever diagnosed (beta coefficient 1.54, 95 % CI 0.99–2.09), and a trend towards a higher number of conditions diagnosed after cancer diagnosis ($P = 0.08$) [17].

The burden of multimorbidity, defined as the concomitant occurrence of ≥ 2 chronic medical conditions in one person, is also of increasing concern in the older cancer population as well as in the general population. A study of Medicare beneficiaries of all ages in the United States showed that 64 % of participants had ≥ 2 conditions whereas 24 % had ≥ 4 conditions [18]. During the period 2000–2020 the number of Americans suffering from multimorbidity is estimated to increase from 60 to 81 million [19]. A Dutch study showed a similar multimorbidity burden in older cancer patients (n = 3,835, mean age 72 years) and in age-, sex-, and practice-matched patients without cancer (n = 11,973) [20]. The prevalence of participants with two chronic conditions was 19.6 % in cancer patients and 19.1 % in non-cancer patients, whereas the prevalence of participants with $\geq$4 conditions was 20.5 % in cancer patients and 20.6 % in non-cancer patients [20].

Despite significant differences in population characteristics, sample size, methods for assessing the presence of chronic conditions and statistical analysis, the available evidence suggests an increase in the prevalence of some disease states and risk factors, e.g. heart disease, respiratory disease, hypertension, hypercholesterolaemia and arthritis, in older cancer patients when compared to older adults without cancer and younger cancer patients. However, the burden of multi-morbidity appears similar in older patients with and without cancer. Little information is available on co-morbidity burden in older cancer patients >80 years, and in patients with different cancer type and severity. Further research is also warranted to ascertain whether there are significant ethnic and/or geographical differences in the prevalence and severity of co-morbid conditions in this patient group.

The assessment of the type and the number of co-morbid states, albeit useful, may not adequately characterize their impact in individual patients. For example, hypertension, particularly when adequately and safely controlled by means of pharmacological and/or non-pharmacological strategies, is a cardiovascular risk factor rather than a disease condition per se. Therefore, the impact of hypertension on measures of self-rated health, functional status and independence is likely to be relatively small if compared to disease conditions such as chronic obstructive pulmonary disease or heart failure. Moreover, the same chronic condition, e.g. diabetes, might exert different effects on health according to its duration, severity, degree of control, and co-existing medical conditions. Finally, considering the impact of different co-existing medical conditions as simply additive does not account for the complex disease-disease, disease-patient and disease-drug interactions. The latter increase the risk of adverse drug reactions and toxicity as well as physical and cognitive decline [21–23].

14.3.2 Impact of Co-morbidity on Cancer Screening and Treatment

The type, severity and number of co-morbid conditions are likely to influence older cancer patients' decisions regarding treatment options and follow up, as well as short- and long-term outcomes. However, the available evidence primarily originates from qualitative and epidemiological studies rather than randomized clinical trials. The latter are unlikely to recruit older cancer patients with significant co-morbidity burden, polypharmacy, and frailty given their generally stringent inclusion and exclusion criteria. Professional groups have recently called for an increased participation of 'real-life' older patients in clinical trials, particularly those involving pharmacological interventions. Although protocol adjustments allowing recruitment of frail older patients seem feasible and justified this group remains largely neglected [23–25].

A recent review has sought to identify factors influencing older cancer patients' decisions regarding treatment from published qualitative studies [26]. Current or previous co-morbidities were factors involved in the decision to decline cancer treatment in seven studies [27–33]. However, these studies were generally small in size, included patients <65 years, and did not demonstrate an independent effect of co-morbidities on decisions regarding cancer treatment. Studies have also investigated the possible impact of co-morbidity and polypharmacy on patient decisions regarding cancer screening. Gross et al. interviewed older adults with ≥ 2 chronic medical conditions and on ≥ 5 prescribed medications [34]. The vast majority of participants (93 %) indicated that the presence of co-morbidities would not affect their screening decisions. After viewing an educational prompt, describing the rationale for screening and its potential benefit in relation to life expectancy, 25 % of patients stated that their current health would affect their decisions, 52 % confirmed that their decisions would not be affected by current health status, whereas the remaining were undecided [34].

Prout et al. [35] assessed the potential impact of age and co-morbidity on specific treatment options in older patients with bladder cancer, using population-based cancer registries. Similarly to other studies, hypertension, heart problems, respiratory disease and arthritis represented the main co-morbid conditions (prevalence >15 %). In patients with bladder invasion, age ≥ 75 years was associated with a significantly reduced number of radical cystectomies. Similar trends were observed for patients with poorer physical status. For the same categories indicating poorer physical status, patients <75 years were 12 times more likely to undergo radical cystectomy than patients ≥ 75 years [35]. Therefore, advancing age, rather than co-morbidity, was a factor influencing treatment options in bladder cancer patients. However, it is not possible to ascertain whether specific treatment decisions were primarily made by patients, carers, or treating physicians.

14.4 Assessing Frailty and Functional Status in Older Cancer Patients

Disease management is based on a number of factors, including disease severity, achievable treatment goals, life expectancy, and co-morbidities as well as individual patient preferences, social circumstances and functional status. Although cancer treatment guidelines primarily focus on objective markers of response patient-centred end-points and frailty are also important, particularly in old age. A related issue is whether traditional cancer end-points, including progression-free survival and overall survival, have similar relevance and significance in frail older patients. The latter group might prioritise other, patient-centred, end-points such as improved quality of life and overall symptom control, e.g. reduced pain, fatigue and nausea. Multiple co-existing medical conditions might impact on key self-rated health measures and overall functioning in this group, regardless of a previous or current history of cancer. Patient-centred end-points should be used in combination with traditional clinical and demographic characteristics when making decisions in relation to cancer screening, management and follow-up.

The comprehensive geriatric assessment (CGA) is routinely performed in the general older population to assess a patient's medical, psychosocial and functional capacities in order to formulate a coordinated plan to maximize health [36]. Based on a multidisciplinary approach and assessment, the CGA includes key 'patient-centred' domains, such as functional capacity, falls risk, cognitive function and mood, nutrition, polypharmacy, social support, financial issues, treatment goals and advanced care preferences. Assessment of these domains allows determining a patient's degree of frailty, with important implications for management planning and follow-up. Performing a CGA has been associated with better clinical outcomes in the general older population, particularly improved functional status (OR 1.75, 95 % CI 1.31–2.35), reduced institutionalization (OR 0.64, 95 % CI 0.51–0.81) and reduced mortality (OR 0.72, 95 % CI 0.55–0.95) [37].

Use of the CGA for the management of older cancer patients is recommended by several key professional societies, such as the US National Comprehensive Cancer Network, the International Society for Geriatric Oncology and the European Organization for Research and Treatment of Cancer [38, 39]. A recent systematic review has assessed the available evidence regarding the use and the impact of the CGA in the management of older cancer patients [40]. Although the feasibility of conducting a CGA was demonstrated in several studies, its impact on treatment decisions and outcomes is less clear. In a study of 1,967 older cancer patients, CGA-related information was available to the treating oncologists for 61 % of patients. In this subgroup, treatment decisions were changed according to the CGA in 25 % of cases [41]. In two similar, albeit smaller, studies the proportion of patients changing treatment plan according to the results of the CGA was 39 and 49 %, respectively [42, 43]. Two further studies have identified older age, living alone, reduced activities of daily living, low body mass index and poor nutrition as CGA components that were independently associated with changes in treatment decisions [44, 45].

Studies have also assessed whether the CGA, or any of its components, is associated with cancer outcomes, including toxicity or other adverse effects related to treatment. Reduced activities of daily living, loss of independence, cognitive impairment, poor nutrition, adverse social circumstances and polypharmacy were independently associated with treatment-induced toxicity in four studies [46–49]. Reduced activities of daily living, impaired mobility and cognitive function, depression, poor nutrition and co-morbidity burden, also predicted mortality in several studies [50–57].

One issue related to the routine use of the CGA in older cancer patients as well as in the general older population is the time and staff resources required to perform the assessments. Simpler, yet robust, tools are being investigated in order to stratify risk and facilitate decision making in this context. A recent systematic review identified published studies on frailty screening methods with the best sensitivity and specificity to predict different CGA components in older cancer patients. Hamaker et al. identified 14 studies investigating 7 screening tools. The latter showed variable degrees of sensitivity and specificity: Vulnerable Elders Survey-13, 68 and 78 %; Geriatric 8, 87 and 61 %; Triage Risk Screening Tool, 92 and 47 %; Groningen Frailty Index, 57 and 86 %; Fried frailty criteria, 31 and 91 %; Barber, 59 and 79 %; and abbreviated CGA, 51 and 97 % [58]. Notably, the tools with the highest sensitivity, Geriatric 8 and Triage Risk Training Tool, also had relatively poor specificity. Therefore, the available evidence questions the routine use of available frailty screening tools to identify older cancer patients benefiting from a CGA for decisions regarding treatment options, follow up and outcomes.

Another limitation of the CGA is the lack of an objective, consistent and quantifiable approach to determine functional status and frailty. This affects its capacity to facilitate cancer treatment decisions and to predict treatment toxicity and overall outcomes. The Multidimensional Prognostic Index (MPI), a recently developed tool based on key components of the CGA, provides a quantifiable index score of between 0 and 1, with higher scores indicating increasing frailty and disability [59]. The total MPI score is obtained by averaging the scores of the following CGA components [59]: Activities of Daily Living [60]; Instrumental Activities of Daily Living [61]; Short Portable Mental Status Questionnaire [62]; Mini-Nutritional Assessment [63]; Exton-Smith Scale, assessing the risk of developing pressure sores [64]; Cumulative Index Rating Scale, assessing the severity of co-morbid conditions [65]; total number of medications; and social support network, assessing whether the patient lives alone, with relatives/partner/friend, or in an institution. Patients are stratified into low (MPI ≤ 0.33), medium (MPI 0.33–0.66) or high (MPI >0.66) risk [59]. The MPI has been shown to independently predict adverse outcomes in older patients in different settings and with specific disease states, e.g. heart failure, chronic kidney disease, dementia and cancer [53, 59, 66–72]. Notably, the MPI demonstrates superior predictive capacity and discriminatory power versus other functional frailty instruments [73]. Giantin et al. [53] investigated the clinical use of the MPI in 160 patients ≥ 70 years with different types of advanced solid cancer, by assessing 6- and 12-month all-cause mortality. In the study population, 60 % of patients had a low MPI (≤ 0.33), 30 % had a medium MPI (0.33–0.66) and 10 % had a high MPI (>0.66). The latter group had a significantly higher risk of death at 6 (HR 8.09, 95 % CI 3.75–14.48, $P < 0.001$) and 12 months (HR 5.66, 95 % CI 2.87–11.16, $P < 0.001$) versus patients with a low MPI. In a model including the MPI, age, gender, co-morbidities, body surface area, depression, cognitive function, chemotherapy treatment and type of cancer the predictive performance (area under the curve) was 0.914 (95 % CI 0.869–0.959) at 6 months and 0.874 (95 % CI 0.819–0.928) at 12 months [53].

Further studies are required to support the clinical use of the MPI in the older cancer population, not only in terms of predicting overall outcomes but also in assisting with treatment decisions and follow up.

Because of their capacity to assess a range of health parameters, including physical and cognitive function, tools such as the CGA or the MPI might also be useful for the assessment of patient-centred end-points during cancer treatment, in addition to traditional outcomes. Recent studies in patients with depression or dementia showed MPI changes during treatment, affecting a number of cognitive, behavioural as well as frailty-related domains [74, 75]. The latter may be particularly relevant in this patient population [23].

14.5 Assessment and Management of Specific Cancer Types in Old Age

14.5.1 Prostate Cancer

14.5.1.1 Epidemiology

As previously discussed, prostate cancer represents the most common type of cancer in older males [10, 11, 76]. The incidence of prostate cancer has increased by 147 % over the last 30 years [10]. The latter finding is at least partly explained by the increasing use, and misuse, of the prostate-specific antigen for cancer screening [77]. Prostate cancer related mortality significantly increases with advancing age, with the highest rates reported in patients >85 years, 790 deaths per 100,000 population [10]. The five-year overall survival of patients with prostate cancer also varies by age, although it is still relatively high in older patients, 88 % in patients 70–79 years and 59 % in patients 80–89 years [10].

14.5.1.2 Impact of Chronic Diseases on Treatment Options and Outcomes

Studies have investigated the effect of co-morbidity in predicting survival in older prostate cancer patients. Fouad et al. [78] identified 561 men (mean age 79 years) with a diagnosis of prostate cancer before death from three databases (death certificates, Medicare and Veteran's Administration). Of them, 42 % died from prostate cancer whereas 53 % died with the disease (the status was undetermined in the remaining 5 %). The prevalence of very serious (index disease severity = 4) and serious (index disease severity = 3) comorbid conditions was significantly higher in patients who died with prostate cancer compared to those who died from the disease (35 % vs. 6 % and 33 % vs. 25 %, respectively). The risk of dying of causes not related to prostate cancer was significantly associated with race (OR 1.8, 95 % CI

1.2–2.7), age at death (OR 2.2, 95 % CI 1.2–3.8) and higher index disease severity scores (OR 5.2, 95 % CI 2.7–10.0) [78]. Common chronic disease conditions in patients who died with prostate cancer versus those who died from the disease were cancer other than prostate (17 % vs. 2 %, $P < 0.001$), ischaemic heart disease (12 % vs. 5 %, $P < 0.05$), heart failure (8 % vs. 1 %, $P < 0.001$), stroke (12 % vs. 5 %, $P < 0.01$) and chronic obstructive pulmonary disease (20 % vs. 8 %, $P < 0.001$). Each of these co-morbidities was also independently associated with an increased risk of dying with prostate cancer than from the disease. Albertsen et al. [79] investigated the impact of co-morbidity burden on overall survival at 10 years in 19,639 older men (age >65 years) with localized prostate cancer, identified using the Surveillance, Epidemiology and End-Results program linked with the Medicare database. Patients included in the analysis received no surgery or radiotherapy within 180 days of diagnosis. The Charlson comorbidity index was measured to assess co-morbidity burden. The latter was considered as confounder, together with tumour grade, stage and age, in survival analyses. Co-morbidity exerted a negative impact on survival. Overall 10-year mortality was 40, 49 and 59 % in patients with 0, 1 or 2 co-morbidities, respectively. Only 5 and 11 % of patients with moderately or poorly differentiated cancer died as a result of the disease. In patients 66–74 years with localized prostate cancer (T2) and Gleason score 8–10, overall 10-year mortality was 61, 77 and 94 % in those with 0, 1 or ≥ 2 co-morbidities, respectively. By contrast, prostate cancer-specific mortality was 24, 9 and 18 %, respectively [79]. Bradley et al. [80] investigated possible differences in prostate cancer treatment and survival according to the presence of co-morbid conditions in 73,563 men identified from a national database during the period 2004–2009. An adapted version of the Charlson co-morbidity index was used to identify co-morbid conditions. The latter were present in 46 % of the study population and included diabetes, heart failure, stroke and chronic obstructive pulmonary disease. The presence of multiple co-morbid conditions was associated with a reduced likelihood of receiving any treatment versus patients without co-morbidities (OR 0.77, 95 % CI 0.73–0.82). Patients with heart failure or multiple co-morbidities had the highest death rate whereas patients with diabetes only or no co-morbidities, had the lowest [80].

The International Society of Geriatric Oncology has published recommendations, in 2010 and 2014, on the management of older patients with prostate cancer [81–83]. The initial reports emphasise that chronological age per se should not determine decisions regarding treatment options in this group [81, 82]. The 2014 report recommends an preliminary general health screening using relatively simple tools such as the Geriatric 8 assessment instrument [84]. The latter includes eight domains: age, food intake, weight loss, mobility, neuropsychological issues, body mass index, number of prescribed drugs, and self-rated health [84]. Based on this assessment, patients would fall into one of the following three management categories: (1) healthy or fit patients, undergoing similar prostate cancer treatment to that offered to younger patients; (2) vulnerable patients with reversible impairment, receiving treatment after medical intervention targeting specific impairments; and

(3) frail patients with permanent impairment, necessitating adapted treatment for prostate cancer [84].

In older patients with clinically localized, high-risk, prostate cancer, the 2014 report recommends that fit and vulnerable patients undergo curative treatment with radiation therapy or radical prostatectomy [84]. Patients in the low-intermediate risk should undergo active surveillance or watchful waiting according to their individual expected survival. In this group, the use of androgen deprivation therapy should be carefully balanced with the increased risk of cardiovascular disease, sexual dysfunction, diabetes, osteoporosis and bone fractures associated with this treatment [85]. Patients with advanced prostate cancer should receive androgen deprivation therapy as first line treatment. Concomitant treatment with supplemental dietary calcium and vitamin D, bisphosphonates or denosumab has been shown to be effective in preventing the detrimental effects of androgen deprivation therapy in this context [85–87].

Although the SIOG professional recommendations represent an important step towards individualization of prostate cancer treatment in older patients a number of issues need to be considered. First, the proposed strategies for patient assessment and management are largely based on clinical judgement and professional opinion rather than evidence. It is unknown whether a risk stratification based on the Geriatric 8 tool leads to better prostate cancer and overall outcomes, reduced treatment-related toxicity, improved patient-centred end-points independent of prostate cancer, e.g. increased food intake or mobility, and better use of available healthcare resources. Second, as previously discussed, a recent systematic review reported that the Geriatric 8 assessment tool, while showing high sensitivity (87 %), also has a relatively low specificity (61 %) for predicting different components of the CGA [58]. Further evidence is therefore required to demonstrate the superior clinical utility of this assessment tool over others in stratifying older prostate cancer patients into different management care pathways. Third, the proposed approach involves a concerted effort by different healthcare staff, including medical oncologists, geriatricians, general practitioners, physiotherapists, nurses, and dieticians. Building these multidisciplinary teams might present challenges, including the need for dedicated clinics, availability of key members, and close liaison with individual patients, relatives, carers as well as other healthcare staff, e.g. surgeons and radiation oncologists.

14.5.1.3 Adverse Effects of Treatment

Available medical treatment options in prostate cancer primarily involve androgen deprivation therapy (ADT), either by bilateral orchiectomy (surgical castration) or by medical orchiectomy. Medical orchiectomy is accomplished by using either gonadotropin releasing hormone (GnRH) agonists, with or without antiandrogens, or GnRH antagonists [88, 89]. A number of short- and long-term adverse effects are commonly observed in prostate cancer patients receiving ADT. They primarily include cardiovascular disease, osteoporosis and bone fractures, and cognitive impairment.

A. Cardiovascular and thromboembolic disease

ADT exerts several adverse metabolic effects, particularly increased fat mass, increased LDL-cholesterol and triglyceride concentrations, insulin resistance and increased incidence of new onset diabetes [90, 91]. However, the evidence for an increased incidence of cardiovascular events in prostate cancer patients treated with ADT is conflicting [92–95]. A meta-analysis of eight randomized controlled trials of ADT versus placebo in 4,141 patients failed to show a significant increase in the risk of adverse cardiovascular outcomes with ADT. The relative risk of cardiovascular mortality was 0.93 (95 % CI, 0.79–1.10) [96]. By contrast, another meta-analysis of eight observational studies in 414,657 patients showed a significant increase cardiovascular risk with ADT. The relative risk of nonfatal cardiovascular events was 1.38 (95 % CI, 1.29–1.48) with GnRH agonists [97]. ADT has also been associated with an increased risk of venous thromboembolic events in several observational studies, with hazard ratios ranging between 1.56 and 1.95 [98–100].

Pending further evidence on the short- and long-term effects of ADT on cardiovascular health in patients with prostate cancer professional groups recommend a thorough cardiovascular risk assessment and management, by means of pharmacological and non-pharmacological interventions, before and during ADT [90]. However, there are some uncertainties regarding the applicability of national and international guidelines on cardiovascular risk management in a population of frailty older patients with cancer [101].

B. Osteoporosis and bone fractures

There is good evidence that ADT leads to a loss of bone mineral density, by 5–10 % in the first year of treatment, and an increased risk of bone fractures in patients with prostate cancer [85]. The reported relative increase in fracture risk ranges between 21 and 54 % [102, 103]. Although treatment with calcium and vitamin D are commonly recommended in prostate cancer patients receiving ADT, no specific randomized controlled trials demonstrating efficacy have been conducted in this population group [104, 105]. By contrast, a number of randomized controlled trials have shown the beneficial effects of bisphosphonates, particularly pamidronate, risedronate and zolendronic acid, on bone mineral density versus placebo in prostate cancer patients [85]. This is further supported by a systematic review and meta-analysis of 15 trials in 2,634 patients, which showed that bisphosphonate therapy was associated with a significant reduction in osteoporosis (RR 0.39, 95 % CI 0.28–0.55) and vertebral fractures (RR 0.80, 95 % CI 0.69–0.94) versus placebo [106].

Denosumab, a humanized monoclonal antibody targeting the receptor activator of nuclear factor-κB ligand, preventing the transformation of pro-osteoclasts to osteoclasts, has been shown to be effective on bone mineral density and risk of fractures in prostate cancer patients treated with ADT. In a study of 1,468 patients, denosumab treatment exerted significant beneficial effects on bone mineral density and reduced the incidence of vertebral fractures versus placebo (RR 0.38, 95 % CI 0.19–0.78) [87]. Positive effects on bone density and fracture risk have also been reported for selective estrogen receptor modulators (SERMs). In a randomized controlled trial in 1,284 prostate cancer patients the SERM toremifene was associated with a significant increase in bone mineral density at the lumbar spine, total hip and femoral neck, and a reduction in the risk of new fractures (RR 0.62, 95 % CI 0.40–0.98) versus placebo [107]. However, toremifene treatment was also associated with an increased incidence of thromboembolic events versus placebo, 2.6 % versus 1.1 % [107].

Several bone health treatment recommendations and management algorithms in prostate cancer patients receiving ADT have been published. They generally involve a thorough baseline and follow-up assessment of bone density and other osteoporosis risk factors as well as treatment with calcium, vitamin D, bisphosphonates or denosumab as first-line options [108–111].

C. Cognitive impairment

The issue of a potential adverse effect of ADT on cognitive function has been widely debated, with several relatively small studies reporting contrasting results [112–114]. More recently, a large retrospective study on 16,888 prostate cancer patients, with 2,397 receiving ADT, demonstrated a significant independent association between ADT and risk of cognitive impairment using a propensity-score matching analysis approach (HR 1.88, 95 % CI 1.10–3.20) [115]. Patients receiving ADT for more than 12 months had the greatest risk of cognitive impairment (HR 2.12, 95 % CI 1.11–4.03). Further longitudinal studies are required to better investigate the short- and long-term effects of ADT on cognitive function.

14.5.2 *Breast Cancer*

14.5.2.1 Epidemiology

Breast cancer is the most common cancer in women and the second most common cancer overall. The lifetime risk of developing invasive breast cancer increases with age, with women ≥ 70 years having the highest 10-year probability risk of 3.8 % [11]. Breast cancer-specific incidence and mortality in women ≥ 70 years are 24.5 and 36.5 %, respectively [116]. As indicated before, the net survival is approximately 90 % in women aged 40–69 years, 81 % in those aged 70–79 years, but only 64 % in those aged 80–99 [10]. Survival is impacted negatively by age at diagnosis, clinical stage and presence of comorbidities.

14.5.2.2 Impact of Chronic Diseases on Treatment Options and Outcomes

The number of co-morbid diseases increases with age in the general population, by 10 % in ages up to 19 years and up to 80 % in people of ages 80 and older [117]. In breast cancer, a constellation of chronic diseases has been reported in 20–35 % of patients. This is anticipated to rise with advancing age [118]. Comorbidities can both influence and complicate the potential treatment options in older breast cancer patients. However, as a result of the under-representation of this patient group in clinical trials, management is reliant on extrapolation of available data, careful geriatric assessment, and close monitoring for potential side effects [119]. Hence, a personalized multidisciplinary care is needed in managing older patients with breast cancer to improve tolerance to systemic treatment and achieve a better outcome [120]. A CGA may provide insights to the patient's overall health status, life expectancy, tolerance to treatment, and may therefore guide clinicians in the decision-making when it comes to balancing risks-benefits with comorbidities and treatment options.

An age-related difference was noted in the treatment of breast cancer in a large population-based study in Netherlands, indicating a less aggressive treatment in older patients [121]. In contrast to younger patients, patients ≥ 80 years were less likely to undergo surgery (95 % vs. 76 %, $P < 0.01$) or breast conserving surgery (54 % vs. 29 %, $P < 0.01$). Axillary dissection was performed less frequently in the presence of comorbidities (78 % in those with ≥ 2 comorbidities vs. 97 % in those without, $P < 0.01$), as did adjuvant radiotherapy (78 % vs. 94 %, $P < 0.01$) [121].

Comorbid conditions adversely affect survival outcomes in breast cancer patients. Mechanisms are either patient- or treatment-related. Patient-related factors include the comorbidity itself, being a contraindication to the desired treatment or reducing the tolerance to treatment due to poor physiological reserve, leading to complications and toxicities. In contrast, treatment-related factors include the treatment itself, i.e. toxic regimen, suboptimal or under-treatment from dose reduction or modification relative to organ function. Breast cancer patients with comorbid conditions have an increased age-adjusted risk of death at one and five years versus patients without co-morbidities, with HR values ranging between 1.60 and 2.34 [122]. Ahern et al. [123], assessing the longitudinal comorbidity in a cohort study of women treated for primary breast cancer over a median follow up of 85 months, observed that a unit increase in the Charlson comorbidity index raises the hazard ratio for all-cause mortality by 1.4-fold, whether accounting for baseline or for acquired comorbidity. In a case-control study of older breast cancer women (median age 76 years) by Schonberg et al. [124], a direct association was found between advancing stage and worse survival after a median follow up of 7.7 years. Women with stage III or IV disease were more likely to die of breast cancer while women with ductal carcinoma in situ or stage I, of cardiovascular disease, similarly to most women without breast cancer [124]. Brandt et al., in a population-based study during the period 1961–1991, showed that age ≥ 80 years was a prognostic factor for poor survival, independent of stage at diagnosis and diagnostic period.

Although there was an improvement in survival rate over time, older patients still had a higher relative risk versus other age categories [125]. In the study of Patnaik et al. [126] on 64,034 breast cancer patients aged ≥ 66 years from the Surveillance, Epidemiology, and End Results (SEER) and Medicare data, patients with stage 1 breast cancer and comorbidities had similar survival rates to patients with stage 2 breast cancer and no comorbidities. The most prevalent comorbidities included previous cancer (16.3 %), diabetes (13.0 %), chronic obstructive pulmonary disease (8.8 %), congestive heart failure (6.5 %), and stroke (4.3 %). Individual comorbidities were associated with a statistically significant increased mortality compared with patients with no comorbidities [126]. Land et al. [127] performed a population-based, stage-specific analysis that revealed an association between comorbidity and survival in 62,591 women diagnosed with early breast cancers in from 1990 to 2008 in Denmark, confirming an increase in all-cause mortality with severe comorbidity.

14.5.2.3 Adverse Effects of Treatment

Available standard systemic treatment options in breast cancer include endocrine therapy, chemotherapy, and anti-Her2 therapy depending on disease biology and comorbidities. However, several chronic conditions could potentially limit available treatment options, reduce treatment tolerance, and exacerbate risk of treatment-related adverse events. The following paragraphs describe the potential impact of common co-morbidities on treatment options.

A. Cognitive impairment

The risk of cognitive impairment increases with age, up to 5 % in persons aged 71–79 years, 24 % in those aged 80–89 years, and 37 % in those ≥ 90 years [128]. The United States Preventive Task Force (USPTF) 2014 did not recommend routine screening for cognitive impairment in older adults lacking signs and symptoms, given the insufficient evidence to assess clinical benefits and harms. However, it acknowledges that decisions should be individualized based on specific patients or situations [128]. In older cancer patients, establishing the presence of cognitive impairment is vital not only in obtaining informed consent, but also in the ability to adhere to complex treatment regimens, manage and report potential toxicities, and attend regular follow-ups.

An increasing number of studies have shown a detrimental effect of adjuvant chemotherapy per se on cognitive function both in cross-sectional and in longitudinal studies [129, 130]. A recent meta-analysis of 27 studies confirmed the presence of a significant association between adjuvant chemotherapy and cognitive impairment, particularly in cross-sectional studies [131]. Another meta-analysis, investigating the evidence on the effect of interventions to manage cognitive impairment in breast cancer patients, showed that pharmacological interventions were generally ineffective. By contrast, non-pharmacological strategies such as cognitive training interventions improved self-reported cognitive function, memory, verbal function and language and orientation/attention whereas physical activity interventions were effective on executive function and self-reported concentration [132].

B. Cardiovascular disease

Cardiovascular disease remains the leading cause of death globally and one of the most common chronic diseases in older patients. The population ageing has led to an increase in global cardiovascular mortality between 1990 and 2013 despite an improvement in age-specific death rates in most regions, specifically in Central and Western Europe [133]. Cardiovascular disease is often associated with other diseases, such as chronic kidney disease and diabetes. Many routine breast cancer therapies have potential adverse cardiovascular effects [134], negatively impacting on quality of life during and after treatment.

Anthracyclines can cause or exacerbate cardiac toxicity, particularly heart failure, both acutely and chronically. The risk is associated with dose and exposure. Older patients have a two-fold risk of developing doxorubicin-induced heart failure versus younger patients, even at relatively low doses [135]. A Cochrane review of seven randomized controlled trials evaluating the duration of anthracycline infusions showed a reduction in heart failure with infusions exceeding six hours compared to shorter duration (relative risk, RR 0.27), with no negative impact on response rate or survival [136]. A review of five randomized controlled trials on epirubicin versus doxorubicin showed a lower incidence of clinical heart failure with epirubicin, while a meta-analysis on the use of liposomal doxorubicin showed a reduction in heart failure risk versus conventional doxorubicin (RR 0.20) [137]. A meta-analysis of dexrazoxane also showed a significant cardioprotective effect (RR 0.29) [138]. The incidence of late onset cardiac dysfunction, increasingly recognized as the survival from breast cancer improves, ranges between 18 and 65 %. Its prevalence rises with time, suggesting a progressive nature of the disease [139, 140]. Older patients at increased risk of cardiotoxicity should be carefully identified and evaluated before treatment with anthracyclines.

Cardiac events from paclitaxel are most commonly due to bradycardia (30 %). However, the incidence of serious cardiac events is low in patients without preexisting cardiac dysfunction [141]. Notably, taxanes can potentiate anthracycline-induced cardiotoxicity by stimulating the formation of doxorubucinol, a toxic metabolite [142]. Fluoropyrimidines increase the risk of endothelial dysfunction and coronary artery vasospasm within two to five days of therapy, lasting up to 48 h. This might trigger acute coronary syndromes, with a reported incidence between 1 and 68 % [143–148].

Of the anti-Her2 agents, trastuzumab has been the most studied. Trastuzumab binding to Her2 has been shown to cause contractile dysfunction via mitochondrial integrity disruption and interference with cardiac myocyte growth, repair and survival [149]. Unlike anthracyclines, trastuzumab-related cardiac dysfunction, ranging from declining left ventricular ejection fraction to overt heart failure, is generally reversible, but the long-term effect is unclear. The risk of cardiac dysfunction is substantially higher when given concurrently with anthracyclines (27 %) versus paclitaxel (13 %) or monotherapy (3–7 %) [150]. A systematic review of randomized trials on adjuvant trastuzumab in patients >60 years showed a 5.2 % pooled incidence of cardiac events [151]. Chen et al. assessed the three-year cardiac event rates (heart failure and cardiomyopathy) after adjuvant chemotherapy and trastuzumab therapy in women aged 67–94 years using the Surveillance, Epidemiology, and End Results-Medicare data from 2000 through 2007. Compared with patients who received neither therapies, there was a 14 % increase in absolute risk for trastuzumab use alone, 23.8 % for trastuzumab and anthracyclines, and 2.1 % for anthracycline use alone [152]. In the NSABP-31 trial comparing doxorubicin and cyclophosphamide (AC) followed by paclitaxel with or without trastuzumab, those in the trastuzumab arm had a 4.1 % cumulative incidence of New York Heart Association class III–IV heart failure and an overall cardiac event incidence of 19 % in three years [153]. The latter occurred more frequently in patients ≥50 years and in patients with marginal post-AC decline in left ventricular ejection fraction. Asymptomatic decrease in left ventricular ejection fraction was the most common cause for trastuzumab discontinuation (14 %) and the cardiac dysfunction was reversible [153]. Similarly, the N9831 trial reported a 5 % reduction in left ventricular ejection fraction and a three-year cumulative incidence of cardiac events of 0.3 % in arm A (AC followed by weekly paclitaxel), 2.8 % in arm B (paclitaxel followed by trastuzumab), and 3.3 % in arm C (paclitaxel plus trastuzumab followed by trastuzumab alone) [154]. Age ≥60 years was associated with increased cardiac events (6.6 %) in the univariate analysis [154]. Cardiac function recovered after trastuzumab discontinuation. Similar results were reported during extended follow-up, with only two additional heart failure diagnoses beyond five years [155]. In the HERA trial, the incidence of trastuzumab-related cardiac dysfunction at 12-month median follow-up was 3.6, and 4.3 % discontinued treatment [156]. Most patients recovered within six months. Early trastuzumab discontinuation could substantially affect overall survival. In a population-based cohort study of 585 women with stage I–III breast cancer (mean age 72 years) and no pre-existing cardiovascular disease, 41 % discontinued trastuzumab treatment early (defined as cardiovascular events within 45 days before the last trastuzumab treatment) [157]. Among these cohorts, 48 % had prior anthracycline, 25 % had prior docetaxel and carboplatin, and 27 % had prior docetaxel and cyclophosphamide. Heart failure, or cardiomyopathy, was the most common cardiovascular event (18.8 %) [157]. Notably, women suffering from cardiovascular events had significantly worse survival, even if they had completed trastuzumab treatment. These results highlight the vulnerability of older patients to cardiotoxicity from adjuvant treatment, with subsequent increased in mortality, regardless of treatment completion status. Developing strategies to prevent and manage cardiac events could impact their overall survival.

Anti vascular endothelial growth factor drugs (anti-VEGF) such as bevacizumab, combined with chemotherapy, are biologically active as first or second line treatment in older patients with Her2 negative locally recurrent or metastatic breast cancer, with significant improvement in progression-free survival but not overall survival [158]. However, anti-VEGF treatment is associated with an increased incidence of hypertension, proteinuria, thromboembolic events and heart failure. In a review of all phase I–III clinical trials published up to December 2008 with approved anti-VEGF therapies, the incidence of grade 3–4 hypertension, cardiac dysfunction and thromboembolism was 9.2, 0.3 and 9.6 %, respectively [159]. The adverse safety profile, together with the relatively high treatment costs, made the use of anti-VEGF drugs prohibitive in older patients with comorbidities.

Aromatase inhibitors, commonly used in postmenopausal breast cancer, also increase cardiovascular risk versus tamoxifen [160, 161]. More than 19,000 patients from seven randomized controlled trials were assessed in a study comparing tamoxifen versus aromatase inhibitors [160]. The latter were associated with an increased risk of cardiovascular events (RR 1.31) and a reduced risk of thromboembolic events (RR 0.53). However, the absolute risks were low, with number needed to harm (NNH) of 189 patients to produce one cardiovascular event, and 85 patients for one thromboembolic event. Similarly, a meta-analysis of more than 30,000 patients from randomized controlled trials confirmed the increased risk of cardiovascular events (OR 1.26, NNH 132) but also showed reduced risk of venous thrombosis (OR 0.55, NNH 79) [161]. The reduced risk of venous thrombosis could be due to the relative increase in risk imparted by tamoxifen [162].

The International Society of Geriatric Oncology has published recommendations for the management of anthracycline-induced cardiac toxicity [163, 164]. Additionally, the European Society for Medical Oncology released clinical practice guidelines for cardiovascular toxicity induced by chemotherapy, targeted agents and radiotherapy (Table 14.1) [165].

C. Type 2 diabetes mellitus

Type 2 diabetes is an independent risk factor for breast cancer [166]. Srokowski et al. reported its negative influence on the choice of chemotherapy regimen, related toxicities, and outcomes. In their cohort study of 70,781 patients aged $\geq$66 years from the SEER-Medicare database, 20.4 % had type 2 diabetes [167]. The latter had reduced odds of receiving anthracyclines (OR 0.78, 95 % CI 0.71–0.87) or taxanes (OR 0.86, 95 % CI 0.75–0.99), and increased odds of any chemotherapy toxicities, including hospitalizations due to chemotherapy toxicity (OR 1.38, 95 % CI 1.23–1.56), infection/fever (OR 1.43, 95 % CI 1.20–1.70), neutropenia (OR 1.22, 95 % CI 1.03–1.45) and anaemia (OR 1.24, 95 % CI 1.05–1.47). Moreover, patients with type 2 diabetes had higher all-cause mortality (HR 1.35, 95 % CI 1.31–1.39) and breast cancer specific mortality than patients without type 2 diabetes, when given chemotherapy (HR 1.20, 95 % CI 1.07–1.35) [167]. In another study of 112 patients $\geq$70 years with early, operable ER-negative breast cancer treated between 2000 and 2010 in China, type 2 diabetes at diagnosis was an independent prognostic factor for overall survival (with the addition of chemotherapy regimen) while chemotherapy was not. This suggests that type 2 diabetes management may be more important than chemotherapy in this group [168].

Table 14.1 Recommendations for management of cardiotoxicity—adapted from SIOG and ESMO [164, 165]

Recommendations	Management	
Rigorous screening for high cardiac risk	Comprehensive patient history and physical examination	Cardiovascular comorbidities and risk factors • Previous exposure to anthracyclines • Previous mediastinal irradiation • Previous or current use of other cardiotoxic drugs • Planned for trastuzumab • Age $\geq$60 years • Comorbidities – Hypertension – Coronary artery disease – Cardiomyopathy – Arrhythmias – Dyslipidemia – Diabetes mellitus – Obesity – Peripheral vascular disease – Smoking – Sedentary lifestyle – Alcohol excess
Not exceeding the recommended cumulative dose	Reduce maximum cumulative dose	Doxorubicin • Max: 450–500 mg/m^2 • Aim: 300 mg/m^2 Epirubicin • Max: 900 mg/m^2 • Aim: <720 mg/m^2 Liposomal Doxorubicin • Max: 900 mg/m^2 • Aim: <900 mg/m^2
Use of alternative, less cardiotoxic therapy	Use of continuous infusion	Aim for at least 6 h
	Avoid concurrent anthracyline and trastuzumab	Sequential anthracycline and trastuzumab
	Use less cardiotoxic formulations	Liposomal doxorubicin
		Epirubicin
		Taxanes
		Capecitabine
		Vinorelbine
		Gemcitabine
	Use cardioprotectant	Dexrazoxane

(continued)

Table 14.1 (continued)

Recommendations	Management	
Regular cardiac function monitoring	Baseline assessment of cardiac function	12-lead ECG
		Echocardiography or Multiple gated acquisition scan (MUGA)
		Cardiac biomarkers[a]
	Serial cardiac monitoring Long-term follow up	Monitor every 2–3 cycles of conventional anthracyclines
		Careful attention to left ventricular ejection fraction drop exceeding 10 %, even if still within normal range
		Cease treatment if left ventricular ejection fraction decreases below the lower limit of normal
Cardiovascular risk reduction intervention	Treatment optimization of pre-existing cardiac dysfunction	Medical management • ACE inhibitors, AII inhibitors, beta-blockers, statins, etc. Lifestyle modification • Smoking cessation, regular exercise, moderate alcohol consumption, diet modification Early recognition and aggressive management of cardiac dysfunction, even when asymptomatic

[a]Biomarkers: troponin and brain natriuretic peptide are experimental, awaiting prospective validation

Taxanes are commonly used in both early and advanced breast cancer. Steroid use, as a premedication to reduce hypersensitivity, could precipitate or exacerbate type 2 diabetes. In a retrospective study on 632 patients given docetaxel-based chemotherapy in Korea, the overall incidence of hyperglycaemia was 13.7 %, 10.9 % in patients without previous type 2 diabetes. The risk for infections was higher with hyperglycaemia, stressing the need for early recognition and optimal glucose management during docetaxel therapy [169]. Moreover, pre-existing type 2 diabetes increases the risk and severity of peripheral neuropathy with taxanes, and predisposes to a slower recovery [170].

D. Renal disease

Older patients with renal impairment are at risk for toxicity when given chemotherapy drugs that are renally excreted, e.g. fluoropyrimidines, cyclophosphamide and bisphosphonates. A dose adjustment is recommended in this context. The cardiotoxicity risk is markedly increased in patients given 5-fluorouracil or capecitabine with intercurrent renal impairment [148]. In a study comparing zoledronic acid with pamidronate, a grade 3–4 increase in serum creatinine concentrations occurred in 0.4 % patients in the zoledronic acid group and in 1.9 % in the pamidronate group after two years of administration [171].

E. Bone health: osteoporosis and osteonecrosis of the jaw

Bone health requires careful evaluation in older patients, particularly those receiving treatment for breast cancer. Age is a non-modifiable risk factor for osteoporosis regardless of bone mineral density [172]. However, in the National Osteoporosis Risk Assessment (NORA) study of >170,000 women aged 50–99 years, a low bone mineral density (T score <−1.0) had a similar relative risk for fracture regardless of age [173]. Risk factors for osteoporosis can be patient-related (i.e. age ≥ 50 years, female gender, personal or family history of fracture, ethnicity, malnutrition, sedentary lifestyle, immobility, falls, alcohol use >2 units/day, and smoking), disease-related (i.e. estrogen deficiency, hypogonadism, nutritional disorders or malabsorption, vitamin D deficiency, chronic liver or kidney disease, endocrinopathies, and malignancy—e.g. breast, prostate, multiple myeloma), or therapy-related (i.e. glucocorticoids, aromatase inhibitors, anti-androgens, thyroxine, proton pump inhibitors, methotrexate, psychotropic agents, antidepressants, and anticonvulsants) [174]. Not surprisingly, older breast cancer patients with pre-existing risk factors are at increased risk of bone loss and osteoporosis, particularly when treated with aromatase inhibitors. For these reasons, tamoxifen is preferred in patients with pre-existing or increased risk of osteoporosis. Tamoxifen conferred a non-significant 19 % reduction in osteoporotic fracture events versus placebo in the NSABP-1 trial, with overall reduction being greatest in women ≥ 50 years [175]. In the cross-sectional analysis of Kwan et al. on 2,157 patients with breast cancer, prior risk factors (11.2 % prior history of osteoporosis, 16.3 % any fracture, and 4.6 % major fracture) had been present for six years or more before cancer diagnosis. The majority of patients were initially treated with aromatase inhibitors although those started on tamoxifen had nearly twice the prevalence of prior osteoporosis, highlighting the clinical consideration of prior bone health history when initiating cancer treatment [176].

Bisphosphonates, selective estrogen receptor modulators, denosumab, plus supplemental calcium and vitamin D are approved for the management of bone loss or bony metastases. Recently, the Early Breast Cancer Trialists' Collaborative Group (EBCTCG) reported the benefit of adjuvant bisphosphonates only in postmenopausal women in reducing the rate of breast cancer recurrence in the bone and improving breast cancer survival [177].

However, bone-modifying agents such as oral bisphosphonates and denosumab have been implicated in osteonecrosis of the jaw (ONJ), a rare but potentially serious complication. In breast cancer, the reported frequency of ONJ ranges from 0.6 to 6.2 % [178]. Review of relevant articles describing the relationship between bisphosphonates and ONJ revealed age ≥ 60 years, female sex, and previous invasive dental treatment as potential risk factors [179]. In a cohort study of 1621 cancer patients treated with zoledronate, ibandronate, and pamidronate, dental extractions and use of dentures were identified as risk factors. The crude ONJ incidence was 3.1 % with breast cancer [180].

Receptor activator of nuclear factor kappa-B ligand (RANKL) inhibitors such as denosumab, are an alternative to bisphosphonates when managing patients at risk for skeletal related events from solid organ metastasis or osteoporosis. Denosumab is widely used because of its superior efficacy to bisphosphonates as well as a more favourable adverse event profile, including manageable hypocalcaemia, reduced nephrotoxicity and acute phase reactions, and ease of subcutaneous administration [181]. However, in a trial on patients with advanced breast cancer denosumab was associated with a non-statistically higher incidence of ONJ versus zoledronic acid (2.0 % vs. 1.4 %, $P = 0.39$) [182].

In summary, patients with breast cancer are at increased risk of ONJ when treated with bone modifying agents, especially in the presence of risk factors. Evidence recommends careful planning and pre-treatment prophylactic dental care to reduce ONJ incidence [181, 183].

F. Arterial and venous thromboembolism

In a retrospective study of 3,283 breast cancer patients treated with tamoxifen, there was an age-associate increase in the risk of thromboembolic events, e.g. deep venous thrombosis, pulmonary embolism, myocardial infarction or cerebrovascular events: 5 % (<45 years), 7 % (45–54 years), 14 % (55–64 years), 19 % (65–74 years), and 27 % ($\geq$75 years) [184]. However, in the NSABP-1 trial on tamoxifen versus placebo, tamoxifen use had no effect on ischaemic heart disease annual rate. It did, however, increase the risk of stroke (RR 1.59), pulmonary embolism (RR 3.01), and deep vein thrombosis (RR 1.6), especially in women >50 years [175]. The ATLAS trial randomized nearly 13,000 women with ER-positive early breast cancer to either five or ten years of adjuvant tamoxifen. The probability of dying from another cause after breast cancer diagnosis, during years 5–14, was 5 % in women <60 years and 20 % in older women. Moreover, there was an increased incidence of pulmonary embolism (RR 1.87) and stroke (RR 1.06) [185]. Age >65 years and prior history of arterial thromboembolism can increase the risk of bevacizumab-associated thromboembolism, especially when combined with chemotherapy [186].

In summary, although improvements in therapeutic options have increased survival in older breast cancer patients, the presence of comorbidities may adversely influence treatment decisions, tolerance, and outcomes. Treatment goals must balance efficacy with toxicity, while controlling the symptoms and maintaining quality of life. The long-term consequences of anti-cancer therapies have become an important issue contributing to morbidity and mortality as survivorship increases.

14.6 Recommendations for Research and Practice

The evidence discussed in this chapter highlights the high prevalence of cancer, as previous or current disease state, in an ever-growing older patient population characterized by significant inter-individual variability in co-morbidity burden, prescribed drugs, homeostatic capacity, physical and cognitive function and social circumstances. Similarly to the general older population, the number of co-morbid conditions increases with age in older cancer patients, although little information is currently available on the impact of disease states on self-rated measures of health as well as functional status. The limited available evidence suggests that the co-morbidity burden may influence decisions regarding cancer screening and treatment options. However, more research is needed to ascertain whether specific disease states and their impact on individual patients' health, rather than patient's preferences or physician's attitudes, independently affect such decisions. Additional knowledge is also required to better identify the pattern of co-morbid states diagnosed specifically after cancer diagnosis and treatment. The latter might also influence decisions regarding cancer management.

Patient-centered end-points, such as measures of self-rated health, functional status and independence are increasingly recognized as factors independently predicting adverse clinical outcomes as well as influencing management decisions in old age. A number of Geriatric Oncology professional societies advocate the use of the Comprehensive Geriatric Assessment (CGA) and other frailty assessment tools for early stratification of frailty and functional status in older cancer patients. As a result of this assessment, patients would be entered into specific management pathways, e.g. active treatment similar to what recommended in younger patient cohorts, medical management of specific co-morbid states before initiating cancer treatment, modified, less-intensive, cancer treatment or palliative care. Although the proposed strategies take into account individual measures of health and functional status, key elements of modern care in old age, additional studies are required to justify their routine clinical use, particularly in regards to acceptance by patients and healthcare staff, adequate resource utilization, reduced treatment-related toxicity, and improvement in traditional cancer outcome measures as well as patient-centred end-points.

References

1. Bongaarts J (2009) Human population growth and the demographic transition. Philos Trans R Soc Lond B Biol Sci 364(1532):2985–2990
2. Mangoni AA (2014) Geriatric medicine in an aging society: up for a challenge? Front Med (Lausanne) 1:10
3. 2011 Census: Population Estimates for the United Kingdom, 27 March 2011 (Internet), 2012. Available from: http://www.ons.gov.uk/ons/publications/re-reference-tables.html?edition=tcm%3A77-270247. Accessed 30 Dec 2015
4. Australia's Demographic Challenges (Internet) (2004) Social Policy Division, The Treasury. Available from: http://demographics.treasury.gov.au/content/_download/australias_demographic_challenges/australias_demographic_challenges.pdf. Accessed 30 Dec 2015
5. Crews DE, Zavotka S (2006) Aging, disability, and frailty: implications for universal design. J Physiol Anthropol 25(1):113–118
6. Quine S, Morrell S (2007) Fear of loss of independence and nursing home admission in older Australians. Health Soc Care Community 15(3):212–220
7. Faria SH (1996) Elders' perceptions about being healthy: being independent. Fla Nurse 44 (7):14–15
8. Marottoli RA, Mendes de Leon CF, Glass TA, Williams CS, Cooney LM Jr, Berkman LF et al (1997) Driving cessation and increased depressive symptoms: prospective evidence from the New Haven EPESE. Established populations for epidemiologic studies of the elderly. J Am Geriatr Soc 45(2):202–206

9. Xue QL (2011) The frailty syndrome: definition and natural history. Clin Geriatr Med 27 (1):1–15
10. Cancer incidence by age: Cancer Research UK, London (2014). Available from: http://www.cancerresearchuk.org/health-professional/cancer-statistics/incidence/age-ref-7
11. American Cancer Society (2014) Cancer facts and figures, Atlanta
12. Hind D, Wyld L, Reed MW (2007) Surgery, with or without tamoxifen, vs tamoxifen alone for older women with operable breast cancer: cochrane review. Br J Cancer 96(7):1025–1029
13. Coebergh JW, Janssen-Heijnen ML, Post PN, Razenberg PP (1999) Serious co-morbidity among unselected cancer patients newly diagnosed in the southeastern part of The Netherlands in 1993–1996. J Clin Epidemiol 52(12):1131–1136
14. Holmes HM, Nguyen HT, Nayak P, Oh JH, Escalante CP, Elting LS (2014) Chronic conditions and health status in older cancer survivors. Eur J Int Med 25(4):374–378
15. Berry NM, Miller MD, Woodman RJ, Coveney J, Dollman J, Mackenzie CR et al (2014) Differences in chronic conditions and lifestyle behaviour between people with a history of cancer and matched controls. Med J Aust 201(2):96–100
16. Keating NL, Norredam M, Landrum MB, Huskamp HA, Meara E (2005) Physical and mental health status of older long-term cancer survivors. J Am Geriatr Soc 53(12):2145–2152
17. Leach CR, Weaver KE, Aziz NM, Alfano CM, Bellizzi KM, Kent EE et al (2015) The complex health profile of long-term cancer survivors: prevalence and predictors of comorbid conditions. J Cancer Surviv 9(2):239–251
18. Wolff JL, Starfield B, Anderson G (2002) Prevalence, expenditures, and complications of multiple chronic conditions in the elderly. Arch Int Med 162(20):2269–2276
19. Care Coordination for People with Chronic Conditions (Internet) (2003) National Academy for State Health Policy. Available from: http://www.partnershipforsolutions.org/DMS/files/Care_coordination.pdf. Accessed 31 Dec 2015
20. Deckx L, van den Akker M, Metsemakers J, Knottnerus A, Schellevis F, Buntinx F (2012) Chronic diseases among older cancer survivors. J Cancer Epidemiol 2012:206414
21. Mangoni AA (2012) Predicting and detecting adverse drug reactions in old age: challenges and opportunities. Expert Opin Drug Metab Toxicol 8(5):527–530
22. Ruxton K, Woodman RJ, Mangoni AA (2015) Drugs with anticholinergic effects and cognitive impairment, falls and all-cause mortality in older adults: a systematic review and meta-analysis. Br J Clin Pharmacol 80(2):209–220
23. Mangoni AA, Pilotto A (2016) New drugs and patient-centred end-points in old age: setting the wheels in motion. Expert Rev Clin Pharmacol 9(1):81–89
24. McMurdo ME, Roberts H, Parker S, Wyatt N, May H, Goodman C et al (2011) Improving recruitment of older people to research through good practice. Age Ageing 40(6):659–665
25. Mangoni AA, Jansen PA, Jackson SH (2013) Under-representation of older adults in pharmacokinetic and pharmacodynamic studies: a solvable problem? Expert Rev Clin Pharmacol 6(1):35–39
26. Puts MT, Tapscott B, Fitch M, Howell D, Monette J, Wan-Chow-Wah D et al (2015) A systematic review of factors influencing older adults' decision to accept or decline cancer treatment. Cancer Treat Rev 41(2):197–215
27. Sinding C, Wiernikowski J, Aronson J (2005) Cancer care from the perspectives of older women. Oncol Nurs Forum 32(6):1169–1175
28. Ciambrone D (2006) Treatment decision-making among older women with breast cancer. J Women Aging 18(4):31–47
29. Sanders T, Skevington S (2004) Participation as an expression of patient uncertainty: an exploration of bowel cancer consultations. Psychooncology 13(10):675–688
30. Verkooijen HM, Fioretta GM, Rapiti E, Bonnefoi H, Vlastos G, Kurtz J et al (2005) Patients' refusal of surgery strongly impairs breast cancer survival. Ann Surg 242(2):276–280
31. Cykert S, Dilworth-Anderson P, Monroe MH, Walker P, McGuire FR, Corbie-Smith G et al (2010) Factors associated with decisions to undergo surgery among patients with newly diagnosed early-stage lung cancer. JAMA 303(23):2368–2376

32. Lim L, Chao M, Shapiro J, Millar JL, Kipp D, Rezo A et al (2007) Long-term outcomes of patients with localized rectal cancer treated with chemoradiation or radiotherapy alone because of medical inoperability or patient refusal. Dis Colon Rectum 50(12):2032–2039
33. Tang SW, Parker H, Winterbottom L, Hassell K, Ellis IO, Morgan DA et al (2011) Early primary breast cancer in the elderly—pattern of presentation and treatment. Surg Oncol 20 (1):7–12
34. Gross CP, Fried TR, Tinetti ME, Ross JS, Genao I, Hossain S et al (2015) Decision-making and cancer screening: a qualitative study of older adults with multiple chronic conditions. J Geriatr Oncol 6(2):93–100
35. Prout GR Jr, Wesley MN, Yancik R, Ries LA, Havlik RJ, Edwards BK (2005) Age and comorbidity impact surgical therapy in older bladder carcinoma patients: a population-based study. Cancer 104(8):1638–1647
36. Stuck AE, Siu AL, Wieland GD, Adams J, Rubenstein LZ (1993) Comprehensive geriatric assessment: a meta-analysis of controlled trials. Lancet 342(8878):1032–1036
37. Bachmann S, Finger C, Huss A, Egger M, Stuck AE, Clough-Gorr KM (2010) Inpatient rehabilitation specifically designed for geriatric patients: systematic review and meta-analysis of randomised controlled trials. BMJ 340:c1718
38. Extermann M, Aapro M, Bernabei R, Cohen HJ, Droz JP, Lichtman S et al (2005) Use of comprehensive geriatric assessment in older cancer patients: recommendations from the task force on CGA of the International Society of Geriatric Oncology (SIOG). Crit Rev Oncol Hematol 55(3):241–252
39. Pallis AG, Wedding U, Lacombe D, Soubeyran P, Wildiers H (2010) Questionnaires and instruments for a multidimensional assessment of the older cancer patient: what clinicians need to know? Eur J Cancer 46(6):1019–1025
40. Caillet P, Laurent M, Bastuji-Garin S, Liuu E, Culine S, Lagrange JL et al (2014) Optimal management of elderly cancer patients: usefulness of the Comprehensive Geriatric Assessment. Clin Interv Aging 9:1645–1660
41. Kenis C, Bron D, Libert Y, Decoster L, Van Puyvelde K, Scalliet P et al (2013) Relevance of a systematic geriatric screening and assessment in older patients with cancer: results of a prospective multicentric study. Ann Oncol 24(5):1306–1312
42. Girre V, Falcou MC, Gisselbrecht M, Gridel G, Mosseri V, Bouleuc C et al (2008) Does a geriatric oncology consultation modify the cancer treatment plan for elderly patients? J Gerontol A Biol Sci Med Sci 63(7):724–730
43. Chaibi P, Magne N, Breton S, Chebib A, Watson S, Duron JJ et al (2011) Influence of geriatric consultation with comprehensive geriatric assessment on final therapeutic decision in elderly cancer patients. Crit Rev Oncol Hematol 79(3):302–307
44. Marenco D, Marinello R, Berruti A, Gaspari F, Stasi MF, Rosato R et al (2008) Multidimensional geriatric assessment in treatment decision in elderly cancer patients: 6-year experience in an outpatient geriatric oncology service. Crit Rev Oncol Hematol 68(2):157–164
45. Caillet P, Canoui-Poitrine F, Vouriot J, Berle M, Reinald N, Krypciak S et al (2011) Comprehensive geriatric assessment in the decision-making process in elderly patients with cancer: ELCAPA study. J Clin Oncol: Official J Am Soc Clin Oncol 29(27):3636–3642
46. Hurria A, Togawa K, Mohile SG, Owusu C, Klepin HD, Gross CP et al (2011) Predicting chemotherapy toxicity in older adults with cancer: a prospective multicenter study. J Clin Oncol: Official J Am Soc Clin Oncol 29(25):3457–3465
47. Extermann M, Boler I, Reich RR, Lyman GH, Brown RH, DeFelice J et al (2012) Predicting the risk of chemotherapy toxicity in older patients: the Chemotherapy Risk Assessment Scale for High-Age Patients (CRASH) score. Cancer 118(13):3377–3386
48. Falandry C, Weber B, Savoye AM, Tinquaut F, Tredan O, Sevin E et al (2013) Development of a geriatric vulnerability score in elderly patients with advanced ovarian cancer treated with first-line carboplatin: a GINECO prospective trial. Ann Oncol 24(11):2808–2813

49. Baitar A, Van Fraeyenhove F, Vandebroek A, De Droogh E, Galdermans D, Mebis J et al (2013) Evaluation of the Groningen Frailty Indicator and the G8 questionnaire as screening tools for frailty in older patients with cancer. J Geriatr Oncol 4(1):32–38
50. Soubeyran P, Fonck M, Blanc-Bisson C, Blanc JF, Ceccaldi J, Mertens C et al (2012) Predictors of early death risk in older patients treated with first-line chemotherapy for cancer. J Clin Oncol: Official J Am Soc Clin Oncol 30(15):1829–1834
51. Maione P, Perrone F, Gallo C, Manzione L, Piantedosi F, Barbera S et al (2005) Pretreatment quality of life and functional status assessment significantly predict survival of elderly patients with advanced non-small-cell lung cancer receiving chemotherapy: a prognostic analysis of the multicenter Italian lung cancer in the elderly study. J Clin Oncol: Official J Am Soc Clin Oncol 23(28):6865–6872
52. Kanesvaran R, Li H, Koo KN, Poon D (2011) Analysis of prognostic factors of comprehensive geriatric assessment and development of a clinical scoring system in elderly Asian patients with cancer. J Clin Oncol: Official J Am Soc Clin Oncol 29(27):3620–3627
53. Giantin V, Valentini E, Iasevoli M, Falci C, Siviero P, De Luca E et al (2013) Does the Multidimensional Prognostic Index (MPI), based on a Comprehensive Geriatric Assessment (CGA), predict mortality in cancer patients? Results of a prospective observational trial. J Geriatr Oncol 4(3):208–217
54. Clough-Gorr KM, Thwin SS, Stuck AE, Silliman RA (2012) Examining five- and ten-year survival in older women with breast cancer using cancer-specific geriatric assessment. Eur J Cancer 48(6):805–812
55. Kim KI, Park KH, Koo KH, Han HS, Kim CH (2013) Comprehensive geriatric assessment can predict postoperative morbidity and mortality in elderly patients undergoing elective surgery. Arch Gerontol Geriatr 56(3):507–512
56. Bo M, Cacello E, Ghiggia F, Corsinovi L, Bosco F (2007) Predictive factors of clinical outcome in older surgical patients. Arch Gerontol Geriatr 44(3):215–224
57. Tougeron D, Di Fiore F, Thureau S, Berbera N, Iwanicki-Caron I, Hamidou H et al (2008) Safety and outcome of definitive chemoradiotherapy in elderly patients with oesophageal cancer. Br J Cancer 99(10):1586–1592
58. Hamaker ME, Jonker JM, de Rooij SE, Vos AG, Smorenburg CH, van Munster BC (2012) Frailty screening methods for predicting outcome of a comprehensive geriatric assessment in elderly patients with cancer: a systematic review. Lancet Oncol 13(10):e437–e444
59. Pilotto A, Ferrucci L, Franceschi M, D'Ambrosio LP, Scarcelli C, Cascavilla L et al (2008) Development and validation of a multidimensional prognostic index for one-year mortality from comprehensive geriatric assessment in hospitalized older patients. Rejuvenation Res 11 (1):151–161
60. Katz S, Ford AB, Moskowitz RW, Jackson BA, Jaffe MW (1963) Studies of illness in the aged. The index of ADL: a standardized measure of biological and psychosocial function. JAMA 185:914–919
61. Lawton MP, Brody EM (1969) Assessment of older people: self-maintaining and instrumental activities of daily living. Gerontologist 9(3):179–186
62. Pfeiffer E (1975) A short portable mental status questionnaire for the assessment of organic brain deficit in elderly patients. J Am Geriatr Soc 23(10):433–441
63. Vellas B, Guigoz Y, Garry PJ, Nourhashemi F, Bennahum D, Lauque S et al (1999) The Mini Nutritional Assessment (MNA) and its use in grading the nutritional state of elderly patients. Nutrition 15(2):116–122
64. Bliss MR, McLaren R, Exton-Smith AN (1966) Mattresses for preventing pressure sores in geriatric patients. Mon Bull Minist Health Public Health Lab Serv 25:238–268
65. Conwell Y, Forbes NT, Cox C, Caine ED (1993) Validation of a measure of physical illness burden at autopsy: the Cumulative Illness Rating Scale. J Am Geriatr Soc 41(1):38–41
66. Pilotto A, Sancarlo D, Panza F, Paris F, D'Onofrio G, Cascavilla L et al (2009) The Multidimensional Prognostic Index (MPI), based on a comprehensive geriatric assessment

predicts short- and long-term mortality in hospitalized older patients with dementia. J Alzheimers Dis 18(1):191–199
67. Pilotto A, Addante F, Franceschi M, Leandro G, Rengo G, D'Ambrosio P et al (2010) Multidimensional Prognostic Index based on a comprehensive geriatric assessment predicts short-term mortality in older patients with heart failure. Circ Heart Fail 3(1):14–20
68. Sancarlo D, D'Onofrio G, Franceschi M, Scarcelli C, Niro V, Addante F et al (2011) Validation of a Modified-Multidimensional Prognostic Index (m-MPI) including the Mini Nutritional Assessment Short-Form (MNA-SF) for the prediction of one-year mortality in hospitalized elderly patients. J Nutr Health Aging 15(3):169–173
69. Sancarlo D, Pilotto A, Panza F, Copetti M, Longo MG, D'Ambrosio P et al (2012) A Multidimensional Prognostic Index (MPI) based on a comprehensive geriatric assessment predicts short- and long-term all-cause mortality in older hospitalized patients with transient ischemic attack. J Neurol 259(4):670–678
70. Pilotto A, Sancarlo D, Aucella F, Fontana A, Addante F, Copetti M et al (2012) Addition of the multidimensional prognostic index to the estimated glomerular filtration rate improves prediction of long-term all-cause mortality in older patients with chronic kidney disease. Rejuvenation Res 15(1):82–88
71. Gallucci M, Battistella G, Bergamelli C, Spagnolo P, Mazzuco S, Carlini A et al (2014) Multidimensional prognostic index in a cognitive impairment outpatient setting: mortality and hospitalizations. The Treviso Dementia (TREDEM) study. J Alzheimers Dis 42 (4):1461–1468
72. Volpato S, Bazzano S, Fontana A, Ferrucci L, Pilotto A (2015) Group MP-TS. Multidimensional Prognostic Index predicts mortality and length of stay during hospitalization in the older patients: a multicenter prospective study. J Gerontol A Biol Sci Med Sci 70(3):325–331
73. Pilotto A, Rengo F, Marchionni N, Sancarlo D, Fontana A, Panza F et al (2012) Comparing the prognostic accuracy for all-cause mortality of frailty instruments: a multicentre 1-year follow-up in hospitalized older patients. PLoS ONE 7(1):e29090
74. D'Onofrio G, Sancarlo D, Addante F, Ciccone F, Cascavilla L, Paris F et al (2015) A pilot randomized controlled trial evaluating an integrated treatment of rivastigmine transdermal patch and cognitive stimulation in patients with Alzheimer's disease. Int J Geriatr Psychiatry 30(9):965–975
75. Pilotto A, D'Onofrio G, Panza F, Copetti M, Cascavilla L, Paris F et al (2012) Treatment of late-life major depressive disorder with selective serotonin reuptake inhibitors improves the multidimensional prognostic index. J Clin Psychopharmacol 32(5):726–729
76. Australian Cancer Incidence and Mortality: Australian Institute of Health and Welfare, Canberra (2015). Available from: http://www.aihw.gov.au/acim-books/
77. Tabayoyong W, Abouassaly R (2015) Prostate cancer screening and the associated controversy. Surg Clin North Am 95(5):1023–1039
78. Fouad MN, Mayo CP, Funkhouser EM, Irene Hall H, Urban DA, Kiefe CI (2004) Comorbidity independently predicted death in older prostate cancer patients, more of whom died with than from their disease. J Clin Epidemiol 57(7):721–729
79. Albertsen PC, Moore DF, Shih W, Lin Y, Li H, Lu-Yao GL (2011) Impact of comorbidity on survival among men with localized prostate cancer. J Clin Oncol: Official J Am Soc Clin Oncol 29(10):1335–1341
80. Bradley CJ, Dahman B, Anscher M (2014) Prostate cancer treatment and survival: evidence for men with prevalent comorbid conditions. Med Care 52(6):482–489
81. Droz JP, Balducci L, Bolla M, Emberton M, Fitzpatrick JM, Joniau S et al (2010) Management of prostate cancer in older men: recommendations of a working group of the International Society of Geriatric Oncology. BJU Int 106(4):462–469
82. Droz JP, Balducci L, Bolla M, Emberton M, Fitzpatrick JM, Joniau S et al (2010) Background for the proposal of SIOG guidelines for the management of prostate cancer in senior adults. Crit Rev Oncol Hematol 73(1):68–91

83. Droz JP, Aapro M, Balducci L, Boyle H, Van den Broeck T, Cathcart P et al (2014) Management of prostate cancer in older patients: updated recommendations of a working group of the International Society of Geriatric Oncology. Lancet Oncol 15(9):e404–e414
84. Bellera CA, Rainfray M, Mathoulin-Pelissier S, Mertens C, Delva F, Fonck M et al (2012) Screening older cancer patients: first evaluation of the G-8 geriatric screening tool. Ann Oncol 23(8):2166–2172
85. Nguyen PL, Alibhai SM, Basaria S, D'Amico AV, Kantoff PW, Keating NL et al (2015) Adverse effects of androgen deprivation therapy and strategies to mitigate them. Eur Urol 67 (5):825–836
86. Smith MR, Eastham J, Gleason DM, Shasha D, Tchekmedyian S, Zinner N (2003) Randomized controlled trial of zoledronic acid to prevent bone loss in men receiving androgen deprivation therapy for nonmetastatic prostate cancer. J Urol 169(6):2008–2012
87. Smith MR, Egerdie B, Hernandez Toriz N, Feldman R, Tammela TL, Saad F et al (2009) Denosumab in men receiving androgen-deprivation therapy for prostate cancer. N Engl J Med 361(8):745–755
88. Saad F, Fizazi K (2015) Androgen deprivation therapy and secondary hormone therapy in the management of hormone-sensitive and castration-resistant prostate cancer. Urology 86 (5):852–861
89. Attard G, Parker C, Eeles RA, Schroder F, Tomlins SA, Tannock I et al (2016) Prostate cancer. Lancet 387(10013):70–82
90. Levine GN, D'Amico AV, Berger P, Clark PE, Eckel RH, Keating NL et al (2010) Androgen-deprivation therapy in prostate cancer and cardiovascular risk: a science advisory from the American Heart Association, American Cancer Society, and American Urological Association: endorsed by the American Society for Radiation Oncology. Circulation 121 (6):833–840
91. Keating NL, O'Malley AJ, Smith MR (2006) Diabetes and cardiovascular disease during androgen deprivation therapy for prostate cancer. J Clin Oncol 24(27):4448–4456
92. Keating NL, O'Malley AJ, Freedland SJ, Smith MR (2010) Diabetes and cardiovascular disease during androgen deprivation therapy: observational study of veterans with prostate cancer. J Natl Cancer Inst 102(1):39–46
93. Saigal CS, Gore JL, Krupski TL, Hanley J, Schonlau M, Litwin MS et al (2007) Androgen deprivation therapy increases cardiovascular morbidity in men with prostate cancer. Cancer 110(7):1493–1500
94. Nanda A, Chen MH, Braccioforte MH, Moran BJ, D'Amico AV (2009) Hormonal therapy use for prostate cancer and mortality in men with coronary artery disease-induced congestive heart failure or myocardial infarction. JAMA 302(8):866–873
95. Alibhai SM, Duong-Hua M, Sutradhar R, Fleshner NE, Warde P, Cheung AM et al (2009) Impact of androgen deprivation therapy on cardiovascular disease and diabetes. J Clin Oncol 27(21):3452–3458
96. Nguyen PL, Je Y, Schutz FA, Hoffman KE, Hu JC, Parekh A et al (2011) Association of androgen deprivation therapy with cardiovascular death in patients with prostate cancer: a meta-analysis of randomized trials. JAMA 306(21):2359–2366
97. Bosco C, Bosnyak Z, Malmberg A, Adolfsson J, Keating NL, Van Hemelrijck M (2015) Quantifying observational evidence for risk of fatal and nonfatal cardiovascular disease following androgen deprivation therapy for prostate cancer: a meta-analysis. Eur Urol 68 (3):386–396
98. Klil-Drori AJ, Yin H, Tagalakis V, Aprikian A, Azoulay L (2016) Androgen deprivation therapy for prostate cancer and the risk of venous thromboembolism. Eur Urol 70(1):56–61
99. Ehdaie B, Atoria CL, Gupta A, Feifer A, Lowrance WT, Morris MJ et al (2012) Androgen deprivation and thromboembolic events in men with prostate cancer. Cancer 118(13):3397–3406
100. Van Hemelrijck M, Adolfsson J, Garmo H, Bill-Axelson A, Bratt O, Ingelsson E et al (2010) Risk of thromboembolic diseases in men with prostate cancer: results from the population-based PCBaSe Sweden. Lancet Oncol 11(5):450–458

101. Bell SP, Saraf A (2014) Risk stratification in very old adults: how to best gauge risk as the basis of management choices for patients aged over 80. Prog Cardiovasc Dis 57(2):197–203
102. Smith MR, Lee WC, Brandman J, Wang Q, Botteman M, Pashos CL (2005) Gonadotropin-releasing hormone agonists and fracture risk: a claims-based cohort study of men with nonmetastatic prostate cancer. J Clin Oncol 23(31):7897–7903
103. Shahinian VB, Kuo YF, Freeman JL, Goodwin JS (2005) Risk of fracture after androgen deprivation for prostate cancer. N Engl J Med 352(2):154–164
104. Cosman F, de Beur SJ, LeBoff MS, Lewiecki EM, Tanner B, Randall S et al (2014) Clinician's guide to prevention and treatment of osteoporosis. Osteoporos Int 25(10):2359–2381
105. Nowson CA, McGrath JJ, Ebeling PR, Haikerwal A, Daly RM, Sanders KM et al (2012) Vitamin D and health in adults in Australia and New Zealand: a position statement. Med J Aust 196(11):686–687
106. Serpa Neto A, Tobias-Machado M, Esteves MA, Senra MD, Wroclawski ML, Fonseca FL, et al (2012) Bisphosphonate therapy in patients under androgen deprivation therapy for prostate cancer: a systematic review and meta-analysis. Prostate Cancer Prostatic Dis 15 (1):36–44
107. Smith MR, Morton RA, Barnette KG, Sieber PR, Malkowicz SB, Rodriguez D et al (2010) Toremifene to reduce fracture risk in men receiving androgen deprivation therapy for prostate cancer. J Urol 184(4):1316–1321
108. Gralow JR, Biermann JS, Farooki A, Fornier MN, Gagel RF, Kumar R et al (2013) NCCN task force report: bone health in cancer care. J Natl Compr Canc Netw 11(Suppl 3):S1–S50; quiz S1
109. Mohler JL, Armstrong AJ, Bahnson RR, Boston B, Busby JE, D'Amico AV et al (2012) Prostate cancer, Version 3.2012: featured updates to the NCCN guidelines. J Natl Compr Canc Netw 10(9):1081–1087
110. Grossmann M, Hamilton EJ, Gilfillan C, Bolton D, Joon DL, Zajac JD (2011) Bone and metabolic health in patients with non-metastatic prostate cancer who are receiving androgen deprivation therapy. Med J Aust 194(6):301–306
111. Lomax AJ, Parente P, Gilfillan C, Livingston PM, Davis ID, Pezaro C (2016) 'First, do no harm': managing the metabolic impacts of androgen deprivation in men with advanced prostate cancer. Int Med J 46(2):141–148
112. Moffat SD, Zonderman AB, Metter EJ, Blackman MR, Harman SM, Resnick SM (2002) Longitudinal assessment of serum free testosterone concentration predicts memory performance and cognitive status in elderly men. J Clin Endocrinol Metab 87(11):5001–5007
113. Green HJ, Pakenham KI, Headley BC, Yaxley J, Nicol DL, Mactaggart PN et al (2002) Altered cognitive function in men treated for prostate cancer with luteinizing hormone-releasing hormone analogues and cyproterone acetate: a randomized controlled trial. BJU Int 90(4):427–432
114. Alibhai SM, Breunis H, Timilshina N, Marzouk S, Stewart D, Tannock I et al (2010) Impact of androgen-deprivation therapy on cognitive function in men with nonmetastatic prostate cancer. J Clin Oncol 28(34):5030–5037
115. Nead KT, Gaskin G, Chester C, Swisher-McClure S, Dudley JT, Leeper NJ et al (2016) Androgen deprivation therapy and future Alzheimer's disease risk. J Clin Oncol 34(6):566–571
116. GLOBOCAN 2012 v1.0, Cancer Incidence and Mortality Worldwide: IARC CancerBase No. 11 (Internet) (2013). Available from: http://globocan.iarc.fr. Accessed on 30 Dec 15
117. van den Akker M, Buntinx F, Metsemakers JF, Roos S, Knottnerus JA (1998) Multimorbidity in general practice: prevalence, incidence, and determinants of co-occurring chronic and recurrent diseases. J Clin Epidemiol 51(5):367–375
118. Sogaard M, Thomsen RW, Bossen KS, Sorensen HT, Norgaard M (2013) The impact of comorbidity on cancer survival: a review. Clin Epidemiol 5(Suppl 1):3–29
119. Biganzoli L, Wildiers H, Oakman C, Marotti L, Loibl S, Kunkler I et al (2012) Management of elderly patients with breast cancer: updated recommendations of the International Society

of Geriatric Oncology (SIOG) and European Society of Breast Cancer Specialists (EUSOMA). Lancet Oncol 13(4):e148–e160
120. Mislang AR, Biganzoli L (2015) Adjuvant systemic therapy in older breast cancer women: can we optimize the level of care? Cancers (Basel) 7(3):1191–1214
121. Janssen-Heijnen ML, Houterman S, Lemmens VE, Louwman MW, Maas HA, Coebergh JW (2005) Prognostic impact of increasing age and co-morbidity in cancer patients: a population-based approach. Crit Rev Oncol Hematol 55(3):231–240
122. Cronin-Fenton DP, Norgaard M, Jacobsen J, Garne JP, Ewertz M, Lash TL et al (2007) Comorbidity and survival of Danish breast cancer patients from 1995 to 2005. Br J Cancer 96 (9):1462–1468
123. Ahern TP, Lash TL, Thwin SS, Silliman RA (2009) Impact of acquired comorbidities on all-cause mortality rates among older breast cancer survivors. Med Care 47(1):73–79
124. Schonberg MA, Marcantonio ER, Ngo L, Li D, Silliman RA, McCarthy EP (2011) Causes of death and relative survival of older women after a breast cancer diagnosis. J Clin Oncol: Official J Am Soc Clin Oncol 29(12):1570–1577
125. Brandt J, Garne JP, Tengrup I, Manjer J (2015) Age at diagnosis in relation to survival following breast cancer: a cohort study. World J Surg Oncol 13:33
126. Patnaik JL, Byers T, Diguiseppi C, Denberg TD, Dabelea D (2011) The influence of comorbidities on overall survival among older women diagnosed with breast cancer. J Natl Cancer Inst 103(14):1101–1111
127. Land LH, Dalton SO, Jensen MB, Ewertz M (2012) Impact of comorbidity on mortality: a cohort study of 62,591 Danish women diagnosed with early breast cancer, 1990–2008. Breast Cancer Res Treat 131(3):1013–1020
128. Moyer VA (2014) Force USPST. Screening for cognitive impairment in older adults: U.S. Preventive Services Task Force recommendation statement. Ann Int Med 160(11):791–797
129. Schagen SB, Hamburger HL, Muller MJ, Boogerd W, van Dam FS (2001) Neurophysiological evaluation of late effects of adjuvant high-dose chemotherapy on cognitive function. J Neurooncol 51(2):159–165
130. Schagen SB, Muller MJ, Boogerd W, Mellenbergh GJ, van Dam FS (2006) Change in cognitive function after chemotherapy: a prospective longitudinal study in breast cancer patients. J Natl Cancer Inst 98(23):1742–1745
131. Ono M, Ogilvie JM, Wilson JS, Green HJ, Chambers SK, Ownsworth T et al (2015) A meta-analysis of cognitive impairment and decline associated with adjuvant chemotherapy in women with breast cancer. Front Oncol 5:59
132. Chan RJ, McCarthy AL, Devenish J, Sullivan KA, Chan A (2015) Systematic review of pharmacologic and non-pharmacologic interventions to manage cognitive alterations after chemotherapy for breast cancer. Eur J Cancer 51(4):437–450
133. Roth GA, Forouzanfar MH, Moran AE, Barber R, Nguyen G, Feigin VL et al (2015) Demographic and epidemiologic drivers of global cardiovascular mortality. N Engl J Med 372(14):1333–1341
134. Gupta D, Verma S, Pun SC, Steingart RM (2015) The changes in cardiac physiology with aging and the implications for the treating oncologist. J Geriatr Oncol 6(3):178–184
135. Swain SM, Whaley FS, Ewer MS (2003) Congestive heart failure in patients treated with doxorubicin: a retrospective analysis of three trials. Cancer 97(11):2869–2879
136. van Dalen EC, van der Pal HJ, Caron HN, Kremer LC (2009) Different dosage schedules for reducing cardiotoxicity in cancer patients receiving anthracycline chemotherapy. Cochrane Database Syst Rev (4):CD005008
137. van Dalen EC, Michiels EM, Caron HN, Kremer LC (2010) Different anthracycline derivates for reducing cardiotoxicity in cancer patients. Cochrane Database Syst Rev (5):CD005006
138. van Dalen EC, Caron HN, Dickinson HO, Kremer LC (2011) Cardioprotective interventions for cancer patients receiving anthracyclines. Cochrane Database Syst Rev (6):CD003917
139. Steinherz LJ, Steinherz PG, Tan CT, Heller G, Murphy ML (1991) Cardiac toxicity 4 to 20 years after completing anthracycline therapy. JAMA 266(12):1672–1677

140. Lipshultz SE, Colan SD, Gelber RD, Perez-Atayde AR, Sallan SE, Sanders SP (1991) Late cardiac effects of doxorubicin therapy for acute lymphoblastic leukemia in childhood. N Engl J Med 324(12):808–815
141. Arbuck SG, Strauss H, Rowinsky E, Christian M, Suffness M, Adams J et al (1993) A reassessment of cardiac toxicity associated with Taxol. J Natl Cancer Inst Monogr 15:117–130
142. Salvatorelli E, Menna P, Cascegna S, Liberi G, Calafiore AM, Gianni L et al (2006) Paclitaxel and docetaxel stimulation of doxorubicinol formation in the human heart: implications for cardiotoxicity of doxorubicin-taxane chemotherapies. J Pharmacol Exp Ther 318(1):424–433
143. de Forni M, Malet-Martino MC, Jaillais P, Shubinski RE, Bachaud JM, Lemaire L et al (1992) Cardiotoxicity of high-dose continuous infusion fluorouracil: a prospective clinical study. J Clin Oncol 10(11):1795–1801
144. Meyer CC, Calis KA, Burke LB, Walawander CA, Grasela TH (1997) Symptomatic cardiotoxicity associated with 5-fluorouracil. Pharmacotherapy 17(4):729–736
145. Van Cutsem E, Hoff PM, Blum JL, Abt M, Osterwalder B (2002) Incidence of cardiotoxicity with the oral fluoropyrimidine capecitabine is typical of that reported with 5-fluorouracil. Ann Oncol 13(3):484–485
146. Kosmas C, Kallistratos MS, Kopterides P, Syrios J, Skopelitis H, Mylonakis N et al (2008) Cardiotoxicity of fluoropyrimidines in different schedules of administration: a prospective study. J Cancer Res Clin Oncol 134(1):75–82
147. Rezkalla S, Kloner RA, Ensley J, al-Sarraf M, Revels S, Olivenstein A, et al (1989) Continuous ambulatory ECG monitoring during fluorouracil therapy: a prospective study. J Clin Oncol: Official J Am Soc Clin Oncol 7(4):509–514
148. Jensen SA, Sorensen JB (2006) Risk factors and prevention of cardiotoxicity induced by 5-fluorouracil or capecitabine. Cancer Chemother Pharmacol 58(4):487–493
149. Yeh ET, Bickford CL (2009) Cardiovascular complications of cancer therapy: incidence, pathogenesis, diagnosis, and management. J Am Coll Cardiol 53(24):2231–2247
150. Seidman A, Hudis C, Pierri MK, Shak S, Paton V, Ashby M et al (2002) Cardiac dysfunction in the trastuzumab clinical trials experience. J Clin Oncol: Official J Am Soc Clin Oncol 20 (5):1215–1221
151. Brollo J, Curigliano G, Disalvatore D, Marrone BF, Criscitiello C, Bagnardi V et al (2013) Adjuvant trastuzumab in elderly with HER-2 positive breast cancer: a systematic review of randomized controlled trials. Cancer Treat Rev 39(1):44–50
152. Chen J, Long JB, Hurria A, Owusu C, Steingart RM, Gross CP (2012) Incidence of heart failure or cardiomyopathy after adjuvant trastuzumab therapy for breast cancer. J Am Coll Cardiol 60(24):2504–2512
153. Tan-Chiu E, Yothers G, Romond E, Geyer CE Jr, Ewer M, Keefe D et al (2005) Assessment of cardiac dysfunction in a randomized trial comparing doxorubicin and cyclophosphamide followed by paclitaxel, with or without trastuzumab as adjuvant therapy in node-positive, human epidermal growth factor receptor 2-overexpressing breast cancer: NSABP B-31. J Clin Oncol 23(31):7811–7819
154. Perez EA, Suman VJ, Davidson NE, Sledge GW, Kaufman PA, Hudis CA et al (2008) Cardiac safety analysis of doxorubicin and cyclophosphamide followed by paclitaxel with or without trastuzumab in the North Central Cancer Treatment Group N9831 adjuvant breast cancer trial. J Clin Oncol 26(8):1231–1238
155. Advani PP, Ballman KV, Dockter TJ, Colon-Otero G, Perez EA (2016) Long-term cardiac safety analysis of NCCTG N9831 (Alliance) adjuvant trastuzumab trial. J Clin Oncol 34 (6):581–587
156. Suter TM, Procter M, van Veldhuisen DJ, Muscholl M, Bergh J, Carlomagno C et al (2007) Trastuzumab-associated cardiac adverse effects in the herceptin adjuvant trial. J Clin Oncol 25(25):3859–3865

157. Wang SY, Long JB, Hurria A, Owusu C, Steingart RM, Gross CP et al (2014) Cardiovascular events, early discontinuation of trastuzumab, and their impact on survival. Breast Cancer Res Treat 146(2):411–419
158. Kumler I, Christiansen OG, Nielsen DL (2014) A systematic review of bevacizumab efficacy in breast cancer. Cancer Treat Rev 40(8):960–973
159. Vaklavas C, Lenihan D, Kurzrock R, Tsimberidou AM (2010) Anti-vascular endothelial growth factor therapies and cardiovascular toxicity: what are the important clinical markers to target? Oncologist 15(2):130–141
160. Cuppone F, Bria E, Verma S, Pritchard KI, Gandhi S, Carlini P et al (2008) Do adjuvant aromatase inhibitors increase the cardiovascular risk in postmenopausal women with early breast cancer? Meta-analysis of randomized trials. Cancer 112(2):260–267
161. Amir E, Seruga B, Niraula S, Carlsson L, Ocana A (2011) Toxicity of adjuvant endocrine therapy in postmenopausal breast cancer patients: a systematic review and meta-analysis. J Natl Cancer Inst 103(17):1299–1309
162. Hernandez RK, Sorensen HT, Pedersen L, Jacobsen J, Lash TL (2009) Tamoxifen treatment and risk of deep venous thrombosis and pulmonary embolism: a Danish population-based cohort study. Cancer 115(19):4442–4449
163. Aapro M (2011) SIOG (International Society of Geriatric Oncology) recommendations for anthracycline use in the elderly. Hematol Rep 3(3s):e6
164. Aapro M, Bernard-Marty C, Brain EG, Batist G, Erdkamp F, Krzemieniecki K et al (2011) Anthracycline cardiotoxicity in the elderly cancer patient: a SIOG expert position paper. Ann Oncol 22(2):257–267
165. Curigliano G, Cardinale D, Suter T, Plataniotis G, de Azambuja E, Sandri MT, et al (2012) Cardiovascular toxicity induced by chemotherapy, targeted agents and radiotherapy: ESMO Clinical Practice Guidelines. Ann Oncol 23(Suppl 7):vii155–vii166
166. Michels KB, Solomon CG, Hu FB, Rosner BA, Hankinson SE, Colditz GA et al (2003) Type 2 diabetes and subsequent incidence of breast cancer in the Nurses' Health Study. Diab Care 26(6):1752–1758
167. Srokowski TP, Fang S, Hortobagyi GN, Giordano SH (2009) Impact of diabetes mellitus on complications and outcomes of adjuvant chemotherapy in older patients with breast cancer. J Clin Oncol: Official J Am Soc Clin Oncol 27(13):2170–2176
168. Jia X, Hong Q, Cheng J, Li J, Wang Y, Mo M et al (2015) Indispensability of chemotherapy in estrogen receptor-negative early breast cancer in elderly women with diabetes mellitus. Diab Technol Ther 17(4):248–254
169. Yoo KE, Kang RY, Lee JY, Lee YJ, Suh SY, Kim KS et al (2015) Awareness of the adverse effects associated with prophylactic corticosteroid use during docetaxel therapy. Support Care Cancer 23(7):1969–1977
170. de la Morena Barrio P, Conesa MA, Gonzalez-Billalabeitia E, Urrego E, Garcia-Garre E, Garcia-Martinez E et al (2015) Delayed recovery and increased severity of Paclitaxel-induced peripheral neuropathy in patients with diabetes. J Natl Compr Canc Netw 13(4):417–423
171. Rosen LS, Gordon D, Kaminski M, Howell A, Belch A, Mackey J et al (2003) Long-term efficacy and safety of zoledronic acid compared with pamidronate disodium in the treatment of skeletal complications in patients with advanced multiple myeloma or breast carcinoma: a randomized, double-blind, multicenter, comparative trial. Cancer 98(8):1735–1744
172. Kanis JA, Johnell O, Oden A, Dawson A, De Laet C, Jonsson B (2001) Ten year probabilities of osteoporotic fractures according to BMD and diagnostic thresholds. Osteoporos Int 12(12):989–995
173. Siris ES, Brenneman SK, Barrett-Connor E, Miller PD, Sajjan S, Berger ML et al (2006) The effect of age and bone mineral density on the absolute, excess, and relative risk of fracture in postmenopausal women aged 50–99: results from the National Osteoporosis Risk Assessment (NORA). Osteoporos Int 17(4):565–574
174. Kanis JA, Borgstrom F, De Laet C, Johansson H, Johnell O, Jonsson B et al (2005) Assessment of fracture risk. Osteoporos Int 16(6):581–589

175. Fisher B, Costantino JP, Wickerham DL, Redmond CK, Kavanah M, Cronin WM et al (1998) Tamoxifen for prevention of breast cancer: report of the National Surgical Adjuvant Breast and Bowel Project P-1 Study. J Natl Cancer Inst 90(18):1371–1388
176. Kwan ML, Lo JC, Tang L, Laurent CA, Roh JM, Chandra M et al (2014) Bone health history in breast cancer patients on aromatase inhibitors. PLoS ONE 9(10):e111477
177. Early Breast Cancer Trialists' Collaborative Group, Coleman R, Powles T, Paterson A, Gnant M, Anderson S, et al (2015) Adjuvant bisphosphonate treatment in early breast cancer: meta-analyses of individual patient data from randomised trials. Lancet 386(10001): 1353–1361
178. Hoff AO, Toth B, Hu M, Hortobagyi GN, Gagel RF (2011) Epidemiology and risk factors for osteonecrosis of the jaw in cancer patients. Ann N Y Acad Sci 1218:47–54
179. Pazianas M, Miller P, Blumentals WA, Bernal M, Kothawala P (2007) A review of the literature on osteonecrosis of the jaw in patients with osteoporosis treated with oral bisphosphonates: prevalence, risk factors, and clinical characteristics. Clin Ther 29(8): 1548–1558
180. Vahtsevanos K, Kyrgidis A, Verrou E, Katodritou E, Triaridis S, Andreadis CG et al (2009) Longitudinal cohort study of risk factors in cancer patients of bisphosphonate-related osteonecrosis of the jaw. J Clin Oncol 27(32):5356–5362
181. Epstein MS, Ephros HD, Epstein JB (2013) Review of current literature and implications of RANKL inhibitors for oral health care providers. Oral Surg Oral Med Oral Pathol Oral Radiol 116(6):e437–e442
182. Stopeck AT, Lipton A, Body JJ, Steger GG, Tonkin K, de Boer RH et al (2010) Denosumab compared with zoledronic acid for the treatment of bone metastases in patients with advanced breast cancer: a randomized, double-blind study. J Clin Oncol: Official J Am Soc Clin Oncol 28(35):5132–5139
183. Dimopoulos MA, Kastritis E, Bamia C, Melakopoulos I, Gika D, Roussou M et al (2009) Reduction of osteonecrosis of the jaw (ONJ) after implementation of preventive measures in patients with multiple myeloma treated with zoledronic acid. Ann Oncol 20(1):117–120
184. Onitilo A, Engel J, Berg R (2011) C-B2-02: Epidemiology of Tamoxifen and Thromboembolism. Clin Med Res 9(3–4):150
185. Davies CPH, Gray R et al (2013) Long-term effects of continuing adjuvant tamoxifen to 10 years versus stopping at 5 years after diagnosis of oestrogen receptor-positive breast cancer: ATLAS, a randomised trial. Lancet 381:805–816
186. Scappaticci FA, Skillings JR, Holden SN, Gerber HP, Miller K, Kabbinavar F et al (2007) Arterial thromboembolic events in patients with metastatic carcinoma treated with chemotherapy and bevacizumab. J Natl Cancer Inst 99(16):1232–1239

Further Reading

187. Hurria A, Balducci L (eds) (2009) Geriatric oncology. Springer Science+Business Media, LLC. doi:10.1007/978-0-387-89070-8_2
188. Extermann M (ed) (2013) Cancer and aging. From bench to clinics. In: Interdisciplinary topics in gerontology, vol 38. Basel, Karger, pp I–VIII. doi:10.1159/000345060

Chapter 15
Chronic Conditions and Cancer at the End of Life

David C. Currow and Jane L. Phillips

Abstract The majority of people diagnosed with cancer are older and therefore are likely to have co-morbidities at the time it is diagnosed and if the cancer progresses to advanced disease. Guidance in the process of managing long-term co-morbidities at the end of life requires clarity about the goals of care for the person's cancer, and for each of his/her co-morbidities. Why was a particular therapy started in the first place? What risk is the therapy mitigating, and does it need to be continued? Very few studies help to inform the process of ceasing medications. For example, with cachexia and its associated weight loss, frequently encountered in advanced cancer, the management of two of the most frequent conditions—hypertension and diabetes—will change. The need for anti-hypertensives will decrease or the person will risk postural symptoms and the need for lower doses of hypoglycaemic agents and liberalised diets will be hallmarks of managing diabetes in order to avoid hypoglycaemia. Mostly, this care is in the setting of multiple co-morbidities, making review a complex and continuing process. Changes in co-morbidities can also directly influence the anti-cancer therapies that are available to patients, because of characteristics of the drug itself or changes in metabolism or elimination. Adjusting chemotherapy in advanced disease also requires careful evaluation of the goals of palliative treatment—are there symptoms that can best be addressed by disease modifying treatments or are there other more direct, better tolerated symptom control therapies available? Not only will there be a need for active management of long-term co-morbidities, but people will need to adjust psychologically to these changes. Modifying the goals of treatment is often the most overt signal to people that their disease is progressing and therefore can be particularly confronting. Such changes will often precipitate, or are an opportunity for, much wider conversations about life, dying and death.

D.C. Currow (✉)
Discipline, Palliative and Supportive Services, Flinders University, Adelaide, Australia
e-mail: david.currow@cancerinstitute.org.au

J.L. Phillips
Faculty of Health, University of Technology Sydney, Ultimo, Australia

B. Koczwara (ed.), *Cancer and Chronic Conditions*,
DOI 10.1007/978-981-10-1844-2_15

Keywords Co-morbid illness · Chronic illness · Diabetes · Heart failure · Chronic obstructive pulmonary disease · Renal failure · End-of-life care

Key Points

1. Clinicians need to actively manage the long term therapies for chronic co-morbid conditions as people experience the systemic changes of advanced cancer, reflected most overtly by cachexia.
2. As function declines and there are measureable systemic changes in muscle mass, fat mass and appetite, it is important to adjust prescribing for long term co-morbidities that may be affected by these changes. Such conditions include hypertension and diabetes as key examples.
3. Most people invest effort and energy in optimally managing their co-morbid illnesses to the best of their ability. Changing the goals of care for such people as systemic changes (weight loss, declining function) dictate the need to adjust these therapies is often a difficult psychological transition to make for patients (and their families).
4. Palliative anti-cancer treatments for symptom control, particularly late in life, need to be considered in the context of the other ways that symptoms can be managed. 'Palliative' chemotherapy must have a specific target symptom that otherwise cannot be well palliated.
5. Co-morbidities will have an increasing impact on whether or not to offer systemic therapies late in life. An adequate assessment of each co-morbidity and its impact on level of function and symptom control is needed in parallel with the assessment of the person's cancer.

15.1 Introduction

Adults with advanced cancer who have other active co-morbidities are at increased risk of adverse outcomes [1]. As cancer advances, its impact on people is dictated in three major ways:

1. The systemic effects of having uncontrolled cancer (most frequently manifest by increasing fatigue, weight loss (of both muscle and fat), loss of appetite and resulting changes in body habitus)
2. Local effects of the cancer (which are most often over-shadowed by the systemic effects of the disease)
3. Psychological transitions associated with these systemic changes. Managing these changes needs to be considered in the context of the person's disease progression, goals and palliative care needs (Fig. 15.1).

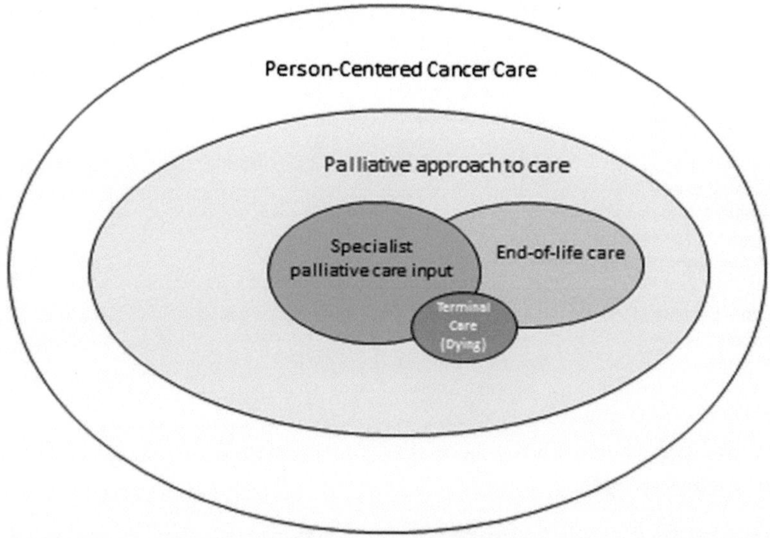

Fig. 15.1 Conceptualising the palliative management of advanced cancer and other co-morbidities

The systemic changes of advanced cancer demand the active management of co-morbid illnesses in order to optimise a person's function and avoid iatrogenic harm. With widespread and sometimes dramatic systemic changes, goals of care need to be reviewed frequently and adjustments made, not only to the goals as function declines, but also to therapies for long term co-morbidities. Such morbidities are frequently encountered in people with advanced cancer as older age is the most prominent risk factor for both cancers and co-morbidities.

In order to adjust therapies for long term co-morbidities, it is necessary to understand in detail why a medication was commenced and the goals of that therapy.

15.1.1 A Framework for Managing Co-morbidities

One proposed framework is to consider the level of prevention being undertaken by prescribing a medication (primary, secondary, tertiary) and the likely timeframes for the onset of problems if the therapy were ceased (Fig. 15.2). Another way to consider this is to quantify the number needed to treat and the timeframes required to avoid an event in order to contextualise the real risk for the specific patient if the medication were to be ceased. This helps clinicians to have an approach to rational deprescribing when there is no evidence that addresses directly ceasing the medication in question.

Therapeutic benefit in context of prognosis	Prevention strategy		
	Tertiary (disease with symptoms)	Secondary (disease with no symptoms)	Primary (no disease)
Potential for short term complications requiring management until death. Independent of prognosis eg glucose lowering drugs	Inflammatory arthritis	Diabetes mellitus	Phenylketonuria
Long term benefits at population level. Ongoing therapy unnecessary in most with shortened life expectancy. Some short term benefits need consideration eg antihypertensive drugs	Pulmonary rehabilitation in chronic obstructive airways disease	Hypertension	Influenza vaccination
Long term benefits at population level. Little short or intermediate term risk of stopping eg cholesterol lowering drugs	Osteoporosis	Hyperlipidaemia	Some aspirin use in elderly people

Key

Treatment likely to be changed later and less in the course of life limiting illness

Treatment likely to be changed earlier and more in the course of life limiting illness

Fig. 15.2 Factors influencing the likelihood of continuing treatment for medical comorbidities in patients with life limiting illness, and examples of conditions in each category. Used with permission from Stevenson et al. [34]

15.1.2 Negotiating Goals of Care

Negotiating goals of care with people who have advanced cancer requires time and conversations that are both honest and respectful. This is often a time of confronting change for patients and especially for their families and friends. Resetting expectations and hence resetting goals is one of the most important conversations that a clinician can have as he/she sees the manifestation of systemic changes of advanced cancer. Although these are often very challenging conversations, especially when first introduced, they are also highly valued conversations by patients and their families. Not having these conversations risks patients making ill-informed decisions about their future, often leading to anger and disappointment regarding the decisions and actions they would prioritised if they had truly known their prognosis.

The process of negotiating goals of care often entails also considering people's fears and concerns: What is my prognosis? How will I die? Will I have uncontrolled symptoms? Who is going to provide care for me? How can I ensure that my wishes are respected even if I am unable to speak for myself? Patients expect that clinicians will be able to brooch these topics (rather than expecting the patient to raise these issues) and answer these questions confidently and sensitively [2]. It is the opportunity to provide information on advanced care planning, and to facilitate these crucial, ongoing conversations.

Many people will also have long term symptoms that pre-date their diagnosis of cancer. These symptoms may require special consideration, especially if they have not previously responded to disease modifying or symptom-focused measures [3].

This chapter is divided into sections on

- Chronic non-communicable diseases
- Communicable diseases
- Multi-morbidities.

It is structured to outline the considerations for key decisions as people face the systemic changes of advanced cancer. The chapter covers major co-morbidities and illustrates how to approach the challenges of managing co-morbidities in advanced cancer. Such a chapter cannot cover all potential co-morbidities, but it can ensure that it illustrates a framework to apply to decision-making from first principles if a particular clinical scenario is not outlined.

15.2 Non-communicable Diseases

Chronic cardiovascular disease in cancer

Managing cancer patients with cardiovascular disease requires consideration of prognosis and the risk factors that are being managed to minimise the impact of cardiovascular disease.

15.2.1 Management with a Prognosis of Months to Weeks

Many people with cardiovascular disease may also be receiving palliative cancer treatment, some of which may cause cardiotoxicity. Cardiotoxicity in this group may manifest as myocardial ischemia, hypertension, arrhythmias, pericarditis or conduction defects that require attention [4]. These people require ongoing monitoring and optimisation of medications to prevent symptomatic decompensated heart failure requiring hospitalisation [5].

People with cardiovascular disease tend to be on a large number of medications. Beyond reviewing medications for dynamic conditions such as hypertension which are likely to change as a result of weight loss, many people will also be taking cholesterol lowering medications. If these are for primary or secondary prevention, there is evidence that these can be safely ceased once a person is identified as having a limited prognosis [6].

15.2.2 Managing Hypertension at the End of Life

Most people will benefit from having their anti-hypertensives reduced or ceased once cachexia is evident. The therapeutic goal should be to avoid any postural symptoms and any ensuing falls. Routine monitoring for this group includes a full assessment, addressing reversible factors and palliating refractory symptoms, irrespective of the underlying cause of the disease (cancer or heart failure).

15.2.3 Symptoms in People with Chronic Cardiac Disease—Pain

Pain in people with heart failure may be related to underlying cancer or heart failure, including refractory (stable) angina especially if there is worsening anaemia, gross edema, immobility or diabetic neuropathy. Key considerations for this group is to avoid if possible medications with anti-cholinergic activity (pro-arrhythmogenic) and, if possible, avoid non-steroidal anti-inflammatory drugs which can increase salt and water retention [7, 8].

15.2.4 Symptoms in people with chronic cardiac disease—breathlessness

Breathlessness: The pharmacological management of breathlessness includes regular, low dose extended release morphine. Benzodiazepines are not recommended, but could be considered if panic is triggering the breathlessness and psychological interventions have not been effective. Supplemental oxygen is unlikely to be of benefit for routine palliation of breathlessness in the absence of hypoxaemia [7, 8]. Non-pharmacological management includes exercise, breathing training, walking aids, psychological interventions, and hand-held (battery operated) fans [7, 8].

15.2.5 Symptoms in People with Cardiac Disease—Edema

Edema is often a major symptom, worsened by hypoalbuminemia late in the course of cancer. Pharmacological management includes diuresis as appropriate, including parenteral diuretics. Non-pharmacological management includes appropriate fluid restriction which may have to be modified across the last months of life, weight monitoring and good skin care [7, 8].

15.2.6 Symptoms in People with Chronic Cardiac Disease—Fatigue

Cancer and heart failure are both multi-system systemic disorders causing skeletal muscle loss, which contributes to both breathlessness and fatigue. The patient's heart failure will be exacerbated by anaemia [5]. which is not uncommon in this group and may worsen fatigue. Non-pharmacological management, if someone still has a reasonable level of function, includes gentle graded exercise. It is also important to consider if people have episodic hypoxia due to sleep disordered breathing such as obstructive sleep apnoea, or central hypoventilation syndromes, or poorly controlled symptoms contributing to the person's fatigue. Other causes of fatigue such as poor nutritional intake, side effects of medications (beta blockers), hypokalaemia, hypothyroidism or depression need to be considered and treated accordingly [7, 8].

15.2.7 Advance Care Planning

Timely advance care planning is essential because patients in this group are at risk of a sudden cardiac death and/or cognitive impairment and need to be provided with an opportunity to plan accordingly [9–11]. Consideration of deprescribing of the cardiovascular medication needs to be sensitively discussed with the patient and undertaken in partnership with their treating heart failure team. Similarly if a plan for deactivation of implantable cardioverter-defibrillator in patients with New York Heart Association functional class IV symptoms had not been previously formulated, this also needs to be devised in partnership with the patient and their team [12].

15.2.8 Management with a Prognosis of Days to Hours

Once the diagnosis is made that prognosis is limited, these patients do not require any further investigations, but rather the focus ought to be on optimising palliative symptom management through careful history and clinical assessment, and effective patient and family communication about the goals of care.

Pharmacological management includes treatments for pain and breathlessness. If the person is on opioids for pain or for breathlessness and is unable to swallow, convert usual opioids to an equivalent subcutaneous dose (eviQ [3] on-line opiate calculator; www.eviq.org.au) [13]. If the person is opioid naïve, small doses of parenteral (subcutaneous or intravenous if there is central access) morphine 1–2.5 mg can be given regularly for pain or for breathlessness.

If the person has heart failure and is unable to swallow, he/she may benefit from subcutaneous frusemide 20–40 mg daily or twice daily; topical nitrates may still be required in the terminal stages of a life-limiting illness for relief of chest pain and oxygen should be given for anyone who is hypoxemic.

Non-pharmacological treatments include elevating the head of the bed if there is any suspicion of heart failure, regular mouth and pressure area care, and reassurance to families and friends about the absolute commitment to providing comfort. If the person has an implantable defibrillator, ensure that it is turned off [12].

15.2.9 How Does Chronic Cardiac Disease Impact on Therapies Directed Against the Cancer?

People who have heart or vascular conditions at the time they are diagnosed with cancer are especially vulnerable to the cardiovascular effects of some cancer treatment (radiotherapy chemotherapy and hormone cancer treatments). Cardiac toxicity is the most common cancer therapy complication, which has increased since the advent of molecularly targeted therapies. The new cancer therapies have contributed to a rise in unexpected cardiac toxicities, especially when added to more conventional chemotherapies [14]. Heart failure is the unfortunate manifestation for many of these toxicities, especially related to anthracyclines [14].

15.2.10 Recalibrating Self-management

The symptom burden associated with cancer and the persons' heart failure necessitates that any self-management plans be reviewed frequently to ensure that they are reflecting the person's changing well-being and that they continue to be helpful.

15.3 Diabetes

Diabetes remains highly prevalent across the community and given that prevalence of diabetes and cancer both increase with age, this is a frequently encountered co-morbidity in the population of people with cancer. With increasing rates of obesity around the world, there is an increasing rate of metabolic syndrome, with increased insulin resistance creating a large group of people with type II diabetes. Sensitively managing diabetes in the setting of advanced cancer requires careful attention to detail and sometimes difficult discussions with patients and their families.

15.3.1 Management with a Prognosis of Months to Weeks

The principles of managing diabetes with a prognosis of months are similar for type I and type II diabetes. Fundamentally, there is a need to adjust goals of care. Avoiding long term micro- and macro-vascular complications ceases to be the primary goal of care as their genesis takes prolonged periods of hyperglycaemia.

The clinical aims when managing diabetes once it is recognised that the person has advanced cancer is to:

- make every effort to minimise the risk of hypoglycemia as untreated hypoglycemia can cause death in minutes,
- reduce the risks of symptomatic hyperglycemia.

The threshold for symptoms from hyperglycemia will vary from person to person but is likely to be above twice the upper limit of blood sugar levels required for glycaemic control.

For people with type II diabetes:

- monitoring can often be relaxed to daily or less frequent if they are stable; and
- dietary restrictions can often be relaxed simultaneously, allowing a wider choice of foods.

The latter is important given that people who are experiencing cancer anorexia cachexia syndrome (CACS) often have reduced appetite and marked changes in food preferences. Allowing a broader range of foods may better support oral intake at a time when this can be difficult. For people with cachexia, the associated weight loss often means that the medications for glycaemic control will have to be reduced markedly in any case.

For people with type I diabetes, a similar approach to management is needed with:

- revised glycaemic controls;
- a relaxing of dietary restrictions (especially in the presence of anorexia); and
- adjustment of insulin doses especially in the presence of marked weight loss.

15.3.2 Management with a Prognosis of Days to Hours

In type II diabetes, oral hypoglycaemic agents are often stopped safely in the last days of life. Ensuring that a small dose of insulin is available for any resultant symptomatic hyperglycaemia is often all that is required. Diet can be liberalised to include anything that a person desires.

In type I diabetes, it is necessary to continue a small (and diminishing) dose of insulin to avoid ketoacidosis. Once more, monitoring can be reduced and diet expanded in order to match the person's rapidly changing metabolic environment.

15.3.3 How Does Diabetes Impact on Therapies Directed Against the Cancer?

There are a number of impacts that diabetes can have on therapies late in life. Most frequently, the challenge is the use of medications that induce diabetes or worsen glycaemic controls. Widespread use of glucocorticoids is the pre-eminent cause of this. (Of note, although often used to stimulate appetite, glucocorticoids also accelerate muscle loss through catabolic pathways at a time when cachexia is already causing profound loss of muscle.) New classes of agents such as ghrelin agonists also cause hyperglycaemia in a small number of people taking them.

15.3.4 Recalibrating Self-management

Most people with diabetes are highly motivated to optimise their care of the condition. For most diabetics, glycaemic control has required major lifestyle changes which need to be maintained daily over many years with incredible attention to detail.

It is likely that many people will have difficulty adjusting to liberalised diet and changed medications as the goals of glycaemic control are shifted from avoiding long term complications of hyperglycaemia to the short term complications of hypoglycaemia as appetite worsens and oral intake and exercise become less predictable. There may well be a time of people feeling very psychologically unsettled with changed goals of care. The ability to adjust to new goals of care and to need to consult health professionals about management that patients have managed for years or decades can be very confronting for patients.

15.4 Renal Impairment/Renal Failure

Mild to moderate renal impairment is frequently encountered in people with advanced cancer. One in 15 people have marked renal impairment reflected in raised serum creatinine when first diagnosed with cancer, but using a more conservative threshold for renal insufficiency, one in two people will have abnormal renal function when diagnosed with cancer using Cockcroft and Gault criteria for calculating creatinine clearance, mostly in the presence of a 'normal' serum creatinine [15]. In the setting of advanced cancer, people with end-stage renal disease include people with:

- Progressive renal failure unrelated to the cancer
- An acute insult (often from the treatment of cancer or cancers such as multiple myeloma) superimposed on, or causing, chronic kidney disease

- Local factors such as post-renal obstruction by a cancer
- A malignancy itself that may be a consequence of previous renal transplantation.

In considering the management of renal failure in the setting of advanced cancer, the underlying insults leading to kidney disease are important only where they are currently remediable because they are worsening renal function.

15.4.1 Management with a Prognosis of Months to Weeks

For most people with renal insufficiency, a prognosis limited to months or weeks may not change the symptoms experienced nor the measures introduced for symptom control. If renal function is stable because of chronic disease that is not progressing, symptom control can continue with careful ongoing review of renal function.

For people on dialysis, symptom control related to advancing cancer can provide some challenges but, by using medications that are short acting, symptoms can be well controlled.

Symptoms from severe renal insufficiency that may co-exist with advancing cancer include (in order of prevalence) fatigue, pruritus, constipation, anorexia, pain, sleep disturbance, anxiety, nausea, restless legs syndrome and depression. On dialysis, the top four symptoms are pain, fatigue, pruritus and constipation [16]. Although many of these symptoms are frequently encountered in other settings, restless legs syndrome is most frequently seen in the setting of renal insufficiency.

Pharmacological management of restless legs syndrome in end-stage renal disease relies on non-ergot dopamine agonists with the more recent approval of gabapentin. Most studies have been underpowered and it is difficult to identify characteristics of either the likelihood of responding to medications or only experiencing toxicities [17]. Non-pharmacological treatments include intra-dialysis exercise including the use of exercise bikes which have collateral benefits of improving aerobic fitness and also patterns of sleep.

15.4.2 Management with a Prognosis of Days to Hours

Part of the challenge of providing excellent care for someone on dialysis and simultaneously facing advanced cancer is the discussion about when dialysis should cease. This conversation requires great skills and empathy. Most patients will have thought about the issue and will expect that their physicians will raise this topic respectfully and confidently. The decision to withdraw dialysis ultimately rests with the patient in consultation with the people that he/she trust to help make decisions like this.

Few data are available about the focus required to provide good symptom control in end-stage renal disease and advanced cancer. Symptom control especially for pain, breathlessness and restless legs will be the focus of the process.

15.4.3 How Does Renal Impairment Impact on Therapies Directed Against the Cancer?

Before initiating systemic palliative anti-cancer therapies, it is important to assess renal function (which diminishes with age), co-morbidities that may affect renal function (such as heart failure), medications that may worsen renal function, medications that may be affected by worsening renal function and hydration status [18]. Approximately one half of all cycles of chemotherapy will require some dose adjustment due to renal insufficiency [15].

Most directly, renal impairment affects the choice and dosing of many systemic therapies for cancer treatment, many of which may be considered even in the setting of advanced cancer.

> Systemic anti-cancer therapies that require dose adjustment in the setting of renal insufficiency include: cyclophosphamide, ifosfamide, docetaxol, vinorelbine, carboplatin, cisplatin, zoledronate, etoposide, topotecan, capecitabine, pemetrexed and methotrexate.

> Systemic therapies that may worsen renal insufficiency include: gemcitabine, carboplatin, cisplatin, oxaliplatin, epirubicin, doxorubicin, paclitaxel, irinotecan. trastuzumab, zoledronate and methotrexate [15, 18].

In people on dialysis, the safe and effective administration of chemotherapy becomes a key consideration. This is a highly specialised area with few data to inform practice.

> Chemotherapy frequently used for treatment in people on haemodialysis where dose adjustment is still needed include cisplatin, oxaliplatin and carboplatin, cyclophosphamide, capecitabine, methotrexate, irinotecan, etoposide, docetaxel, and vinorelbine [19].

For people with cancer and renal insufficiency, careful consideration of the most appropriate analgesic is also required as morphine and its derivatives (codeine) are not recommended for people with severe (stage 5) kidney disease (calculated creatinine clearance of less than 10 mL/min) due to accumulation of active metabolites and opioid toxicity. Buprenorphine, fentanyl, hydromorphone or oxycodone are preferred opioids in severe kidney disease [20].

15.5 Liver Impairment/Liver Failure

Hepatic impairment may be due to:

- Infiltration of the liver with cancer
- Obstruction to the biliary tree by cancer including local lymph nodes
- Long term disease

Globally, the most common non-malignant causes of hepatic impairment include viral hepatidities (although the burden of disease will change with increasing immunisation rates against hepatitis B and highly effective treatments now available for hepatitis C) and alcohol. The ability to metabolise some drugs and the liver's synthesising function for key proteins can have a major influence on the therapeutic choices in late stage disease.

Symptoms manifest as a result of worsening hepatic impairment include fatigue, pain, itch, ascites and progressive cognitive impairment. Cognitive impairment can be frustrating for the patient and his/her family.

15.5.1 Management with a Prognosis of Months to Weeks

Fatigue is commonly experienced by people with advanced cancer, and is more pronounced in the presence of co-existing liver disease. While the mechanisms driving fatigue in both cancer and liver failure continue to be poorly understood, anaemia, medications (i.e. anti-histamines, anti-emetics, anti-depressants and analgesics) and anorexia all contribute to this debilitating symptom. As sarcopenia is more pronounced in this population, with 15–50 % of patients with cancer and 30–45 % with liver failure having CT defined sarcopenia, it is likely to play a role [21]. Managing fatigue in this population is predominately focussed on non-pharmacological interventions, such as:

- Promoting physical activity;
- Spacing activities;
- Reserving energy for important and enjoyable activities;
- Accessing assistance with instrumental activities of daily living; and
- Nutritional support.

Managing pain in the presences of liver failure requires careful consideration of the analgesic type and dose. Paracetamol use in the context of chronic alcohol use can lead to unexpected toxicity, while more cautious titration of codeine and morphine is needed to avoid precipitating encephalopathy or coma. Non-steroidal anti-inflammatory medications should also be avoided in this population.

Persistent itch is another distressing symptom that is challenging to manage. Whilst there is no universally effective medication a number of drugs are often trialled [22]. Non-pharmacological interventions such as avoiding soap, shampoo and hot water on the skin, and using bath oil, a soap substitute and soothing lotions and avoiding vaso-dilating food and drinks (e.g. coffee, alcohol and spices) provide some comfort.

Ascites may be due to either cancer, liver failure or a combination of both [23]. If the underlying cause of the ascites cannot be managed, then symptom management becomes the goal of treatment. Abdominal paracentesis is indicated if it is causing pain, breathlessness or nausea and vomiting, and only if the coagulation profile permits. Diuretics need to be ceased for 24 h immediately prior to and after paracentesis.

Assess and manage any post-paracentesis adverse effects such as hypovolaemia, hypotension, renal dysfunction, perforated viscus, peritonitis or fistula formation. Patients with ascites due to liver failure, who have had abdominal paracentesis where more than five litres has been drained may benefit from concentrated albumin replacement therapy. If not already in place, sodium restriction and oral diuretics need to be initiated [23]. The use of ACE-inhibitors and angiotensin receptor blockers in patients with chronic liver failure and ascites maybe harmful, so their use in this population needs careful consideration [23].

Liver failure is associated with changes in central neural transmission that result in:

- Alterations in behaviour
- Cognitive dysfunction
- Mood disorders
- Sleep disturbances (inversion of the day/night cycle).

which impact on patients' quality of life [24]. People with advanced chronic liver disease frequently develop hepatic encephalopathy that causes a wide spectrum of neuropsychiatric symptoms from subclinical neurological or psychiatric abnormalities through to coma [25].

Cognitive changes due to liver failure will be exacerbated in the presence of delirium and/or cerebral secondaries. These distressing and debilitating symptoms severely affect the lives of patients and their families. In addition to initiating early advance care planning conversations in this population, patients and families need to be made aware of the reasons for any cognitive impairment and supported to cope with these changes.

15.5.2 Management with a Prognosis of Days to Hours

Managing gross ascites is a potentially common problem for this population. If abdominal paracentesis is contra-indicated, the discomfort and breathlessness associated with gross ascites is best addressed through the use of opioids. If SC opioid administration is required, care needs to be taken to ensure that the SC cannula is not located in an oedematous area. Anti-emetics often need to be maintained to manage a hypomotile gut or a squashed stomach and to minimise nausea and vomiting.

15.5.3 How Does Hepatic Impairment Impact on Therapies Directed Against the Cancer?

Markers of hepatic impairment sufficient to suggest dosing changes in chemotherapy include raised bilirubin or the presence of ascites due to liver dysfunction [18]. The impact of hepatic impairment on drug metabolism is far more difficult to predict from hepatic function tests than renal impairment using creatinine clearance [26, 27]. Further, severe renal impairment is likely to alter medications with hepatic metabolism through a number of mechanisms acting on the liver.

Chemotherapy likely to require dose adjustments in the setting of hepatic impairment include: docetaxel, paclitaxel, doxorubicin, epirubicin, gemcitabine (in the presence of hyperbilirubinaemia), irinotecan (hyperbilirubinaemia), erlotinib, sorafenib, and vinorelbine [26]. Imatinib may cause hepatic dysfunction and should be ceased without rechallenge if this occurs [26].

15.6 Advanced Respiratory Disease

Obstructive lung disease is highly prevalent in resource rich, and even more so in, resource poor countries. Smoking remains the world's primary cause of obstructive lung disease. As this is also the most frequent lifestyle choice related to lung cancer, many people with lung cancer have co-existing symptomatic chronic obstructive pulmonary disease. It means that for many people diagnosed with lung cancer, breathlessness on exertion or while carrying out the activities of daily living will already be part of everyday life.

Less frequently, chronic lung disease is caused by restrictive diseases, most frequently related to idiopathic pulmonary fibrosis, connective tissue diseases or occupational exposures. For those, particularly with occupationally related lung disease, smoking rates are relatively higher than the population in general, often leading to severe breathlessness.

15.6.1 Management with a Prognosis of Months to Weeks

The management of respiratory diseases themselves is unlikely to change greatly even when advanced cancer creates a limited prognosis. As such, the major implication for people with co-existing cancer and chronic respiratory diseases relates to symptom management.

As cancer worsens, breathlessness also tends to worsen. As such, focus on the symptom of chronic breathlessness once the underlying causes have been optimally treated is the focus of care. As noted in the section on heart failure, non-pharmacological and pharmacological approaches are need for most people. Many clinicians are concerned about introducing regular, low dose oral extended release morphine, but there is good evidence that this safely relieves breathlessness even in people with co-existing chronic obstructive pulmonary disease (COPD) [28, 29].

Pain is frequently encountered in late stage respiratory disease, and its genesis is usually multifactorial. Adequate treatment of pain is necessary to optimise quality of life in the setting of advanced cancer. Musculoskeletal pain is a major source of discomfort, especially with weight loss which includes loss of muscle. Both regular paracetamol and non-steroidal anti-inflammatory medications have a key role to play in optimising analgesia for people with cancer and respiratory disease.

Fatigue is frequent, especially as people expend greater proportions of diminishing energy on the activities of daily living. Pacing such activities is a management plan, but is very difficult to put into practice for many people. Other manifestations of fatigue include leg tiredness that for many people is more likely to limit exertion than breathlessness [30].

Unfortunately, many people with advancing cancer and respiratory disease find themselves in a cycle of breathlessness leading to anxiety, reducing the person's exercise which, in turn, leads to more deconditioning and worsening breathlessness. This cycle is understandable and, with advancing disease is often very difficult to break.

15.6.2 Management with a Prognosis of Days to Hours

In the terminal stages of advanced cancer, breathlessness and fatigue are two symptoms that tend to worsen (in contrast to almost all other symptoms). Contributing factors include loss of muscle mass and, in some people, disease progression of intra-thoracic malignancy. Few interventions are likely to reduce fatigue predictably and, in people with worsening breathlessness, increasing reliance on pharmacological interventions will be required if the symptom is troublesome to the patient. As noted in the cardiology section, if anxiety is a major component of breathlessness then there may be a place for an anxiolytic such as a benzodiazepine.

15.6.3 How Does Respiratory Impairment Impact on Therapies Directed Against the Cancer?

Rarely does respiratory impairment limit the treatment of cancer. Breathlessness may, however, be sufficiently troublesome that people may choose not to attempt or continue disease modifying therapies.

15.7 Neurological Conditions

Chronic neurological conditions rarely have a direct implication for treatment of advanced cancer. Major issues can arise with progressive neurological diseases where cognition, mobility or swallowing are affected. Of particular concern is:

The ability to make informed decisions about treatment (and assimilate the implications of not pursuing a particular path (in order to ensure that the consent is truly informed).

The ability to take medications orally is important for:

- Acute symptom control related to cancer treatments
- Anti-cancer treatments
- Symptom control for co-existing diseases.

Mostly, there are parenteral variants that are able to ensure excellent anti-cancer therapies and good symptom control.

15.8 Mental Health Concerns

15.8.1 Management with a Prognosis of Months to Weeks

The prevalence of depression for people with advanced cancer is no different for that of the general public. However, it is often under-diagnosed and under-treated in people with advanced cancer. Patients with mild to moderate depression need to be provided with access to counselling and support, while those with a major depression will need treatment with anti-depressants. Any pharmacological treatment needs to be considered alongside potential drug-drug interactions, altered pharmacokinetics due to hepatic or renal impairment and the impact of cachexia, and monitored accordingly [31]. Variations in withdrawal syndromes and the washout period before a new anti-depressant can be initiated are based on specific anti-depressant drug type (i.e. SSRIs, tricyclics and MAOIs).

Any deprescribing of long term antipsychotics needs to be discussed with the patient and their usual psychiatric team and appropriate monitoring and psychological support provided.

15.9 Communicable Diseases

15.9.1 HIV/AIDS

Certain cancers are more common in people living with HIV, and the risk of developing cancer is amplified when their infection is poorly controlled (low CD4 count). Cancers such as Kaposi sarcoma, Non-Hodgkin lymphoma and cervical cancer are all AIDS defining cancers [32].

15.9.2 Management with a Prognosis of Months to Weeks

Managing the needs of this population is complex and requires an integrated multi-disciplinary team approach. Anti-retroviral treatment needs to be maintained in this population as it helps prevent the development of opportunistic infections and allow for the use of standard cancer treatments. However, ongoing antiretroviral treatment is associated with potential adverse effects than need to be prevented or managed [31].

Despite, the social progress made since HIV was initially identified, a person living with HIV may experience social stigma and isolation, marginalisation and be estranged from their family of origin. Advance care planning in addition to providing people living with HIV and cancer with an opportunity for reconciliation with others, provides an opportunity for conversations about appointing a power of attorney and/or enduring guardian who can make financial and clinical decisions, when the person is no longer able to.

15.9.3 Management of HIV with a Prognosis of Days to Hours

In additional to usual palliative care, the most important intervention is to maintain anti-retrovirals for as long as possible or until the person is unable to swallow, to prevent the latent development of opportunistic infections.

15.9.4 How Does HIV Impairment Impact on Therapies Directed Against the Cancer?

Antiretroviral use is associated with numerous drug interactions which are too numerous and complex to list. However, an evidence based point of care resources is available to assist clinicians identify these interactions [33].

15.10 Multi-morbidity

Most patients with advanced cancer have more than one co-morbidity. Currently, there are few data about how to manage several co-morbidities in a coordinated and logical way. Most clinical decisions are made using guidance for a particular co-morbidity and few take into account the impact of other co-morbidities. Even fewer data are available about the role of how to safely prioritise the management of several co-morbidities in the clinical setting of advanced cancer. For example, in the setting of marked cachexia with co-existing heart and renal failure, the balance of clinically conflicting goals of achieving adequate renal perfusion and adequate blood pressure, while minimising left sided heart failure becomes more challenging as cancer advances.

15.11 Future Direction for Research and Practice

The rational management of multi-morbidities in general is in its infancy. How to provide scientific rigour around how to do this in the setting of advanced cancer is at an even more fundamental level. Fully understanding the underlying pathophysiology of cachexia and identifying ways to reverse it or slow its progression requires much more work.

Deprescribing studies in large populations are necessary to ensure that the timing of dose decrements or cessation are based on the best available evidence. These studies can be undertaken but there is too little commitment from funding bodies to provide resources for these fundamentally important works.

References

1. Bayliss EA, Reifler LM, Zeng C et al (2014) Competing risks of cancer mortality and cardiovascular events in individuals with multimorbidity. J Comorbidity 4(1):29–36
2. Clayton JM, Hancock KM, Butow PN et al (2007) Clinical practice guidelines for communicating prognosis and end-of-life issues with adults in the advanced stages of a life-limiting illness, and their caregivers. Med J Aust 186(12):S77–S108
3. Currow DC, Clark K, Kamal A et al (2015) The population burden of chronic symptoms that substantially predate the diagnosis of a life-limiting illness. J Palliat Med 18(6):480–485
4. Rushton M, Clark R, Brideson G, Damarell R (2015) The effectiveness of non-pharmacological interventions for the management of cancer treatment-induced cardiotoxicity: a systematic review protocol. JBI Database Syst Rev Implementation Rep 13(5):53–73
5. Hunt SA, Abraham WT, Chin MH et al (2005) ACC/AHA 2005 guideline update for the diagnosis and management of chronic heart failure in the adult: a report of the American College of Cardiology/American Heart Association task force on practice guidelines (writing committee to update the 2001 guidelines for the evaluation and management of heart failure). American College of Cardiology. Available at: http://www.acc.org/clinical/guidelines/failure//index.pdf

6. Kutner JS, Blatchford PJ, Taylor DH Jr et al (2015) Safety and benefit of discontinuation statin medications in the setting of advanced life-limiting illness. JAMA Int Med 175(5):691–700
7. Gadoud A, Jenkins SM, Hogg KJ (2013) Palliative care for people with heart failure: summary of current evidence and future direction. Palliat Med 27(9):822–828
8. Phillips JL, Johnson M, Currow DC (2015) Heart failure and palliative care: are we there yet? Cardiol Today 5(1):13–16
9. Goodlin SJ (2009) Palliative care in congestive heart failure. J Am Coll Cardiol 54(5):386–396
10. Vogels RL, Scheltens P, Schroeder-Tanka JM, Weinstein HC (2007) Cognitive impairment in heart failure: a systematic review of the literature. Eur J Heart Fail 9(5):440–449
11. Australian Health Ministers' Advisory Council (2011) A national framework for advance care directives. Available online at: www.ahmac.gov.au. AHMAC (Sep 2011)
12. NSW Agency of Clinical Innovation (2014) NSW guidelines for deactivation of implantable cardioverter defibrillators at the end of life. NSW Health, Sydney
13. Cancer Institute NSW (2010) eviQ: Cancer treatments online. https://www.eviq.org.au/. Accessed on 25 May 2010
14. Jarkowski A, Glode AE, Spangenthal EJ, Wong MK (2011) Heart failure caused by molecularly targeted therapies for cancer. Pharmacotherapy 31(1):62–75
15. Launay-Vacher V, Oudard S, Janus N et al (2007) Prevalence of renal insufficiency in cancer patients and implications for anticancer drug management: the renal insufficiency and anticancer medications (IRMA) study. Cancer 110(6):1376–1384
16. Murtagh FE, Addington-Hall J, Higginson IJ (2007) The prevalence of symptoms in end-stage renal disease: a systematic review. Adv Chronic Kidney Dis 14(1):82–99
17. Giannaki CD, Hadjigeorgiou GM, Karatzaferi C et al (2014) Epidemiology, impact, and treatment options of restless legs syndrome in end-stage renal disease patients: an evidence-based review. Kidney Int 85(6):1275–1282
18. Lichtman SM, Wildiers H, Launay-Vacher V et al (2007) International society of geriatric oncology (SIOG) recommendations for the adjustment of dosing in elderly cancer patients with renal insufficiency. Eur J Cancer 43(1):14–34
19. Janus N, Thariat J, Boulanger H et al (2010) Proposal for dosage adjustment and timing of chemotherapy in hemodialyzed patients. Ann Oncol 21(7):1395–1403
20. Australian Adult Cancer Pain Management Guideline Working Party (2014). Cancer pain management in adults. Cancer Council Australia, Sydney (2015)
21. Peterson SJ, Braunschweig CA (2016) Prevalence of sarcopenia and associated outcomes in the clinical setting. Nutr Clin Pract 31(1):40–48
22. Beuers U, Boberg KM, Chapman O et al (2009) EASL clinical practice guidelines: management of cholestatic liver diseases. J Hepatol 51(2):237–267
23. Runyon BA (ed) (2012) Management of adult patients with ascites due to cirrhosis: update 2012. American Association for the Study of Liver Disease. _documents/141020_Guideline_Ascites_4UFb_2015.pdf
24. D'Mello C, Swain MG (2014) Liver-brain interactions in inflammatory liver diseases: implications for fatigue and mood disorders. Brain Behav Immun 35:9–20
25. https://www.aasld.org/sites/default/files/guideline_documents/hepaticencephenhanced.pdf
26. Field KM, Michael M (2008) Part II: Liver function in oncology: towards safer chemotherapy use. Lancet Oncol 9:1181–1190
27. Verbeek RK (2008) Pharmacokinetics and dosage adjustment in patients with hepatic dysfunction. Eur J Clin Pharmacol 64(12):1147–1161
28. Ekstrom M, Nilsson F, Abernethy AP, Currow DC (2015) Effects of opioids on breathlessness and exercise capacity in chronic obstructive pulmonary disease. A systematic review. Ann Am Thoracic Soc 12(7):1079–1092
29. Ekström MP, Bornefalk-Hermansson A, Abernethy AP, Currow DC (2014) Safety of benzodiazepines and opioids in very severe respiratory disease: national prospective study. BMJ 348:g445
30. Wilcock A, Maddocks M, Lewis M, England R et al (2008) Symptoms limiting activity in cancer patients with breathlessness on exertion: ask about muscle fatigue. Thorax 63(1):91–92

31. Therapeutic Guidelines (2010) Palliative care (version 3 ed). Therapeutic Guidelines Limited, Melbourne
32. American Cancer Society (2014) HIV infection, AIDS, and cancer. http://www.cancer.org/acs/groups/cid/documents/webcontent/002295-pdf.pdf
33. HIV Drug Interactions http://www.hiv-druginteractions.org
34. Stevenson J, Miller C, Abernethy AP, Currow DC (2004) Managing comorbidities in patients at the end of life. Br Med J 329(7471):909–912

Further Reading

35. Olver I (ed) (2010) The MASCC textbook of cancer supportive care and survivorship. Springer, Berlin
36. Clark K, Currow DC (2007) Emergencies in palliative medicine (Ch 9). In: Walsh D et al (eds) Textbook of palliative medicine. Elsevier, Oxford University Press
37. Cherny NI, Fallon MT, Kaasa S, Portenoy R, Currow DC (eds) (2015) Oxford textbook of palliative medicine 5th ed. Oxford University Press, UK

MIX
Papier aus verantwortungsvollen Quellen
Paper from responsible sources
FSC® C105338

If you have any concerns about our products,
you can contact us on
ProductSafety@springernature.com

In case Publisher is established outside the EU,
the EU authorized representative is:
Springer Nature Customer Service Center GmbH
Europaplatz 3, 69115 Heidelberg, Germany

Printed by Libri Plureos GmbH
in Hamburg, Germany